THE ELEMENTS OF
Nursing

NANCY ROPER, after spending 15 years as a nurse teacher, became a freelance writer and lecturer. She is the author of *Principles of Nursing in Process Context* (4E 1989) and a research monograph *Clinical Experience in Nurse Education* (1976). Over 30 years ago, she became the Editor of *Churchill Livingstone Nurse's Dictionary*, now in its 16th edition, and *Churchill Livingstone Pocket Medical Dictionary*, now in its 14th edition. She spent 4 years at the Scottish Office as its first Nursing Research Officer. Her international experience includes consultancies with the World Health Organization in Europe and the Eastern Mediterranean Region.

WINIFRED LOGAN, previously head of the Department of Health and Nursing at Glasgow College (now Glasgow Caledonian University), was Executive Director of the International Council of Nursing from 1978–80. She had already worked in Canada and the USA, and is a graduate of Columbia University, New York. Further international work includes serving as a WHO consultant in Malaysia and Iraq; and as the first Director of Nursing Services in the Ministry of Health, Abu Dhabi. At a national level she held a senior post in the Department of Nursing Studies, University of Edinburgh, and later was Nurse Education Officer at the Scottish Office, as well as serving on various national nursing and academic committees.

ALISON TIERNEY is now a Reader in the Department of Nursing Studies at the University of Edinburgh, having been Director of the Nursing Research Unit for 10 years until 1994. She is one of the UK's most experienced nurse researchers and, through her research, she continues to maintain close links with providers and users of health and nursing services. At the national and international levels, she has contributed to the strategic development of research in nursing, particularly through active membership of the Royal College of Nursing (RCN) and as the RCN's representative on the Workgroup of European Nurse Researchers (WENR).

The authors can be contacted at their publisher's address:
Churchill Livingstone, 1–3 Baxter's Place, Leith Walk, Edinburgh, Scotland EH1 3AF.

THE ELEMENTS OF

Nursing

A model for nursing based on a model of living

Nancy Roper

MPhil RGN RSCN RNT

Winifred W. Logan

MA DNS(Educ) RGN RNT

Alison J. Tierney

BSc(SocScNurs) PhD RGN

FOURTH EDITION

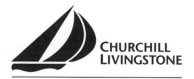

CHURCHILL
LIVINGSTONE

NEW YORK EDINBURGH LONDON MADRID MELBOURNE SAN FRANCISCO TOKYO 1996

CHURCHILL LIVINGSTONE
An imprint of Harcourt Publishers Limited

 is a registered trademark of Harcourt Publishers Limited

First edition 1980
Second edition 1985
Third edition 1990
Fourth edition 1996
   Reprinted 1998
   Reprinted 1999

ISBN 0 443 05201 8

British Library of Cataloguing in Publication Data
A catalogue record for this book is available from the British Library.

Library of Congress Cataloging in Publication Data
A catalog record for this book is available from the Library of Congress.

For Churchill Livingstone:

Commissioning Editor: Ellen Green
Project Manager: Valerie Burgess
Project Development Editor: Mairi McCubbin
Design Direction: Judith Wright
Project Controller: Derek Robertson
Copy editor: Carolyn Holleyman
Sales Promotion Executive: Hilary Brown

The
publisher's
policy is to use
**paper manufactured
from sustainable forests**

Printed in China
EPC/03
NPCC/03

Contents

Preface to the Fourth Edition

Since *The Elements of Nursing* was first published in 1980, new editions have been prepared at five-year intervals. Even with extensive updating, textbooks seldom have an indefinite life and, in the fast-changing field of nursing and health care, it is important that books which were once innovative are not recycled beyond their useful life. With the ever-increasing emphasis on the multi-professional nature of health care, and the increasingly influential voice of 'the new nursing' we had to ask ourselves if *The Elements of Nursing* — with its underpinning model for nursing — could be considered to have had its day.

But the growing emphasis on multidisciplinary practice, both in community and hospital settings, does not mean that the individual disciplines no longer need their own identity and body of knowledge. On the contrary, it is more important than ever for nursing to have a clear view of its particular contribution to health care. The model for nursing which is presented in *The Elements of Nursing* is entirely in keeping with present-day thinking, which advocates greater emphasis on the individuality of patients/clients, health promotion and care in the community.

In any case, we were persuaded to take on the task of preparing a fourth edition of the book because critical feedback from nurse educators indicated that, with updating, it would remain a useful book for beginning nursing students and they wished to see it retained. Further more, *The Elements of Nursing* has a strong and growing international following, especially in other European countries and in the developing world, where indigenous nursing literature is still scarce.

However, we have taken account of the UK's broadened nursing curriculum, which in the first eighteen months (the Common Foundation Programme) requires an introduction to the nursing of adults and children, as well as people with learning disabilities and those who have mental health problems. The terms referring to the various areas of nursing have changed over time, and the terms in current usage are used throughout the text.

The number of Sections in the book has been reduced to two. Section 1 comprises three chapters: the first retains the title 'Nursing in health and illness' but it is updated to include an overview of the changes in health care systems and how nursing is responding to the resultant challenges. Chapter 2, 'a model of living', provides the basis for our model for nursing which is presented in Chapter 3. The model is, in effect, the core material of this textbook. Section 2, entitled 'Nursing and the Activities of Living', is really an expansion of Chapter 3 and in each of its 12 Chapters the text has been rearranged and strengthened to reflect the five concepts of our model for nursing. The content of each has been extensively revised and the references updated, wherever possible including research literature, but older references which are still relevant have been retained.

In keeping with the changed style of publishing, appropriate material is presented in this new edition in bullet points and boxes. The boxes in some instances highlight a point made in the text; in others they summarize factual information; and in yet others they give a brief account of a related piece of research.

The Prefaces from the first three editions of this book have been retained so that readers can understand the original purpose of the book and how it has developed over time.

Of course, a conceptual model for nursing cannot capture all of the complexities of the discipline. Our model offers beginning students a means by which they can conceptualize nursing to guide their practice and, as they gain experience, they will be able to adapt it to particular circumstances. Deliberately, the model is broad and flexible so that it can accommodate any further changes in nursing, whether these are imposed by governmental health care systems or introduced by nurses themselves.

Finally, we acknowledge our thanks to all those nurses who have shared with us their interpretation and use of our model, which has further refined our thinking. We hope that this new edition will continue to provide a useful text for beginning students and their teachers in this and other countries.

Winifred Logan would like to thank teaching and library staff at Tayside College of Nursing and Midwifery for their helpfulness during preparation of this Fourth Edition.

Edinburgh 1995   N.R. W.L. A.T.

Preface to the Third Edition

This third edition of *The Elements of Nursing*, as before, is essentially for beginning nursing students. It is not a comprehensive text in the sense of covering all aspects of nursing knowledge and practice required in the course of a basic education programme; rather, it encourages a logical mode of thinking about nursing in the framework of a model for nursing. An immediately obvious change to the third edition is the title. It has been extended to include, 'a model for nursing based on a model of living'. It would seem that a number of potential readers did not appreciate that *The Elements of Nursing* used the framework of a model for nursing, and the extended title should help to draw attention to this important feature of the book.

The presentation of the book itself has been rearranged and its content substantially revised and updated. Section 1 has been changed. Its introductory chapter emphasizes the link between nursing and health — a point which is stressed increasingly by the World Health Organization. The content of the second chapter is new. It includes a discussion, albeit brief, of some of the other internationally well-known models for nursing, in order to provide an understanding of the context in which the Roper, Logan and Tierney model can be considered.

Section 2 has been considerably altered; the objective here being to present the Roper, Logan and Tierney model more clearly, incorporating some of the refinements which have been made since the last edition. It commences with a chronological account of the background to the model showing how it developed from research and a review of the literature.

Subsequently, the model of living and the model for nursing are discussed sequentially — in the previous editions they were separated by three brief chapters introducing some concepts from biology, psychology and sociology. Perhaps this was appropriate when the first edition was published 10 years ago, but increasingly nursing students are expected to study the biological and social sciences as foundation subjects, so these three chapters have been omitted. Instead the third edition emphasizes more than previously, the application of such knowledge in the context of 'Factors influencing the ALs', a component of the model. For purposes of clarification too, there are minor alterations in the diagrams of the models, to emphasize the relationships between the components. It is in Section 2 also that we describe how the model relates to the practice of nursing — in 'Individualising nursing' — and proforma are provided as a suggested method for documenting nursing data.

Section 3, as before, consists of 12 chapters, one devoted to each of the 12 Activities of Livings (ALs), the main component of the model. All of these chapters have been extensively revised, obviously to update the content but also to reflect the five components of the model more clearly than in the second edition. The first half of each chapter discusses the nature of the AL, mainly in the context of 'healthy living'; the second half provides selected examples of the problems related to the ALs which can be caused by illness.

We have welcomed feedback about the two previous editions of the book, and consider all comments as a means of helping us to refine our thinking; a number of changes in the third edition reflect such feedback. It is appropriate to comment here on two recurring criticisms. A number of readers have been concerned about the apparent lack of provision in the model for consideration of the individual's spiritual needs. Obviously we had not made it sufficiently clear that sociocultural factors (related to each of the 12 ALs) include spiritual, religious and ethical considerations — and this remains the case. We do not see spiritual needs standing on their own (any more than physical needs or sociocultural needs) but firmly related to the individual's ALs because this is how they are manifest. A second area which continues to cause concern is the relevance of the AL of expressing sexuality in a model for nursing. In the first edition, the term was certainly a novel inclusion in a nursing context although it is now used frequently in the mass media, and increasingly in the nursing literature. However, it is still used too narrowly. We hope we have emphasized its broad application to femininity/masculinity in general and have clarified that, as with any AL, individual circumstances will dictate whether or not it is a relevant subject for consideration.

Also on the subject of feedback, it is appropriate to mention that *The Elements of Nursing* is becoming increasingly well-known in other countries, especially in Europe and more recently in Australia. As a result, a number of translations of the book into other languages has been undertaken.

Of course, no one model can be all-embracing; indeed a challenging feature of any model is that it suggests growing points for further thinking and refinement about the discipline. And no single text can possibly exhaust discussion of something so complex as a conceptual framework for nursing, and its application in practice. We hope this third edition provides a clearer account of the model and a further analysis of those concepts which, we believe, comprise the elements of nursing.

Edinburgh 1990   N.R. W.L. A.T.

Preface to the Second Edition

This second edition of *The Elements of Nursing* retains the format of the original text and, as before, is essentially for beginning nursing students. The fact that the first edition has been positively received, in particular because of its focus on a model for nursing (which incorporates the process of nursing), reassured us that there is still a need for an introductory text of this kind. However, we wish to emphasize that this book is not intended as 'comprehensive'; the expectation is that it will be complemented by other nursing texts and literature from other disciplines such as human biology, psychology and sociology. Our extended use of reference in this edition is intended to encourage students to read widely and, especially, to take account of research as a basis for nursing practice.

The contents of the book are basically as outlined in the preface of the first edition. Section 1, 'Nursing and health care', is still introductory but has been revised, updated and re-arranged.

In Section 2, the chapters on the 'Model of living' (Ch. 2) and the 'Model for nursing' (Ch. 6) have been re-written for purposes of clarification and to incorporate refinements of the model which are the result of giving considerable further thought to our original ideas in the course of writing *Learning to Use the Process of Nursing* (1981), and to undertaking a project which is described in *Using a Model for Nursing* (1983). The middle chapters of Section 2 — 'Biological aspects of living' (Ch. 3), 'Developmental aspects of living' (Ch. 4) and 'Social aspects of living' (Ch. 5) — have been minimally revised and have been retained to provide beginning students with a brief overview of material which is relevant as a background to Section 3.

Section 3 consists of 12 chapters (Chs 7–18), one devoted to each of the 12 Activities of Living, the main focus of the model. All of these chapters have been substantially rewritten, obviously to update material but also to reflect the components of the model more clearly than in the first edition.

Section 4, consisting of one short chapter (Ch. 19), is new to this edition. One of the current major criticisms about nursing models is that although they may be of theoretical interest, there is difficulty in using them in the real world of nursing. This chapter therefore has been added to help readers to appreciate how the Roper/Logan/Tierney model can be applied in practice. To give some guidance for documentation, we discuss the proforma which developed out of the project of the third book *Using a Model for Nursing* (1983).

No one model can be perfect and no single text can possibly exhaust discussion of something as complex as a conceptual framework for nursing and its application to practice. We hope, however, that this new edition provides a clearer account of our model and a further analysis of those concepts which comprise the elements of nursing.

Edinburgh 1985   N.R. W.L. A.T.

Preface to the First Edition

It has been said and written scores of times that every woman makes a good nurse. I believe on the contrary, that the very elements of nursing are all but unknown

FLORENCE NIGHTINGALE

We planned and wrote this book because of our conviction that the degree of complexity and specialization of nursing today makes it more necessary than ever for the elements of nursing to be identified and understood. Today's nursing students right from the start of their education programme need to become familiar with those elements common to all branches of nursing and relevant to all patients.

Consequently we examined the core of knowledge required by nurses and we have presented it within a model for nursing which is based on a model of living. The model for nursing incorporates the process of nursing so that together they provide a conceptual framework for the book. It is hoped that this framework will assist learners to develop a way of thinking about nursing which will help them to provide effective and compassionate nursing for people of whatever age who have various problems and who are in different health care settings. In addition, as nursing experience is gained, this way of thinking should facilitate the acquisition of new and specialized knowledge.

In Section 1 the reader is encouraged to think about the meaning of health and illness and how a health care system develops within a country. Nursing's contribution to health care is examined and the section ends with a consideration of the educational preparation needed by today's nurses.

The two models — the model of living and the model for nursing — are described in Section 2. Both models focus on 12 Activities of Living (ALs): maintaining a safe environment; communicating; breathing; eating and drinking; eliminating; personal cleansing and dressing; controlling body temperature; mobilizing; working and playing; expressing sexuality; sleeping; and dying. All Activities of Living have biological, developmental and social dimensions and so a chapter is devoted to each of these aspects of living within this section. Finally there is a discussion of the process of nursing, showing how this concept is used as a framework for the analysis of each of the Activities of Living.

This analysis of the 12 ALs makes up the 12 chapters in Section 3 of the book. In the first part of each chapter there is a description of the nature of the activity, the purpose of the activity, factors influencing the activity and body structure and function required for the activity. Guidelines are given on assessing an individual's performance of the activity. The second part of each chapter contains discussion of possible patients' problems associated with that AL. For example, among the problems discussed relating to the AL of eliminating are those arising from lack of privacy in the ward; dependence due to limited mobility or confinement to bed or psychological disturbance; urinary incontinence; urinary catheterization; and anxiety associated with investigations of the urinary and defaecatory systems. Emphasis is placed on the problems as experienced by the patient, and related nursing activities are therefore presented as assisting the patient to solve, reduce or prevent problems which interfere with everyday living. Each chapter has a summary chart which shows how this problem-orientated approach is used in applying the process of nursing to the AL. Although a chapter has been devoted to each AL, in reality the activities are interrelated and it must be remembered that a problem with one can produce problems with any or all of the other ALs.

At the end of each chapter there are two lists, one of References and the other of Suggested Reading. Relevant research reports are included in both. Most of the listed articles and books contain references which will guide the reader who wishes to gain further information about a particular topic.

In the process of writing this book we were constantly clarifying and extending our thinking about nursing. All three of us feel that we now have a better understanding of the elements of nursing and a greater awareness of their complexity, which we hope we have conveyed to the readers of this book.

Edinburgh 1980   N.R. W.L. A.T.

Foreword to the First Edition

Professional practice is in constant need of review and refinement if it is to adapt to new demands and advances in knowledge. One of the most significant advances in nursing in recent years has been the move towards replacing ritualized and institutionalized approaches with those that are rationally planned and individualized.

The teaching of nursing in the past was often based on body systems, disease entities and procedures. The emphasis is now changing to one that concentrates on the essential nature of nursing action and the principles which underlie practice.

The authors of *The Elements of Nursing* have done a great deal to help us in this direction. They have given a model for nursing based on activities of living and incorporating the process of nursing. Components of the nursing function are analysed and guidelines are given for assessing the patient's functional abilities in each activity of living. A theoretical framework for assessment and nursing care evolves. The result is a unique amalgam of theory drawn from biological and behavioural sciences which should equip a nurse to function on a sound scientific basis.

The book begins with a quotation from Florence Nightingale:
'. . . the very elements of nursing are all but unknown.' The authors have accepted the professional challenge of those words and, 120 years later, they have done much to identify those elements of nursing which should help us towards rational, individualized nursing practice. I believe there is in their work a basis for innovation and improved quality of performance to which we all aspire.

January, 1980   McFarlane of Llandaff

A model for nursing based on a model of living

Nursing in health and illness

> It has been said and written scores of times that every woman makes a good nurse. I believe on the contrary that the very elements of nursing are all but unknown.
>
> Florence Nightingale (1859)

These words were written over a century ago but the profession continues to refine its ideas about 'the elements' of nursing. This is not surprising. Nursing exists to serve society and, as social conditions and health care needs change, nurses' roles and nursing practices continue to alter in response to the changes.

Since the start of the 1980s, nursing has been in an almost constant state of rapid change. Throughout the Western world, health care systems have been undergoing radical reform, and these reforms have far-reaching implications for all of the health care professions but, perhaps, especially for nursing in view of its size and the range and cost of its services.

Changes in nursing, of course, are not shaped by external forces alone. Indeed, many of the developments of the 1980s and 1990s have resulted from the profession's *own* desire for innovation and change in practice, and for commensurate improvements in nurse education. Some nurse leaders (e.g. Salvage, 1992) consider that, taken together, all of the changes which have occurred add up to 'a movement'; and this they describe as the 'New Nursing'. This new ideology (see Box 1.1) essentially represents a modern-day attempt to answer the age-old question, 'What is nursing?'

What is nursing?

FAMILY NURSING

History reveals that sick people required and received care long before nursing became an organized occupation; indeed, in the Western world until the end of the last century family members or domestic staff usually nursed the sick in their own homes, and hospitals were used only for paupers or grossly mentally deranged people. The family is the oldest, and still the most used 'health care service' in the world. Indeed, there is new recognition of the reliance of formal health services on the family, and patients are discharged from hospital as soon as they can be cared for at home.

It is still the custom in some countries elsewhere in the world to admit the family members to hospital with the patient, complete with bedding and cooking utensils so that they can attend to the sick relative's everyday living activities while the nurses carry out specific treatments associated with the disease condition.

HOSPITAL NURSING

Undoubtedly, however, during the last century nursing has been most associated in the eyes of the public with care of the sick, especially in hospital. As nurses have become increasingly involved with the curative, technical treatments provided by medical staff they have come to occupy a strategic position in the hospital sector of the health service. Nurses are the link between what are often stressful, complicated technical procedures associated with treatment of the disease condition and the maintenance of everyday bodily and mental functions which are so critical to the patient's comfort and so important to him as a person.

Admittedly, looking back at the major professional developments in nursing in the Western world during the 20th century, it would appear that they have been associated mainly with the 'sickness' services. However, knowledge about disease processes, developments in biological and social sciences, increasing sophistication in technology and a better-educated public have produced a new awareness about health care services in general, and there is increasing public interest in individual, family and community health.

The hospital-based, disease-orientated health care system, and nursing within that system, has been questioned. Nurses along with other health professionals now see the importance of putting increasing emphasis on maintaining health, preventing sickness, enhancing self-help and promoting maximum independence according to the individual person's capability. Care in the community is now considered to be preferable wherever possible, and the interface between health and illness is no longer so clearly defined.

COMMUNITY NURSING

However, on analysis, nursing has not only been associated with people who are ill. There are specially trained nurses who work in the community and are involved, almost exclusively, with people who are well.

Midwives (or the alternative title used in different countries) monitor the health status of pregnant women, the majority of whom are healthy while undergoing a normal physiological experience; midwives also facilitate development of the skills required for breast feeding, parenting, inclusion of the new baby into the family and so on.

Health visitors (or equivalent title) provide a service to pre-school children and their families; they have encouraged uptake of immunisation, and the promotion and maintenance of health as well as the prevention of accident and illness.

School nurses have carried out a similar function for children during the period of formal education, and occupational health nurses have provided a comparable service for adults throughout their working lives. Increasingly, too, they are concerned with helping older people to retain a healthy lifestyle.

So, the idea of nurses nursing well people outside hospital is not new even although 'care in the community' has been presented in the context of recent health service reforms as if it were a 'new' idea. Indeed, Florence Nightingale was calling for nursing to reform itself along these very same lines more than a century ago! (See Box 1.2.)

Over 100 years later, the World Health Organization promoted an ambitious worldwide campaign — 'Health for all by the year 2000'. To begin to understand this international endeavour, in which nurses are involved, all students of nursing are required to examine and develop their concept of 'health' so that not only will it inform their personal style of living, but will also influence their concept of nursing practice in relation to healthy as well as ill people. So, first of all, can health be defined?

What is health?

Perhaps the people of the ancient world were much more aware of maintaining health than we are now. In Ancient Greece, there is little doubt that the pursuit of excellence, encapsulated in the Platonic ideal, required a sound mind in a sound body; both contributing to the good of the soul. In Plato's *The Republic* it is declared that:

> *'. . . in a well-run society each man . . . has no time to spend his life being ill and undergoing cures . . . there's nothing worse than this fussiness about one's health . . . it is tiresome in the home, as well as in the army or in any civilian office.'*

Perhaps a 'good' state of health was possible in the heyday of the Greek city state. Some time later, Galen (AD 130–201), the celebrated physician, accepted that health in the abstract was an ideal state to which no one attained, yet he found difficulty regarding as unhealthy, all who did not function perfectly. He therefore was prepared to overlook small ailments and to consider health as a state of reasonable functioning and freedom from pain.

These are obviously old ideas about health, but they are being reaffirmed by the World Health Organization, health professionals and members of the lay public in many countries — health is not an absolute quantity but a concept which is continually changing with the acquisition of knowledge and changing cultural expectations.

WHO DEFINITION OF HEALTH

Probably the best known definition of health appears in the Constitution of the World Health Organization (1946): -

> *'Health is a state of complete physical, mental and social well-being, and not merely the absence of disease or infirmity.'*

When WHO defined health in this way, however, it was genuinely believed that there was a clear distinction between health and ill-health. Thus, in the early 1940s when Lord Beveridge, the well-known British economist, was helping to plan the National Health Service in the UK, it was assumed that there was a strictly limited quantity of illness which, if treated, would be reduced. Indeed the planners expected that the annual cost of the health service would decrease as treatment reduced the incidence of illness, and people were transferred from the 'ill' category to the 'healthy' category. With the advantage of hindsight, this interpretation of health is too simplistic and it has become accepted by most people that there is no such clear-cut distinction between health and ill-health.

HEALTH-ILLNESS CONTINUUM

In the first place, in strictly scientific terms, it is not possible to demonstrate a cut-off point between an individual's healthy state and diseased state (OHE, 1971). For a range of biochemical and physical observations which can be made on the individual, there is a continuous distribution curve for the population as a whole, for example for haemoglobin levels or blood pressure readings. The distribution of measurements ranges smoothly from those for the obviously healthy to those for the obviously diseased; and there is a substantial overlap area in the middle where one cannot objectively draw definite conclusions from the measurements.

In fact it is probable that for many measurements the optimum varies from person to person so that correcting an abnormality by treatment, and bringing the measurement to some average value, would be unnecessary. Thinking about health and illness as *relative* states provides a construct in the form of a health-illness continuum.

LAY PERCEPTIONS OF HEALTH

It is, however, a purely subjective judgement on the part of individuals whether they feel well or unwell, and this to some extent is dependent on prevailing attitudes. Formerly, for example, deafness, lack of teeth and failing sight were accepted as an inevitable part of the ageing process whereas now, corrective treatment is the expectation and considered as a right.

Also, sophisticated procedures such as renal dialysis and transplant surgery offer the possibility of restoration of health to people who, even 10 years ago, were resigned to an incurable illness and an early demise. There are less dramatic ways in which an increasing number of people are being transferred back to health by such treatments as permanent medication for a specific disorder; a special diet for life; a technological implant such as a pacemaker and so on.

As a result of advances in medical technology, and public knowledge of these through the media, lay expectations of 'better health' (at least in Western society) are ever-increasing. Even so, some people will insist that they are 'healthy' despite quite severe illness or disability. On the other hand, people with no detectable illness may persist in considering themselves to be 'unhealthy' because they feel 'unwell'.

The *subjective* element, therefore, limits the value of visualizing health and illness as a continuum, with health at one end, and illness at the other.

HEALTH AS COPING

A growing number of writers and practitioners now consider that the health status of individuals is dependent on their ability to adapt to, and cope with, challenges they meet throughout life. In fact, they say that those who feel well and live in a way which they find socially and economically satisfactory may be considered 'healthy' even though they have a significant disability such as a physical or mental disability or a disease.

Coping behaviours resulting in health/wellness, or maladaptive behaviours resulting in illness, are often learned within the family, and are strongly influenced by attitudes, values and beliefs about health.

PERSONAL RESPONSIBILITY FOR HEALTH

Although in industrialized countries the individual has come to be so dependent on the state and in particular, on the health services provided, it is fascinating to note a resurgence of interest in the notion of personal responsibility for health. Health professionals are having to reconsider ordinary people as self-providers of health and health care.

Self-care is a term that is used increasingly to denote health care activities which include health caring services of the family, extended family, friends, lay volunteer groups, mutual and self-help groups, religious organizations, and in some instances, a whole neighbourhood. Self-care is, of course, the dominant form of health care for most of the world's rural people in developing countries.

Several factors have been suggested as sources of Western societies' increasing awareness of self-care and its potential, and Levin summarized them as long ago as 1981:

- in the industrialized nations, the massive shift in disease patterns during the last 50 years to almost a trebling of the incidence of chronic diseases when lay caring is a partnership with professional resources
- an erosion of professional mystique; and the public's awareness of rights and of options
- the public's awareness of alternative health care strategies
- a change in public attitudes to disease prevention

and health promotion involving personal lifestyle and collective action
- the public's awareness of the economic implications of health care.

Levin claimed that this was an exciting period in the transition of health planning from a professional/industrial to a social model and concluded: 'we shall need a new conceptual vocabulary free of the we/they dichotomy'.

CURRENT HEALTH TARGETS

Changes in the way in which health is now being conceptualized are reflected in current approaches to health promotion and current health targets, nationally and internationally.

At a nursing conference held in 1988 to discuss the targets for the WHO programme 'Health for All by the Year 2000', participants were reminded that the targets are based on 'the premise that health is not the mere absence of disease but the opportunity to create well being and realize human potential' (Nath & O'Neill, 1988). The targets take full account of the fact that promoting health and helping to prevent illness are not the prerogative of the 'health care' professionals. There are many other agencies concerned with providing requisites which contribute to health, such as housing, sanitation, education and safe transportation systems. A whole network of professionals, medical and non-medical, is available to assist patients and their families (see Fig. 1.1).

Nevertheless, the main responsibility for promoting health and preventing illness falls to a country's health service and, throughout Europe, Government health departments have translated the objectives of the WHO programme into national targets. In 1991 the UK's Department of Health published 'The Health of the Nation' (DoH, 1991a). This document emphasizes that the major gains in health in the foreseeable future will result from change in personal lifestyles and, specifically, in relation to smoking, diet, exercise and safe sexual practices. Known causes of significant ill-health and premature death are also targeted (Box 1.3).

While some of the targets of the UK's Health Department are concerned with promotion of *health*, others are focused specifically on causes of *ill-health*. It is important, therefore, having considered the concept of health, to ask the question 'What is illness?'.

What is illness?

From time immemorial, man has sought to explain illness, and beliefs regarding its cause have determined the role of the sick person, the role of the healer and the system of care provided.

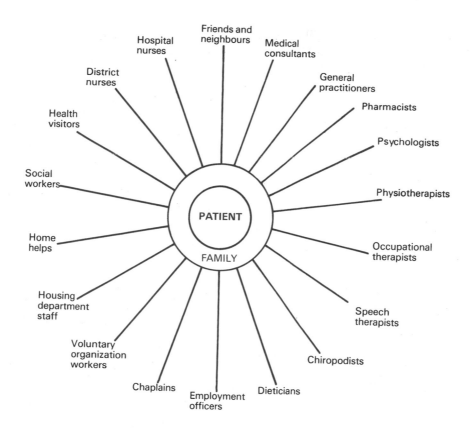

Fig. 1.1 Some members of the team who assist the patient and family

Box 1.3 UK targets for health promotion and improvement

- The need for people to change their behaviour in relation to:-
  - smoking
  - diet and alcohol
  - exercise
  - sexual activity
- Areas in need of improved health services:-
  - health of pregnant women, infants and children
  - rehabilitation for people with a physical disability
- Measures to reduce deaths from:-
  - coronary heart disease
  - stroke
  - cancers
  - accidents
- Measures to tackle causes of substantial ill-health, including:-
  - diabetes
  - asthma
  - mental illness

DoH (1991a) *The Health of the Nation.* Department of Health, HMSO, London.

AN HISTORICAL PERSPECTIVE

Primitive man attributed illness to evil spirits and sought to drive them out by practising witchcraft or assuaging their wrath by some sacrificial gift. Centuries later, the ancient civilizations — Egypt, Babylon, India, China, Greece, Rome — still thought of illness as a supernatural phenomenon. The healer might be a magician or a priest-physician or a god, and the care might be offered, for example, in a Greek temple of healing or a Roman military hospital.

With the advent of the Christian era, the sick received care from deaconesses; or from members, male and female, of religious orders; or during the Crusades, from members of the prestigious Order of the Knights Hospitallers of St John of Jerusalem; or under the feudal regime, from the lady of the manor. Care was given with Christian compassion and as illness was sometimes considered to be a just retribution for sinful word or deed, the care included concern for the soul as well as for relief of bodily distress.

In Europe, there was an historical watershed around 1500 and the long period of domination by the feudal system and by the Church was replaced by a great up-surge of new ideas, new discoveries and new inventions. It was during this post-Renaissance period that there were also great advances in man's knowledge about diseases and their treatment. The human body was studied in detail anatomically and physiologically, much of this investigation being made possible by the invention of the microscope.

SCIENTIFIC DISCOVERIES

From the evidence produced by historical researchers, it can be detected that down through the centuries there have been isolated attempts to use a scientific approach in determining the cause of disease, but it was not until the 19th century that the focus moved away to any extent from magical techniques, religious practices and folk medicine.

More reliance began to be placed on methods demanding systematic, objective, verifiable observations about the course of a disease and its treatment. Knowledge acquired through science was not considered to be static; there was the expectation that observations and conclusions would be constantly re-examined in an attempt to evolve more effective treatments for illness.

By the mid-19th century, the experiments of Pasteur were demonstrating the growth of microorganisms but when, in 1843, Holmes published a paper in the USA entitled, 'The Contagiousness of Puerperal Fever', the whole idea of infection was ridiculed by many learned contemporaries and continued to be so, even though objectively corroborated by Semmelweiss in Austria in 1867. This 'germ theory' however was given practical application by Lister in Scotland who started the use of substances called antiseptics, and subsequently used the 'aseptic method' which transformed the course of surgery.

More sophisticated surgery became possible after Morton gave the first demonstration of the use of ether as an anaesthetic in Boston, Massachusetts, in 1846, and Simpson employed chloroform the next year in Edinburgh, Scotland. By the early 1900s, many of the microorganisms causing the commonly occurring infectious diseases had been isolated, and this process has continued, a contemporary example being identification of the human immunodeficiency virus (HIV) which causes AIDS. Each discovery has provided yet another stimulus for the development of agents which inhibit or destroy specific pathogens in the human body, and these advances have contributed to the growth of the pharmaceutical industry.

CAUSES OF ILLNESS

But not all illness is caused by microorganisms which produce infectious diseases.

- *Inflammation* Some pathogenic microorganisms cause other infections which produce inflammation of, for example, body organs such as the bronchi (bronchitis). The body response of inflammation

can also be produced by allergy, extremes of cold or heat, chemicals and friction; and it can be acute or chronic.
- *Trauma* Trauma, too, can remove people from a health to an illness status either temporarily or permanently; it causes many types of wounds involving tissue and even a whole organ: and trauma can also cause sprains, fractures and paralysis, particularly of the limbs.
- *Insects* Insects can be carriers of disease; the bites of fleas, lice, mosquitoes and ticks can transmit to man a variety of diseases.
- *Congenital abnormality* Some people of course are in an illness category because of congenital abnormality of body structure or function and this can be hereditary. Such an abnormality can also be acquired and the condition may be familial.
- *Degenerative processes* There can also be degenerative processes in the tissues thereby changing their structure and function.
- *Malignancy* Malignancy can cause local tissue destruction and, by metastasis (i.e. spread), invade other tissues: carcinoma refers to malignant tumours of epithelial tissue and sarcoma to malignant disease of connective tissue.

For all of these illness conditions there is an agreed international classification of medical diagnoses, use of which provides statistical data for investigating patterns of disease throughout the world (epidemiology).

PREDISPOSING FACTORS

However, it is no longer sufficient to concentrate only on the pathophysiological factors of disease. It is necessary to consider the *social factors* which contribute to the development of health problems, including poverty and overcrowding; the *cultural factors* which determine individual lifestyles such as food preferences, and customs surrounding the treatment of critical events such as birth, illness and death; the *environmental factors* including the effects of water and air pollution, poor sanitation and industrial hazards; and the *psychological factors* including the impact of past experiences and personality on mental health.

These sociocultural, economic, environmental and psychological factors can be just as important as physical factors in creating circumstances which predispose to illness. Knowledge about these many variables can influence the care provided for the individual during an illness episode. For more general purposes, such knowledge is vital for an understanding of the aetiology (i.e. causation) of any specific illness. It is only possible to take measures to *prevent* a particular illness if the full picture of its aetiology is understood.

CHANGING PATTERNS OF ILLNESS

Over time, there are continual changes in patterns of illness, both within and between countries. This results from the successful prevention of diseases (e.g. tuberculosis) and even the wholescale eradication of others (e.g. smallpox) which, in the past, were major causes of ill-health and death; and, of course, the appearance of new conditions (e.g. HIV/AIDS) as well as an increasing prevalence of others (e.g. senile dementia) also serve to alter the overall pattern.

Worldwide, the major causes of ill-health and death today are:-

- heart disease
- stroke
- cancers
- accidents.

However, at least in the Western world, one of the most significant shifts in the overall picture of ill-health is the ever-increasing amount of *age-related chronic illness*. At the beginning of this century, average life expectancy in countries such as the UK was around 50 years, with few people living to the age of 60 or beyond. Now, with the average life expectancy at birth being over 70 years, age-related illnesses (e.g. stroke, arthritis, hip fracture and dementia) are on the ascendancy. The ever-increasing health care needs of ageing populations are one important reason why health care systems throughout the Western world are currently in the throes of radical reform.

Why are health care systems under reform?

During this century, even in developing countries, the tendency in health care has been to provide increasingly specialized services which, at vast expense, have focused on ever more elaborate techniques for diagnosing disease; on providing hospitals to house the expensive equipment and the people being treated; and on using advances in medical technology to prolong the lives of newborn babies and people of all ages who, in the past, would not have survived. This method of providing care has been described as a 'disease-based, hospital-based, medical-based model of health care' providing the greatest good, achieved at high expense, for the minority of people. The great disparity between the high cost of care in these systems and the low health benefits are now widely recognized.

SHIFTING THE BALANCE OF CARE

As a result, in many countries, providers of health services are now recognizing that greater emphasis should be given, once again, to community-based health care.

THE CONCEPT OF PRIMARY HEALTH CARE

The World Health Organization promoted the concept of Primary Health Care (PHC) (WHO, 1978) whereby the greatest good can be achieved at low expense for the greatest number of people (see Box 1.4).

It was emphasized by WHO that such services must be easily accessible to individual families in the community, by means available to them, and at a cost which that community and country can afford. PHC is presented as a practical approach to achieving an acceptable level of health throughout the world and 'for developing countries it is a burning necessity'.

Discussing PHC nearly a decade later, Powell (1986) wrote that, despite some success, there are formidable obstacles in the form of politicomedical controversy when trying to redistribute power from the top to rural power. He maintained, nevertheless, that 80% of health problems can be solved at primary (non-hospital) level.

So important is the concept of Primary Health Care for nurses, that the International Council of Nurses in collaboration with the World Health Organization published a booklet, 'The role of the nurse in PHC' (1979), which describes how nurses can contribute in practice to the promotion of primary health care.

Community care developments

While the specific objectives of PHC are perhaps most geared to the needs of developing countries, the essential concept is equally pertinent to the 'developed' world. In recent years, there have been significant developments towards shifting the balance of care from hospitals to the community in countries such as the UK.

In 1989, the UK Government issued a White Paper on community care, called 'Caring for People' (HMSO, 1989) and new legislation based on this became effective in

---

Box 1.4 Primary Health Care (PHC)

Key elements suggested by WHO:-
'Promotion of proper nutrition and an adequate supply of safe water; basic sanitation; maternal and child care, including family planning; immunization against the major infectious diseases; prevention and control of local endemic diseases; education concerning prevailing health problems and the methods of preventing and controlling them; appropriate treatment for common diseases and injuries.'

Box 1.5 Key objectives of the reform of Community Care in the UK

- To promote the development of domiciliary, day and respite services to enable people to live in their own homes wherever feasible
- To ensure that service providers make practical support for carers a high priority
- To make proper assessment of need and good case management the cornerstone of high quality care
- To promote the development of a flourishing independent sector alongside good quality public service
- To clarify the responsibilities of agencies and so make it easier to hold them to account for their performance
- To secure better value for taxpayers' money by introducing a new funding structure for social care.

Smith S 1993 All Change (The Community Care Act). Nursing Times 89 (3): 24–26

Box 1.6 Containing the costs of health care

The health care systems across Europe are financed and operated differently, but address the same needs and face common challenges. Over the years the national health systems and governments of European countries have been wrestling to satisfy two seemingly conflicting demands. On the one hand, there is the constant political pressure to provide every citizen with ever better access to higher quality of care. On the other, there is the imperative to keep costs at a level the nation and its taxpayers can afford. Resolving this conflict poses a key challenge for health care systems in all industrialized countries. Across Europe national governments are issuing demands for action and change.

Andersen Consulting (1993) *The Future of European Health Care.* A study by Andersen Consulting in co-operation with Burson-Marsteller. London.

1993. Key objectives of the reform of community care are shown in Box 1.5.

In practice, this means that responsibility for planning care in the community has shifted from health care workers to social services' staff (i.e. mainly social workers) although co-operation between health and social service agencies is vital. Although systematic 'needs assessment' and 'case management' (since re-termed 'care' management) may be new features of the reformed system, the transfer of elderly people and people with learning disabilities or mental health problems from hospitals to the community has been Government policy for more than 20 years.

Some critics believe that this policy has contributed to social problems, such as homelessness; and, of course, shifting the balance of care from hospitals to community cannot be achieved successfully without adequate finance.

CONTAINING COSTS OF HEALTH CARE

Shifting the balance of care from hospital to community obviously has cost implications and, without added money, this means that extra funding to extend care in the community must be drawn from funds previously allocated to the hospital sector of the health service. However, irrespective of the new ideology, the objective of containing the overall costs of health care has been a driving force behind the radical reform which health care systems throughout the Western world (including Britain's National Health Service) have been/are undergoing. This very point was made in a report on health care in ten European countries which was published in 1993 (Andersen Consulting, 1993) — see Box 1.6.

Health care funding

The need for overall cost containment exists irrespective of variation in the *way* in which health care systems are financed. In the UK, the National Health Service has been financed almost entirely from general taxation and, on its introduction in 1948, the British public was promised comprehensive health care free of charge at the point of delivery. Other health care systems are funded through direct and/or indirect taxation or state and/or personal schemes of insurance or, increasingly, a combination of methods.

The *amount* of funding tends to reflect a country's overall economic status and/or the value its Government places on health. The usual way of calculating how much a country spends on health is in terms of the proportion of what the country produces — i.e. its Gross Domestic Product (GDP). The European average is about 8% of GDP (with Spain and the UK among the lowest spenders), considerably lower than the USA's level of health care spending (see Fig. 1.2). The very high level of spending in the USA, yet without provision for all of the population, was the main reason why that country entered the 1990s with its President intent on achieving major health care reform.

The costs of nursing

Since nurses are the largest single group of health care

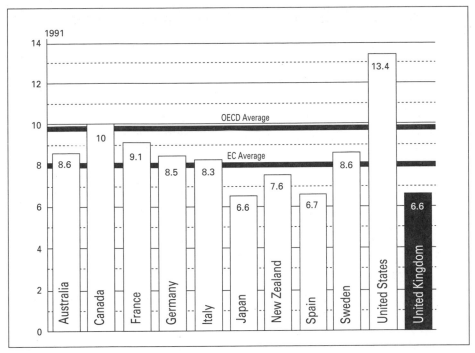

Fig. 1.2 Health care spending. Reproduced with kind permission from RCN 1994 NHS Expenditure-The Facts. Royal College of Nursing, London

workers, their salary costs are generally the largest single item of expenditure in the budget of a health care system. In the UK, nurses' wages have accounted for over 40% of the overall NHS budget.

Not surprisingly, therefore, the costs of nursing are coming under increasing scrutiny in the course of health service reforms. Understandably, there are fears that Governments will seek to cut nursing costs, for example by replacing experienced qualified nurses with inexperienced support workers. There is some evidence, however, that a richer 'skill mix' (i.e. a higher ratio of qualified nurses to unqualified nursing staff) actually produces better outcomes for patients at a lower overall cost (RCN, 1994). It is crucial that the nursing profession continues to gather evidence that nurses *are* cost-effective.

Increasing emphasis on cost-effectiveness

This evidence is crucial because of the increasing emphasis which Governments are placing on the *cost-effectiveness* (and not simply the costs) of health care. This is particularly so in relation to the hospital sector of health services because, as already explained, it is in this sector that costs have escalated but now need to be contained if the shift towards care in the community is to be realized and adequately financed.

In the UK, the Government recognized the need for improved management of the NHS and, in 1984, replaced management by health care professionals with a system of general management (i.e. professional managers).

Box 1.7 Self-government for hospitals

'The Government believes that self-government for hospitals will encourage a stronger sense of local ownership and pride ... It will stimulate the commitment and harness the skills of those who are directly responsible for providing services. Supported by a funding system in which hospitals can flourish, it will encourage local initiative and greater competition. All this in turn will ensure a better deal for the public, improving the choice and quality of services offered and the efficiency with which those services are delivered.'

HMSO 1989 *Working for Patients* (Government White Paper on the Reform of the NHS). London.

Then, to further increase cost-effectiveness and financial accountability in the hospital sector of the health service, the reforms of the British National Health service, announced in the Government's 1989 White Paper, 'Working for Patients', paved the way for the transfer of hospitals to self-governing status as 'NHS Trusts' (see Box 1.7).

The notion of 'competition' is central to the NHS Reforms. For purposes of creating an 'internal market' for health care, the functions of 'purchasers' (i.e. those who *buy* the services) and 'providers' (i.e. those who *provide* the services) have been split. Thus, health authorities, fund-holding GPs (general practitioners, i.e. family doctors) and health insurance companies have become purchasers of health care. Hospitals, community units and private sector facilities (e.g. independent hospitals and nursing homes) are the providers.

In a competitive market, providers have to 'win' contracts and, to do this, they must be able to demonstrate to purchasers the cost-effectiveness and quality of their services. Thus, activities such as costing, clinical audit and quality assessment are increasingly important activities in provider units. The concept of a market system has been introduced in the UK and other industrialized countries to many areas of the public sector, not just to health care. In theory, a market achieves greater cost-effectivess through the pressures of competition and by responsiveness to the needs and demands of the consumers. It remains to be seen whether this model works for health care.

IMPROVING QUALITY AND CHOICE FOR CONSUMERS

It has to be said that these radical health care reforms of the 1990s are not only concerned with increasing cost-effectiveness. 'Putting patients first' was a key theme in the UK Government's proposals for reform of the NHS (see Box 1.8).

'In short', this section of *Working for Patients* concluded, 'every hospital in the NHS should offer what the best offer now. These improvements will bring greater appreciation and recognition from patients and their families for all the care that the Health Service provides.'

Box 1.8 Putting patients first

A key objective of the NHS reforms is:-

'. . to give patients, wherever they live in the UK, better health care and greater choice of the services available.' (p 3)

The Government believes that each hospital should offer patients (pp 6–7):-

- appointments systems which are reliable and reduce waiting times in outpatient clinics
- quiet and pleasant waiting areas with proper facilities for children and for counselling worried parents and relatives
- clear information leaflets about the facilities available and what patients need to know when they come into hospital
- clearer, easier and more sensitive procedures for making suggestions for improvement and, if necessary, complaints
- once in hospital, clear and sensitive explanations of what is happening with regard to practical matters (e.g. where to go, who to see) and to clinical matters (e.g. on the nature of an illness and its proposed treatment)
- rapid notification of the results of diagnostic tests
- a wider choice of optional extras and amenities for patients who want to pay for them (e.g. single rooms, personal telephones, TVs) and a wider choice of meals

HMSO 1989 Working for Patients, London.

How is nursing managing the changes and challenges?

It was pointed out, right at the beginning of this chapter, that *change* has been a hallmark of nursing's development over time. The growing emphasis on health and community care, and the current reforms of health care systems, have required further change and present new challenges for nursing.

In many respects, however, nursing is already well prepared to participate in the reformist strategies which Governments have been introducing. As already discussed, nursing has long been involved in care in the community and, over time, the profession has increased its attention to prevention of illness and promotion of health while maintaining its key position in the hospital sector of health services.

Accountability has become a well understood concept in nursing and the goal of improving the quality of care

has been high on the nursing profession's own agenda for a long time now. Throughout the 1980s, in the UK and in many other countries, this was expressed in the activity of setting quality standards for nursing; and reflected in the increasing use of quality assurance methods and an expansion of research by nurses into issues of quality. By the beginning of the 1990s, nurse researchers were starting to address seriously the complexities of identifying and measuring the outcomes of nursing; practising nurses were acquiring the skills of clinical audit; and, in addition, they were becoming concerned with the costs of health care through involvement in the new arrangements of devolved clinical budgeting.

Perhaps most importantly, the nursing profession is well prepared for the so-called reformist strategy of 'putting patients first', as the British Government chose to describe one of its key objectives for the NHS Reforms. Nurse-led developments in nursing practice which grew throughout the 1980s were directly concerned with moving the emphasis away from 'tasks' and finding a way of *individualizing nursing*. The culmination of this movement has been described, as mentioned right at the start of the chapter, as the 'New Nursing' (Box 1.1).

It is not possible to discuss in detail here all of the dimensions of this 'movement' in nursing. By way of introduction to this book, however, it is important to explain the changes which have taken place in the way nursing is *organized* (i.e. from preoccupation with tasks to a focus on patients); how, in relation to that, the introduction of the 'nursing process' provided a *systematic method* for individualizing nursing; and how an understanding of individualized nursing can be formed and developed through the process of *conceptualization*.

CHANGES IN THE ORGANIZATION OF NURSING CARE

'Putting patients first' is certainly not compatible with the traditional method of organizing nursing around tasks.

Task allocation, sometimes called 'job assignment' was based on the industrial concept of 'division of labour'. Applied in nursing, this meant that patient care was fragmented into a series of jobs, these assigned to different nurses of different grades. Thus, a hierarchy of tasks and staff was created and, for patients, there was fragmentation of care and no continuity of carer. Indeed, patients were subordinated to the system rather than central to it. Dissatisfaction with this method of organizing patient care led to the introduction of more patient-centred systems.

Patient-centred systems of organising nursing care include *patient allocation* (in which each nurse is allocated a small number of patients to look after during a whole work shift) and *team nursing* (in which a ward's nursing staff divide up into teams, each taking responsibility for the total care of a sub-group of the patients).

Primary nursing can perhaps be described as the ultimate patient-centred nursing system. The key feature here is that one nurse ('the primary nurse') assumes individual responsibility for an individual patient. Theoretically, this responsibility extends over the entire period during which the patient requires nursing although, in practice, there has to be delegation to others ('the associate nurses') during periods of absence from the ward. The potential benefits of primary nursing for patients are obvious: there is both continuity of care and carer.

These various methods of organizing nursing are illustrated in Figure 1.3 in the order described.

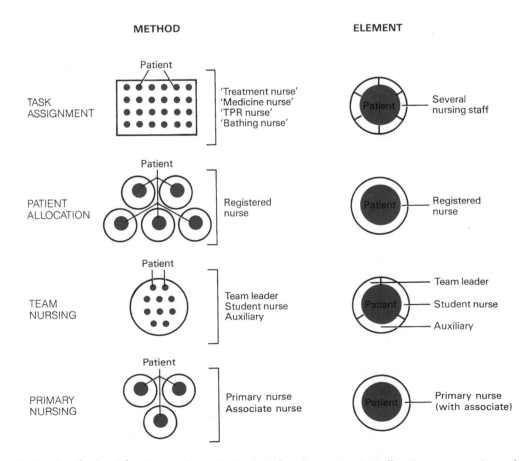

Fig. 1.3 The organizational method and the element of organization in task assignment, patient allocation, team nursing and primary nursing.

Although it is true to say, in the UK at least , that 'task assignment' was almost exclusively practised in the 1960s in the context of hospital nursing, it should not be forgotten that community nurses have always operated in a patient-centred fashion by virtue of the nature of their work. Nor should it be forgotten that 'task assigment' has not entirely disappeared: in some instances it may be the only feasible way of ensuring basic standards of nursing within the limits of available staffing.

The staffing requirements of 'primary nursing', if fully operated, are stringent. It is generally believed that only a fully qualified nurse is competent to act as a primary nurse. Insufficient numbers of nurses, or a low proportion of qualified staff in the ward nursing team, are the reasons most often given for the system breaking down or for not attempting to operate primary nursing. It has to be said that, even into the 1990s, firm evidence of the cost-effectiveness of primary nursing was still lacking (see Box 1.9).

Nonetheless, despite the lack of scientific evidence of its operational benefits, the philosophical imperatives of primary nursing remain relevant. Much can be learned about the original thinking behind primary nursing from the writings of early pioneers such as Zander (1980) in North America and Pearson (1988) in the UK. There is no doubt that the concept of primary nursing responds to the directive of 'putting patients first'; and it embodies all of the ideals of *individualized nursing*.

Box 1.9 Primary nursing

Thomas and Bond (1991) undertook a comprehensive review of research on primary nursing and concluded that '*despite the plethora of studies attempting to evaluate primary nursing, there is little consensus as to whether, and under what circumstances, primary nursing results in improved outcomes*'.

However, this may be because of weaknesses in the research rather than a weakness of primary nursing and Thomas and Bond drew attention to the former in concluding their review.

'*The vast majority of studies (on primary nursing) are flawed by an absence of operational definitions, and a failure to recognize the multidimensionality of the concept, as well as a failure to control other relevant variables, to the extent that findings have little validity and cannot be generalized.*'

Thomas L H, Bond S 1991 Outcomes of nursing care: The case of primary nursing. International Journal of Nursing Studies 28 (4): 291–314

THE INTRODUCTION OF A SYSTEMATIC APPROACH TO INDIVIDUALIZING NURSING

While systems of nursing (i.e. patient allocation, team nursing and primary nursing) provide a means of creating the *conditions* for individualizing nursing, they do not, on their own, provide a *method* for doing so.

The introduction of the 'nursing process' provided the means for patient-centred systems of nursing to be operationalized in a systematic way. Universally, the term 'nursing process' is recognized as describing a systematic approach to nursing which comprises a series (or cycle) of steps (or stages) which, most commonly, are referred to as assessing, planning, implementing and evaluating.

Background

It is interesting to note that, although commonplace nowadays, the term 'nursing process' had only recently been introduced into the UK when the first edition of this book (published in 1980) was in early stages of preparation in the mid-1970s. Some 15 years or so earlier, however, the idea of the nursing process had been introduced into the North American literature by nurse theorists writing about the development of conceptual frameworks for nursing.

Perhaps because of its origins and attendant jargon, the notion of the nursing process was greeted with suspicion by British nurses and when first introduced, it met with considerable resistance. Perhaps a more sympathetic view might have been taken had the nursing process been seen less as an American import and an apparent threat, and more as a vehicle for advancing the expression of interest in putting into operation the developing systems for individualizing nursing. Much was written about the introduction of the nursing process and interested readers are referred to Walton's (1986) comprehensive review of nursing process literature published over the initial period.

Development

In spite of the initial resistance, the nursing process gained remarkably rapid recognition at a formal level for, in 1977, the professional registering body of the UK (then the General Nursing Council, now the United Kingdom Central Council) decreed that 'the nursing care of patients should be studied and practised in the sequence of the nursing process' (Dickinson, 1982).

Development of the nursing process in terms of practice was given enormous impetus when the Regional Office of the World Health Organization decided to incorporate it into the European Medium Term Programme for Nursing/Midwifery and 23 participating centres across 11 countries, including the UK, collaborated in this multinational study which commenced in 1983. Reports arising from the venture have been published in the form of an overall summary from WHO under the title 'People's Needs for Nursing Care' (WHO, 1987) with separate accounts of the work undertaken in specific countries (e.g. Farmer's 1985 report pertaining to Scotland).

This ambitious programme did much to encourage discussion and a sharing of ideas about the nursing process at an international level; and, although aspects of its implementation are peculiar to local practice circumstances, the essential ideas which are encapsulated in the term 'nursing process' are universal, as is the case so often in nursing.

Essential ideas

The essential ideas are, in fact, not new in nursing even if the term 'nursing process' was considered as such; the 'good nurse' has always used it. Often, however, nurses did not analyse or explicate what they were doing in terms of a process or steps within it, nor did they document information in an ordered and comprehensive manner.

Because nurses had not explained or recorded nursing, there was no tangible evidence of the intellectual aspect of the process to the onlooker who saw only the observable behaviour of the nurse. Thus, for the onlooking learner in particular, no wonder it was difficult to appreciate and understand the often rapidly executed mental activity which determined the experienced nurse's actions. The process involved was neither explained nor documented and, frequently, the results of the nurse's actions were neither evident nor systematically evaluated.

The value, then, in envisaging the nursing process as something new — even recognizing that the 'good nurse' had always endeavoured to provide individualized and systematic nursing — lay, and still lies, in its emphasis on strengthening evaluation and on making explicit the intellectual as well as the behavioural components of nursing.

Attention to the intellectual or 'thinking' aspects of nursing has been much neglected and, in a sense, this failing is perpetuated when nurses view the nursing process essentially in 'doing' terms (notably the activity of documentation) rather than in terms which emphasize the process as simply a logical mode of thinking. Viewed in these terms, it becomes easier to accept that 'the process' is not peculiar to nursing; a systematic approach through assessing, planning, implementing and evaluating could be (and is) applied equally in doctoring, in teaching and in studying, irrespective of the discipline.

Perhaps if the nursing process initially had been understood essentially as a mode of thinking rather than a method of doing (... 'doing assessments' ... 'doing care plans' ... and so on), then many of the problems encountered and misunderstandings perpetuated might have been avoided.

Problems and misunderstandings

Problems and misunderstandings there have been and still continue to be over the nursing process; letters and articles in the nursing press over the years attest to that. Initial concerns were not confined only within nursing circles either; the scepticism and hostility felt by some doctors towards the nursing process was voiced publicly at one stage in the debate, most notably in a prominent journal paper by a medical professor (Mitchell, 1984) although many of those criticisms could be contested (Tierney, 1984).

But, even within nursing and among those who supported the introduction of the nursing process, it was generally accepted that the way in which this concept was introduced, at least into the UK — in haste, and adopting a 'top-down' or 'power-coercive' change strategy (Walton, 1986) — led to many of the misunderstandings and difficulties.

Certainly, with the benefit of hindsight, the introduction of the nursing process approach could have been better managed. It should have been realized more quickly that it would be impossible to instantly introduce a truly individualized system of nursing into practice settings which still operated an essentially 'task-oriented' rather than 'patient-centred' approach. It later became recognized that the nursing process is only wholly feasible in the context of practice which is organized on a basis of patient allocation, team nursing or, best of all, primary nursing.

Over recent years, the nursing process has not been a subject of such controversy. In the main, the activities of assessing planning, implementing and evaluating have become embedded in everyday nursing practice. More is said about each of these activities later in the book. As long as the nursing process is not applied in a dogged, linear fashion, its essential ideas still have a place in nursing today; there is nothing essentially incompatible between the *process* of nursing and more recent developments, such as the growing interest in 'managed care' (Laxade & Hale, 1995).

Relationship to nursing models

The nursing process is neither a 'philosophy' nor a 'theory' although it was not infrequently described as such in the early days of its introduction. The process on its own is in vacuo; it has to be used in the context of a conceptual framework — a nursing model.

This book, The Elements of Nursing, describes — and

is built around — *a model for nursing based on a model of living*. Before the development of our model is outlined, and the model is described, some introductory comments about nursing models, and theoretical development in nursing more generally, may be helpful.

THEORETICAL DEVELOPMENT IN NURSING

When people think about nursing, they tend to think of it as a very *practical* activity. As long ago as 1859, Florence Nightingale was writing *Notes on Nursing*, and deploring the fact that nursing was considered to be little more than the administration of medicines and the application of poultices!

It is curious that, even today, many people consider nursing to be simply a series of practical tasks carried out by the nurse. Undoubtedly practical skills are a very important aspect of nursing, but this restrictive interpretation does not take account of the thinking processes which are involved in the complex activities of assessing, planning and evaluating; and nor does it acknowledge the knowledge and attitudes which must be acquired for implementing individualized nursing in many different circumstances and for patients/clients from different age groups and backgrounds.

So, despite Nightingale's early recognition of the need for a combination of intellectual skills and practical skills, nursing remained for a long time at a practical level only rather than developing, simultaneously, a theoretical perspective on which to base its practice.

Developing nursing knowledge

Interestingly, the need for theoretical development in nursing was recognized initially more by nurse educators than by nurses in practice. Meleis (1991), in her account of the development of theoretical nursing, describes how North American nurses in the 1950s recognized the difficulty of designing improved nursing curricula in the absence of any clear conceptual view of the nature of the 'discipline' of nursing. They recognized, too, that without ongoing research, nursing knowledge would remain stagnant and nursing practice could not develop with the advantage of theoretical understanding.

The importance of research

From the 1950s onwards, research activity and theory development began to grow, initially mainly in North America but, gradually, in other parts of the world too. Many of those nurses who engaged in these 'academic' pursuits in the early days were regarded with considerable scepticism by practising nurses. Over the years, however, the need for research in nursing has become

accepted universally. The value of the knowledge which has been generated through research and scholarship in nursing over the past three decades should become clearly evident in this book which draws on up-to-date knowledge.

Knowledge, however, in any discipline, is always nothing more than provisional. Research and scholarship must be an ongoing, inherent activity. There are many definitions of research, but most emphasize the basic point that research is concerned with generating knowledge in a systematic and scientific way (Nolan & Behi, 1995). In the USA, there is now a very strong research infrastructure and a well-funded national nursing research agenda. Few other countries are at such an advanced stage, but in many countries nursing research activity is now extensive and better co-ordination and use of research is gradually being achieved through the development of *strategy* for nursing research. The UK is one of several countries which now has a national Strategy for Research in Nursing, Midwifery and Health Visiting (DoH, 1993) — see Box 1.10.

This UK strategy for research in *nursing* followed the publication of a Research and Development Strategy for the NHS as a whole (DoH, 1991). It is clear that, in the current climate of reform in the health services, research has become an explicitly valued activity; and, indeed, there is the expectation that *all* aspects of health care should be soundly based on the best possible scientific knowledge.

Box 1.10 Nursing research strategy

The Taskforce concluded that the particular needs which exist within nursing, midwifery and health visiting include:-

- the integration of nursing, midwifery and health visiting issues and researchers from these fields within the new organisational structures for R&D in the NHS;
- targeted investment in research education and training for nurses, midwives and health visitors;
- the identification of an enhanced range of sources and types of funding for research in nursing;
- an improvement in the dissemination and implementation of research and development in nursing.

Recommendations are made which address each of these needs.

DoH (1993) Report of the Taskforce on the Strategy for Research in Nursing, Midwifery and Health Visiting. Department of Health, London.

The need for theory

While the legitimate application of the findings of particular research studies may be limited (i.e. not generalizable beyond the setting of the study or the particular patient group in question), *theory* has potentially wider applications. A theory is a generalizable explanation of a phenomenon. Psychology, for example, has theories of behaviour; education draws on substantiated educational theories, and so on. In its own theoretical development, nursing has drawn on the theories of these and other disciplines, including the biological sciences.

Theory is important in underpinning research and in providing a way of explaining the meaning of the findings of research. It is also useful in providing a 'language' for the communication of nursing knowledge, and the labels and definitions for phenomena: therefore, nursing practice can be explored and explained through the use of common concepts.

Concepts such as 'pain', 'grief', 'stress', 'quality of care', 'patient satisfaction', 'discharge planning' and so on, to name but a few, are concepts which have been reviewed and researched in nursing. A common understanding of the nature and dimensions of such concepts allows researchers and practising nurses to communicate with each other — and, importantly, also with health care professionals from other disciplines. Thus, over time, the knowledge base of nursing practice is clarified and extended. It is also important to have some means of understanding how individual concepts, and clusters of concepts, relate together, i.e. some overall view of nursing. This really brings us back to the question which was asked at the very beginning of this chapter, 'What is nursing?'

The value of an overall conceptual framework

Attempts to answer this question, and identify nursing's key concepts, led North American nurse theorists of the 1960s and 1970s to devise conceptual *models* for nursing.

What use is a model? The advantage of using models is perhaps more obvious if one uses the analogy of a physical model which depicts a concrete reality such as a car, or the plan for a new housing development; or in anatomy, a model of the lungs or an ear. They are made up of three-dimensional parts and can be handled, taken apart and reassembled. Models of a discipline are more abstract and although they cannot be touched as such, they can be seen diagrammatically and can be mentally arranged and re-arranged.

They are also made up of parts although in this instance, symbolized by a word or a set of words — a concept. And just as importantly, a model indicates the relationships between the parts. Of course, models are not peculiar to nursing; they can be, and are, used in any discipline. However, two nurse authors (Riehl & Roy, 1980) provide a useful working definition of a nursing model as:

'. . . a systematically constructed, scientifically based and logically related set of concepts which identify the essential components of nursing practice, together with the theoretical bases of these concepts and the values required for their use by the practitioner . . .'

How are models devised? It is important to realise that conceptual models are not made up of a few transient thoughts, hastily put together; they are developed carefully and systematically, sometimes as a result of research, and may involve months or years of observing nursing practices, and thinking about why, as well as how, nursing is carried out.

Models are not set in marble, however; they are constructed in the knowledge that they are essentially a basis for further thinking about the discipline. As new, scientifically tested theories are produced to explain observed practice, the model may be modified, or improved, or enlarged or even discarded — as it should be if it is no longer useful. In fact, if one looks at the writings of some model-builders in nursing, over a period of years, the developments in their thinking can be identified both as alterations in the diagrams they present of their model, and from explanations in the accompanying text.

How is theory used in a model? A model is not a theory. However, theory can assist the construction of a model. Although a discipline will identify some knowledge which is unique to itself, theories from other disciplines are sometimes included in a model, albeit applied in a specific context. Stevens (1979) made the point that all disciplines have areas '. . . where the inquiries and answers of one field overlap with another'. Thus 'borrowed theories' become 'shared knowledge' when transferred into nursing. Most of the model-builders in nursing acknowledge the use of theories from other disciplines.

What value are nursing models? Fawcett (1984) considered that the development of conceptual models, and labelling them as such, was an important advance for the discipline of nursing. To make her point she quotes Reilly (1975):

'We all have a private image (concept) of nursing practice. In turn, this private image influences our interpretation of data, our decisions and our actions. But can a discipline continue to develop when its members hold so many differing private images? The proponents of conceptual models of practice are seeking to make us aware of private images, so that we can begin to identify commonalities in our perception of the nature of practice . . .'

Conceptual models for nursing, then, are the formal presentations of images of nursing. They consist of the main concepts which identify the essential components of the discipline; show the relationships between the concepts; and may introduce already established theories from other disciplines which are applicable to nursing.

A model is not just an intellectual aid; it can be useful for nursing practice, education, management and research. In practice terms, a model can provide a framework for what the nurse does and how she does it; in education, it can provide a framework which organizes the curriculum — the knowledge, skills and approach which are necessary for learning to practise; in management, it can outline the common goals to be achieved; in research, a model can provide guidance about what should be studied in order to extend nursing knowledge and thus improve practice.

What kinds of models have been devised? Of the early North American nursing models, Orem's '*self-care*' model is one of the best known (Orem, 1971): it depicts nursing as assisting individuals to their optimal level of self-care. Roy (1970) centred her model around the concept of '*adaptation*'. Rogers (1970) focused on the concept of '*environment*' and the nursing client (i.e. patient) in interaction with that environment. And so on. For a full understanding of the various models which have been devised, the original publication and later refinements need to be studied. By way of introduction, and quick resumé, there are texts which provide summary accounts of nursing models (e.g. Aggleton & Chalmers, 1986; Meleis, 1991).

What do different models have in common? It is reasonable to expect that, although different nursing models are devised from different paradigms, they have some common features in their portrayal of nursing. Kuhn (1977) coined the phrase 'metaparadigm' to describe the global concepts of a discipline. By the mid 1980s, there was general agreement (e.g. see Fawcett, 1984) that the metaparadigm concepts shared by nursing models are:

- person
- environment
- health
- nursing activities/process.

The model for nursing which is described in this book predated the articulation of this metaparadigm but it does, in fact, address all four of the main concepts. Our model for nursing is based on a model of living and its development is described in the following chapter.

REFERENCES

Aggleton P, Chalmers H 1986 Nursing models and the nursing process. Macmillan, London
Andersen Consulting 1993 The Future of European Health Care. A study by Andersen Consulting in co-operation with Burson-Marsteller. London
Beardshaw V, Robinson R 1990 New for Old? Prospects for Nursing in the 1990s. King's Fund Institute, London
Dickinson S 1982 The nursing process and the professional status of nursing. Occasional Paper, Nursing Times 78(16) June 2
DoH 1991a The Health of the Nation. Department of Health, HMSO, London
DoH 1991b A Strategy for Research and Development in the NHS. Department of Health, London
DoH 1993 Report of the Taskforce on the Strategy for Research in Nursing, Midwifery and Health Visiting, Department of Health, London
Farmer E S 1985 On introducing a systematic method for the practice and study of nursing: A report of the Scottish component of the WHO (Euro) multinational study of needs for nursing care in two selected groups of patients. Nursing Research Unit, Department of Nursing Studies, University of Edinburgh
Fawcett J 1984 Analysis and evaluation of conceptual models of nursing. F A Davis, Philadelphia
HMSO 1989 Caring for People: Community Care in the Next Decade and Beyond. Departments of Health and Social Security, London
HMSO 1989 Working for Patients (Government White Paper on the Reform of the NHS), London
Kuhn T 1977 Second thoughts on paradigms. In: Suppe F (ed) The structure of scientific theories. University of Illinois Press, Chicago
Laxade S, Hale C A 1995 Managed care: an opportunity for nursing. British Journal of Nursing 4(5): 290–294 and 4(6): 345–350
Levin L 1981 Self-care in health: potentials and pitfalls. World Health Forum 2(2): 177–184
Meleis A 1991 2nd ed. Theoretical nursing: development and progress. Lippincott, Philadelphia
Mitchell J 1984 Is nursing any business of doctors? A simple guide to the 'nursing process'. Nursing Times 80(19) May 9: 28–32
Nath U R, O' Neill P 1988 International networks: report from the first Pan-European Nursing Conference. Nursing Times 84 (28) July 13: 21
Nightingale F 1859 Notes on nursing. Duckworth, London (reprinted 1952)
Nolan M, Behi R 1995 What is research? Some definitions and dilemmas. British Journal of Nursing 4(2): 111–115
Orem D 1971 Nursing: concepts of practice, McGraw-Hill, New York
Powell D 1986 Hospitals for health. Nursing Times 82 (49) December 3: 30–32
RCN 1994 NHS Expenditure — The Facts. Royal College of Nursing, London
Reilly D 1975 Why a conceptual framework? Nursing Outlook 23: 566–569
Riehl J, Roy C 1980 Conceptual models for nursing practice, 2nd edn. Appleton-Century-Crofts, New York
Rogers M 1970 An introduction to the theoretical basis of nursing. F A Davis, Philadelphia
Roy C 1970 Adaptation: A conceptual framework for nursing. Nursing Outlook 18 (3): 42–45
Skeet M 1988 Florence Nightingale — a woman of vision and drive. World Health Forum 9: 175–177
Smith S 1993 All change (the Community Care Act). Nursing Times 89 (3): 24–26
Stevens B 1979 Nursing theory: analysis, application, and evaluation. Little, Brown, Boston
Thomas L H, Bond S 1991 Outcomes of nursing care: The case of primary nursing. International Journal of Nursing Studies 28 (4): 291–314
Tierney A 1984 Defending the process. Nursing Times 80(2) May 16: 38–41
Walton I 1986 The nursing process in perspective: a literature review. University of York, York
World Health Organization 1946 Constitution. World Health Organization Geneva (Definition of health)
World Health Organization/UNICEF 1978 Primary health care. World Health Organization, Geneva, p 7

2

A model of living

If a model can be said to have a birthplace, then the Roper, Logan and Tierney model is indisputably an Edinburgh one — all three of the trio are graduates of the University of Edinburgh.

Nancy Roper had long been concerned about the adjectives used to categorize nursing. Students had to be allocated to various wards to gain experience in gynaecological, orthopaedic, medical, surgical and so on. There were also broader classifications — children's nursing, mental handicap nursing and psychiatric nursing. The common denominator was 'nursing'. So in 1970 she started a research project to investigate whether or not there was an identifiable 'core' of 'nursing' because if it existed then nurses in the adjectival areas could identify the additional knowledge, skills and attitudes required for 'nursing' people with a gynaecological condition and so on.

There was a library search for other projects related to identification of a 'core', but none had been conducted in clinical areas. A Patient Profile was used to collect data from patients in all clinical areas to which one college of nursing allocated its students:

- a general hospital
- a maternity hospital
- a psychiatric hospital
- 12 community districts.

The 774 profiles were analyzed and the results revealed that there was a 'core' which related to everyday living activities; hence the idea to base a model for nursing on a model of living. However the original Roper models (1976) were enlarged and regrouped to produce the Roper, Logan and Tierney models and the result of this work was first published in 1980 as 'The elements of nursing'. Subsequent refinements were included in the second edition (1985) and the third edition (1990).

To encapsulate the complexities of 'living' in a model which is simple enough to be meaningful is, of course, impossible. The model of living presented here is only an attempt to identify the main features of a highly complex phenomenon, and to indicate relationships between the various components of the model (Fig. 2.1). As indicated in Figure 2.1, there are five main components (concepts) in our model, namely:

Activities of Living (ALs)
Lifespan

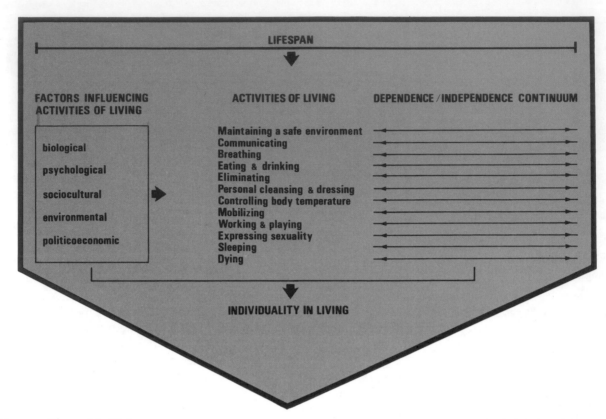

Fig. 2.1 Diagram of the model of living

Dependence/independence continuum
Factors influencing ALs
Individuality in living.

In the following text, each of these components will be discussed in turn.

Activities of Living

A model of living must offer a way of describing what 'living' means. If asked to describe what everyday living involves, most people — irrespective of their age and circumstances — would mention activities such as eating and drinking, working and playing, and sleeping. If prompted, they would probably agree that breathing, communicating and eliminating are also activities which are an integral part of living, even if at times they may be hardly aware of performing them. All of these activities, and others — such as maintaining a safe environment, and personal cleansing and dressing — collectively contribute to the complex process of living. They are *activities of living*.

It is this concept which is used as the focus of our model of living; and a set of Activities of Living (ALs), 12 in number (Fig. 2.2), makes up the main component of the model as they describe the person who is central to it.

The term 'Activity of Living' (AL) is used as an all-

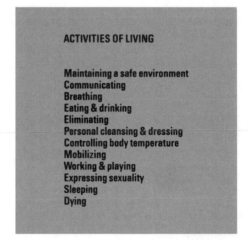

Fig. 2.2 Activities of Living

embracing one. *Each* 'Activity' has many dimensions; indeed it could be thought of as an overall activity composed of a number of particular activities, rather as a compound is made up of a number of elements. The more one analyses the Activities of Living the more one realizes just how complex each one is. Compounding this complexity is the fact that they are so closely related. For example, communicating is related to many of the other ALs: just imagine eating and drinking, working and playing, and expressing sexuality without communicating! And breathing is essential for all of the ALs. So only for the purpose of description and learning can they be separated, and here only a brief description of each AL is necessary by way of introduction.

MAINTAINING A SAFE ENVIRONMENT

In order to stay alive and carry out any of the other activities of living, it is imperative that actions are taken to maintain a safe environment. In fact, each day, many activities are carried out with this purpose although, because they are such a routine part of everyday living, they are performed almost without conscious effort. For example, steps are taken to prevent accidents in the home by guarding fires, by keeping poisonous substances in a safe place, and ensuring that carpets are in good condition and trip-free.

Every day, too, precautions are taken to prevent accidents when travelling and while working and playing. Maintaining a safe environment on the roads and the workplace is not only a shared responsibility of individuals but also, through action and legislation of the government.

Some people, in addition to ensuring their own personal safety, engage in activities — such as campaigning for nuclear disarmament or action to prevent pollution of the environment — which they consider will help to ensure for future generations an environment which is as safe as possible.

COMMUNICATING

Human beings are essentially social beings and a major part of living involves communicating with other people in one way or another. Communicating not only involves the use of verbal language as in talking and writing, but also the non-verbal transmission of information by facial expression and body gesture. Communication of this type also provides the vehicle for transmission of emotions: long before a baby has acquired verbal skills, feelings such as pleasure and displeasure can be communicated to others. Communication through touch is equally subtle although less frequently used except in intimate personal relationships and here, as in verbal language, there are distinct cultural differences.

By its very nature, the activity of communicating permeates the whole area of interpersonal interaction and human relationships which are such a fundamental and important dimension of living.

BREATHING

The very first activity of a newborn baby is breathing. The ability to do this is vital since by this action the cells of the body will receive from the air, oxygen which was previously supplied from the mother's blood. But, thereafter, breathing becomes an effortless activity and people are

not consciously aware of performing it until some abnormal circumstance forces it to their attention. Oxygen is absolutely essential for all body cells; there is irreversible damage to the brain cells when they are deprived of it, even for a few minutes. Consequently all other ALs — and life itself — are entirely dependent on breathing.

EATING AND DRINKING

A baby is born with the ability to suck and swallow so that nourishment can be obtained without which survival and growth are impossible. Human life cannot be sustained for long without eating and drinking so this activity, like breathing, is absolutely essential. Eating and drinking is also a time-consuming activity since apart from the time spent eating meals, food itself has to be procured and prepared. The way meals are taken, and the food and drink selected, reflect the influence of sociocultural factors on this AL. For most people, eating and drinking are pleasurable activities but the fact that great numbers of people in the world die daily from starvation serves as a reminder of the essential nature of this AL.

ELIMINATING

We have chosen to describe urinary elimination and faecal elimination together because, although two distinct body systems are involved, there is no good reason to separate them in the context of an Activities of Living framework. The essential nature of this AL is such that in infancy elimination occurs as a reflex response to the collection of urine in the bladder and faeces in the bowel. The acquisition of voluntary control over elimination and independence in this AL are important milestones of development in the early years of life.

Eliminating, like eating and drinking, is a necessary and integral activity of everyday life. However, interestingly, whereas eating and drinking and many other ALs are performed in the company of others, elimination is regarded as a highly private activity. Throughout the world people are socialized into eliminating in private and this contributes to many strongly held attitudes and taboos which are associated with this Activity of Living.

PERSONAL CLEANSING AND DRESSING

Cleanliness and good grooming are commended in most cultures, whatever the particular standards and norms. Apart from taking pride in their appearance, people have a social responsibility to ensure cleanliness of body and clothing. The term 'personal cleansing' was deliberately chosen in preference to 'washing' because in addition to handwashing, body washing and bathing, the activities of perineal hygiene and care of the hair, nails, teeth and mouth are also carried out. In relation to dressing it is interesting to appreciate that clothing not only fulfils the function of protection of the body but also reflects important aspects of culture and tradition; has sexual associations; and is a medium of non-verbal communication.

CONTROLLING BODY TEMPERATURE

Unlike cold-blooded animals whose body temperature is subject to the temperature of the external environment, man is able to maintain the body temperature at a constant level irrespective of the degree of heat or cold in the surrounding environment. The heat-regulating system is not fully sensitive at birth but, once its function is established, the temperature of the human body is maintained within a fairly narrow range. This is essential for many of the body's biological processes and also ensures personal comfort in continually varying, sometimes dramatically changing, environmental temperatures. Human tissue cannot survive very long when subjected to extremes of heat or cold; trauma and even death can occur from either heatstroke or hypothermia.

Although body temperature is essentially self-regulating, people have to perform certain deliberate activities to avoid the hazards and discomforts of heat or cold. Therefore activities such as adjusting the temperature and ventilation of the surroundings in a building; varying the amount and type of clothing and regulating the amount of physical activity are all carried out with the objective of helping to control body temperature.

MOBILIZING

Although a rather clumsy word, 'mobilizing' seemed more explicit than 'moving' to describe the capacity for movement which is one of the essential and highly valued human activities. The devastating effects — physical, psychological, economic and social — of any serious long-term limitation on movement bear witness to this fact.

The AL of mobilizing includes the movement produced by groups of large muscles, enabling people to stand, sit, walk and run as well as groups of smaller muscles producing movements such as those involved in manual dexterity or in facial expressions, hand gesticulations and mannerisms; all of which are part of non-verbal communication.

The relationship of mobilizing to other ALs should be readily apparent; behaviour associated with the ALs of breathing, eating and drinking, eliminating, working and playing and so on, all involve movement.

WORKING AND PLAYING

When not sleeping most people are either working or playing; play has been described as the child's work. Usually for most adults working provides an income from which, after essential costs are met, leisure activities are financed. The activities of working and playing can have very different meanings for different individuals. The old adage 'one man's work is another man's play' illustrates this well; for example, one person might earn an income as a market gardener by growing flowers and vegetables whereas, for another, this might be a hobby.

For most people, the sense of belonging to work and leisure groups, the satisfaction from challenge and achievement, and the prevention of boredom, are all important aspects of this AL. Both working and playing can be seen to have positive and negative effects on personal health and well-being. Because both involve physical and mental activity, each can contribute positively to physical and mental health. Conversely, enforced lack of working (as in unemployment or retirement) or insufficient playing may contribute to physical or mental ill-health.

EXPRESSING SEXUALITY

So important is the subject of 'sex' in life today that it cannot be ignored and the publicity associated with the current AIDS epidemic has made it less of a taboo subject . . . but how were we to describe this as an Activity of Living? The specific activity which tends to be directly associated with sex is sexual intercourse. Of course this is an important component of adult relationships — and essential for the continuation of the human race — but there are also many other ways in which human sexuality is expressed.

An individual's sex is determined at conception and throughout the lifespan sexuality is an important dimension of personality and behaviour. Femininity and masculinity are reflected not only in physical appearance and strength but also in style of dress; in many forms of verbal and non-verbal communication; in family and social roles and relationships; and in choices relating to work and play.

SLEEPING

It may seem strange to describe sleeping as an 'activity' until it is realized that body processes do not stop being active during sleep. All living organisms have periods of activity alternating with periods of sleep. In human beings this is a 24-hour rhythm of sleeping and waking. Babies spend the major part of the time asleep and even most adults spend up to one-third of their entire lives sleeping and so, in terms of time alone, this is an important AL. It is an essential one too; growth and repair of cells take place during sleep and sleep enables people to relax from, and be refreshed to cope with, the stresses and demands of everyday living. Without adequate sleep people suffer discomfort and distress, and a variety of ill-effects result from accrued sleep deprivation.

DYING

The inclusion of 'dying' in our list of ALs has been questioned: for example, it has been pointed out that it seems illogical without also including 'being born'. Death is what marks the end of life just as the event of birth marks its beginning. However, the concern is not solely with the event of death, but rather with the process of dying. It could be said that the process of living is a fatal one and certainly, in the process of dying, all the ALs are affected and eventually cease with death. In describing 'living' it seems essential to acknowledge that death is the only really certain thing in life. The whole of a person's life is lived in the light of the inevitability of death, for some people overshadowing living and for others giving positive meaning to life. And of course people do not live only in anticipation of their own eventual death, but also in the knowledge that loved ones will die. It has been said that 'grief is the cost of commitment' in our lives. Grieving is the activity inextricably linked with dying, through which a bereaved person comes to terms with the death of a loved one and finds the courage to begin living fully once more.

Even from such a brief description of the 12 ALs, it is clear that conceptualizing 'living' as an amalgam of 'activities' is a helpful way of beginning to think simply yet constructively about the complex process of living. All of the ALs are important, although obviously some have greater priority than others; the AL of breathing is of prime importance. However, the order in which the ALs are listed does not reflect an order of priority because, according to circumstances, a person's priorities change. Also, as previously mentioned, although the 12 ALs are described separately, they are very closely related to each other. Indeed, although the ALs are presented as one component of the model, they should not be thought of in isolation since they are affected by the other components and these too are closely related to each other. Nevertheless, in their own right, each of the components contributes another dimension of 'living', as the following discussion will show.

Lifespan

It is easy to appreciate why a lifespan is included as one component of the model of living. 'Living' is concerned with the whole of a person's life and each person has a *lifespan*, from birth to death.

The lifespan is represented in the diagram of the model by a line, arrowed to indicate the direction of movement along it from birth to death (Fig. 2.3).

Most countries have local Registry Offices where

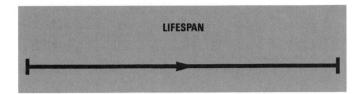

Fig. 2.3 The lifespan

births and deaths have to be recorded. From these data both local and national birth and death rates can be calculated, as well as 'expectation of life at birth by sex', which in the UK in 1994 was 80 years for females and 75 for males (Central Statistical Office, 1994). The age structure of a society can also be ascertained, for example the number of people at work and paying taxes relative to those on retirement pension.

There are usually statutory ages for entering and leaving school and retiring from work. Ageism, namely discrimination on grounds of age, is causing concern in western societies. It may occur when people as early as in their thirties are unsuccessfully seeking further employment after they have been made redundant from their previous job.

As a person moves along the lifespan there is continuous change and every aspect of living is influenced by the biological, psychological, sociocultural, environmental and politicoeconomic circumstances encountered throughout life.

Dependence/independence continuum

This component of the model is closely related to the lifespan and to the ALs. It is included to acknowledge that there are stages of the lifespan when a person cannot yet (or for various reasons, can no longer) perform certain ALs independently. Each person could be said to have a *dependence/independence continuum* for each AL. As shown below (Fig. 2.4), the term 'total dependence' and 'total independence' are used to describe the poles of the continuum and the arrows indicate that movement can take place in either direction according to circumstances. We define independence as 'ability to achieve the AL to a per-

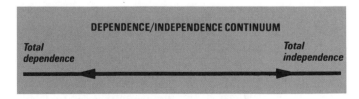

Fig. 2.4 Dependence/independence continuum

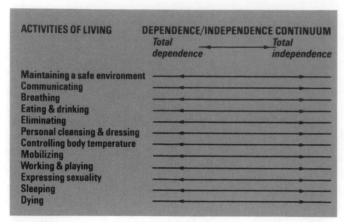

Fig. 2.5 Dependence/independence continuum related to the ALs

sonally and socially acceptable standard without help'.

To emphasize that the dependence/independence continuum relates to each of the ALs — for on its own the concept is too global to be meaningful — the continuum appears in the diagrammatic representation of the model of living alongside each of the 12 activities (Fig. 2.5).

A person's position could be plotted on each continuum (at either pole or somewhere between) to provide an impression of the degree of dependence/independence in respect of the 12 ALs. If repeated at intervals of time, any obvious change in direction or movement along the continua would become apparent.

Comparing the dependence/independence status of people at different stages of the lifespan illustrates the close links between these two components of the model. Newborn babies are dependent on others for help with most of the ALs. From this state of almost total dependence, each child according to capacity can be visualized as gradually moving along the continuum towards the independent pole for each AL.

From collected data there are statistical averages for the age at which independence is achieved for particular ALs. However there are always exceptions; by no means everyone has the capacity or opportunity to achieve or retain independence in all of the ALs. Not all children are born with the potential for 'total independence', whether as a result of severe physical or learning disability, or both. In such circumstances, progress during infancy and childhood cannot be measured against normal developmental milestones and the goal is maximum independence in the ALs according to the capacity of the individual child.

Even in adulthood, there are circumstances which can result in dependence in one or more of the ALs: obvious examples are illness and accident. Dependence may be on help from other people or on special aids and equipment: for example, a wheelchair which provides 'aided independence' for the AL of mobilizing. Indeed, in a broader context even healthy able-bodied adults are dependent

on others for their so-called 'independence' in many of the ALs: for example, for the AL of eating and drinking there is dependence on people such as the farmer, fisherman, factory worker and shopkeeper and on various types of equipment and a supply of safe water and heat which aid preparation and cooking of food and drink.

There is, therefore, no absolute state of 'independence' in the ALs. The concepts of 'dependence' and 'independence' are really only meaningful when considered as relative to one another, hence the reason for presenting these ideas in our model of living by means of a dependence/independence *continuum*. Change in dependence/independence status for one AL can, because the ALs are so closely related, cause change in status for one or more of the others.

The dependence/independence status of an individual in relation to ALs is not linked only to lifespan, it is also closely associated with the factors which influence ALs.

Factors influencing the ALs

So far, three components of the model have been described — the Activities of Living, the lifespan, and the dependence/independence continuum. However although everyone carries out Activities of Living (at whatever stage of the lifespan and with varying degrees of independence) each individual does so differently. To a large extent these differences arise because a variety of factors have influenced/are influencing the way a person carries out ALs, and these 'factors' form the fourth component of the model.

It would be possible to devise a long list of the different factors: for example, biological, intellectual, emotional, social, cultural, spiritual, religious, ethical, philosophical, environmental, political, economic and legal factors.

However, one of the intentions when creating a model is that it should not seem excessively complicated, so the factors influencing the ALs are described in five main groups — biological, psychological, sociocultural, environmental, and politicoeconomic factors (Fig. 2.6). It must be noted, however, that intellectual and emotional are subsumed under psychological factors; that spiritual, religious, philosophical, and ethical are subsumed under sociocultural factors because for this model of living it is considered that such values and beliefs often find expression within a particular cultural view; and legal are subsumed under politicoeconomic factors.

The factors are deliberately focused on the Activities of Living. It would be possible to focus them on the individual as a total entity discussing in general terms the effects of the five groups of factors on lifestyle, but this is

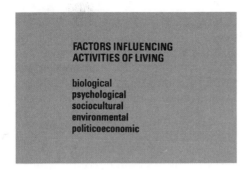

Fig. 2.6 Factors influencing the ALs

too global. In preference, discussing them as they influence each of the 12 ALs highlights the individuality in living.

The factors, the ALs, the lifespan, the dependence/independence continuum are interlinked, and the five factors themselves are interlinked. Each factor involves a huge area of human knowledge and students will have specific textbooks and study related to these topics in other parts of the curriculum. At this stage, however, for the purposes of discussion, a few general points will be made about each factor separately.

BIOLOGICAL

For the purposes of this model of living, the term biological relates to the human body's anatomical and physiological performance. This is partly determined by the individual's genetic inheritance and although the influence of heredity is usually more obvious in facial appearance and physique, it also affects each person's overall physical performance. The individual's physical endowment is important in its own right, but it is inextricably linked with other factors — psychological, sociocultural, environmental and politicoeconomic.

Not only are the biological factors interlinked with these others; as a group, the factors are related to the other components of the model. Even in a healthy person for example, the body's physical ability varies according to age (i.e. the lifespan component of the model), and influences the degree of dependence possible to the individual (i.e. the dependence/independence continuum), so inevitably the factors influence the person's individuality in living and affect the way each person carries out the ALs. Despite the phenomenal physical growth of the fetus in utero, a newborn baby is far from biological maturity and unlike most animals, there are many years of further growth before reaching the physical competence and independence synonymous with young adulthood in the human. At the other end of the lifespan, the physical ability of the older person is gradually deteriorating and there may be an insidious loss of independence. It is logical to expect therefore that the biological

state of the body has an important contributing influence on the individual's ALs throughout the lifespan. However, it must be emphasized that it is only for the purposes of discussion that biological factors are singled out; it is the overall consideration of the person which is important and other factors are involved.

PSYCHOLOGICAL

Psychological factors cannot be considered in isolation; they are related to biological and also to sociocultural, environmental and politicoeconomic factors. As well as being related to the other four factors, psychological factors are related to the other components of the model. They influence living throughout the lifespan, especially intellectual and emotional development, and have a bearing on the person's level of independence; so inevitably they influence the person's individuality in living, and affect the way each person carries out the ALs. In Chapters 4–15 specific examples are given to indicate the influence which psychological factors can have on individual ALs; here, to provide a background to Chapters 4–15, a few general points are made about their influence on a number of ALs.

Intellectual aspects

The term 'cognitive development' is often used to refer to the process of acquiring intellectual skills — thinking, reasoning and problem-solving — which are essential for physical survival and affect all Activities of Living. The process by which people obtain information about themselves and their environment begins as a baby. Via the sense organs, the baby perceives stimuli such as pressure, pain, warmth, cold, taste, sound, changes in light intensity and various visual images. At first, the response to many of these stimuli may be simply a reflex action, because highly differentiated responses are not possible until the cerebral cortex grows and conceptual processes begin to develop.

It is important to remember that sensory deprivation, for example, visual or hearing impairment may result in delayed intellectual development and that this can affect almost every AL. It is just as important to remember that lack of stimulation during the early years of life at home and at school, can retard intellectual development. Indeed the neglected child, even with a genetic inheritance which would promise high potential, has less opportunity to develop intellectually and emotionally thereby affecting ALs such as maintaining a safe environment, communicating, and working and playing.

Intellectual development continues in childhood and early adolescence, by means of formal education and the pursuit of personal interests and leisure. In late adolescence, there is usually a more marked differentiation between individuals, and this can affect decisions about advanced studies and choice of job or career. Establishment in an occupation is one of the major tasks during adulthood and the significance of the AL, working and playing is paramount.

During the ageing process, overall intellectual functioning becomes gradually less efficient and may cause problems with Activities of Living, for example, there may be difficulty with communication because the senses are less acute; maintaining a safe environment in the home may be less easy as memory fails; opportunities for fulfilling the AL of working and playing may be reduced, and boredom or loneliness may result. However, an enhancing environment can help to sustain even an elderly person's intellectual status making it possible to remain independent for the majority of ALs, thus facilitating residence in the community rather than resorting to care in an institutional setting.

Emotional aspects

Like intellectual development, emotional development is closely related to lifespan and the growth of independence in the relevant ALs. The need for love and belonging is crucial in young children; and from a stable and close relationship in infancy, the child can grow with self-confidence and a feeling of worth. The development of personality is one of the outcomes of emotional development which influences, for example, the AL of communicating in the model of living. Early sex-related behaviour patterns tend to be strengthened and the child often models on the parent of the same sex, sometimes through the AL of playing. Parents are significant in influencing emotional development, and the acquisition of norms and moral standards are part of communicating in the model of living.

Emotional development during the teens is closely related to the biological changes of puberty. Emotional relationships with parents undergo change and adolescents begin to assert their individuality and independence, at first for the 'playing' part of the AL of working and playing and eventually for working; and they may resist adult authority and advice.

During young adulthood, there are usually important emotional relationships associated with courtship and setting up house with a partner (usually of the opposite sex) and the rearing of children; all associated with the AL of expressing sexuality. Consequently late adulthood may bring with it major emotional readjustments when grown-up children leave home; there may often be an experience of tremendous loss although there may also be a new sense of freedom to enjoy the 'playing' part of the AL, working and playing.

For the older person there may have to be many emo-

tional adaptations related to the physical effects of ageing and sometimes declining intellectual ability which can influence ALs such as maintaining a safe environment, communicating and expressing sexuality. There are reduced opportunities for emotional and social relationships as family and friends in their peer group die, which influences the bereavement and grieving part of the AL of dying in the model.

There are individual differences. There are marked variations in the capacity for intellectual development; and enormous differences related to the general ability to cope with the emotional demands of life events. And, of course, this intellectual and emotional development takes place not only within the family; it develops in the context of the society and culture where the individual lives.

SOCIOCULTURAL

For the purposes of the model of living, the term sociocultural subsumes spiritual, religious and ethical aspects of living. Sociocultural factors are closely related to the biological and psychological factors already discussed, and also to the environmental and politicoeconomic factors which will be introduced subsequently.

As well as being related to the other four factors, sociocultural factors are related to the other components of the model. They influence living throughout the lifespan and have a bearing on the person's level of independence, so inevitably they influence the person's individuality in living and affect the way each person carries out the ALs. In Chapters 4–15 specific examples are given to indicate the influence which sociocultural factors can have on individual ALs; here, to provide a background to Chapters 4–15, a few general points are made about their influence on a number of ALs.

Culture

Within every society there is some kind of organization of people into groups and of activities into institutions. The social organization may be simple, as in a nomadic tribe or it may involve a highly elaborate network of groups and specialised structures, as in technologically advanced countries. *Culture* is the word used in sociology to refer to the way of life of a particular society, and cultural differences exist in even the most basic of everyday living activities.

Within the last few decades, however, a host of circumstances including emigration and the movement of refugees has accelerated a mixing of cultures so that within recognized national boundaries, a multicultural society is becoming more common. This introduces a fascinating diversity yet also holds the seeds of conflicting interests and potential unrest. Cultural idiosyncrasies related to the various ALs are mentioned in later chapters.

Spirituality, religion and ethics

An aspect of living which is a reflection of culture, and which is sometimes overlooked, is *spirituality*. It is defined broadly as 'that which inspires in one the desire to transcend the realm of the material'. Discussing this definition, Labun (1988) maintains that it could refer to religion as well as more philosophical orientations to belief and meaning in life. The characteristics of the spiritual self, she goes on, in combination with those of the emotional and physical self respond to situations as a totality. As far as orientation to belief and meaning in life are concerned, these are reflected in *ethical* standards and manifest themselves in 'being true to oneself', as well as in behaviour to other people.

Organized *religions* can be considered as specific manifestations of spirituality, and are often closely linked to culture. In fact, for someone who feels alone and deprived of social networks which would give meaning to existence, religion can sometimes supply an identity, as well as communal links around religious observances.

A religion's influence on group and individual behaviour can be considerable; indeed, where there is religious unity in a society, the culture and religion are almost inseparable. Religion can influence ALs such as eating and drinking, eliminating, personal cleansing and dressing, and expressing sexuality. However, secular groups such as humanists facilitate their members' expression of spirituality in a number of ways which can affect an adherent's Activities of Living just as forcibly as a recognized religion.

Community

As well as belonging to a society and sharing its culture, every person is a member of a *community*. The kind of community in which people live greatly affects the quality of their lives; even their personal safety is to a large extent dependent on the maintenance of safety in the community at large; for example, in its schools and transport systems, at work, and in the provision made for the observance of law and order.

Role

The concept of *role* is helpful in describing the part an individual plays in society. There are many different social roles and each carries very specific expectations and makes specific demands on the individual. From birth, a male baby may occupy the roles of son, brother and grandson and these differ from the daughter, sister and granddaughter roles of a female baby. These are examples of 'ascribed' roles, i.e. those allocated to people at birth according to their sex and existing kinship network. Others are 'achieved' as a result of personal choice and endeavour, for example occupational roles.

Status

Even such fundamental roles as man or woman and child or parent have to be learnt. One of the important functions of the family is the socialization of children, the process whereby they are taught and learn about the characteristics, expectations and responsibilities attached to the whole range of social roles. In general, there are differences in the degree of *status* attached to particular roles, and in the importance attributed to 'ascribed' as compared to 'achieved' roles.

Relationships

In any society, each individual has his own unique network of *relationships*. Initially, this emerges from the kinship network into which the person is born, and it comprises relationships with members of the nuclear family and the extended family, then in adulthood to relationships arising from marriage, childbearing and an occupation. During adult life, a person's network continually changes and expands; in old age, there is a gradual retraction in the number and variety of social relationships.

Social groups

However, an individual does not interact only with another individual. Cooperation plays an important role in a complex society and to this end a great deal of social interaction takes place within *social groups*. An individual begins life as a member of the most generic social group, the family. Thereafter, individuals spend their entire lives joining and leaving various groups which exist in society to serve a multitude of functions: social, occupational, recreational, educational, political and religious. In general, membership of groups is extremely important for the fulfilment of love and belonging needs and the development and enhancement of self-esteem. Those individuals not strongly integrated with social groups may suffer from social isolation and become lonely and depressed, even sometimes suicidal.

Social stratification/social class

Almost every society, in addition to a set of social institutions, has some form of *social stratification* which delineates the role and status of its various groups. Social stratification results from a layering process which creates units described as *social classes*. A social class is a group of people who have in common certain social, economic and occupational characteristics which determine their relative social status within society. There are different systems of class used throughout the world. In industrialized countries, the class system is often based on occupational grouping and in the UK the Registrar General's Social Class Scale is used to categorize social class according to occupation (p. 316). In general, people still tend to think of three social classes — 'upper', 'middle' and 'working' class — and to attribute to each a stereotyped set of characteristics.

The concept of social class is useful in order to understand the variations in lifestyles of different social groups. For example, it is known that methods of child-rearing and the value placed on education vary between socioeconomic groupings. Power and status in society are also related to social class, those of the 'upper' socioeconomic groupings usually having greater political power and social influence. Whether or not there is the opportunity for social mobility later in life, the classification of a child is determined at birth according to the father's social position. In this and many other matters, it is the social institution of the family — even although nowadays in Western countries, the 'family' has come to have a much wider interpretation — which determines and shapes an individual's personal process of socialization, and therefore influences most of the ALs which interact to produce individuality in living.

However, although sociocultural factors have a considerable influence on ALs, individuals in a society are also influenced by the physical environment in which they live.

ENVIRONMENTAL

Environmental factors cannot be considered in isolation; they are related to biological, psychological and sociocultural, as already mentioned, and also to politico-economic factors which will be discussed later. As well as being related to the other four factors, environmental factors are related to the other components of the model. They influence living throughout the lifespan and have a bearing on the person's level of independence; so inevitably they influence the person's individuality in living, and affect the way each person carries out the ALs. In Chapters 4–15 specific examples are given to indicate the influence which environmental factors can have on individual ALs; here to provide a background to Chapters 4–15, a few general points are made about their influence on a number of ALs. In this text the environment is conceptualized in a broad dimension and includes all that is physically external to people.

Atmospheric components

As far as the individual is concerned, the atmosphere is perhaps the most obvious and immediate environmental factor. It has many components, for example:

- *Organic and inorganic particles*
  The atmosphere is in contact with exposed skin and outer garments on which it deposits inorganic matter such as particles which are the products of combustion, and the removal of these substances relates this factor to personal cleansing and dressing. Such particles can also be inhaled thereby relating it to the AL of breathing. In addition, the atmosphere contains organic matter in the form of pollen, pathogenic microorganisms, and vectors such as flies and lice. These can affect several ALs. Pollen can influence breathing by causing hay fever; microorganisms can settle on to food and cause food poisoning thus affecting the AL of eliminating and, if there is a fever, the AL of controlling body temperature. Vectors, particularly flies, can cause food poisoning by depositing pathogens directly on to food; and lice can infest skin and clothes, thus relating atmospheric factors to the AL of personal cleansing and dressing.
- *Light rays*
  Light rays are transmitted via the atmosphere; they can be from the sun providing daylight; from an electrically- or gas-operated apparatus which provides light when natural lighting is inadequate or absent; from technological apparatus such as batteries, and from burning candles. Light rays not only stimulate the sense of sight in normal eyes, but also provide the ambience for such varied ALs as communicating, for example, for hearing-impaired people to maximize the visual input to a conversation; or for eating and drinking when soft lighting can be relaxing and even romantic; or for working in mines which depend on artificial lighting; or for 'playing' in places such as discos to enhance the excitement of dancing; or for expressing spirituality in cathedrals and churches where candles are lit to meet various spiritual objectives.
  Of course, the sun's rays also provide the earth with energy and heat, some of which are absorbed by the earth and some radiated back into space. However, gases in the atmosphere (carbon dioxide, methane, chlorofluorocarbons) absorb some of this energy forming a blanket which returns additional heat to the earth — the greenhouse effect. Some of the sun's rays — ultraviolet — may burn exposed skin or, after long exposure, may even cause cancer and many people require to take preventive action by applying screening lotion or wearing clothes which cover the skin — a relationship to the AL of personal cleansing and dressing.

• *Sound waves*

Sound waves are also transmitted by the atmosphere and in various ways, can influence different ALs. For example, those produced by speech are an essential part of communicating for most people. Those produced by professional vocalists could be said to relate to the AL of working, while for the majority of people, singing would involve the AL of playing. Sound waves may, of course, contribute to an emergency warning such as a fire alarm which would certainly influence the ALs of mobilizing, and maintaining a safe environment.

Although the obvious AL affected by atmospheric components is that of breathing, atmospheric components and characteristics can be seen to influence several ALs and there are many other examples. The temperature and humidity may well relate to ALs such as controlling body temperature, working and playing, and sleeping. Atmospheric turbulence in the form of gale force winds, thunder storms or hurricanes are likely to modify the ALs of maintaining a safe environment, and working and playing. The rarefied atmosphere at high attitudes, particularly the reduced oxygen content, not only affects breathing but, because it lowers metabolism, less energy is available for the ALs of mobilizing, and working and playing.

Clothing

Clothing can be considered as an environmental factor which is in immediate contact with non-exposed skin and it provides a further association with personal cleansing and dressing. People modify clothing in relation to controlling body temperature which can be influenced by atmospheric temperature. Clothing is also a part of the non-verbal dimension of the AL of communicating and is an aspect of the AL of expressing sexuality.

Household environment

Solid objects in the home are part of the environment and they range from eating utensils to cooking apparatus, refrigerators, washing machines, television sets, furniture and furnishings. To ensure that such equipment is conducive to healthy living, including the prevention of accidents, many countries have evolved consumer councils or similar organizations to set minimum standards of quality and safety; indeed many countries have legal requirements to regulate their manufacture and sale.

Vegetation

Not only internal household objects, but the vegetation in our environment should be conducive to healthy living.

Gardening may be a work activity for some people, but a leisure activity for others. The crops, trees and foliage which can be an important economic facility or may be purely aesthetic, should all facilitate healthy living. They should not be contaminated by, for example, the use of toxic herbicides or the fumes produced by vehicular traffic when crops are adjacent to motorways.

Buildings

Buildings are an essential part of the environment and can influence several ALs. They need to be free from hazard so that their occupants can continue the AL of maintaining a safe environment. They should also be adequately ventilated so that inside atmospheric conditions do not unduly influence body temperature by causing it to rise or fall outwith the range of normal — an important factor both at home, at school and at work.

In any consideration of buildings, of course, housing is of primary importance to the individual and can have a direct effect on ALs. The availability of a safe, effective water supply and waste disposal system can affect the ALs of cleansing and dressing, and eliminating, not to mention the AL of eating and drinking; the adequacy of play areas inside and out-of-doors obviously is an advantage for the optimal physical and psychological development of children; high-rise blocks of flats with unreliable lifts can deter occupants from venturing outdoors if they are elderly or disabled thus affecting the AL of mobilizing.

These few examples highlight the importance of an individual's living environment, but of course, environmental factors do not exist in isolation.

POLITICOECONOMIC

For the purposes of this model of living, the term politicoeconomic factors subsumes aspects of living which have a legal connection; frequently political and/or economic pressure and action is reflected in legislation. Again, politicoeconomic factors do not stand alone.

As well as being related to the other four factors just discussed, politicoeconomic factors are related to the other components of the model. They influence living throughout the lifespan and have a bearing on the person's level of independence, so inevitably they influence the person's individuality in living, and affect the way each person carries out the ALs. In Chapters 4–15 specific examples are given to indicate the influence which politicoeconomic factors can have on individual ALs; here, to provide background to Chapters 4–15 a few general points are made about their influence on some selected ALs.

The state, the law and the economy

In the modern world, every citizen is the subject of a state.

The citizen is legally bound to obey the orders of the state and to a large extent, the individual's Activities of Living are influenced by its norms. These norms are the laws, and the state has the power to enforce the law on all who live within its frontiers.

The state is the apex of the modern social pyramid and has supremacy over other forms of social groupings, so, in general terms, the state regulates human activities of living. For example in relation to the AL of mobilizing, traffic regulations are enforced by the state; and in relation to the AL of eating and drinking, there are laws controlling the type and amount of food additives permitted in food processing, and also regarding the cleanliness of premises where food is prepared which, in addition, involves the AL of maintaining a safe environment.

However, the state is dependent on the economic system which underlies the legal order; only limited social progress is possible when a state has a precarious economic base.

The influence of the state

The state has involvement, in varying degrees, with an enormous range of interests, some personal, for example, the statutory requirement to register births, marriages and deaths; and others corporate, for example, the provision of national and local parklands for the leisure and enjoyment of all.

The power of the state is considerable. But if individuals are sufficiently outraged, they can register disapproval and examples of disapproval can be found in, for example, the suffragette movement, the pacifist movement, and opposition to the use of nuclear power; the contention being that when individuals suspect their rights are being threatened, they will question the state.

In a modern democratic society, individuals consider that, for example, they have rights associated with their Activities of Living: the right to a safe environment; the right to work in order to earn a livelihood; the right to leisure; the right to health; the right to education; the right to freedom of speech, freedom of association and so on. But while making such demands, citizens have to accept that rights and freedoms carry with them social responsibilities. They do not have licence to do what they like; they have freedom to act responsibly within the law and appreciate that other people have equal rights to carry out their various Activities of Living.

The influence of the individual in the state

Of course the individual may not always be immediately conscious of personal political power vis-á-vis the state, but the combined efforts of individuals working as a group can have a profound effect. In the vast modern state, associations have come to assume considerable im-portance; indeed some focus on their ability to translate the results of their efforts into legislation, for example, employers' associations and trades unions. And many small voluntary groups, pioneering minority causes, may highlight issues which are precursors to legislation. Of course all associations are not directly relevant to the state; they may be formed for the purposes of sport or for aesthetic pursuits, and add considerably to the variety and quality of daily life.

The welfare state

In varying degrees, the modern state is a welfare state, virtually ensuring for all citizens a minimum level of protection against social risks. The interpretation of 'minimum' is a political decision and is influenced by the country's economic status and level of affluence. Gradually, however, claims against the national budget have come to cover the entire lifespan, for example, for maternity grants at birth; for child allowances; for general education and higher education; during unemployment; for pensions at retirement; and finally for death grants. All groups in society have come to have considerable dependence on the state. However, in periods of economic recession, it becomes more immediately apparent that a national budget is finite, that competing claims have to be arranged in some order of priority, and that in the process, certain demands, albeit worthy, will be unmet.

In fact, quite apart from periods of recession, many countries in the Western world are finding the welfare state concept insatiable in terms of cost. They are reappraising selected health and social services which have been free or offered at token cost and seeking to put some of the financial responsibility back to the individual and/or family.

The interdependence of states

In the modern world, the state is not concerned only with its own citizens. Each state is one among many and some of the most important current issues are problems which are external to the individual state. It has come to be realized that it is necessary to have regulations between states in the form of international laws; rapid economic and political changes make it unsatisfactory to leave individual states to make decisions in isolation on matters which are really of international concern.

The world is now interdependent in a large array of matters related to, for example frontiers, tariffs, marketing, labour laws, monetary markets, shipping channels and flight paths, as well as for health regulations; and in varying degrees these affect each state and eventually the individual's ALs. Indeed some of the politicoeconomic issues have ethical considerations such as the unequal distribution of food — a basic necessity for living; in many wealthy countries there is a superabundance, and in others the economic level of the state is so fragile that its citizens are undernourished and sometimes starving.

World interdependence, in fact, appears to be leading the United Nations Organization into a controversial sphere — the right to humanitarian intervention (Sullivan 1993). This is a revolutionary concept in world affairs. It is not mentioned in the Charter of the UN, indeed any sort of intervention 'direct or indirect, individual or collective' in the domestic jurisdiction of another state is explicitly banned. Yet the world seemed to applaud when, in the name of the UN, a 'benevolent' army of occupation entered Iraq following the Gulf War to protect the Kurds; went to Somalia in 1993; or was sent as a peace-keeping force to the former Yugoslavia — all attempts at maintaining a safe environment for the people involved or avoiding a spillover of violence to neighbouring countries.

In the post-Cold War world, calls on the UN increasingly result from the collapse of nation states, ethnic conflict, major humanitarian disasters or a combination of these. It is one thing to introduce a peace-keeping force between two consenting parties, but quite another to inject a peace-keeping force into civil war situations without invitation from the warring factions, and with little prospect of bringing pressure to bear on the opposing parties.

In fact, the UN lacks the money and trained manpower to enforce humanitarian operations everywhere they might be needed in the world, but the issue is creating international controversy and sometimes, acrimony.

These few examples indicate that this vast interdependence has actually created a world community in political, economic, and to some extent, legal terms, operating alongside the national and local structures which have a more obvious influence on the individual's Activities of Living.

In this section, the five factors (biological, psychological, sociocultural, environmental and politicoeconomic) that can influence the ALs have been outlined. But, as indicated in Figure 2.1, all four concepts in the model of living contribute to the fifth concept, namely, individuality in living.

Individuality in living

Our model of living attempts to provide a simple conceptualization of the complex process of 'living'. However, the concern of the model is with living as it is experienced by each individual and this fifth and final component — *individuality in living* serves to emphasize this point.

The Activities of Living were selected as the main component of the model and, although every person carries out all of the ALs, each individual does so differently. In terms of our model, this individuality can be seen to be a product of the influence on the ALs of all the other components, and the complex interaction among them. Each person's individuality in carrying out the ALs is, in part, determined by stage on the *lifespan* and degree of *dependence/independence*; and is further fashioned by the influence of various biological, psychological, sociocultural, environmental and politicoeconomic *factors*.

A person's individuality can manifest itself in many different ways, for example in:

- *how* a person carries out the AL
- *how often* the person carries out the AL
- *where* the person carries out the AL
- *when* the person carries out the AL
- *why* the person carries out the AL in a particular way
- what the person *knows* about the AL
- what the person *believes* about the AL
- the *attitude* the person has to the AL.

The idea that this component of the model — individuality in living — is a product of the other components, is conveyed in the way it is depicted in the diagram of the model of living (Fig. 2.1). The other four components combine to produce the unique mix which determines individuality.

Again, it must be emphasized that the diagram of a model is merely an aide-memoire and, indeed, has little meaning without explanation. Although each of the five components was described separately, the fact that they are closely related was emphasized; the relationships are portrayed in the diagram both by position and the addition of arrows. In other words, the whole model is more than simply the sum of its parts.

Given our emphasis on the individual person as central to our model of living, ipso facto, a family has to be viewed as a collection of individuals, so their individuality may also have to be considered. For thinking about and providing a milieu congenial to healthy living for a larger group of people such as 'a community', our proposed model of conceptualizing living is a pertinent basis, because, as we have described them, the concepts are broad and can have wide application. The Roper, Logan and Tierney model for nursing is based on this model of living, and both were developed from a research project, as mentioned at the beginning of this chapter.

REFERENCES

Central Statistical Office 1994 Social Trends 24. HMSO, London
Labun E 1988 Spiritual care: an element in nursing care planning. Journal of Advanced Nursing 13 (3): 314–320
Roper N 1976 Clinical experience in nurse education. Churchill Livingstone, Edinburgh
Sullivan S 1993 A right to intervene? Newsweek CXXI (3) January 18: 6–8

A model for nursing

A model for nursing

We believe that our conceptualization of nursing based on a model of living captures the 'core' of nursing (p. 19). It is an indisputable fact that people who are in need of the nursing part of the health service for whatever reason and wherever they are located, have to go on 'living'. The rationale is that a similar mode of thinking engendered by the two models will encourage minimal disturbance of the pattern of living while a person requires nursing, unless of course, the person needs help with learning to cope with a different pattern. Figure 3.1 illustrates comparison of the main concepts in both models. They differ only in the fifth. The objective in conceptualizing living according to the first four components in the model of living is to identify each person's individuality in living, and this is the basis of our conceptualization of nursing. Individualizing nursing is accomplished by application to practice of the concept of the process of nursing comprising four stages as shown in Figure 3.2.

Our model for nursing is, we believe, sufficiently broad and flexible to be used as a framework for the process of nursing in any area of professional practice, and as a means of appreciating the underlying unity of the various branches of the profession. However, even more importantly, the person who enters the nursing service is central to the model, and the nursing required can be tailored to the individual's circumstances and not imposed by the nurses.

Certainly, the model appears simple — as simple as the model of living on which it is based. This is not to suggest that either 'living' or 'nursing' are simple processes because, of course, they are not. However, we believe that to be useful, a model should be readily understood, and in the case of nursing, directly relevant and applicable to practice. There is no necessity for a model to exhaust

MODEL OF LIVING	MODEL FOR NURSING
12 Activities of Living (ALs) Lifespan Dependence/independence continuum Factors influencing the ALs Individuality in living	12 Activities of Living (ALs) Lifespan Dependence/independence continuum Factors influencing the ALs Individualizing nursing

Fig. 3.1 Comparison of the main concepts in the model of living and the model for nursing

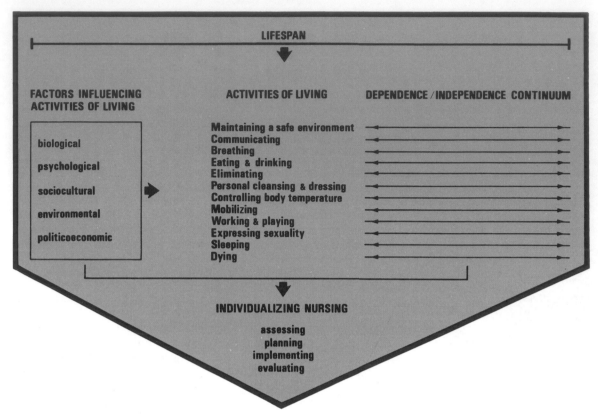

Fig. 3.2 Diagram of the model for nursing

every aspect of the subject and, indeed if its presentation is excessively complicated by detail, its application to practice is unlikely to be readily apparent, however interesting and academically respectable it may be. Deliberately our model seems uncomplicated, but, as John Ruskin said, 'it is far more difficult to be simple than to be complicated'. Our model is offered as an overall framework to assist learners to develop a way of thinking about nursing in general terms, which then can be utilized in practice as a means of developing individualized nursing.

However, here it is necessary to state the assumptions on which our model for nursing is based.

Assumptions on which the model is based

As already said, the selected concepts and their relationships in a nursing model are a means of interpreting the discipline of nursing. It is not surprising, therefore, that creators of models give considerable attention to the assumptions which underlie their approach to the discipline; Fawcett (1984) considered that creators of models for nursing should make their assumptions explicit because they are indicative of the authors' values and their special points of emphasis. The authors of the Roper, Logan and

Tierney model make the following assumptions:

- Living can be described as an amalgam of Activities of Living (ALs)
- the way ALs are carried out by each person contributes to individuality in living
- the individual is valued at all stages of the lifespan
- throughout the lifespan until adulthood, the individual tends to become increasingly independent in the ALs
- while independence in the ALs is valued, dependence should not diminish the dignity of the individual
- an individual's knowledge, attitudes and behaviour related to the ALs are influenced by a variety of factors which can be categorized broadly as biological, psychological, sociocultural, environmental and politicoeconomic factors
- the way in which an individual carries out the ALs can fluctuate within a range of normal for that person
- when the individual is 'ill', there may be problems (actual or potential) with the ALs
- during the lifespan, most individuals experience significant life events which can affect the way they carry out ALs, and may lead to problems, actual or potential
- the concept of potential problems incorporates the promotion and maintenance of health, and the

prevention of disease; and identifies the role of the nurse as a health teacher, even in illness settings
• within a health care context, nurses work in partnership with the client/patient who, except for special circumstances, is an autonomous, decision-making person
• nurses are part of a multiprofessional health care team who work in partnership for the benefit of the client/patient, and for the health of the community
• the specific function of nursing is to assist the individual to prevent, alleviate or solve, or cope positively with problems (actual or potential) related to the ALs.

The language of the assumptions is reflected in the model for nursing (Fig. 3.2) and, as has been said, it is based on the model of living.

The way of thinking about 'living' generated by the model of living will now be transferred to nursing in the following discussion of each of the five components. Only an outline is provided in this chapter because the next section of the book comprises 12 chapters (Chs 4 to 15), one devoted to each of the ALs, in which more detailed discussion of the five components of the model is presented in the context of nursing.

Activities of Living (ALs)

As in the model of living, the ALs are considered as the main component of the model for nursing and they are illustrated in Figure 3.3.

The ALs are the focus of the model because they are central to our view of nursing and characterise 'the person' who is central to the model. Nursing is viewed as helping people to prevent, alleviate or solve, or cope positively with problems (actual or potential) related to the ALs. Recognition of the fact that people's problems may be actual or potential means that nursing not only responds to existing problems but is also concerned with preventing problems, whenever possible. A summary of the nursing function is provided in Figure 3.4.

In Chapters 4 to 15, there is discussion of assessing people in the particular AL, followed by identifying people's actual and potential problems using four categories:

• change of dependence/independence status
• change in habit of carrying out the AL
• change in mode of carrying out the AL
• change of environment and routine on carrying out the AL.

Each chapter ends with a summary discussion of planning and implementing nursing activities and evaluating outcomes.

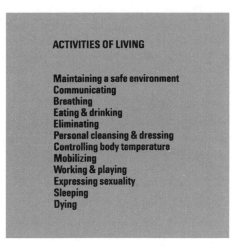

Fig. 3.3 The Activities of Living

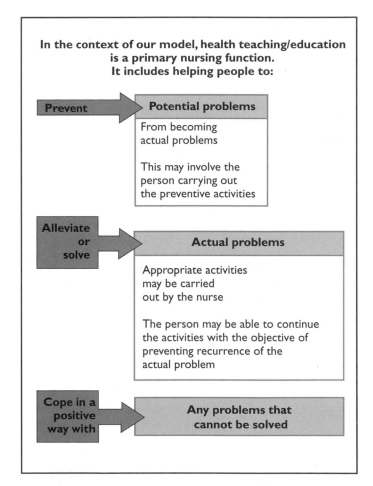

Fig. 3.4 Summary of the nursing function

So far, only a brief outline of the ALs has been provided in the context of the model of living (pp. 20 to 23). In the context of the model for nursing, the remainder of this section offers some comments on the ALs collectively.

USE OF THE CONCEPT OF AL

In our early work in the late 1970s we searched for comprehensive and widely accepted descriptions of nursing. One of the well-known pioneers in this quest was Virginia Henderson (1969) who described 14 'components' of what she termed 'basic nursing care'. Roper (1976) in her research monograph used the term 'Activities of Daily Living' (ADLs), which at that time seemed appropriate, but it was also in the vocabulary of occupational therapists. After lengthy debate we selected and named 12 'activities' then realised that 'daily' was not applicable to all of them, so we coined the term 'Activities of Living' (ALs).

However, we cannot stress too strongly that our concept of each AL includes the other components of our model, and the interaction of these results in individuality, even when people are brought up in a particular group, of which there are many in today's multicultural society.

We deliberately chose to use the concept of ALs in preference to 'basic human needs', a concept which has been widely used in nursing, based on Maslow's analysis of human motivation. He identified several levels of human need: satisfaction of basic physiological needs provided motivation to rise through the levels of safety and security, love and belonging, then to self-esteem and to self-actualization. To some extent, this thinking is relevant to the concept of ALs but, unlike needs, ALs have an advantage for a nursing model in that they are observable and can be explicitly described, and, in some instances, objectively measured. It is not easy for the nurse to assess needs as such; it is less difficult (although still not easy) to describe a person's behaviour in relation to ALs.

Naming the ALs

The terms we chose to name the ALs also merit comment. Although anxious to avoid jargon, finding suitable names for some of the activities was difficult. The names of the 12 ALs were selected in an attempt to be consistent in emphasizing their active nature (therefore, 'eliminating' rather than 'elimination') and their comprehesiveness (for example, though 'washing and dressing' is the more common term, we decided on 'personal cleansing and dressing' because it is all-embracing of the various activities subsumed within that AL). As a consequence, some of the names may seem rather strange at first but we believe that familiarity with the 12 ALs should result in acceptability of our deliberately and carefully chosen terms.

The set of 12 ALs is unique to our model. Many of the activities are contained in other lists, but in addition, our list contains some activities (such as 'expressing sexuality') which have not always been included alongside the more obvious activities (such as 'eating and drinking') despite the fact that they are integral to the process of living and, therefore, relevant in the context of nursing.

COMPLEXITY OF THE ALs

The fact that each AL is highly complex because it subsumes a variety of activities was a point mentioned in discussion of the AL component of the model of living (p. 20). The point is worth reiterating here because it explains why, in the context of nursing, there is such diversity in people's problems and related nursing activities associated with each of the 12 ALs. This will become apparent from discussion of nursing and the ALs in Section 2 of the book (Chs 4 to 15).

RELATEDNESS OF THE ALs

The relatedness of the 12 ALs was also commented on (p. 20) and this too is an important consideration in the context of nursing. In the course of obtaining information (by assessment) about any one AL, the nurse is likely to find out a great deal about other closely related ALs. For example, discussion of eating and drinking habits leads naturally to description of eliminating habits. A problem with one AL may well cause problems with one or more of the others: for example, mobilizing difficulties are likely to cause problems with other ALs, such as 'personal cleansing and dressing' and 'working and playing'.

On the other hand, when applying the model in practice, the identified problem of, for example, pain, could be placed on the Nursing Plan in more than one AL. If the pain can be identified as being specific to the AL of eating and drinking, or eliminating, or mobilizing, it would be recorded with that specific AL. If it were generalized pain, it would be recorded under the AL of communicating because pain is a subjective phenomenon experienced via the nervous system, which in our model is allocated to the AL of communicating.

To repeat, a model should be flexible; it is not a rigid straitjacket. It is intended merely as a tool which can be useful to the nurse in practice.

PRIORITIES AMONG THE ALs

Although every AL is important in the process of living, some are more vital than others. The AL of breathing must be considered as of prime importance because it is essential for all the other ALs and, indeed, for life itself. The notion of priorities among the ALs was briefly mentioned in discussion of the model of living (p. 23) and in the context of nursing is an extremely important consideration.

With the exception of the AL of breathing, there is no fixed order of priority among the ALs because, depending on the individual's choice and prevailing circumstances, priorities among the ALs alter. On the whole, however, those activities which are vital to survival and safety take precedence over others and, in nursing, this principle certainly applies in circumstances of acute mental and physical illness and any condition which is considered to be life-threatening.

RELEVANCE OF THE ALs

Closely associated with the order of priority among ALs is the notion of relevance. Although the 12 ALs all have relevance to nursing, not all of them are necessarily relevant to all patients or to any one patient all of the time. For example, although it takes up much time in ordinary life, consideration of the AL of working and playing will not be relevant during a period of critical illness. Or after a myocardial infarction, the AL of expressing sexuality will have a low priority, but quickly the person is usually concerned about general appearance and before discharge from hospital may wish information about whether and when it will be safe to resume sexual relations again. However, for a woman having a mastectomy many aspects of that same AL may assume great importance, both pre- and post-operatively and in the longer term too.

What is important is for nurses to be aware that different circumstances create different priorities and, therefore, to apply common sense and professional judgement (which comes from knowledge and experience) in making decisions about the relevance of the ALs for any particular person: any one, or indeed several, may not merit consideration at all; or may merit consideration only at certain points in a person's nursing plan.

ALs AND THE INDIVIDUAL PERSON

After this more generalized discussion of the ALs, it is pertinent to focus further discussion on a particular person. The way in which each person deals with each AL is influenced by:

- stage on the lifespan
- level of dependence/independence and methods of coping with dependence
- factors which have influenced/are influencing individual lifestyle, categorised as:
  — biological
  — psychological
  — sociocultural
  — environmental
  — politicoeconomic

and these will now be discussed sequentially, in a nursing context.

Lifespan

The reason for including a lifespan as one component of the model of living has previously been explained (p. 23). Of course, all people do not live through all stages of the lifespan; some die at birth, and some otherwise healthy people die prematurely, for example as a result of accident, disease, natural disaster or war. So although each individual has a lifespan from birth to death, its length is variable.

Collection of statistics, usually at national level, allows life expectancy to be predicted (p. 23). The infant mortality is used as an audit index in comparing health services in different countries. And the age range of people dying from particular diseases or road traffic accidents can guide the activities of for example the Health Education Authority.

In a nursing context, the lifespan (Fig. 3.5) serves as a reminder that nursing is concerned with people of all ages: that an individual may require nursing at any stage of the lifespan, from birth to death. So relevant is the concept of the lifespan to nursing that some branches of the profession, and some professional qualifications, are linked specifically to certain stages of the lifespan: for example, midwives are concerned with the prenatal stage, birth and the immediate postnatal period; paediatric nurses and health visitors with the stages of infancy and childhood; and 'care of the elderly' is the current official category for 'nursing' elderly people.

Taking account of a patient's age — the fact which identifies the stage of the lifespan involved — has always been recognised as important in nursing. It influences all phases of the process of nursing — assessing, planning, implementing and evaluating — and is an important consideration in individualizing nursing.

The following brief comments on each of the main stages of the lifespan help to illustrate the relevance of this component of the model for nursing.

INFANCY

The first moments of life after birth are crucial and, here too, midwives play a vital role. They ensure, for example, that the AL of breathing is satisfactorily established; that there is immediate opportunity for communication

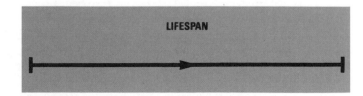

Fig. 3.5 The lifespan

between mother and baby; that the baby is dried and kept warm to prevent problems with the AL of controlling body temperature; and so essential to life is the AL of eating and drinking, that the midwife may encourage the mother to suckle her baby at the breast very soon after the birth. Helping the mother to learn to feed and care for her baby is a major concern of postnatal nursing, for after all the baby is totally dependent on the mother in respect of almost all the ALs.

Throughout the first year of life, even the most healthy babies remain vulnerable to the hazards of infection and injury and susceptible to a variety of problems with the ALs, for example, hypothermia, malnutrition and dehydration. In all countries with a developed health care system, child health services are afforded a high priority and nursing makes an important contribution to efforts aimed at achieving ever lower rates of infant mortality and morbidity.

There are of course some babies and young children who, for a variety of reasons, require nursing in a neonatal unit or children's hospital. Their nursing is provided by specially qualified nurses who, in addition to knowing about treatment of disease, require an in-depth understanding of the normal processes of development in the early years of the lifespan. This is essential for nursing to be tailored to the very different needs and abilities of young children of different ages; and to prevent the experience of hospitalization from adversely affecting the child. There is now widespread acceptance of the need to avoid the adverse effects of separation and for this reason parents are encouraged to visit freely (p. 337) and take an active part in nursing their baby or young child.

Some young children have the misfortune to suffer from chronic illness or a fatal disease or a condition which results in long-term physical or learning disability. Frequent readmission to hospital and, in some cases, long-term hospitalization or community nursing support may be necessary. In such cases nurses play a very significant part in the child's early years of the lifespan.

CHILDHOOD

Childhood tends to be a period of relatively good health for the majority, with death an unusual occurrence. In the Western world the single most important cause of death in this age group is accidents (p. 77).

Serious illness is rare too. Apart from transient illness, such as respiratory infections or the infectious diseases of childhood, the majority of children have little need for medical treatment or nursing. The exceptions are those children with a chronic illness or long-term physical or learning disability. For nurses involved in their care, whether in hospital or the community, one of the important considerations is to provide nursing in such a way

that there is minimal interference with normal development in this stage of the lifespan, such as progress at school; involvement in family life and friendships; and increasing independence in all of the ALs.

However, even 'well' children come into contact with nursing through the school health service. Like health visitors with the younger age group, school nurses are primarily concerned with the monitoring of growth and development, and the early identification of problems: for example, defects of hearing, sight, and speech. The monitoring role of school nurses can include the daily activities of children with chronic bowel conditions (p. 212), those with stomas (p. 223) or with asthma (p. 155). Above all, the role includes health education; children are introduced in a positive way to dental and oral hygiene; a well balanced diet with minimal sugar; prevention of infestation; sex education in the context of relationships and safe sex. In some instances school nurses provide treatment, but equally important is their referral of children and parents to an appropriate source of help.

Increasingly, health education is viewed as more than simply information giving, and through discussion, debate and experimentation, children are being encouraged to appraise their personal health practices and to develop positive health values at an early age.

Unfortunately there has to be a warning — nurses in contact with children (and infants) whether at primary level, in Accident and Emergency Departments or in children's wards need to be aware of the possibility of child abuse. There is a national policy (DHHS, 1988) but some authorities have opted for a local policy and the result can be patchy 'some areas picking up incidents of abuse that others may miss' (Laurent, 1991).

ADOLESCENCE

During this stage of the lifespan, the dominant feature is puberty. Sex education in school and at home during the years of childhood helps to prepare the adolescent to anticipate and cope with the associated physical and emotional changes. However for those who have been abused and 'kept the secret' (as often demanded by the perpetrator), increasing knowledge and experience during adolescence can give rise to severe feelings of guilt and lack of self-worth, and indeed the person may be scarred for life.

Many of the problems which can arise in adolescence are related to physical and psychological aspects of sexual development. Some adolescents experience severe emotional or psychological problems, such as depression or anxiety, which require psychiatric treatment; some require treatment for drug dependence (p. 329); some may benefit from psychosexual counselling; some need treatment for sexually transmitted disease. Many adolescents use family planning centres for advice about contraception and selection of contraceptives; and girls who do become pregnant may seek an abortion or require obstetric care. Thus it can be seen that a variety of nurses come into contact with adolescents — psychiatric nurses, nurse counsellors, school nurses, nurses who work in genitourinary clinics, and those in family planning services, gynaecology and midwifery.

For all of these nurses, an understanding of adolescence is essential. They are unlikely to deal effectively and sympathetically with an adolescent's problems, whatever they may be, in the absence of an appreciation of the emotional turbulence of this stage of the lifespan and of other features, such as a teenager's changing relationship with parents, the pressures of school and worries about future employment.

Appreciating these difficulties and remembering that adolescence is a period of transition, with fluctuation between the desire for adult independence and regression to child-like dependence, is certainly essential for nurses involved with adolescents who require hospital or home care, whether short- or long-term. Adolescence is, like childhood, a stage of the lifespan when serious illness is uncommon. For those affected that fact must make illness or incapacity harder to accept when it occurs; for example, an adolescent who becomes physically disabled following an accident or an adolescent with diabetes mellitus.

Even short-term hospital care of an adolescent presents the nurses with a considerable challenge. On the one hand there may be the desire to be talked to and treated as an adult but, on the other hand, the circumstances may well precipitate some regression to child-like behaviour. This may be manifest in signs of fear and anxiety, or in a desire for parental closeness; or perhaps in a reluctance to accept responsibility and independent decision-making.

The swings of mood common in adolescence may make for difficulties in the nurse-patient relationship and ambivalent feelings towards authority may be projected on to nurses and doctors. Self-consciousness about physical development and relationships with members of the opposite (or same) sex may cause the adolescent person to experience considerable embarrassment in some physically intimate nursing activities; for example, those related to the ALs of personal cleansing and dressing, and eliminating.

The nursing of adolescents, whatever the circumstances, requires sensitivity and knowledge of 'normal' developments in this stage of the lifespan. Whereas many health authorities provide specialist services, for children and elderly people, very few such facilities exist for adolescents. One such service resulted from a nurse carrying out a mental health survey in senior schools (Woods, 1990).

ADULTHOOD

In discussion of development during the lifespan, adulthood is sometimes described as comprising three stages — young adulthood, the middle years and late adulthood. Here, all three stages are discussed together.

It is easy to appreciate the necessity of adapting nursing to the very specific needs and abilities of children of different ages. Adults of different ages also have special requirements, but because of their independence in the ALs and their ability to communicate their needs and desires, there is not the same need to adapt nursing so specifically to age as there is with children. It is also the case that the parameters of 'normal' are very much wider in adulthood, resulting in much greater diversity in lifestyle, abilities and attitudes than among children of a certain age. Appreciating the diversity, however, is helpful because it warns against making assumptions, pointing to the need to collect relevant information about each adult person as an individual.

However, there are two dominant areas of concern for all adults, namely, work and family life. Both are directly affected by illness and hospitalization and, therefore, individualized nursing must take account of the adult patient's work and family circumstances. In some instances these circumstances may be directly related to the person's need for nursing: for example, a person who has suffered an accident at work; or a person requiring family planning advice.

Therefore, work and family life not only bring adults into direct contact with nursing but are directly affected, often disrupted, by illness and hospitalization. There are, too, direct links between work and family life and health and ill-health.

Early adulthood is considered to be a stage of relative stability, with both physical fitness and intellectual ability at their peak. Apart from those young adults who are continuing to cope with a life-long physical or learning disability, serious ill-health is uncommon and the death rate is low although the AIDS epidemic currently affects this group most severely. Apart from AIDS, the more common conditions include bronchitis, peptic ulceration, gall bladder disease, alcoholism, back injury and psychiatric illness, particularly depression. With advancing age into the middle years of life, ill-health becomes more common. There is a sharp increase in the death rate in late adulthood with three conditions responsible — heart disease, cancer and stroke.

Knowing the causes of morbidity and mortality in the various stages of adulthood gives some idea of the reasons why adults come into contact with the health care system, and with nurses. And this knowledge can be used by nurses, as well as other members of the health team, to encourage a healthy lifestyle, such as taking adequate exercise; eating a well-balanced diet and avoiding obesity;

Box 3.1 The healthy adult lifestyle

- Take adequate exercise
- Eat a well-balanced diet
- Avoid obesity
- Sensible drinking of alcohol
- Do not drink and drive
- Do not smoke.

taking alcoholic drinks in moderation; avoiding driving after drinking; and abstaining from cigarette smoking (Box 3.1).

Social, environmental and economic, as well as personal problems can contribute to adults not responding to these encouragements and continuing their 'health threatening' behaviour. It is therefore important to avoid a victim blaming culture (Caraher, 1994; Jacob, 1994), when in fact the social and political systems may be contributing to behaviour which may prevent achievement of some of the targets set by the government in *The Health of the Nation* (DoH, 1991a). Bearing this in mind, health education (DoH, 1991a) is one means of encouraging adults to adopt a more healthy lifestyle and there are many ways in which nurses can contribute to this effort in both their professional and civic roles.

When adults do succumb to illness there are usually two dominant areas of concern, namely work, and family life, whatever the cause or prognosis of the current ill-health problem.

OLD AGE

Nowadays many more people are living longer. Especially in the Western world, elderly people now make up a larger proportion of the total population than ever before; in the UK, it is estimated that by the year 2000 there will be a million more people aged 85 or over, with proportionately fewer people to look after them. It is predicted that by the year 2000, there will be a million fewer in the 16–24 age group so that the needs of the elderly are now a matter of concern to many groups, not least to nursing.

Despite the legitimately increasing concern, however, it should be kept in perspective because the majority of people in this last stage of the lifespan do manage to remain in their own homes, often totally independent (sometimes referred to as the healthy elderly). Contrary to the somewhat gloomy predictions about the ageing West, the marketing people see a flourishing market where 'maturity sells'; the increasingly affluent and healthy older person, they predict, will alter not only money markets but also fashion and taste. Much can be

done, for example by the health visitor, to promote and maintain health in this group of citizens although there will, inevitably, be some in need of assistance with some of the ALs.

The fact that ill-health is more common in this stage of the lifespan than in any other is reflected in the numbers of elderly patients in the wards of general hospitals. To some nurses this comes as something of a surprise and it certainly would seem to contradict the belief that old people are the concern only of the specialist services for care of the elderly. All nurses, (with certain obvious exceptions such as paediatric nurses) nowadays require extensive knowledge of the process of ageing; a sympathetic understanding of the needs of older people; and a positive attitude towards their care and rehabilitation. Individualized nursing is as necessary for an older person as for a child or a young adult — even more so it might be argued, for there is a longer established individuality in living!

When physical or mental disability is such that an elderly person can no longer stay at home, or cope within a community care setting, placement in a 'continuing care unit' may be the only solution. In such a setting, the primary aim is to help the person to maintain what independence there still is in the ALs and, of course, to provide an atmosphere and environment which is like 'home' as far as is humanly possible. Long-stay care of the elderly wards have not enjoyed a good reputation on the whole and, while inadequate conditions are certainly to blame, staff attitudes probably contributed to the unnecessary routinization and institutionalization which prevailed. Ageism, discrimination solely on the criterion of 'being old', has been investigated among nurses and others who provide a service in these areas (Slevin, 1991; Treharne, 1990). The emphasis nowadays on individualized nursing, through the process of nursing method (which is incorporated in this model) offers a way of enabling people in long-stay units to continue their individuality in living.

The inevitable preoccupation of old people with death is something which should always be borne in mind by nurses who are involved with the elderly. In Western society most people die in old age and skilled and sensitive nursing may help a person to come to the very end of the lifespan, to the event of death, in comfort and with the greatest possible dignity.

In this overview of the relationship between stages of the lifespan and nursing, various ALs have been mentioned. The specific effects of the lifespan on each of the 12 ALs are described in Chapters 4 to 15; and from that it will be apparent how a patient's age is a relevant consideration in all phases of the process of nursing. Therefore, the lifespan component of our model for nursing is closely related to the AL component, as it is to the dependence/independence continuum which will now be discussed.

Dependence/ independence continuum

The reason for including the dependence/independence continuum in the model of living was described (p. 23). The concept of dependence/independence has been widely utilized in nursing and, as a component of the model for nursing, is related directly to the 12 ALs (Fig. 3.6).

There is also a close link between this component of the model and the lifespan. Nursing for newborn babies acknowledges their total dependence in respect of almost every AL whereas children's nursing must take account of the fact that the early years of the lifespan are associated with increasing independence in the ALs. Some children do not have the capacity to acquire this independence, to the same extent or at the 'normal' rate, either due to physical or learning disability. Where nurses are involved in care of such children, whether at home or in an institutional setting, the objective is an individualized programme for the acquisition of maximum independence for each AL.

For any child, an episode of illness or injury as a result of accident will not only affect the level of independence already achieved in the ALs but may also require a stay in hospital. Young children are very easily upset by any change in environment or alteration to their daily routine. For example, a child who has recently achieved independence in certain personal cleansing activities, or who is able to dress without help, is likely to be confused if the nurse washes or dresses him. On the other hand, children may be very distressed if expected by the nurses to exercise a degree of independence in the ALs which has not

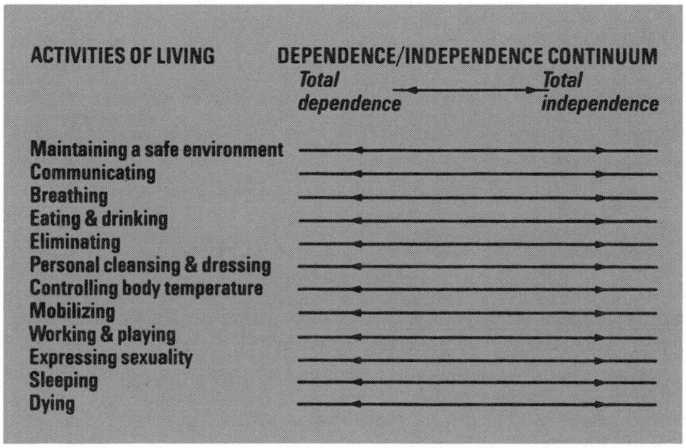

yet been acquired: for example, being expected to use the toilet when still at the stage of using a potty; or being given a game to play or books to read which are beyond their level of comprehension. It is obvious that nurses require to have detailed information about what each child can and cannot do independently in relation to each AL so that the nursing plan is tailored to the individual child, as well as to the circumstances of his illness or injury.

For the majority of people, independence is a central feature of adulthood. When for any reason there is enforced dependence, for example as a result of illness or injury, many people find this hard to cope with. If the period of dependence in relation to any or all of the ALs is to be only temporary, for example following a surgical operation, it is likely to be more easily tolerated. However if the circumstances mean that there will be some residual dependence in some of the ALs, the person needs time and support to adjust and to begin to cope with the changed dependence/independence status.

And, of course, disabled adults are just as likely to suffer from the many conditions which bring the nondisabled into hospital. So, when nursing adult patients who are physically disabled (or who have loss or impairment of sight, hearing or speech), nurses need to have detailed information about their dependence/independence status for each AL. It should not be automatically assumed that because people have, for example, a physical disability, they will necessarily be dependent on the nurse. They may well wish to continue to use the coping mechanisms, aids or equipment — 'aided' independence — which have enabled them to remain independent in the ALs outwith the hospital, and nurses should ensure that this is made possible and that relevant information is provided on the nursing plan.

Even for the most able people, independence in the ALs is generally acquired over a long period of time. In old age the loss of independence can be equally gradual and it is seldom for all of the ALs. The AL of mobilizing is often one of the first affected and because movement is required to perform many other activities, this may result in loss of independence in some of the other ALs. The elderly person may be reluctant to bath and careful questioning may elicit that it is due to fear of falling. Difficulties with personal cleansing and dressing activities may in fact be due to problems with mobilizing. There are now many gadgets available to help elderly people with such difficulties and provision of these may permit a person to retain independence, albeit 'aided' independence in these activities. It is worth repeating a point made in the context of the model of living that old age does not necessarily bring about loss of independence, and there is seldom dependence for all ALs.

As already mentioned the age structure of western societies is changing and with a significant relative in-

ACTIVITIES OF LIVING	DEPENDENCE/INDEPENDENCE CONTINUUM
	Total dependence ←——————→ Total independence
Maintaining a safe environment	
Communicating	
Breathing	
Eating & drinking	
Eliminating	
Personal cleansing & dressing	
Controlling body temperature	
Mobilizing	
Working & playing	
Expressing sexuality	
Sleeping	
Dying	

Fig. 3.6 Dependence/independence continuum related to the ALs

crease of those in their 80s and 90s, more provision is being made in the community for assisting elderly people to remain healthy and active, and retain optimal independence. Clubs are available to encourage exercise, recreational games and handicrafts which, as well as encouraging physical and mental activity, also provide a social reason for meeting, and help to reduce the loneliness which often accompanies living alone. Especially in Western cultures with a nuclear family structure, more and more elderly people do live alone and currently there is a trend to provide what is termed 'sheltered housing', often purpose-built, where elderly individuals or couples, who are becoming less able physically, can retain their own home; however each is connected via an intercom system to a warden's flat where someone is constantly on call. Usually these are small developments, organized by local authorities, or by voluntary agencies or sometimes as private enterprise; and as far as possible they are integrated into other local housing so that they do not form ghettos. They are a form of 'sheltered independence'.

An important skill in nursing is developing professional judgement in relation to people's abilities and never depriving them, however old, of independence in those ALs for which they are capable. There is, of course, a fine line between this and misjudgement in demanding independence when a person is incapable of so being.

It is, equally, a skill in nursing to know when a person is in a state of dependence, or should be helped to accept that this is necessary. Although the emphasis in nursing is generally on encouraging people to achieve or regain maximum independence in the ALs, there are circumstances (for example, unconsciousness or severe illness) when people are totally dependent on nurses. There are other circumstances when, although people may desire to be independent, this is not in their best interests. At certain times (for example, immediately postoperatively), in certain illnesses (for example, severe respiratory conditions) and for other reasons (for example, immobilization in traction), it is important for the person to move as little as possible and for energy to be conserved. Such people may need to be helped to accept that their dependence is necessary and their distress is likely to be lessened if nurses carry out activities on their behalf in a willing manner and in a way which does not offend the person's dignity and self-esteem.

Therefore, sometimes nurses help people towards independence in the ALs and, at other times help them to accept dependence. The dependence/independence continuum in the model for nursing, as in the model of living, is arrowed to indicate that movement can take place along it in either direction — an important dimension of the concept of dependence/independence in the context of nursing. A very important aspect of nursing is assessing a person's level of independence in each of the ALs and judging in which direction, and by what amount,

they should be assisted to move along the dependence/independence continuum; what nursing assistance they need to achieve the goals set; and how progress in relation to these goals will be evaluated.

This discussion of the dependence/independence continuum as one component of the model has been presented in general terms. In later chapters of the book (Chs 4–15) the concept is discussed more specifically in relation to each of the 12 ALs. In each case there is a section which identifies causes of change in people's dependence/independence status, and some of the related nurse-initiated interventions.

Factors influencing the ALs

In the model of living (p. 24), this component was introduced to explain why there are many individual differences in the way the ALs are carried out. As described there, the various 'factors' which influence the ALs were categorized into five main groups and in the model for nursing this component is similarly presented (Fig. 3.7).

It is worth repeating that there are innumerable aspects of the five factors; and worth emphasizing that those selected for mention in this book are chosen because of their relevance to nursing, or because they provide a context for the discussion of nursing.

As already indicated, the five factors influence each of the ALs and are related to the other components of the model — the lifespan and the dependence/independence continuum. The five factors themselves are interrelated, and, when assessing a patient/client it may be difficult to make a clear cut distinction between the influence of biological as against psychological factors; or between sociocultural and politicoeconomic factors. Despite the overlap, however, the five factors are mentioned separately at this stage, high-lighting some general points which are related to health and illness in a nursing context.

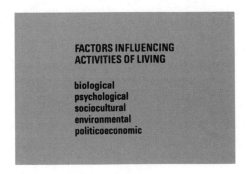

**FACTORS INFLUENCING
ACTIVITIES OF LIVING**

biological
psychological
sociocultural
environmental
politicoeconomic

Fig. 3.7 Factors influencing the ALs

BIOLOGICAL

It is essential that nurses should have knowledge of biological factors and how they influence ALs. In the model for nursing therefore, the status of the individual, in anatomical and physiological terms, is introduced to indicate how this helps nurses to understand, assess, plan and implement relevant nursing interventions and evaluate the effects. There is no attempt to cover biology comprehensively in this textbook; human biology must be studied as a separate subject which contributes (along with other subjects in the nursing curriculum) to an understanding of human beings in health and illness.

To provide a context for discussion of the biological factors, however, it is worth commenting on the nomenclature of various body systems and indicating how we relate them to our model.

Like all living creatures, the human body is made up of cells, about 10^{16} in number. In the human, although the cells are similar in structure, certain clusters of cells have become specialized to deal with specific activities, for example, those dealing with gaseous exchange of oxygen and carbon dioxide in the lungs; and the cells secreting hydrochloric acid in the stomach to assist with the digestion of foods. Knowledge about these clusters of cells, or tissues, has grown enormously during this century partly because of increasing technical and technological sophistication in monitoring and measuring cellular activity.

At one stage in the development of such knowledge, the anatomists and physiologists categorized body tissues which seemed to interact structurally or functionally into body systems and labelled them separately, for example, the skeletal, muscular, respiratory and circulatory systems. As knowledge developed, the interrelationship of these systems became even more obvious and terms came to be used such as musculoskeletal, genitourinary and cardiopulmonary systems. More recently, certain tissues with highly specialized functions have been identified which previously had not been considered as systems and reference is made in the literature to, for example, the immunological system; the temperature-controlling system; the reticuloendothelial system; and the biorhythm system related to sleep control.

Obviously the human body is a highly complex organization of cells and tissues with many interrelated systems, so it is only for the purposes of learning and discussion that systems can be considered separately.

Given the complexity and the interrelationships, it is difficult to juxtapose just one body system with each AL, for example, although it's main function is related to the AL of mobilizing, the musculoskeletal system is involved in many of the ALs.

One of the objectives in presenting our model for nursing is to help students to integrate, in this instance biological factors, into the AL framework, particularly when the nursing documentation in use reflects our model. Therefore to assist students to see the relationship of biological factors to ALs, we have matched a body system with an AL when relevant, for example, the cardiopulmonary system with the AL of breathing; the lower alimentary and urinary systems with the AL of eliminating; the musculoskeletal system with the AL of mobilizing; and this is illustrated in later chapters when each AL is discussed separately (three of the ALs are so generalized that they have not been matched to a specific body system namely; maintaining a safe environment; working and playing; and dying).

The term 'biological factors', however, can cause a problem when mentioned in a nursing context. Some people still jump to the conclusion that it refers only to pathology. Unquestionably, nursing is associated partly with physical dysfunction and disease, particularly in emergency situations, but nursing is also concerned with the promotion and maintenance of health, and the prevention of disease.

Promoting and maintaining health

Irrespective of the setting – home, clinic, hospital – the nurse has innumerable opportunities for introducing aspects of health teaching which aim to maintain the body in a biologically healthy state. In fact, currently, in many industrialized societies, considerable amounts of money are used by governments via the mass media to extol physical health and fitness as a way of life, and the nurse as a health professional should not find it too difficult to reinforce the message. It should be borne in mind, however, that any discussion of promoting and maintaining health can provoke controversy, indeed some people pose the question 'what right do health promoters have to intervene in the lives of other people?' The nurse must gauge the appropriateness of introducing such topics – and know when to desist!

The biological state of the body is not static of course; it is constantly changing. Even during sleep, the cells are perpetually active, and hormonal and chemical substances are regulating the body's internal environment to maintain homeostasis. It is not difficult to appreciate that for various biological functions there is a range of normal in terms of individual differences; and this is corroborated using physiological measurements although even these vary with age, for example, at rest a newborn baby has a pulse rate of 140 beats per minute and the normal rate for a young adult would be 70 beats per minute. It is within the range of normal that the body functions physically to its optimum.

Preventing disease

Of course nurses are also involved in the process of preventing physical disease when, for example, explaining or participating in immunization programmes and it is important for students to understand the physiological changes which occur in the body in the process of acquiring immunity so that people do not succumb to physical diseases which have the potential to cause dysfunction in one or more ALs.

Physical disease

The individual may, however, succumb to physical disease or trauma and this may necessitate nursing the person at home or in hospital during a brief episode of illness, or perhaps during the course of a long-term dysfunction or perhaps during the process of dying. Some of the causes of physical dysfunction are genetic in origin and some seem to start in a manner, not always understood, within the body's own internal environment, for example, autoimmune disease and idiopathic (no known cause) disease. As would be expected, when there is physical dysfunction in any tissue, the body does not remain passive; it reacts physiologically in a number of ways in an attempt to maintain equilibrium, via reactions collectively referred to as defence mechanisms (p. 69). It is particularly in relation to disease and medical diagnosis that nurses collaborate closely with medical staff; and some nursing interventions, for example the administration of most medications, are doctor-initiated.

Many diseases have been identified and rigorously researched and there is an internationally agreed Classification of Diseases which provides a yardstick, nationally and internationally, for the collection of epidemiological data about the incidence of disease and causes of death.

In all these instances — for the maintenance of health, prevention of disease, care during episodes of disease and during the process of dying — it is crucial for nurses to have a knowledge base of human biology so that they can understand normal structure and function, and so that they can comprehend the cause of dysfunction (in so far as it can be identified) and how it affects the individual's Activities of Living.

However, as already indicated, Activities of Living entail infinitely more than the body's biological structure and function; even basic survival would not be possible without intellectual and emotional abilities — the psychological factors.

PSYCHOLOGICAL

It is essential that nurses should have knowledge of psychological factors and how they influence ALs. In the model for nursing, therefore, psychological factors are introduced to indicate how this knowledge helps nurses to understand, assess, plan and implement nursing interventions, and evaluate the effects. There is no attempt to cover the discipline of psychology comprehensively in this textbook. General points only are made at this stage to show how this type of knowledge (along with other subjects in the nursing curriculum) contributes to an understanding of human beings as manifest in their various Activities of Living. More specific examples of the application of psychological concepts to each AL are made in Chapters 4–15.

Intellectual development

In relation to impaired *intellectual* development, nurses may come in contact with children or adults who are mentally disabled because of a genetic disorder such as Down's syndrome. It is important, therefore, for nurses to know about genetics in order to be able to understand the principles of genetic counselling and the significance of diagnosis in utero via amniocentesis, ultrasound or in some instances, maternal blood sampling.

Knowledge is also required in order to ensure that a person who has a mental disability (learning difficulty) is treated essentially as a healthy person, although pathologically slow in developing intellectual skills and the many other skills which are dependent on intellect. And if a suitably stimulating environment is provided based on what such people *can* do rather than what they cannot do, it is usually possible to promote an optimum level of intellectual and emotional growth for each individual. Deprived of stimulation, the mentally disabled person may be grossly impaired and the effect on ALs is readily observable, for example in poor communication skills; difficulty with eating and drinking in a socially acceptable manner; problems with toileting; and incapacity for work and leisure activities.

Carefully staged education and stimulation of the intellect using an individualized plan is of major importance when someone has learning difficulties so that full use is made of the person's abilities, no matter how limited. There are many skills besides intellectual acumen which lead to a happy and fulfilling life. Reality must prevail, however, when discussing expectations with the parents of such children at the time of diagnosis.

Emotional development

Impaired *emotional* development is perhaps less easy to identify. The crucial mother-infant relationship was mentioned earlier: how it nurtures the growth of self-worth and how it influences the way in which the individual will eventually deal with emotions such as happiness, anger, fear, anxiety, stress; all of which can influence the AL of communicating. Each individual learns to adopt coping mechanisms and for some people even apparently large amounts of stress are viewed as challenging, exciting and stimulating rather than predisposing to avoidance tactics.

Psychological stressors are often associated with major life events and for some people may cause extreme anxiety. These significant life events may occur at various points on the lifespan; they may be developmental in nature such as weaning, toilet training, puberty or they may be associated with incidents in living such as changing school, job or house; marriage and divorce; childbearing; death of family members and friends. The anxiety may affect the performance of several ALs. In any of these situations the nurse may be asked for advice, and through counselling may help to prevent exacerbation of the cause, or assist the person to develop/maintain coping mechanisms until the cause of anxiety is removed or alleviated — and the person returns to a pattern of ALs which is acceptable to the individual.

It is sometimes said that psychological stressors involve the 'fight or flight' mechanism. For the purposes of survival, man is capable of an extreme response to perceived danger — an identifiable cause of fear. Activated by the autonomic nervous system and the secretion of certain hormones, there is an increase in heart rate and flow of blood to the muscles; a rise in blood pressure; an increase in depth and rate of respiration. The body is physiologically prepared for fight or flight.

There are many life experiences which are less dramatic, however, and the physiological response is less intense, yet the person will describe a feeling of anxiety which may not have an identifiable cause. Because it is unpleasant, the individual may try consciously, or sometimes subconsciously, to avoid it. A range of coping mechanisms to reduce anxiety to a tolerable level can be manifest in observable behaviour and are important aspects of living; in psychological and psychiatric literature they are recognized as denial, fantasy, projection, rationalization, regression, and withdrawal to name but a few.

When, however, the stress is of great intensity and long duration, especially in a susceptible person who has not developed effective coping mechanisms, general systemic changes may occur and cause what are sometimes called psychosomatic disorders such as coronary heart disease, asthma, and ulcerative colitis. Apart from adverse physical sequelae, some studies have shown that when an individual feels unable to alter the stressful circumstances, it leads to a feeling of hopelessness, and eventually pathological depression, categorized as a psychiatric disorder.

The effect on ALs can be far-reaching. For example in a person who is pathologically depressed, there may be withdrawal from communicating unless pressed to respond; disinterest in eating and drinking; difficulty with eliminating such as constipation; disinclination for work or leisure activities; disruption of the sleeping rhythm and so on depending on the severity of the depressed state.

It is important, therefore, for nurses to have knowledge of psychological factors which influence ALs. It is important when dealing with a healthy person because even coming in contact with a nurse for advice on health, or for immunization to prevent illness, may induce anxiety. How much more so when the person comes into hospital. Not only is the individual anxious about the cause of admission; the strange environment also requires psychological adaptation to the disruption of normal patterns of living such as eating and drinking, eliminating, and sleeping.

The nurse must be sensitive to individual differences in the speed of adaptation to anxiety-producing circumstances. Slower adaptation is probably more evident at the extreme ends of the lifespan, and will require especially careful handling in our multiethnic society if the person belongs to a sociocultural group with which the nurse is less familiar.

SOCIOCULTURAL

It is essential that nurses should have knowledge of sociocultural factors and how they influence ALs. In the model for nursing, therefore, social, cultural, spiritual, religious and ethical factors are introduced to indicate how this knowledge helps the nurse to understand, assess, plan and implement nursing interventions, and evaluate the effects. As already stated, there is no attempt to cover the disciplines of sociology and anthropology in this textbook. General points only are made at this stage to show how this type of knowledge (along with other subjects in the curriculum) contributes to an understanding of human beings as manifest in their various Activities of Living. More specific examples of the application of sociocultural concepts to each AL are provided in Chapters 4–15.

Health status: effect on role

Different systems of health care throughout the world show that culture influences the way societies deal with health and illness. Deep-rooted cultural beliefs and traditions affect an individual's behaviour when ill — for example, responses to pain vary according to ethnic origin. Also cultural factors influence the way people treat others who are ill so that some types of disability and certain diseases carry a degree of stigma in some societies. The mentally disabled may be shunned or feared even today because of the legacy of the view once held that this was inflicted on people as punishment for their sins. Sociocultural factors are therefore important in understanding an individual's health behaviour and people's varied responses to illness and hospitalization.

Of particular interest to those involved in the delivery of health care is what happens to an individual's *role and status* when they become ill. Talcott Parsons, a sociologist, described this phenomenon as long ago as 1966 in what he termed the '*sick role*'. He pointed out that most societies exempt a sick person from some of their usual obligations and responsibilities as long as they fulfil a corresponding obligation to seek medical care and cooperate in the process of getting well. In many parts of the world there is in fact legislation to ensure that the sick are given special entitlements; for example, there are government schemes which provide the employee with sickness leave along with protection from financial hardship caused by loss of earnings.

However, as more recent writers have pointed out, there are many social implications of illness not considered in Parson's analysis. It does not acknowledge the subjectivity involved in defining 'health' and 'illness' or take account of the fact that some sick people will not get 'well' and others may not wish to cooperate in attempts to restore them to health.

Certainly, assuming the role of 'patient' involves many role changes: for example, a young mother is expected to receive rather than give care; the managing director usually responsible for many employees becomes the responsibility of others; and the lawyer and the labourer are treated as equals despite occupying quite different social positions in real life.

Health status: effect on relationships

It is not just roles which change during illness or hospitalization, but also *relationships*. For example, the doctors' high social status is still reflected in the way some patients/clients tend to behave subserviently to them, submitting to their authority and accepting their advice unquestioningly. Such behaviour also serves to reinforce the traditional asymmetrical doctor-patient relationship. In fact, throughout the whole health care system there is an elaborate set of expectations and rules about the kinds of interaction considered to be appropriate between members of different health care professions and between professionals and patients, although this is changing rapidly.

Health status and social class

There is also an important correlation between social class and health status. In general, there are differences in the types of illnesses that affect members of different social classes. For example statistics show that heart disease is more prevalent among professional people, and respiratory conditions are more common in less advantaged socioeconomic groups. Not only are there differences in morbidity, there are also differences in mortality rates; a baby born into a less advantaged home is more likely to have a lower birth weight and more likely to die

in the first week of life, and there are strong links between social deprivation and premature adult mortality (Eames, 1993).

There is also an apparent correlation between social class and response to illness. The best possible use of health services tends to be made by members of upper socioeconomic groupings; others often fail to take advantage of provisions such as child health or family planning clinics. Sociologists have made a considerable contribution to for example, the analysis of inequalities in health, thus assisting health professionals to understand certain aspects of the aetiology of illness and some determinants of health.

Health status and religion

The influence of *religion* on individual behaviour in relation to health and illness is a particularly fascinating aspect of the sociocultural factors, religious doctrines often dictating a very circumscribed lifestyle (Neuberger, 1987). Nurses must be aware of these practices so that every person's religious and spiritual needs may be appreciated.

Many religions have regulations affecting eating and drinking habits which will affect nursing activities. Orthodox Jews, for instance, consider every meal a religious rite and must eat specially prepared 'kosher' food at all times. Muslims consider the pig an unclean animal and observe total fasting throughout the daylight hours in the month of Ramadan. Of great importance to Hindus is cleanliness as bathing renders one not only physically, but spiritually clean; traditionally the right hand is used for clean tasks only, the mouth is rinsed out after each meal and the anal region is washed after defaecation. Expressing sexuality is yet another activity of living sometimes influenced by religious beliefs and customs: limitations on family planning are imposed on Roman Catholics and Jews, and the Muslim religion prohibits free mixing socially of the sexes.

A person's religious beliefs may also influence his attitudes to health and health care and sometimes may present an obstacle to care and recovery. It is well-known that Jehovah's Witnesses are not allowed to accept a blood transfusion (Finfer et al, 1994) and that Christian Scientists believe in the healing of illness by spiritual means.

In fact, religious and cultural differences may actually discourage the use of health services by people from ethnic minorities especially when there is also a language barrier (Haggan, 1994). Discussing this deterrent, Richardson et al (1994) quote the Race Relations Code of Practice in Primary Health Care (DoH, 1992) which reports that services in the UK 'have not been sufficiently sensitive to the full range of racial, religious and linguistic diversity' and they go on to describe a research project which sought to solve some of the problems.

Whatever the circumstances, the nurse offers care to people without regard to creed, race or colour; and the nurse's function, generally speaking, is to provide an environment in which each person can continue to live by the principles which guide their behaviour.

For many people, however, religion provides a source of hope and comfort during illness. Sometimes, as in the Roman Catholic church, special sacraments may be offered to the sick and the dying. Baptism, thought by some to be necessary for a person's salvation, is carried out for any infant in danger of death or for a stillborn child (or fetus). The Sacrament of the Anointing of the Sick (formerly known as Extreme Unction or Last Rites) is often performed for a Roman Catholic during illness to aid healing and give moral strength or as a preparation for death. In general, for the dying and the bereaved, religion often assumes a role of great importance, and this subject is returned to in Chapter 15.

In fact religion, as a social institution, plays a key role in determining attitudes and customs on matters of life and death in nearly every existing society, regardless of whether the members actively practise the religion. In a multiracial society, some knowledge about a variety of religious faiths is a prerequisite for acceptance of diversity in attitudes and behaviour.

Health status and spirituality

A concept which is more encompassing than organized religion is *spirituality,* interpreted as a 'search for meaning' in one's life; it involves theistic and non-theistic approaches which can apply to agnostics and atheists as well as to followers of recognized religious persuasions. People who declare themselves agnostics or atheists may still require what Labun (1988) calls spiritual care. Discussing 'Spiritual care: an element of nursing care planning', Labun maintains that during illness, a person with no defined religious belief may wish to explore feelings, values and life with another person; perhaps a close friend, family member or a religious person, or perhaps with the nurse as the person most available, and most aware of the patient's thoughts and feelings. Labun concludes, however, that further exploration of the topic of spirituality is needed before nurses will be able to utilize this potential in a nursing plan.

Nurses need to consider carefully their own value judgements and accept that a personal belief system may not coincide with a client's system of beliefs and values. It is important to acknowledge that, for example, death may not be fearful for an unbeliever, nor for unbelieving relatives, and that secular forms of funeral services may be desired by those who profess atheism or agnosticism.

It is interesting that the effect of religion and spirituality on mental health has prompted the American Psychiatric Association, for the first time, to include religious and spiritual problems in the next edition of the Diagnostic and Statistical Manual of Mental Disorders (DSM-IV) under a broad section 'Other conditions that may be a focus of attention'. The Manual considers it can be used:

> '. . . . . . when the focus of clinical attention is a religious or spiritual problem. Examples include distressing experiences that involve loss or questionning of faith; problems associated with conversion to a new faith; or questions of other spiritual values which may not necessarily be related to an organized church or religious institution . . . . .'

The Deputy Medical Director of the APA enlarged that there is a need to be more systematic and inclusive with the category of conditions not considered mental disorders but which might be a reason for a person to consult with a mental health professional (Charatan, 1994).

Health status: ethical aspects

Inevitably, as it is dealing with human beings, health care has *ethical* aspects. Since the compilation of the Hippocratic Oath in 420 BC, doctors have attempted to arrive at common principles of ethics in health care, but nurses and other health professional groups have also sought common principles to guide their practice, for example the International Council for Nurses has devised a Code for Nurses. In essence, such codes concern themselves with, for example, duty to do good and no harm; respect for life and human dignity; justice to individuals such as non-discrimination on the basis of race, sex, religion, political affiliation, social standing, disability and mental disorder; equal opportunity in terms of access to resources including preventive and treatment services; duty to protect the vulnerable. The acceptance of such principles and putting them into practice will depend on the individual's culture and type of experience, and the kinds of criteria used for interpreting, applying and justifying them. One instance of such a dilemma relates to the controversy over emergency resuscitation. Should this technique be used in every instance when breathing and heart rate appear to have ceased? Or are there some instances when the individual should be allowed to die with dignity instead of attempting to prolong an existence where there is no longer any quality of life? This moral dilemma is discussed on p. 159.

In this section, some of the concepts associated with sociocultural aspects of nursing have been mentioned in order to provide background to the discussion of their influence on each of the ALs in Chapters 4–15.

ENVIRONMENTAL

As in the model of living, environmental factors cannot

be considered in isolation in the model for nursing. They are related to biological, psychological and sociocultural factors which have already been described, and also to politicoeconomic factors which will be discussed later. They are necessarily related to the other components of the model for nursing; for instance a person's stage on the lifespan will influence the type of relevant environmental information required when assessing, planning, implementing and individualizing a nursing plan. The same applies regarding a person's status on the dependence/ independence continuum. Knowledge from other parts of the curriculum needs to be synthesized into a nursing context so that the environment can be manipulated to achieve people's optimal level of independence for carrying out their ALs. Chapters 4–15 provide specific examples of how environmental factors can influence a particular AL; here, to provide a background to Chapters 4–15, a few general points are made about their influence on a composite of ALs.

Atmospheric components

If one particularizes to health, there are many components which are relevant, for example:

- *Organic and inorganic particles*
  Atmospheric pollutants can be both particulate inorganic and organic matter as, for example, in dust, and the minimization of dust is an important contribution to the prevention of infection in the home, at the clinic and in hospital. The organic matter can be in the form of pathogenic microorganisms, some of which cause specific infectious diseases. To give just one example of their influence on ALs — whooping cough will affect the AL of breathing and the accompanying fever will affect the AL of controlling body temperature.

  Other pathogens cause inflammation, for instance in the intestinal tract as happens in food poisoning; they can settle directly from the atmosphere onto food, or they can be transferred to food by vectors (particularly flies), or by unclean hands. The three ALs which are most likely to be influenced are eating and drinking, eliminating and controlling body temperature. There are many nursing implications, but one prime example is the importance of handwashing (to remove both resident and transient flora) before handling food, after visiting the toilet and after handling excreta.

  Other atmospheric pollutants (see p. 76) although less specific may also contribute to ill-health.
- *Light rays*
  Nurses should remember that what may seem

normal lighting can, for some people, be excessive and distressing. It can be tiring for people who are ill, and prevent them from resting and relaxing or even sleeping; and it can be particularly disturbing for people who have photophobia or who are dying.

However light has many positive uses in a health context, for example, to assist in the examination of body orifices. Light from an auroscope is used to examine the external auditory canal which can reveal conditions interfering with hearing, and thereby communicating. Similarly, an ophthalmoscope is used to examine the eye, with the objective of identifying conditions which interfere with sight; also associated with communicating. Yet another example is the bronchoscope for investigating the bronchi when a person is experiencing problems related to breathing.

Light can now be transmitted through flexible glass fibres (fibreoptics), indeed the use of fibreoptics has resulted in the development of 'minimal access' or 'minimally invasive' surgery (Royston et al, 1994) or keyhole surgery, as well as extending the scope of diagnostic techniques. 'Keyhole' procedures are much less invasive, can sometimes be performed on a day basis, and may require only a local anaesthetic.
- *Sound waves*
  Noise needs special consideration in a nursing context (p. 90). It scarcely requires research to show that noise in hospital wards interferes with sleeping and ipso facto with resting and relaxing. But noise can also be intrusive and interfere with communicating when, for example, a nurse and a patient are discussing sensitive information. And it can lessen the concentration (a dimension of communicating) necessary to relearn, for example, mobilizing skills.

Clothing

Clothing in a nursing setting influences the same ALs as in the model of living (p. 29) and it is now accepted that once patients are ambulant for several hours, the donning of daytime attire has a rehabilitative effect. Personally-marked clothing systems have been introduced in most long-stay wards, and particular emphasis is placed on the use of personal underwear to maintain patients' self-respect and self-esteem.

And a consideration of bedclothes is important in nursing. More obviously they can influence the AL of controlling body temperature but they are also associated with the AL of maintaining a safe environment — microorganisms adhere to the scales of the skin's outer layer and are continually being shed on to the sheets. When disseminated into the atmosphere during bed-making, they can be a cause of hospital-acquired infection (p. 94).

Nursing environment

Objects in many forms are legion in a nursing environment. They include all those already mentioned in a person's home. Also included are special items of furniture, furnishings, equipment and the many aids to mobilizing: collectively they give some idea of the many ALs which can be influenced by them.

Another example is the presence of flowers and plants brought by visitors, communicating to patients, emotions such as love and affection, belongingness, being valued as a person and so on. They are also aesthetically pleasing and may promote a response which, for some people, borders on spirituality.

Buildings

The buildings which are relevant in a nursing context are the person's home, nursing homes, clinics, health centres and hospitals. People's homes are relevant on two scores; firstly, should a member of the family require nursing services at home because of illness, the suitability of the physical layout of the rooms in relation to the problematic ALs needs consideration, as well as the availability of lay helpers, usually family members. If the person is very breathless and the house is on two floors, it may be advisable to put the bed in a room which is on the same floor as the toilet/bathroom. Discussion with the family will help them to make appropriate decisions about how ALs such as personal cleansing and dressing, and eliminating will be carried out.

Secondly, if ill in hospital, it is appropriate to discuss with patients, before discharge, relevant details about the physical layout of their home related to the affected ALs, for example, the availability of the toilet if the person has been prescribed diuretics.

Environmental facilities available at clinics and health centres can certainly influence several ALs. Clients with an increased frequency of micturition will need to have easily accessible toilets, clearly labelled. Inaccessibility for people with mobilizing problems may deter them from seeking help. Inadequate provision for pushchairs, cycles and cars can deter a wide range of people from seeking help, for example, parents with young children, as well as disabled drivers of cars, and they may be seeking help with a variety of ALs.

Hospitals just like other buildings reflect the period in which they were constructed. When older hospitals were built, many patients remained in bed for most of the day, so their bathing and toilet facilities are inadequate to cater effectively for the needs of today's mobile patients. The same applies to storage space for clothes. For medium and longstay patients, it is important to be able to store several sets of daytime clothes in order to allow for decision-making regarding general appearance. Matching clothes to mood also helps to prevent conditions such as boredom and institutionalization (p. 326). In older hospitals, too, adequate and pleasant surroundings for ambulant patients' leisure activities, and for eating and drinking are often at a premium; these environmental factors can influence, for example, the ALs of communicating, eating and drinking, and working and playing.

The need for finance to upgrade older hospitals or pay for new buildings and equipment which provide a suitable environment for attending to ALs is one example of the link between environmental and politicoeconomic factors.

POLITICOECONOMIC

It is essential that the nurse should have some knowledge of politicoeconomic (including legal) factors and how they influence ALs. In the model for nursing, therefore, political, economic and legal factors are introduced to indicate how this helps nurses to understand, assess, plan and implement nursing interventions, and evaluate the effects. There is no attempt to cover these disciplines in this textbook. General points only are made at this stage to show how this type of knowledge (along with other subjects in the nursing curriculum) contributes to an understanding of human beings as manifest in their various activities of living. More specific examples of the application of politicoeconomic concepts to each AL are provided in Chapters 4–15.

Health and economic status

Conventionally, health is considered to be the responsibility of the health professions and they are credited with improvements in health and the fight against disease. They deserve some of the accolade. It is often overlooked, however, that the major determinants of health are firmly rooted in prevailing political, economic and social realities. The economic status of the mass of the population in a country undoubtedly affects living conditions and Activities of Living, which in turn influence health and the incidence of illness.

It is difficult to appreciate just how precarious life could be for the masses in the Western world only 100 years ago. For example, in the 1880s life expectancy (one indicator of health status) for a male child in the UK at birth was 41 years, and for the female was 45 years. As the result of continuing industrialization, the population was still adapting to the new urban way of life and experiencing new economic problems created by the growth of industry and decline in agriculture. The hastily built towns with poor planning, overcrowding, unsafe water supplies (AL of eating and drinking) and inadequate sanitation (AL of eliminating) were not conducive to the maintenance of health, and the long hours of work (AL of working) for low wages in poorly ventilated factories and mines, with unguarded machinery, accounted for crippling disabilities due to accidents (AL of maintaining a safe environment) and a lowered resistance to many of the prevalent infections. However, this began to change.

Health and political/legal activity

In the late 19th century there was an enormous sanitary reform movement which, with political support, culminated in the UK in the 1875 Public Health Act. The UK was not alone in the field of health reform. Around this time most other industrialized countries were taking similar legal action, indeed there was beginning to be international cooperation in an attempt to control the various pandemics; national boundaries were no barrier to the spread of infection.

Around the same period, too, in a number of industrialized countries, there was considerable political activity, which, along with the wealth which accompanied the economic industrial boom was focused to improve housing; provide safer food; create facilities for better education. As a result of these better living conditions there was a decline in the incidence of several killer infections and the health status of the masses began to improve even before the discovery of specific preventive and curative measures in the form of immunization and pharmaceutical products. In factories, working conditions were also improved.

Health in industrialized countries

Much of the industrialized world's economic success which was reflected in environmental reform and improved health was associated with acts of parliament. National parliamentary action, however, was sometimes precipitated by the work of voluntary organizations, often working at a local level, not on a nationwide basis. Voluntary organizations did a considerable amount to improve health and well-being, for example by providing free milk for children (the AL of eating and drinking) or warm clothes (the AL of personal cleansing and dressing); or free contraceptives (the AL of expressing sexuality) to mothers who did not have the finance to support yet more children. When responsibility for making basic provision for such activities of everyday living was taken over by the government, it was possible to contribute to the promotion of health on a national scale. It is fascinating to compare the current position in the so-called developing countries.

Health in developing countries

When the United Nations Organization was established in 1945, many of the developing countries had the same major objectives as the industrialized countries cherished a century before — to develop the economic and social status of their peoples. The major emphasis was on economic development and investment in modern science and technology. An important economic asset in any country of course, is the health of the work force, but during the 1970s, the World Health Organization (WHO) — the health agency of the United Nations Organization — was showing increasing concern about the lack of improvement in the health status of the world's poorer, mainly rural, population. It began to be realized that not only the conventional health professionals were involved in health; it required an integrated approach at government level from, for example, housing, public works, agriculture and education. Even more significantly, the community-based preventive and health promotive services needed the active participation of the people; and to achieve this, political will and cooperation were needed at national and local levels.

It is worthwhile to note WHO's 12 indicators for monitoring and evaluating its Global Strategy for Health for All by the year 2000 (World Health Assembly, 1981). It is remarkable how these minimal requirements reflect the state of affairs in industrialized countries about a century ago; and there is a strong politicoeconomic flavour to the indicators. The first evaluation of the 1981 Strategy was carried out in 1985 and some modifications were made prior to the evaluation in 1991 when 151 out of WHO's 186 member countries completed reports covering 5200 million people in the world (World Health Organization 1993: 8).

Health and the world economy

Of course it is a rare nation that is economically self-sufficient nowadays. Countries and governments are economically interdependent and inexorably intertwined politically. The economic interdependence of richer and poorer nations was graphically described in 'North-South; a programme for survival' — the Brandt Report, produced in 1980 — and it is tempting to think that in the intervening years, progress has been made in some areas.

The ending of the 'Cold War' which dominated international affairs for four decades certainly gave opportunities for a widespread discussion about democracy and development. In Europe, however, the threat of war was replaced by the threat of an uncertain future including hostilities between ethnic and religious groups; and internationally, an economic recession made it difficult for developing countries to benefit from a potentially more peaceful world where, theoretically, less money would be allocated to military expenditure and more spent on health and economic development.

Inevitably health and development are also linked with population trends (Box 3.2) and the estimated poverty level. Recent studies by the World Bank, the United Nations and the OECD indicate that the number of people living below poverty level has increased because of the rapid growth in population, so even an increased food output has had no significant effect on their nutritional status (World Health Organization, 1993). Other studies in Europe and N. America have found that the elderly, typically, account for 30–40% bed days in hospitals and of visits to general practitioners; quite disproportionate to their percentage of the population.

However, even if population trends were ideal, the fragile world economy is not helped by the fact that the West is moving out of an industrial economy to a bio-technological economy where robots are already doing the routine, manual chores at the work place and even in the home.

Politicoeconomic influences affecting the individual's health

Clearly the economic and social circumstances of an individual's community and the political will of the state exert a considerable influence on the lifestyle and health status of the individual and the family unit; and this will vary from country to country. As an example, in the UK, in the formal health service as such, political and economic circumstances influence the legal provision. Parliamentary Acts enforce the registration of qualified practitioners such as nurses and doctors; for example, the

Nurses, Midwives and Health Visitors Act of 1992 regulates the nursing profession and the preparation of its future practitioners. The UK Central Council for Nurses, Midwives and Health Visitors (UKCC), funded by the government, issued for example, the Code of Professional Conduct for a Nurse, Midwife or Health Visitor (UKCC, 1992). This is a directive, not a guideline.

Parliamentary Acts and legal requirements do not influence only the practitioners in the health service; patients are also involved. Patients with certain types of disorders are protected by the law, for example the Mental Health Act 1983 focuses on the rights of mentally ill people especially regarding consent to treatment. Although not mandatory, the Patient's Charter (DoH, 1991b) outlined 'specific standards which the government looks to the NHS to achieve as circumstances and resources allow'. It was sent to every household in the UK and certainly has done much to raise clients' expectations of the Service, although in a National Consumer Council poll, only 24% of the sample recalled seeing a copy (Cohen, 1994).

In the UK, too, as well as having government regulations related to the practice of the professional groups employed, and to certain groups of patients, the health service itself is a nationalized institution, funded by government and influenced by the economics of the national budget. Of necessity, the financial allocation to health is finite, yet with technological advances making cure possible for increasingly esoteric disorders, the demand for the relevant expensive treatment is prodigious and cannot always be met, thereby creating considerable ethical dilemmas for both professionals and politicians (Redmayne & Klein, 1993). Most industrialized countries have similar regulations for similarly organized health services, and for the professional staff who work in them.

So to understand the patient's circumstances, and the nurse's legal duties and responsibilities, the nurse must have background knowledge of the political and economic factors which can, potentially, influence the individual's Activities of Living; and also influence the nurse's professional interventions in helping individuals to practise their Activities of Living in a manner acceptable to the individual and the community.

Individualizing nursing

Individualizing nursing is accomplished by using the process of nursing which involves four phases — assessing, planning, implementing and evaluating (Fig. 3.8). 'The process' is neither a 'model' nor a 'philosophy' as it is sometimes described but simply a method of logical thinking and it needs to be used with an explicit nursing

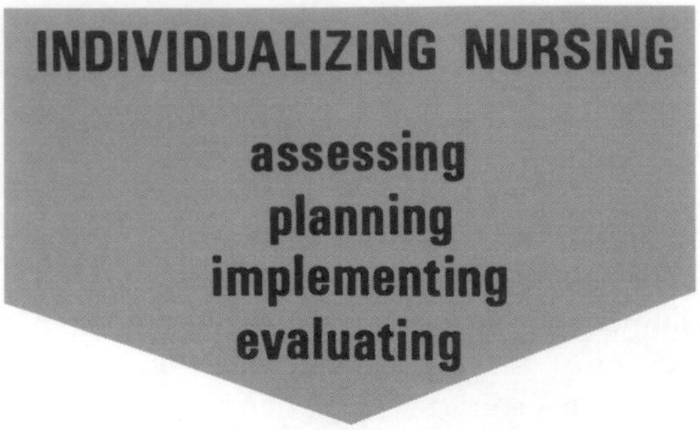

INDIVIDUALIZING NURSING

assessing
planning
implementing
evaluating

Fig. 3.8 Individualizing nursing

model. This is the rationale for incorporating the process into our model for nursing.

We have already stated the rationale for using the model of living as a basis for our model for nursing, and the patient's individuality in living should be borne in mind in all four phases of the process.

Throughout the process the patient should wherever possible be an active participant: for example, making decisions about continuing to carry out certain activities of living and perhaps agreeing to modify others in the interests of health and recovery from illness. Encouraging a sense of personal responsibility for health, and protecting autonomy even in illness, increasingly are seen as important principles in modern health care, hence the emphasis on viewing the person as a 'consumer' and an active participant. Of course participation may not be possible in the case, for example, of a child, a confused or an unconscious person. In these instances family members or significant others may participate in decision-making on behalf of the patient, possibly carrying out some of the activities, as is usually the case when people are nursed in their own homes.

Patient participation demands a somewhat radical approach to nursing by both patients and nurses. To take patients first — in the past the majority accepted what happened to them while they were in the health care system, assuming that the doctors and nurses 'knew best'. With social changes which have occurred in the last few decades, particularly the influence of the mass media, more and more patients are knowledgeable about what is happening to them and wish to be involved in discussions and decisions about their health and treatment. However, there are still people who are not sufficiently assertive to indicate their desire to be so involved and others who do not wish to be so (Tmobranski, 1994; Waterworth & Luker, 1990), and these variations need to be recognized and acted on accordingly by the nurse. There is evidence that this also applies in psychiatric services (Glenister, 1994).

Patient participation has repercussions in nursing which also require recognition. For example, the introduction of a policy allowing self-medication has obvious advantages for patients in terms of independence and preparation for discharge home; but, at the same time, this policy alters the nurse's role to one of teacher and supervisor rather than administrator of drugs (Davis, 1991; Thornett, Heaseman & Bentley, 1994). Careful planning and cooperative teamwork, particularly with the pharmacist is essential (Cottrell, 1990; Hancock, 1994). A medication discharge planning programme measured the effect on re-admissions (Schneider et al, 1993).

Having made some general comments about the process of nursing, some more specific commentary is provided on each of the four phases involved. Although the process is described as comprising four phases, this is merely for the purpose of description and discussion. The implication in describing four phases is that they are carried out sequentially but in reality all four phases are interactive. It is important for nurses to realize this from the outset so that thinking will not be rigid and compartmentalized because, in practice, the process operates naturally and flexibly with continuous feedback.

ASSESSING

The word 'assessment' has been adopted for the first phase of the process of nursing by the majority of nurses. However, we think that over-use of the word assessment encourages the idea that it is a once-only activity and we prefer to use 'assessing' to encourage recognition of the ongoing nature of the activity. There is some dubiety about what assessment includes, so it is necessary to clarify our use of the word; it includes:

- collecting information from/about the person
- reviewing the collected information
- identifying the person's problems
- identifying priorities among problems.

The information will be gained by observing, interviewing, examining, measuring and testing as appropriate: data gained at the initial assessment form a baseline against which further information can be compared. It is likely that as rapport with the person is established, more information will be volunteered and, indeed, new and supplementary information becomes available to the nurse in the course of each contact with the person.

The primary source of information about the person is the person. However, secondary sources such as health records and family members are important and especially so in the case of children and disoriented, unconscious or severely mentally ill or disabled people. Information volunteered by the person is classified as subjective, whereas other types of information, such as data from measurement, are objective. The use of objective measures is becoming more common in nursing, partly an outcome of nursing research, and some of the available tools are mentioned in the later chapters of this book; such as Norton's scale for assessing patients' risk of developing pressure sores (p. 248).

In building up a data base for each person, the initial assessment is of great importance although, as has been said, this is only the beginning and not the end of assessing. The first meeting of nurse and patient may be in the person's own home, a nursing home, at the health centre or during admission to hospital, (whether as an emergency or from the waiting list). In hospital, it may well be that after the patient has been greeted, he is shown his bed, introduced to nearby patients and shown the toilet and bathroom facilities. The rationale for this is that it gives the person time to settle and become composed before the nurse returns at a suitable time to carry out the 'initial assessment'. However, the person may be so ill that such civilities become irrelevant and only absolutely essential information is ascertained before the nurses proceed to carry out essential treatment.

At whichever location, assessing should ideally be carried out as early as possible in the person's stay in the health service. In reality it is often not possible to collect extensive information within a few hours of admission to hospital, and McFarlane & Castledine (1982) illustrate a 'first stage history format' which they say 'provides enough information for the nurses to start looking after the patient', then it is followed as soon as possible by using a more detailed second stage format. There are however some topics about which information must be collected early. Any bleeding or injury would of course be assessed immediately; information about pressure sores or any bruises is essential; it is *customary* to record the temperature, pulse and respiration (see p. 271), blood pressure (see p. 157) and the result of testing a specimen of urine. It is also necessary for the staff to know of any sensitivities, allergies and any medicines which are currently being taken. All of this information is important to record whatever the location.

Many employing authorities now provide specific stationery on which the information from nursing assessment is written. Beginning nurses may be confused by the various names which are used for it — nursing assessment form, patient assessment form, nursing Kardex, nursing history and patient profile. Whatever the name and format, the objective is to record two different sorts of information: for our purposes, one we call the patient's 'biographical and health data', and the other is 'Activities of Living data' which are concerned with the individual's usual routines and current problems. We designed suitable forms for recording these two different sorts of data; they are illustrated in Appendix 1, and how they are used for assessing patients is explained below. The information is useful, whatever type of stationery is supplied.

Biographical and health data

The person's biographical and health details include such obvious items as name, sex, age, next of kin and usual place of residence. This list is deceptively simple! But even these apparently straightforward items must be carefully collected.

Surname The custom in Western countries is to use the surname of the family, or in the case of a married woman, the husband's family name; but this is not so in all cultures and nurses may need to seek expert help so that the 'correct' surname is recorded.

First name Likewise it used to be customary to talk about 'Christian' names but with changing social mores the word 'Forename' or 'First name' is now widely used. Increasingly nurses are directed to ask patients what form of address they prefer as some people use a name other than the one on their birth certificate, and use of the familiar one can help them to retain their sense of personal identity.

Use of first names has become widespread in the last decade at all levels of the health service, particularly between nurses and patients. The subject has been aired in several letters to the editor of the two weekly nursing journals (Sears, 1994). Semi-structured interviews were conducted on 103 convalescing inpatients revealing that a 'substantial minority' were against the use of first names (Nursing Standard, 1994; Nursing Times, 1994-Editorial).

Marital status Another sometimes complicated item is the patient's marital status and nurses should be sensitive to the fact that there may be embarrassment over mentioning separation or divorce or partner status.

Home address Beneath that item, the form asks for the patient's address and it is becoming more common to record the type of living accommodation — information which is particularly relevant to community nurses on relief duty when visiting patients in their own homes, and indeed for hospital nurses so that they know for instance whether the patient will need to climb stairs at home. Noting the 'mode of entry' to the home may be necessary information for the community nurse who needs to know how to gain entry when, for example, the patient is unable to go to the door. Knowing who else resides with the patient may also be relevant information in certain circumstances.

At this time of high unemployment and redundancy, there are people housed in 'bed and breakfast' accommodation. Local authorities provide hostels where homeless people can sleep overnight. There are refuges where battered wives can live temporarily and so on. This is merely a reminder that not all people live in a house and those using the aforementioned 'address' may well be in need of the nursing service (Gaulton-Berks, 1994).

Next of kin and significant others 'Next of kin' requires to be known for legal purposes and, usually, as the person to be contacted if the patient's condition is giving rise to concern. However, a person who is separated from a spouse may wish to name a partner or, perhaps, an alternative contact as may also be necessary if the next of kin is abroad. In contrast, it is important to know about 'significant others' in terms of the person's social network and sources of support. A 'significant other' may be a person of the same sex, whether or not they reside at the patient's residence. It is usual to record any specific support services being used such as meals-on-wheels or visiting by community nurses as on discharge, arrangements for their resumption may have to be made.

Occupation This is a useful piece of information. From a health point of view it may have contributed to the person's health problem, for example an injury sustained at work, or in other instances there may be implications for return to former employment, for example when an accident causes paraplegia.

Religious beliefs and practices Recording of information about religious beliefs and practices is essential if they have implications for nursing, such as the provision of a special diet. The recording of recent significant life events (in the context of the patient's beliefs) may sometimes be relevant because illness can follow a life crisis such as bereavement which may impede recovery. In any event it will be important for the nurse to be aware of, and sympathetic to, any major recent events in the life of the person.

Current health problems and reason for admission It is useful, too, to know the person's and the family's perception of the person's current health problem. Asking the person about the reason for admission/referral can give an indication of the person's level of understanding or it can reveal a lack of knowledge; for example, that an 'operation' is scheduled, when in fact it is an investigation. Alongside this the actual reason for admission/referral can be stated and some additional medical information recorded about the person's diagnosis, past history and any allergies. It is usual to record the address and telephone number of the person's own doctor and consultant.

Discharge planning Making plans for discharge acknowledges the importance of health teaching, rehabilitation and discharge planning even from the beginning. This is particularly important for elderly people in acute wards and the recommendations from a research project are contained in Box 3.3 (King & Macmillan, 1994; Tierney et al, 1993).

So, this outline gives an idea of the sort of information which might be collected at the initial assessment. These biographical and health data are unlikely to change and will be useful and, therefore, should be available to all nursing staff whether the person's stay in the health service is long or short.

Box 3.3 Recommendations for discharge of elderly people from acute wards

- There is an increasing need to assess the discharge requirements of elderly patients in all acute wards
- Assessment information must be fully and accurately recorded
- Standard proforma need to have sufficient space to accommodate the recording of the complex needs of elderly people
- Comprehensive, detailed assessment is required as soon as possible after admission as a basis for discharge planning
- Use of standardized instruments for recording physical and mental function would aid assessment and documentation
- Multidisciplinary documentation would be of great benefit for staff and patients
- Interviewing and information-gathering skills need a higher educational profile in nursing.

Assessing ALs

The second part of assessment focuses on the person's ALs — the individual's usual routines and current problems. Use of the ALs for assessment is central to our model for nursing. Data collected about them in the context of the five influencing factors outlines each person in his or her entirety. Those who will nurse the person need to know about usual routines — importantly what the person can and cannot do independently — and whether or not there are any problems or discomforts associated with any AL; if so, whether these have been experienced previously and if this is the case, how they have been coped with (Appendix 1). The following outline provides only an introduction to assessing the ALs because each is developed more comprehensively in its particular chapter in Section 2.

The form (Appendix 1) on which AL assessment information is recorded is deliberately without ruled spaces for each AL so that the nurse can use the space to best advantage for each particular patient, ordering the data in terms of the most problematic ALs first or whatever seems the most appropriate order in the circumstances. A few other general comments about the documentation of AL data and related people's problems will be made following a brief comment on assessing each of the 12 ALs.

- *Assessing ability to maintain a safe environment* is of particular importance if the person is physically disabled or has a learning disability. The nurse needs to know whether or not the person appreciates the dangers in the environment and knows how to prevent accidents. Assessing the level of safety in the home is an important responsibility of the nurse who visits elderly people or families with young children.

• *Assessing communicating skills* is necessary in order to discover the person's level of communication and this is important whether in the home, health centre or hospital. It is very important for nurses who have an extensive technical vocabulary to remember that not all people will be familiar with nursing and medical terms, however ordinary or straightforward they seem to staff.

The nurse should observe whether the person is reticent or forthcoming when talking about home and health problems. It is sometimes possible to discern from the conversation whether the person is gregarious by nature or shy. It may be necessary to gather specific information about one of the sensory organs if the nurse suspects a deficiency or dysfunction which is affecting the person's AL of communicating. Finally, when assessing this AL, any general information about the person's pain should be sought and recorded. The rationale for linking pain with the AL of communicating is based on the fact that pain is a subjective experience, its presence and degree is communicated to us by the person's verbal and non-verbal behaviour. Additional data about pain which affects specific ALs (e.g. abdominal pain affecting the AL of eating and drinking) can be recorded at that AL.

• *Assessment of breathing* may involve counting the number of respirations per minute. For the majority of people, however, it is simply a case of the nurse noting whether there is an apparent breathing difficulty and asking whether there is the problem of a cough or breathlessness. In turn, this may offer an opportunity to discover whether or not the person smokes and if so how much. The Health of the Nation (Department of Health, 1992) recommends that a 'smoking history' is taken for each person contacting the health service. The nurse should attempt to discover the person's perception of the multiple ill-effects of smoking and whether or not help with giving up or reducing smoking would be welcomed.

More detailed assessment of breathing is necessary when a patient is unconscious, still under the effects of an anaesthetic or suffering from a disease affecting the cardio-pulmonary system. It should be noted that information about haemorrhage (other than bleeding related to a specific AL; e.g. vaginal bleeding would pertain to the AL of expressing sexuality) should be recorded under the AL of breathing on the basis that the cardiopulmonary system is related to this AL.

• *Assessing eating and drinking routines* is relatively easy because most people enjoy talking about this AL. When nursing underweight and overweight people it is especially important to talk with them about what they eat, as well as when and how much. Nurses will need information about how disabled people manage this activity. When the person complains of discomfort associated with eating or drinking, more specific assessment will be required.

• *Assessing a person's eliminating habits* is a nursing function even though admission to the health care system may not have been associated with bowel or urinary dysfunction. But there may well be a persistent problem with, for example constipation and this may be elicited from the assessment. Many people find it embarrassing to talk about elimination and the nurse needs to broach the topic with sensitivity and phrase the questions carefully and clearly to avoid embarrassment yet elicit information.

• *Assessing personal cleansing habits and dressing* is possible by observing the result of these activities; ill-cared-for clothes may be an indication of financial hardship or a lack of self-esteem which can characterize exhaustion or mental illness. The nurse may discover unhygienic practices, for example related to cleaning teeth or lack of handwashing after visiting the toilet. With this knowledge the nurse can plan to include relevant teaching in the nursing plan. It should be noted that assessment of the AL of personal cleansing and dressing should include an assessment of the patient's skin status (including signs of bruising which could be from abuse) and an assessment of the person's risk of developing pressure sores. The rationale for including this here is on the basis of the link between the integumentary system and the AL.

• *Assessing control of body temperature* usually involves taking the temperature with a thermometer on admission and regular measurement may become necessary if the person is suffering from pyrexia or hypothermia. There are other ways of assessing this AL — observation may reveal flushing of the skin, excessive perspiration, the presence of goose flesh, shivering, and excessively hot or cold hands and / or feet.

• *Assessing mobilizing* may only involve observing that the person does not appear to have any problems. But later observation might reveal, for example, stiffness of the joints on rising after sleep, a common occurrence for the older person. People who have persistent back pain often adopt a characteristic posture to minimize low back movement. Other mobilizing problems are usually self-evident and nurses need to know how the person copes with them and detailed information should be obtained on this from physically disabled people so that nursing can be planned to enable maximum independence to be retained.

• *Assessing working and playing routines* is an essential part of an initial assessment. By the way the person talks about these activities, the nurse will gather what is considered challenging and what boring. The physical conditions at the person's place of work may have contributed to the accident or illness which has necessitated admission to hospital. On the other hand, difficulty in social relationships because of personality problems or mental illness may be revealed or suspected, and difficulties inherent in enforced unemployment would be important to know about for people in that situation.

• *Assessing the AL of expressing sexuality* involves observing how people express their gender in a general way, for example, in mode of dress, use of cosmetics and so on. Specific assessment is not usually necessary or appropriate unless the person's problems or potential problems are somehow associated with sex and reproduction; most people find it embarrassing to talk with strangers about this private AL. However, the observant nurse will perceive cues which are expressions of sexuality, or indicators of anxieties related to the AL of expressing sexuality. With sensitivity the nurse can create an atmosphere in which people feel able to discuss sex-related problems and diseases and a detailed assessment may become necessary in certain circumstances.

• *Assessing sleeping routines* at an early stage is important so that nurses have information on which to base nursing activities aimed at promoting sleep. People are not usually admitted to hospital because of a sleep problem as such, but adequate sleep is important for progress towards recovery, whatever the reason for admission and promotion of sleep requires knowledge of the person's usual routines and use of medication, if any.

• *Assessing the needs of the dying* is a very important role of the nurse in hospital and in the community. Although we included the AL of dying in our list of 12 ALs, 'assessing' only becomes essential when the diagnosis and prognosis indicate that the person's death is probable in the immediate or near future. However, constant sensitivity and acute observation are necessary to recognize whether or not the person wants to talk about the many aspects associated with death, dying and bereavement. Much more is discussed about assessing the needs and problems of the dying in the chapter on the AL of dying (Ch. 15).

Assessing is not a once-only activity and additional data will be collected as the nurses have further opportunity to observe people and talk with them in the course of their nursing. Whether additional data is obtained and recorded on a daily basis or less frequently will depend on factors such as the person's condition, length of stay in hospital, or frequency of visits in the case of a person at home.

And, equally, the amount and type of information collected about the ALs will vary according to different circumstances and, in some, information about all of the ALs may not be relevant. Assessing therefore is not a rigid routine carried out at a particular time and in a set pattern; it is an ongoing activity and one which requires to be tailored to the circumstances of the individual person.

Assessing is just as applicable to people who are in the health care system for surveillance or maintenance of health as for those who are in hospital for investigation and/or treatment of illness. Some nurses think that the identification of patients' problems is not applicable to health maintenance and promotion, but in healthy living the aim is to avoid potential problems from becoming actual ones and the process of identifying potential problems with the ALs is the same as that involved in the identification of actual problems.

Whatever the health/illness status, while collecting information about the person's ALs the nurse will necessarily take account of the stage on the lifespan, one of the components of the model. There is a reminder on our proforma (Appendix 1) to consider the person's 'Previous routines' and it is necessary to remember that these will have been fashioned by biological, psychological, sociocultural, environmental and politicoeconomic factors — another component of the model. The nurse is reminded of the dependence/independence continuum of the model by the heading 'what can/cannot be done independently'. And there is a prompt 'previous coping mechanisms' to remind the nurse that if there are problems or discomforts with any of the ALs, enquiry should be made about how these have been coped with.

In summary then, the objective in collecting information about the ALs is to discover:

• previous routines
• what the person can do independently
• what the person cannot do independently
• previous coping behaviours
• what problems the person has, both actual and potential, with relevant ALs.

Identifying people's problems

Identifying the person's problems is the final activity of the assessing phase of the process of nursing. In many cases, the presence of *actual* problems (such as pain, bleeding, anorexia, pyrexia) will be obvious to the person and to the nurse. But it has to be remembered that there can be a 'nurse-perceived problem' of which the patient is not aware (raised blood pressure being an obvious example); and, also possible, a 'patient-perceived problem' (such as a particular worry) of which the nurse is not immediately aware. Being alert to these possibilities will ensure that they are explored in the course of assessment.

When it comes to identifying *potential* problems, the nurse's greater knowledge of factors which predispose to ill-health, and are complications of illness and treatment, make it possible to collect information which the person may not volunteer without prompting. It is the concept of potential problems which also highlights the aspects of nursing which are concerned with the maintenance and promotion of health.

A statement of the person's problems, as ascertained

from the nursing assessment, is increasingly being referred to as 'a nursing diagnosis'. In an article entitled 'Can nurses diagnose?' Marks-Maran (1983) says that the garage mechanic tells her that he has 'diagnosed' what is wrong with her car; he is not afraid of the word 'diagnosis'. A reluctance to use this term in nursing, at least in the UK, may be for the reason that 'diagnosis' is traditionally the doctor's role. But, in fact, a nursing diagnosis is a description of the problems which people experience with ALs, whereas the medical diagnosis is usually concerned with pathological changes. Returning to Marks-Maran's article, she states that a person with one medical diagnosis may have several nursing diagnoses.

The development and classification of nursing diagnoses has advanced in recent years, particularly in North America where there is an extensive literature and Gordon (1979) is still regarded as a classic reference. Roper (1988) considers that medical vocabulary should be avoided when recording people's problems (nursing diagnoses) which should be written from the patient's perspective of how everyday living is being affected by the problem.

However, research in the early 1990s is revealing differences in interpretation of the words 'assessment' and 'nursing diagnosis', and classification of the latter is being questioned. So, in this uncertain state of knowledge related to nursing diagnosis, we continue to prefer the idea of 'patient's problems with the ALs'. The proforma (Appendix 1) provides space for each problem identified from assessment to be listed, alongside the related AL, and specified as 'actual' or 'potential' (by noting 'p' against the latter).

Having reached this stage, all that remains before proceeding with planning is to decide on the relative priority among the problems. It hardly needs to be said that life-threatening and health-threatening problems take precedence over other less immediate or less important problems and, among these, the priority will be decided in collaboration with the person and maybe with the family. The person's priority may not always be the same as the nurse's, and this must be taken into account for it will affect motivation and cooperation. The priority of problems can be indicated on the form by arranging the problems in order or, alternatively, numbering their priority.

PLANNING

The second phase of the process of nursing is planning, and it reflects our definition of nursing. The objective of the plan is:

- to prevent identified potential problems from becoming actual ones
- to solve actual problems

- where possible, to alleviate those which cannot be solved
- to help the patient cope positively with those problems which cannot be alleviated or solved
- to prevent recurrence of a treated problem
- to help the person to be as comfortable and pain-free as possible when death is inevitable.

Setting goals

To achieve this, a goal has to be set for each actual and potential problem (in collaboration with the person whenever possible and maybe with the family) with a distinction made between short-term and long-term goals. Instead of the word 'goals' some nurses prefer 'objectives' or 'patient outcomes'; it is a matter of preference.

Goals should be achievable within a person's individual circumstances, otherwise there is the danger of disheartenment. Whenever possible, goals should be stated in terms of outcomes which are able to be observed, measured or tested so that their subsequent evaluation can be accomplished. Whenever feasible, a time/date should be specified alongside a goal to indicate when evaluation should be undertaken. So the nurse (along with the person when relevant) sets a goal and estimates when it might be achieved just as the traveller decides on a destination and, according to the mode of travel, estimates the time of arrival. But, it needs to be said, such travelling is considerably less complicated and more certain than nursing!

Preparing a nursing plan

Before nursing plans can be written, or recorded on a computer, account has to be taken of existing resources which in a nursing context may be equipment, personnel and physical environment: and available support services may have to be considered when a person is being nursed at home. Possible alternative nursing interventions may be determined by the availability of resources and influenced by the person's expressed preferences.

A plan is then made of all the proposed nursing interventions to achieve the goals, stated in sufficient detail so that any other nurse, on reading it, would be aware of the plan of nursing. There is no argument against a recorded plan being essential since no one nurse can be on duty throughout the 24 hours. Social changes such as decreased working hours, and an increase in both annual leave and use of part-time staff, have made it essential for nurses to develop the skill of communicating by recording adequate nursing plans. If such social trends continue, it may well be that the nursing plan will assume even greater importance as a means of communication between nurses. And furthermore, assessing a person and recording a nursing plan helps the nurse to know the person which aids the establishment of a satisfactory nurse/patient relationship, the unique basis of the nursing contribution to a person's health care.

The Nursing Plan which is part of the proforma for use with the model is shown in Appendix 1. There is a section for noting nurse-initiated interventions (i.e. those derived from problems with ALs) and another section which is for medically-prescribed interventions (e.g. prescriptions for pain management). Explanation of these sections of the Nursing Plan is provided below.

Nursing Plan related to ALs   The Nursing Plan on page three of our document (Appendix 1) is related to the ALs and it forms the right side of the double fold. This positioning is deliberate so that the problems, both actual and potential, identified at the initial assessment, do not need to be written again. Opposite the problems the goals are written, together with the 'Nurse-initiated interventions' to achieve these; and there is a column in which to record the result of 'Evaluation'.

The Nursing Plan may have nursing interventions at an AL even although there is not a specific problem stated. For example when the person does not have a problem with the AL of personal cleansing and dressing but has a particular preference for a shower rather than a bath. Noting this fact will alert nurses reading the Plan to the person's preference and deter them from initiating an alternative form of intervention. Similarly, a disabled person may not have a problem as such with the AL of mobilizing as long as aids which are relied on remain available; noting details of the person's requirements for aided independence will avoid unnecessary dependence on the nursing staff as well as frustration for the person.

The Nursing Plan is just that — a *plan* which tells nurses what to do and when. Extra information should only be recorded:

- when a goal has been achieved
- when the nursing intervention has to be changed to achieve the already set goal
- when, for any reason, the goal has to be modified
- when the date for evaluation has changed
- if the person develops other problems. Other day-to-day information about the person should be recorded in the Patient's Nursing Notes and proforma for these kinds of recordings are usually devised locally.

Nursing Plan derived from medical/other prescription   We have discussed so far the nurse-initiated nursing interventions related to ALs, but clearly there are nursing interventions which are derived directly from medical prescription and, increasingly, from the prescriptions of other members of the health care team such as the dietitian or physiotherapist. Although some such prescriptions may be charted separately (e.g. prescribed drugs on the person's medicine chart), others are not, and it was

for this reason that we decided to add this fourth page to the nursing proforma.

Inclusion of these nursing interventions does not mean a return to the 'medical model', a term which does not appear in the medical literature. Nursing is a collaborative activity and it irrefutably includes interventions arising from medical prescription, but thereafter they are nursing interventions and in the domain of our model as helping to solve or alleviate people's problems.

At the bottom of this part of the Nursing Plan is a space for 'Other Notes'. The information which could be recorded here might be about the time and place of clinic appointments; arrangements for transport to and from these clinics; and particulars about the loan of equipment, such as a walking frame for the patient to use at home. These examples alert the nurse to the fact that planning is necessary for the patient's discharge (p. 54). Discharge planning starts at the initial assessment as acknowledged on our suggested form for biographical and health data (Appendix 1). However, there is no constraint on the type of relevant information which nurses may record in the space for 'Other Notes'.

Here it is appropriate to mention that in some in-patient areas there is experimentation with multi-disciplinary records and D'Sa (1995) describes one such development.

Summarizing the planning phase of the process — it involves writing a nursing plan which contains the following information:

- stated goals for each problem
- a date on which the goals are expected to be achieved
- the nursing interventions (and patient participation) to achieve the goals.

The objective of the nursing plan is to provide the information on which systematic, individualized nursing can be based and implemented by any nurse, but preferably by the primary nurse or her associate.

IMPLEMENTING THE NURSING PLAN

Implementing the plan of nursing is the third phase of the process of nursing. Traditionally, nursing has been associated with 'doing', so nurses have little difficulty in knowing how to go about this phase of the process. It is, however, being recognized increasingly that it is both helpful and necessary for nurses to make explicit the thinking and decision-making which underlie and explain the nursing interventions which they carry out.

Activities which could be described as 'nursing interventions' are many and varied. For any one person it is likely that the number and range of nursing activities which are carried out will far exceed those specifically listed in the Nursing Plan. It is likely that the Plan will include all the essential and important 'main' interventions but, alongside carrying out these particular, specified activities, the nurse will be doing many other things as well.

In carrying out nursing interventions, the nurse draws on an amalgam of skills — from listening, talking and observing to helping and, perhaps, deliberately not helping — in her contact with the person over time. It may be that some of the 'unplanned' or apparently 'unimportant' interventions of this kind seem to merit recording. Such a record can be made on the 'daily report' on the person. The proforma for use with the model does not contain a section for these purposes and we suggest the use of a separate sheet or document which could be called 'Patient's Nursing Notes'. These would contain information supplementary to the Patient Assessment Form and Nursing Plan. Such information could be helpful for purposes of evaluating nursing intervention both ongoing and summative.

EVALUATING

It is difficult to justify planning and implementing nursing interventions if the outcome cannot be shown to have benefited the person in some way. Hence, the fourth phase of the process of nursing — evaluating — is crucial and, in turn, it provides a basis for ongoing assessment and planning as the person's circumstances and problems change.

The evaluating phase of the process has caused difficulties for nurses. This is not surprising because evaluation is an extremely difficult and complex matter and this is true not only in respect of nursing. Put simply, the objective of evaluating is to find out whether or not (or to what extent) the goals which were set have been (or are being) achieved. In this sense, evaluation is of the type known as 'outcome evaluation'. The skills which are used in evaluating are essentially similar to those used in assessing — observing, questioning, examining, testing and measuring. Whereas they are used in assessing to provide baseline data, in evaluating they are used to discover whether or not the set goals are being or have been achieved: in other words evaluating involves comparison against an objective.

Goal achievement in effect cancels the nursing intervention. However, it may be necessary to ask the question 'Was the goal set too low?' and a reconsideration of the original goal setting might answer this question. In the absence of complete goal achievement the nurse might ask:

- is it partially achieved and is more information needed before reconsidering whether or not to continue the intervention?

- is the problem unchanged/static and should the nursing intervention be changed or stopped?
- is there a worsening of the problem and should the goal and the planned nursing intervention be reviewed?
- was the goal incorrectly stated or inappropriate?

All of these possibilities rest on the assumption that the goal was achieved or not, solely by the nursing intervention and, in many instances, this cannot be assumed. Nurses need to recognise that the contribution by other health workers in a multidisciplinary team inevitably influences and interacts with their own intervention and, indeed, it is seldom possible to isolate out the nursing intervention and, therefore, directly and unequivocally link the 'outcome' with 'input'. Thus, the evaluating phase of the nursing process is beset with complexities and an important challenge for the future in nursing will be to improve and extend our evaluation skills.

We advocate documentation in process format, illustrated in Figure 3.8. The objective when using the phases of the process is to individualize nursing. Individualizing is a dynamic process and Figure 3.9 illustrates this, using our model for nursing as a conceptual framework.

As a postscript, conceptualizing nursing in the way proposed in this chapter, and documenting it in process format with the objective of individualizing nursing need not be the only goal. Documentation can give greater job satisfaction; nurses can only work one shift in each 24 hours; on return to duty they can read about what has happened in their absence thereby contributing a sense of continuity and participation. Documents can be so worded that they:

- are a part of a monitoring programme related to the quality of nursing service
- provide factual information to managers when, because of staff shortages, items in the 'planned nursing' had to be omitted
- provide factual information to managers when a second best nursing intervention had to be planned because of lack of resources
- provide information which can be used in defence of patient's complaints in a legal context
- help nurses to describe nursing's contribution to the total health care programme, particularly important when submitting an application for adequate financial resources
- provide substantiation for adequate remuneration for nursing personnel.

In conclusion, it must be stated that the preceding text advocates documentation of nursing practice. The quality and accuracy of nursing documents have long been a cause for concern and the UKCC (1993) states the standards required for records and record keeping (Eiloart &

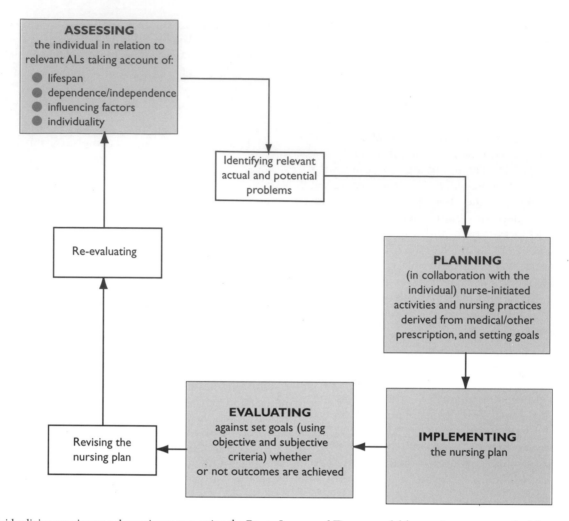

Fig. 3.9 Individualizing nursing as a dynamic process, using the Roper, Logan and Tierney model for nursing as a conceptual framework

Cooper, 1994). This brings with it the ambiguity and un-certainty related to the subject of confidentiality which nurses have to consider (Burley, 1991). This concept includes others, particularly those of accountability, dis-closure and non-disclosure as well as personal liability. 'Patients' have a legal right to inspect and have copies of their health records which are kept in manual form (Dimond, 1991; Little, 1990; Tingle, 1991). Increasing use of computers will compound these issues and offer a challenge to nurses to comply with the Data Protection Act, Section 21 (1984) and provide a nursing service which is 'in the best interests' of those requiring it (Robinson & Robinson, 1990).

Because the 12 ALs are the main focus of the model, each AL will be discussed in a separate chapter in Section 2. Of course it is only for the purpose of discussion and learning that each AL is considered separately; in reality they are closely related.

REFERENCES

Burley D 1991 Dilemmas in practice. Nursing 4 (43) October 10–23: 27–28

Caraher M 1994 Nursing and health promotion practice: the creation of victims and winners in a political context. Journal of Advanced Nursing 19: 465–468

Charatan F 1994 Psychiatrists in US put religion in diagnostic manual. British Medical Journal 308 (6931) March 19: 740

Cohen P 1994 Passing the buck? Nursing Times 90(13) March 30: 28–29

Cottrell N 1990 The view from the pharmacy. Nursing Times 86 (43) October 24: 55–57

Central Statistical Office 1994 Social Trends 24. HMSO, London

Davis S 1991 Self-administration of medicines. Nursing Standard 5 (15/16) January 9: 29–31

DoH 1991a The health of the nation. HMSO, London

DoH 1991b The patient's charter. HMSO, London

DoH 1992 William Waldegrave launches Code of Practice on Primary Health Care for Members of Ethnic Minorities. Press Release H92/42 DoH, London

DHSS 1988 Working together: A guide to arrangements for interagency co-operation for the protection of children from abuse. HMSO, London

Dimond B 1991 A question of access. Nursing Standard 6 (4) October 16: 18–19

D'Sa S 1995 Multidisciplinary bedside notes: an experimentation in care. Nursing Times 91 (12): March 22: 46–47

Eames M, Ben-Shlomo Y, Marmot M 1993 Social deprivation and premature mortality: regional comparison across England. British Medical Journal 307 (6912) October 30: 1097–1102

Eiloart L, Cooper S 1994 How to implement an audit to improve records. Nursing Times 90 (35) August 31: 48–50

Fawcett J 1984 Analysis and evaluation of conceptual models of nursing. F A Davis, Philadelphia

Ferguson K 1991a Health education in psychiatry, Part 1 Nursing Standard 5 (42) July 10: 33–35

Ferguson K 1991b Health education in psychiatry, Part 2 Nursing Standard 5 (43) July 17: 37–39

Finfer S, Howell S, Miller J, Willett K, Wilson-MacDonald J 1994 Managing patients who refuse blood transfusions: an ethical dilemma. British Medical Journal 308 (6941) May 28: 1423–1426

Gaulton-Berks L 1994 Homeless but not helpless. Nursing Times 90 (15) April 13: 53–55

Glenister D 1994 Patient participation in psychiatric services: a literature review and proposal for a research strategy. Journal of Advanced Nursing 19: 802–811

Gordon M 1979 The concept of nursing diagnosis. Nursing Clinics of North America 14: 487–496

Haggan V 1994 Cultural challenge. Nursing Times 90 (15) April 13: 71–72

Hancock B 1994 Self-administration of medicines. British Journal of Nursing 3 (19) October 27-November 9: 996–999

Henderson V 1969 The basic principles of nursing care. International Council of Nurses, Geneva

Jacob F 1994 Ethics in health promotion: freedom or determinism? British Journal of Nursing 3 (6): 299–302

King C and Macmillan M 1994 Documentation and discharge planning for elderly patients. Nursing Times 90 (20) May 18: 31–34

Labun E 1988 Spiritual care: an element in nursing care planning. Journal of Advanced Nursing 13 (3): 314–320

Laurent C 1991 Spotting trouble in A & E. Nursing Times 87 (19) May 8: 56–57

Little S 1990 Let the patients know. Nursing Times 86 (11) March: 14: 18

Marks-Maran D 1983 Can nurses diagnose? Nursing Times 79 (4) January 26: 68–69

McFarlane J, Castledine G 1982 A guide to the practice of nursing using the process of nursing. Mosby, St Louis, ch. 4

Meleis A I 1993 Theoretical nursing development and progress. Lippincott, New York

Neuberger J 1987 Caring for people of different religions. Lisa Sainsbury Foundation, London

Nursing Standard 1994 Patients divided over first name terms. Nursing Standard 8 (30) April 20: 15

Nursing Times 1994 COMMENT Use of first names (Editorial). Nursing Times 87 (33) August 14: 3

Redmayne S, Klein R 1993 Rationing in practice: the case of in vitro fertilisation. British Medical Journal 306 (6891) June 5: 1521–1523

Richardson J, Leisten R, Calviou A 1994 Lost for Words. Nursing Times 90 (13) March 30: 31–33

Robinson H, Robinson K 1990 Square pegs into round holes. Nursing Times 86 (41) October 10: 71–72

Roper N 1988 Principles of nursing in process context. Churchill Livingstone, Edinburgh

Roper N 1976 Clinical experience in nurse education. Churchill Livingstone, Edinburgh

Roth S, Brown M 1991 Advocates for health. Nursing Times 87 (21) May 22: 62–64

Royston C, Lansdown M, Brough W 1994 Teaching laparoscopic surgery: the need for guidelines. British Medical Journal 308 (6935) April 16: 1023–24

Schneider J K, Homberger S, Booker J, Davis A, Kralicek R 1993 A medication discharge planning programme. Clinical Nursing Research 2 (1) February: 41–53

Sears C 1994 Familiarity breeds presumptuousness. Nursing Standard 8 (26) March 23: 36

Slevin O D'A 1991 Ageist attitudes among young adults: implications for a caring profession. Journal of Advanced Nursing 16: 1197–1205

Jones K 1990 Positive health. Nursing 4 (22) November 8–21: 18–19

Thornett S, Heaseman N, Bentley D 1994 An evaluation of self-administration of medicines on a rheumatology ward. Journal of Clinical Nursing 3 (2) March: 74–75

Tierney A J, Closs S J, Hunter H C, Macmillan M S 1993 Experiences of elderly patients concerning discharge from hospital. Journal of Clinical Nursing

Tingle J 1991 For the record. Nursing Times 87 (38) September 18: 18–19

Tmobranski P H 1994 Nurse-patient negotiation: assumption or reality? Journal of Advanced Nursing 19: 733–737

Treharne G 1990 Attitudes towards the care of the elderly. Are they getting better? Journal of Advanced Nursing 15: 777–781

UKCC 1993 Standards for records and record keeping. UKCC, London

United Kingdom Central Council 1992 Code of Professional Conduct for the Nurse, Midwife and Health Visitor. UKCC, London

Waterworth S, Luker K A 1990 Reluctant collaborators: do patients want to be involved in decisions concerning care? Journal of Advanced Nursing 15: 971–976

Woods M 1990 Counselling services for adolescents. Nursing Standard 4 (21) February 14: 17–19

World Health Assembly 1981 Global Strategy for Health for All. WHO Chronicle 35 (4): 118–142

World Health Organization 1993 Implementation of the Global Strategy for Health for All by the Year 2000. 8th Report. Vol 1. WHO, Geneva

Young A 1995 Record keeping. (Law Series: 3) British Journal of Nursing 4(3): February 9–22: 179

ADDITIONAL READING

Bond J, Bond S 1994 Sociology and health care, 2nd edn. Churchill Livingstone, Edinburgh

Thompson I E, Melia K M, Boyd K M 1994 Nursing ethics, 3rd edn. Churchill Livingstone, Edinburgh

Tschudin V 1992 Ethics in nursing: the caring relationship. Butterworth-Heinemann, Oxford

Section 2

Nursing and the Activities of Living

4

Maintaining a safe environment

The AL of maintaining a safe environment

Every day people are engaged in many activities with the specific purpose of maintaining a safe environment, whether at home or at work or at play or travelling. In order to maintain health, both personal and public, much energy has to be directed at maintaining an external environment which is as safe as possible, not only for the present but for future generations to inherit.

Throughout history, man has been concerned with controlling the external environment or adapting to its vagaries. To an amazing degree man has conquered the dangers inherent in the physical environment and has devised methods of protecting his family, his property, his crops and his livestock. Nowadays most humans no longer live in constant threat of danger, although there are powerful natural forces such as earthquakes, floods and drought which they are impotent to control despite the availability of sophisticated technology. The fact that this is the case is illustrated by events in recent history, such as earthquakes in Japan in 1995, devastating forest fires in Australia in 1994, the virtually annual floods in the Indian subcontinent in the wake of the monsoon rains, and the continuing drought in parts of the African continent which have taken the lives and livelihood of countless people. It should not be forgotten either that in this so-called era of peace, there are wars going on in many parts of the world which means that some people are living in an unsafe environment and in constant danger.

Even under normal circumstances, however, people throughout the world are still exposed to a variety of environmental hazards which jeopardize their safety, health, happiness and, indeed, survival. Increasingly too, in this age of technological and scientific advancement, there are yet new hazards to contend with — such as the risks associated with radiation, chemical waste, the illicit use of drugs and modern war weaponry — and these, in contrast to natural forces, have been created by man himself.

There are many dimensions to the AL of maintaining a safe environment and obviously only some major categories can be discussed in this text. As so many different activities contribute to maintaining a safe *external* environment, the section on 'Environmental Factors' will be appropriately longer when discussing the various concepts of our model — lifespan, dependence/independ-

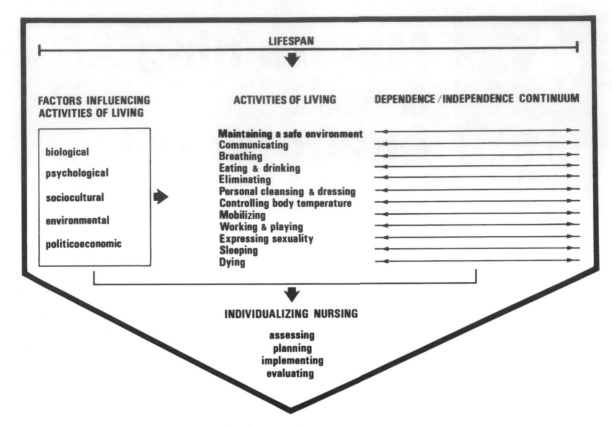

Fig. 4.1 The AL of maintaining a safe environment within the model for nursing

ence, factors affecting the AL, and individualizing nursing — for the AL of maintaining a safe environment (Fig. 4.1).

Lifespan: relationship to the AL of maintaining a safe environment

The inclusion of the lifespan as one component of the model serves as a reminder that living is a lifelong process, from birth to death. Safety is a basic human requirement for survival, development, health and self-fulfilment at every stage of the lifespan.

Childhood and adolescence

During prenatal existence, a safe environment is provided by the mother's uterus, but from the moment of birth, a baby becomes instantly exposed to all the hazards in the external environment and is totally dependent on adults for the provision of a safe environment in which to thrive and survive. For young babies, choking and suffocation are major death risks; and protection from accident, infection, and excessive heat or cold is of vital

importance. When they become more active and curious, crawling babies and toddlers are increasingly vulnerable to accidents in the home; and falls, burns, scalds and accidental poisoning are major causes of injury and death at this stage of the lifespan.

In contrast, school-age children are most at risk to hazards in the outdoor environment, particularly on the roads and in the school playground. Once at school, children cannot be under constant adult surveillance and learning about safety, risk management, and personal responsibility for maintaining a safe environment is an important dimension of their education.

During adolescence, bicycle accidents and sporting injuries become more common and, although more aware of danger, rebelliousness or over-confidence may result in lack of consideration for personal safety and the safety of others.

Adulthood and old age

For young adults, hazards in the work environment become an added area of responsibility in the AL of maintaining a safe environment and the degree and type of danger vary according to the nature of the work. Adults, especially when they become parents, seem to develop an increasing sense of responsibility concerning safety and may become involved politically over issues of personal, local or national safety, for example, safe road crossings outside schools, and local dumping of nuclear waste.

The process of ageing, which involves a gradual deterioration of physical and intellectual ability and loss of acuity of the senses, inevitably results in lessened ability to carry out the many activities involved in the AL of maintaining a safe environment. Elderly people become more prone to falls because of arthritic joints or dizziness, they are vulnerable to pedestrian accidents due to lessened acuity in sight and hearing, and are at risk from fire hazards. Maintaining a safe environment during the final stage of the lifespan may involve dependence on others and on safety aids, and requires renewed awareness of the hazards which are ever-present in the external environment.

Dependence/ independence in the AL of maintaining a safe environment

There are several different aspects of the concept of dependence/independence which are incorporated in the model, and can be considered in relation to the AL of maintaining a safe environment.

Independence and age

The general principle that dependence/independence status is closely linked with an individual's point on the lifespan has just been outlined. Broadly speaking, there is dependence in the early stages of the lifespan; independence during adulthood; and the likelihood of at least some degree of dependence again in old age.

Without question, babies are totally dependent on others for the maintenance of a safe environment and require to be protected from accidents, fire, infection and pollution. Young children are also to a very great extent dependent on adults for their safety. They do not have either the mental or physical equipment to be able to carry out the many complex activities involved in the AL of maintaining a safe environment. Neither do they have any real appreciation of the hazards in the environment or a well-developed understanding of the concepts of safety and personal responsibility for maintaining safety.

Throughout adolescence, such attributes develop, but although more independent, people of this age-group are still dependent on adult guidance and surveillance. In contrast, adults are expected to assume independence for maintaining a safe environment and are involved in doing so in the home, at work, at play and while travelling.

In old age, there may be the will to retain independence in this AL but circumstances and the effects of the process of ageing may force an elderly person to be dependent on others, at least to some degree. Financial constraints may limit maintenance of safety in the home: for example, an old person may not be able to afford to replace worn carpets or an ageing electricity system and both are potential causes of accident. In addition, loss of acuity of the senses — particularly impaired sight and hearing — will reduce an elderly person's awareness of danger, for example when crossing roads or when cooking in the kitchen. Even if the senses are acute, physical frailty reduces the ability to take the necessary quick action to avoid accidental injuries, such as those caused by falls or burns.

Independence and disability

Although independence in the AL of maintaining a safe environment is the norm during adulthood, it is important to recognize that not all adults have this capacity. Unquestionably, people with less severe learning difficulties should engage in all the activities of the community where they live, but those who have more profound learning difficulties cannot be expected to cope independently with every aspect of this AL. They are encouraged and educated to engage in a wide range of activities such as cooking, shopping and so on, but their dependence on others for safety is especially important to recognize. An important part of any social skills programme for them involves tuition about safety in all aspects of everyday living.

Similarly, although many physically disabled adults are extremely independent in their everyday lives, the AL of maintaining a safe environment is one aspect of living with which they may need some assistance. In addition to dependence on people, someone who is physically disabled will almost certainly be dependent on aids and equipment; for example a specially equipped bathroom to minimize the risk of falling while bathing or using the toilet, and special safety gadgets in the kitchen to ensure that cooking can be accomplished without the risk of being cut or burned.

For those who have a mental illness, too, there may be periods of their lives when they are dependent on others for their own safety. Voices may be instructing an individual to indulge in self-harm or to injure others during an acute psychotic phase; or a depressed person may be too lethargic to observe care when crossing a busy road, perhaps leading to personal harm or even fatalities involving others.

Another group of people who are unlikely to achieve full independence for maintaining a safe environment in adulthood are those who are visually disabled. To a remarkable extent, these people do cope with the many hazards to personal safety which exist, but they are likely to be more vulnerable in an unfamiliar environment. Therefore, while they may be independent in their own homes, dependence on others may be necessary in other settings, for example when out of doors or when travelling by public transport. It is interesting to reflect on the value of a guide dog to a blind person as an aid to independence in the AL of maintaining a safe environment.

Is independence a mirage?

People who are mentally, physically and visually disabled have been described in terms of their 'dependence', the inference being that 'independence' is enjoyed by intelligent, able-bodied adults in relation to the AL of maintaining a safe environment. However, it is worth pausing to question whether 'independence' in this AL is actually attainable by any adult person, irrespective of mental and physical ability. The fact is that no individual has complete independence in this AL. Irrespective of personal efforts to maintain safety, all people are exposed to dangers — natural forces as well as man-made hazards — which are inherent in the environment and which the individual is impotent to control or eliminate.

Equally important, the safety of any individual is dependent on the safe behaviour of others. People can take every precaution to avoid accidents while travelling, but cannot guarantee their safety because there are others who drive dangerously, or there are conditions such as poor visibility and icy roads, and these factors are outside their control. Similarly, a person can attempt to avoid infection by washing hands before handling and eating food, but nevertheless, is dependent on others as to whether or not the food itself was free of pathogenic microorganisms when it was purchased.

There are numerous other examples supporting the idea that complete independence in the AL of maintaining a safe environment is just impossible. Every individual is dependent on others — other ordinary individuals as well as people with special responsibilities for maintaining a safe environment who include, for example, politicians, town planners, public transport personnel, employers and manufacturers, firefighters, safety officers and police.

Factors influencing the AL of maintaining a safe environment

The AL of maintaining a safe environment is, by nature, multidimensional and therefore, not surprisingly, many different factors play a part in influencing the way indi-

viduals carry out the activities involved. In keeping with the relevant component of the model, the factors involved are discussed under the following headings — biological, psychological, sociocultural, environmental and politico-economic factors.

BIOLOGICAL

If a person is to carry out the AL of maintaining a safe environment, many of the recognized biological systems are involved. No one system is readily aligned as in the case of the AL of eating and drinking, for example, which is readily associated with the upper alimentary system. However, for maintaining a safe environment, acuity in all of the five senses is obviously important because external safety hazards are identified by means of vision, hearing, touch, smell and taste.

Any impairment associated with the senses, therefore, will make a person less able to identify hazards in the environment and, consequently, more likely to have an accident. For example, impaired vision and impaired hearing are obvious limitations on safety as a pedestrian, making such simple tasks as crossing a road a hazardous undertaking. Impairment can be of the sensory receptor, or of the pathway carrying the impulse to the brain, or of the brain's interpreting ability. Even if there is no impairment in an individual's ability to become aware of a hazard to safety, there may be some reason which prevents taking the necessary avoiding action. A physically disabled or ill person or a frail elderly person are obvious examples of people who may be physically unable to avoid accidental injury in certain circumstances.

Apart from specific anatomical and physiological disabilities which may make it less easy for the individual to maintain safety, there are many external agents in the environment which can cause injury and disease. However the body has several biological internal mechanisms for combating the adverse external conditions which are an inevitable part of living. For instance, the body has many reserve capacities which ensure that vital functions can continue even when an organ is injured or diseased; there is more lung tissue than is normally required, there is reserve liver tissue, there are two kidneys, eyes and ears. Apart from this 'over-provision' there are other mechanisms.

Physical barriers and secretions

Parts of the skeleton act as an internal physical barrier and are protective; the hard bony skull protects the brain; the vertebral column protects the spinal cord; and the ribs protect the lungs and heart. The intact skin acts as a barrier between the internal and the external environment which contains many potentially harmful agents. The filtering of lymphatic tissue enables the tonsils and adenoids to trap pathogens. The cilia in the respiratory tract hasten the exit from the body of possibly harmful foreign material. By reflex action — a mechanism of the nervous system — the threatened hand is instantly withdrawn and the threatened eye closed. The eye is further protected by the constant secretion of tears.

The inflammatory process

Inflammation is another internal defence mechanism and is a reaction of living tissue to agents in the external environment such as infection, injury and irritants. Regardless of the cause, the reaction is similar. A substance, histamine, is produced by injured cells; it causes capillaries in the area to dilate thus bringing greatly increased amounts of blood to the site of injury and producing the cardinal features of inflammation (Box 4.1). These features are protective since they usually induce rest and aid healing. Furthermore inflammation is frequently accompanied by fever and an increased temperature is unfavourable to the survival of some microorganisms. There comes a point, however, when inflammation is no longer a defence and the body may succumb to infection.

The process of tissue repair

As inflammation subsides and damaged tissue cells are cleared away in the blood, repair begins in one of two ways:

- *repair by first intention* occurs when there is replacement by cells identical to those which were damaged. The best example is a surgical incision, which is sutured and heals without complication of infection. Only a small amount of new tissue is required to fill the gap.

Box 4.1 Cardinal features of inflammation

REDNESS AND HEAT
When inflammation occurs on or close to the skin surface, it appears red and feels warm to the touch

SWELLING
Capillaries dilate, become more permeable and allow fluid to escape into the tissues causing swelling

PAIN
The swelling produces pressure on sensory nerves causing pain

LOSS OF FUNCTION
To minimize pain, the person attempts to keep the affected part as still as possible

---

- *repair by second intention* occurs when a considerable amount of tissue has been lost and the wound edges cannot be approximated; a mass of new tissue is required to fill the gap. First, the damaged tissues are sealed with tissue fluid and blood, which clots. Then blood vessels invade the clot and connective tissue cells from the blood enter the clot and form fibroblasts. At this stage the healing area is reddish in appearance and is referred to as granulation tissue. The fibroblasts are then converted to fibres which, when they contract, draw the wound edges together. As the process proceeds many blood vessels become nipped and the scar tissue changes in colour from red to white which can take many years.

The healing process is completed when epithelium grows in from the edge and covers the granulation tissue. The skin and the tissue in the digestive tract heal quite rapidly; bone takes longer; and the cells of the brain and spinal cord, once damaged, cannot be replaced, although recent scientific developments indicate that the regrowth of nerve cells may be possible in the not too distant future.

The rate of healing is influenced by several factors:

- *degree of injury* is pertinent; the repair process takes longer when extensive areas of tissue have been damaged.
- *nutritional state* of the tissues is important; substances such as protein and vitamin C are essential for rapid healing. Protein is needed for the formation of new tissue and vitamin C for the maturation of fibrous tissue.
- *blood circulation*, particularly any occlusion of blood flow, delays healing by depriving the cells of nutrients and oxygen, so vital to tissue repair.
- *age* can affect the rate of healing which is usually more rapid in younger than in older people. This is partly due to the decreased circulatory effectiveness in the elderly.
- *infection* inevitably delays wound healing because the pathogenic microorganisms destroy tissue.

The process of immunity

Immunity is another type of internal defence mechanism usually arising in response to an infection. The basic response to infection is inflammation (see above); another response is related to immunity. The body reacts to the entry of any foreign materials (antigens) by developing substances called immune bodies. Immune bodies which destroy microorganisms are called antibodies and those which destroy toxins produced by microorganisms are called antitoxins. For purposes of brief description, the process of immunity can be classified into four main

---

Box 4.2 Types of immunity

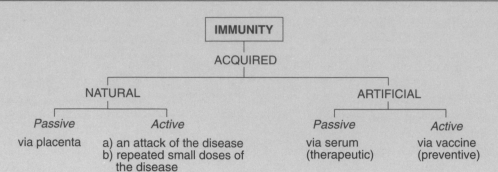

Natural passive immunity. Antibodies and antitoxins circulating in the pregnant woman's blood are passed via the placenta to the fetus. This inherited, natural, passive (the baby has not produced it) immunity to, for example, measles and whooping cough usually lasts only for a few months after birth. Thereafter, the baby is vulnerable to such infections and this is borne in mind when organizing immunization programmes for the child.

Natural active immunity. This type of immunity can be naturally acquired in two ways both of which involve the production of antibodies:

- By having an attack of the infectious disease the body is stimulated to produce appropriate antibodies not only to assist recovery but also to provide a sufficient quantity to remain in the blood for a longer period, sometimes throughout life, for example after an attack of rubella
- By being exposed to repeated small doses of the infecting agent. The amount is insufficient to cause

the classical signs and symptoms of the disease but is sufficient to stimulate the body to produce antibodies which remain in the blood throughout life. Many adults have developed an immunity to tuberculosis in this manner.

Artificially initiated active immunity. This is produced by injecting a small dose of the antigen into the body and allowing time for the person to produce antibodies himself, which then remain in the body for a variable time. It may be short-term, for example as a protection against influenza, or almost life-long, for example against diphtheria. The antigen can be a modified toxin called toxoid and it stimulates the body to make antitoxins.

Artificially initiated passive immunity. This is produced by injecting ready-made antibodies (usually developed in the blood of another human or in a horse serum and suitably treated for injection purposes). This technique is only used when a person is dangerously ill and his own blood would not have time to develop the antibodies. It can be life-saving.

---

types (Box 4.2) although the subject will be discussed in more detail in another part of the curriculum.

The phenomenon of shock

The body responds to both physical and emotional trauma by a phenomenon known as shock. When it occurs, the body defences immediately try to compensate.

Basically shock is a state of circulatory failure and is discussed on p. 158.

All of these mechanisms — physical barriers and secretions, the inflammatory process, the process of tissue repair, the process of immunity and the phenomenon of shock — are anatomical and physiological body defence mechanisms against injury and disease which are protective, and are an attempt to prevent further damage. However, there are other non-biological factors which are just as important in maintaining a safe environment.

PSYCHOLOGICAL

Intellectual impairment

Intellectual processes are involved in learning about maintaining a safe environment and in carrying out the many activities involved. Therefore, people who suffer from intellectual impairment may be unable to acquire adequate knowledge and respond quickly and appropriately to a threat to safety. For this reason, people with severe learning difficulties depend on others for protection and surveillance and, similarly, parents and teachers accept responsibility for the safety of children in their care.

Attitude, personality and temperament

Attitude to safety and prevention is important and it is desirable that people develop a concept of safety and an awareness of their personal responsibility in maintaining a safe environment, for themselves and for others. Undesirable attitudes do not help such as thinking that accidents, fires and infection happen only to others and hoping that someone else will do the campaigning about pollution issues.

Personality and temperament play a part in the attitudes people hold about maintaining a safe environment and affect their efficiency in carrying out the activities involved. Mood is also an important factor. Angry people may become aggressive and violent, possibly causing injury to themselves or to others; and 'non-accidental injury to children' and also to a spouse and to the elderly are increasingly recognized as serious current social problems. Depressed people may endanger their own safety because tiredness, lethargy and loss of motivation and self-confidence result in a lack of attention to maintaining a safe environment. Worried and preoccupied people are also vulnerable to accidents, perhaps especially on the roads, either as drivers or pedestrians.

Confidence plays a part in maintaining safety. The over-confident driver or motorcyclist may overtake without due caution, thus increasing the risk of causing a road traffic accident. Conversely the under-confident person may be hesitant to predict danger or to react to it with sufficient purpose or determination. Therefore, both over-confidence and under-confidence may play a part in creating an environment in which accidents happen more readily.

Stress

The individual's level of stress is known to be important in relation to maintaining a safe environment. Some writers use an engineering analogy and point out that the words 'stress', 'strain', 'tension' and 'pressure' are used when the load becomes too great and a breaking point is reached; it is the point where the strain is so great that metal ceases to bend and it snaps. Hans Selye, who pioneered the stress concept in the 1950s, concluded that stress was the wear and tear on the body in response to stressful agents. These he called 'stressors' and said that they could be physical, physiological, psychological or sociocultural.

Biological stressors have already been mentioned. Psychological and sociocultural stressors are frequently associated with life events/crises and can often cause intense feelings of fear and anxiety. Life events can be developmental in nature: weaning, toilet training and puberty are examples that characterize all people's lives. Others are the periods of inevitable stress and anxiety which although varying in degree and pleasurability/sadness do surround incidents like changing school, job or house; getting married or divorced; child bearing; and death of loved ones.

Psychological stressors are known to be important

contributory factors in relation to accidents among all age groups and the potentially harmful effects of psychological stressors at work are discussed on p. 313.

Emotional abuse

Injury, however, is not always accidental, and it is not only physical. The emotionally devastating effects of non-accidental injury (NAI), especially to children, has been receiving dramatic media coverage because of its apparently increasing prevalence.

Children In their 1993 Annual Report, the National Society for the Prevention of Cruelty to Children (NSPCC) estimated that in the UK, three to four children die each week following abuse and neglect. In the year 1992–3, there were 14 624 requests for their services in the following categories:

- sexual abuse   28%
- physical abuse   27%
- neglect   19%
- emotional abuse   6%
- other   20%

and there were 33 512 requests for advice, support or counselling on a wide range of matters relating to children.

The plight of abused children (whether physically, emotionally, or sexually) is a tragic and sensitive story which apparently often goes undetected because the mother, fearing reprisals or removal of the children, does not report abuse by her husband/partner or visiting male relative; in many instances having suffered violence herself from him. Children who have been abused may grow up feeling they are worthless and may have difficulty forming happy relationships. In fact Eaton (1994) maintains that 'one quarter to one half of psychiatric in-patients were abused as children'. As a community mental health nurse she is working full-time with adult survivors of sexual abuse using group therapy and individual counselling. According to the NSPCC, research has shown that abused children may also be more likely to turn to alcohol, drugs or crime, and may be more likely to abuse their own children.

Abuse is not necessarily associated with economically disadvantaged families. People who abuse children come from all social backgrounds, all walks of life, and are of different races and cultures. In an attempt to determine causes, a previous NSPCC Report asked workers involved with families to indicate factors they thought precipitated child abuse, and the one recorded most frequently was a problem in the marriage, particularly in cases of emotional and sexual abuse. The specific problem of sexual abuse in children and rape in women will be mentioned in more detail in the AL of expressing sexuality (p. 352).

The NSPCC, one of several child care voluntary agencies, carries out research and produces literature to educate parents, children and the general public about child abuse, including the problem of abuse of children with disabilities. It also operates the National Child Protection Helpline.

Women Women are also subject to abuse. According to a 1991 United Nations document:

*'A woman's right to be free from
danger and fear for her personal
safety within the home, the workplace
and society is likely to be the toughest
battle women will wage in the 1990s.'*

Commenting on various agencies in different countries which are concerned with women's rights, Trevelyan (1994a) reported that women are subjected to violence the world over and many are powerless to do anything about it. For most, abuse begins at home with husbands, fathers, brothers and uncles. She goes on to suggest that, in many societies, abuse arises because women have low status and are trapped in a vicious circle of economic dependence by fear for their children's lives as well as their own; and are ignorant of their legal rights. Trevelyan gives some useful UN and UK addresses which provide information about the problem, and in a second article (1994b) takes a closer look at how a society's traditions can affect the health and well-being of its female members.

However, women themselves sometimes abuse children according to the child safety charity Kidscape (White, 1992) and of the reported instances, most female abusers were mothers, although also included were grandmothers and babysitters. Abusing women tended to come from 'chaotic abusive backgrounds' with emotional, physical or sexual violence being part of their experience. They often had low self-esteem and tended to feel very alone.

Elderly people While the problems of child abuse and violence against women have been much publicized, abuse of the elderly — sometimes called granny-bashing — has more recently become a subject of attention. Although acknowledged that it is difficult to find a suitable definition for elder abuse, the Social Services Inspectorate (1993) suggest a useful guideline:

'abuse may be described as physical, sexual, psychological or financial. It may be intentional or unintentional, or the result of neglect. It causes harm to the older person either temporarily or over a period of time.'

Discussing the problem as long ago as 1986, Garrett considered that many families began their caring commitment for older relatives with genuine concern and sympathy but became overwhelmed by the task, so the relationship soured, resulting in harm to the old person.

Garrett went on to indicate that the harm may not only be physical but may include mental and social suffering such as neglect (withholding e.g. food, fluid, washing facilities, or overmedicating); exploiting (often financial e.g. misappropriation of pensions, savings, jewellery); psychological abuse (ridicule, humiliation, removal of decision-making); and even sexual abuse including rape and not always against female elderly.

Emphasizing the problem in 1994, Kingston and Penhale recognize the same manifestations and exhort nurses to improve their understanding of elderly abuse so that they can participate effectively in multidisciplinary assessments and care; the problem is too complex for the attention of one agency alone.

It must be borne in mind, however, that an increasingly dependent elderly person, cared for at home, may be a heavy burden on a carer who has other family commitments including children, or who also may be obliged to continue paid employment. The stress on the carer can be considerable and such circumstances, of course, are not helped by low income and poor, overcrowded housing. When indications of abuse are identified, a supportive programme to relieve pressure on the family may be appropriate and Kingston and Penhale summarize some of the options (Box 4.3). Nevertheless it is occasionally necessary to remove the elderly person to hospital, temporarily or permanently, and in certain circumstances, this may be the only possible action.

However, at a symposium launching a new group 'Action on Elderly Abuse', one of the speakers warned against professionals 'taking over' the decision-making. He stressed the importance of 'empowering older people' to take decisions affecting their own lives and also warned against alienating carers from professionals (Laurent, 1993).

Box 4.3 Non-accidental injury: elderly people at home

Kingston and Penhale (1994) suggest the following options to alleviate abusive situations in the home:

- Respite care (or short-term care) and adult placement schemes
- Day care
- Home care support
- Carer support groups
- Aids/adaptations to the home
- Nursing support (physical and mental health staff)
- Continence advice/aids
- Counselling and relationship work, family therapy
- Rehousing
- Use of refuges.

Disabled people People with disabilities, too, may be victims of non-accidental injury. Reporting a community research study about adult abuse, the Nursing Times News (1994) quoted that the groups defined as most at risk were not only older people, but also other age groups who had chronic mental illness, learning difficulties and physical disabilities — all groups who are vulnerable and less able to assert their rights.

Self-harm Self-mutilation is another form of non-accidental injury. It is not new, indeed although in the Western world it is regarded as a sign of mental illness, it is seen in some societies as a social or cultural norm (Rayner, 1994). In his discussion of the subject Ferry (1994) uses four categories:

- self-injury that is cultural
- self-injury related to mental illness
- self-injury and personality disorders
- self-injury and learning disabilities

and emphasizes that treatment has to be individually planned, implemented and evaluated.

According to a consultant psychiatrist in the UK, however, it is on the increase and the 100 000 cases per year which come to the notice of the medical profession are an underestimate of the size of the problem (Crewe, 1993). Self-harm usually starts in adolescence, may persist into the late twenties and thirties, and occurs mostly in females (a 10:1 female/male ratio). It takes many forms, for example, cutting parts of the body — arms, legs, breasts — with carving knives or razor blades, and is a common way of 'ridding oneself of the badness inside'. Or it may take the form of excessively hot baths designed to redden or blister the skin 'to rid oneself of dirt'. Characteristically, self-harmers do not feel the pain and seem to be on a high after the mutilating act.

Surprisingly it is not a cry for attention; it is a private ritual and harmers go to great lengths to hide their scars. Nor is death the intention; it is a way of coping — 'you're in control and no one can take it away', quotes Crewe. Self-harming seems to go with low self-esteem; hatred of the body; feeling horrible about sex; the need to dissociate feeling from experience. The person is in need of psychiatric help. O'Dwyer et al (1991) discussing the problem in adolescents, emphasize the need for staff in Accident and Emergency Departments to be more vigilant about detecting instances of self-mutilation and they highlight the necessity of incorporating the skills of the on-call child psychiatrist before discharging the teenager.

The issue of non-accidental injury — to children, women, the elderly, the disabled, the self — although mentioned under psychological factors, obviously also has physical, sociocultural, environmental and politico-economic aspects and is another reminder that although in this textbook, the five factors are dealt with separately for the purposes of discussion, in reality they are closely related.

The complexity of psychological factors involved in the AL of maintaining a safe environment means that publicity campaigns and health education programmes must go beyond simply imparting information about safety, realizing that people often know what they should and could do, and yet do not act on their knowledge. Health education programmes in schools can contribute towards the development of a concept of safety and a responsible attitude towards maintaining a safe environment. In the same way, publicity campaigns and advertising and television documentaries can disseminate knowledge about safety, and attempt to change attitudes and behaviour in a positive way.

SOCIOCULTURAL

Each culture has a unique interpretation of the concept of 'safety' and what is deemed to be responsible, 'safe' behaviour by individuals. This is true largely because the problems associated with maintaining a safe environment are different in different parts of the world.

Societal differences

The most obvious differences are apparent when comparing problems in so-called developing societies with those which confront the industralized societies. There are obviously wide differences in the provision of social amenities and social services. The structure of the society, too, may vary from a large extended family system where care for all dependants — the young, the elderly, the mentally disabled, the ill — is shared, to the small nuclear family, typical of the Western world, where often the state has taken over some of the traditional caring activities of the family, with their attendant safety aspects.

Within any one society also, there are internal differences in relation to the problems of maintaining a safe environment and the particular kinds of hazards to which certain groups of people are exposed. There are social class differences as is apparent in the RSPA Fact Sheet (1994), especially in relation to childhood mortality; those in less advantaged socioeconomic groups, for example, are more likely to have a fatal accident in the home.

Social disorder

Across social boundaries, however, an increasingly disturbing feature of modern living is the prevalence of social disorder. It is not new; throughout history it has had varying degrees of prominence as a problem yet has seemed relatively 'containable' in social terms. Now, however, there is mounting anxiety about the rising tide of crime, purposeless thuggery and vandalism, much of it accompanied by violence.

Understandably there is considerable public alarm when innocent people are murdered for no known reason, for example the violent and fatal attack on a mother walking with her child in a London park; or the killing of an elderly woman walking to morning church in a quiet English hamlet; or the series of motiveless murders in Florida involving harmless overseas tourists. Some areas have acquired a reputation as being particularly dangerous. Certain large housing estates, known to have violent inhabitants, have even been singled out as 'no-go' areas, where milk floats, postmen and repair men venture at their peril. On the other hand, upmarket housing developments are now heavily protected by high gates, guards and video cameras, although even modest householders, in city and quiet rural areas alike, are resorting to burglar alarms on their homes and cars, or organizing Neighbourhood Watch schemes. In various ways, legally and illegally, more people are arming themselves against potential attackers at home, in the street, and even in recreational settings.

Perhaps it is even more disturbing to learn that it is not only adults who are perpetrators of violence. Violence in schools has reached alarming dimensions. A spokesman for one of the UK trades unions maintains that 3000 teachers per week experience physical aggression of some kind from pupils. There is also violence between pupils and much concern about related bullying, a form of 'peer abuse' (Dawkins, 1995). People were stunned, however, when two 11-year-boys murdered a 2-year-old in 1993 after luring him from his mother's side in a shopping mall.

Apart from threats to the safety of individuals or small groups of people, great turmoil can be created at international events. There is always grave concern for the safety of both competitors and spectators at meetings such as the Olympic Games when terrorists, sometimes representing minority and almost unknown groups, stage (or threaten) an attack to wreak revenge or to gain publicity for their cause. And for similar reasons, highjackings involving aircraft, ships or cars are not uncommon. International publicity for terrorist causes is inevitable, too, when they claim responsibility for incidents such as the explosion at the World Trade Centre, New York in 1993, and in London's financial centre in the same year involving enormous economic damage as well as fatalities and injuries to people. Even irreplaceable masterpieces are not exempt; Italy's Uffizi Gallery was shattered by a car bomb in 1993.

In the work setting, too, incidents involving violence are becoming increasingly common and are discussed in more detail in the AL of working and playing (p. 315).

Quite apart from identifying the perpetrators, there is now much more public demand for support to the victims of violent crime. In addition to medical prescription, victims require emotional support and reassurance which is not necessarily available from sources such as the family. They also require information about compensation; help with approaches to the Criminal Injuries Compensation Board, social services, crime prevention officers, and legal advice centres; and practical help to repair or recover property following robbery.

It is becoming increasingly recognized that many people who are victims of violence suffer persistent adverse symptoms, now recognized as post-traumatic stress disorder (PTSD). Ravenscroft (1994) quotes the American Psychiatric Association who identify PTSD as:

'. . . a clinical syndrome best described as the development of characteristic symptoms following psychological traumatic events which are considered to be outside the range of normal human experience.'

The APA provide diagnostic criteria (Box 4.4). Clancy and McVicar (1993) explored the sociopsychophysiological subjectivity of stress and quote three aspects mentioned by Lazarus:

- individuals differ in their reactivity to stress
- stress is determined by the perception of a stressful situation rather than by the situation itself
- the extent of stress depends partly on the capabilities of the individual to cope.

Not only victims suffer; rescuers at stressful events may also require support, and Hodgkinson and Stewart (1991) underscore the need for helpers to be debriefed by experienced counsellors. Bamber (1994) provides a review of literature on PTSD and describes how their unit set up a team to provide support for emergency staff. Castledine (1993) explores what nurse aiders can do in disaster situations so that they are prepared to help in a variety of ways at the scene; at relief headquarters; at casualty clearing stations; at hospitals; and at mortuaries.

Spirituality and disorder

It seems sacrilegious to link religion with disorder but certain cults, ostensibly associated with religion and spirituality have been exposed as contributing to a form of social disorder. Group suicides at Waco, Texas in 1993 when most of a cult group died in a blazing inferno, and the murder of members of the Solar Temple in Switzerland in 1994 captured international attention, but initially these cults appear 'normal' and responsible, and provide trainees with pleasant experiences. According to Jerram (1994) cults are often religious but can have political, psychotherapeutic or New Age beliefs, and their aim is to advance the leadership's goals which are often financial but may also be sexual or criminal. When adherents are 'rescued' from new style cults or leave them —

Box 4.4 Diagnostic criteria for post-traumatic stress disorder

A. *The person has experienced an event that is outside the range of usual human experience and that would be markedly distressing to almost anyone; for example, serious threat to life or physical integrity or serious threat to one's child*

B. *The traumatic event is persistently re-experienced in at least one of the following ways:*

- Recurrent and intrusive distressing recollections of the event
- Recurrent distressing dreams of the event
- Acting or feeling as though the traumatic event were recurring, including flashbacks when waking or intoxicated
- Intense psychological stress at exposure to events that symbolize or resemble an aspect of the traumatic event

C. *Persistent avoidance of stimuli associated with the trauma or numbing of general responsiveness (not present before the trauma), as indicated by at least three of the following:*

- Efforts to avoid thoughts or feelings associated with the trauma
- Efforts to avoid activities or situations that arouse recollections of the trauma
- Inability to recall an important aspect of the trauma (psychogenic amnesia)

- Markedly diminished interest in significant activities, such as a hobby or leisure-time activity
- Feeling of detachment or estrangement from others
- Restricted range of affect; for example, inability to experience emotions such as feelings of love
- Sense of a foreshortened future, such as not expecting to have a career, more children or a long life

D. *Persistent symptoms of increased arousal (not present before the trauma), as indicated by at least two of the following:*

- Difficulty falling or staying asleep
- Irritability or outbursts of anger
- Difficulty concentrating
- Hypervigilance
- Exaggerated startle response
- Physiological reactivity on exposure to events that resemble an aspect of the traumatic event; for example, breaking into a sweat

Adapted from American Psychiatric Association criteria. (DSM – IV)
(Ralph and Alexander (1994). Reproduced by kind permission of the Nursing Times where it first appeared with 'Borne under stress' on 23 March 1994.)

'walkaways' — exit counselling is often required or even 'de-programming', and mental health nurses may be involved in helping them to help themselves.

Disorder allegedly linked to a cult took a new and frightening direction in 1995 when a nerve gas was used in Tokyo's underground railway system, ostensibly to destroy 'enemies' of the cult. Hundreds of commuters were affected and some died.

ENVIRONMENTAL

It is obvious that environmental factors exert a far-reaching influence on this AL; indeed the concept of safety has no real meaning unless it is considered in relation to the environment.

Over recent decades, legislation in the UK has done much to improve environmental conditions and in 1990, for the first time, a Government White Paper set out a comprehensive survey of all aspects of environmental concern 'from the street corner to the stratosphere, from human health to endangered species'. The survey documents action already taken, and outlines future plans and goals.

Action in the UK alone, however, is not enough. Environmental problems do not recognize national boundaries. Rainforest destruction, soil erosion, desertification, global warming, depletion of the ozone layer, drought, and the loss of plant and animal species have implications for the whole world and require international cooperation.

It is not possible to mention all environmental concerns in this text, but four major areas have been selected and their health implications highlighted:

- preventing pollution
- preventing accidents
- preventing infection
- preventing fire.

Preventing pollution

One major environmental issue which has a significant effect on health is pollution.

Drinking water   Preventing the pollution of drinking water by untreated excrement, for example, has long been recognized as a basic health concern. Nowadays, in most industrialized countries, national measures to ensure safe water are taken for granted, but in several developing countries, polluted water is a major cause of diarrhoeal disease, often with high mortality rates. Unfortunately, urbanization, industrialization, affluence and technological advances have created new types of hazard, for example, air pollution, waterway pollution, lead pollution and noise pollution.

Air Admittedly, air pollution has been brought under control over many populous areas as a result of smoke control measures and legislation associated with Clean Air Acts. However, the chemical fallout from industry and agriculture has produced many unseen air pollutants, which are damaging not only to human health — linked to ills ranging from leukaemia to heart disease — but are implicated in the formation of 'acid rain'.

Acid rain is produced mainly by sulphur dioxide and oxides of nitrogen in the air which come, for example, from power stations and other plant burning coal, oil or gas; and from motor vehicles. It has been blamed for devastating large tracts of forest, killing fish in lakes and damaging plants, habitats and buildings (White Paper, 1990). Inevitably acid rain (when in cloud form) can travel over long distances so international collaboration is needed to control this threat to the environment.

Even conditions beyond the earth's immediate environment can affect human beings. The sun's rays provide the earth with energy and heat, some of which is absorbed by the earth and some radiated back into space. However, gases in the atmosphere (carbon dioxide, methane, chlorofluorocarbons — CFCs) absorb some of this energy forming a blanket which returns additional heat to the earth. The rate of warming is thought to be faster now than for the last 10 000 years (the greenhouse effect). It is estimated that this could change the weather in ways which threaten food production; alter patterns of disease; submerge low-lying coasts; and precipitate the migration of these coastal inhabitants (White Paper, 1990) thereby affecting a number of ALs. International measures are being taken to control this global warming by reducing the man-made production of these gases from sources in the home, agriculture and industry.

Nevertheless, it is worth noting that there are other schools of thought about the *intensity* of the global warming. The US National and Oceanic Atmospheric Administration, which has used the most extensive survey of global temperatures ever conducted, has found no evidence of a warming trend over the last 14 years (Evans-Pritchard, 1993).

CFCs are also implicated in depleting the stratospheric ozone layer, the layer which absorbs all ultraviolet C and a proportion of ultraviolet B from sunlight before it reaches the earth's surface. Concern for man is raised because increased exposure to ultraviolet B is closely linked to skin cancer which is an increasingly common problem (p. 255).

Waterways Not only the air we breathe but the natural waterways of the world are endangered. Disposal of industrial waste into rivers and seas is a major source of water pollution. Coastal waters have suffered most, yet they play the most important role in the chain of life as that is where the majority of marine species spend at least part of their lives, for example in the North Sea many fish have been found to suffer from skin infections, deformed skeletons and tumours. Not only that, sea birds are often the victims of oil spills. Human bathers, too, risk viral hepatitis, skin reactions and oral thrush. However, during the last decade, a United Nations Organization programme has been coordinating the work of environmentalists to halt the scale of pollution, although political will by individual governments is also essential if the fragile ecosystem is to be preserved.

Lead One pollutant which has attracted considerable concern in recent years is lead. Lead occurs widely in nature, in the soil and in the water. In compound form it has come to be used in paint as a pigment, in plastics as a stabilizer and in petrol as an anti-knock agent. Lead has long been used by man and its toxic properties recognized. Severe lead poisoning is a cause of intellectual impairment. It is widely known that there are harmful effects from inhalation of outfall from a lead works; for children who ingest it by licking lead-painted toys; and for families whose drinking water is supplied through lead pipes. Some local authorities have removed lead pipes from the water supply system; and others have provided financial grants to enable house owners to do likewise.

More recently, concern has shifted to the more insidious problem which affects the entire population — pollution of roadside areas by leaded petrol. Fall-out from exhaust emissions is not only directly inhaled, but can be ingested because lead settles on the hands and on vegetables, crops and fruit growing near roadsides. In many countries there has been a phased reduction in the lead content of petrol; lead-free petrol is on sale at a lower price; and there are indications of a move towards the obligatory use of lead-free petrol for all vehicles.

However, even unleaded petrol produces end products that are air pollutants and there is mounting pressure to reduce the number of vehicles using the roads. The provision of additional public transport facilities is one suggestion especially in urban areas, and there is a race among car manufacturers to design Zero Emission Vehicles (ZEVs) such as electrically powered cars.

Noise An entirely different kind of problem in modern living is 'noise pollution' and that term is increasingly being used to describe the problem of excessive noise. Everyone does not regard noise in the same way. Latin and Anglo-Saxon temperaments are at variance about what would constitute an acceptable noise level; and young people do not seem to be so intolerant of noise as their elders. However, an environment in which people cannot sleep adequately because of excessive noise cannot be considered a safe environment. People who live near noisy factories, close to flight paths near airports, and in the proximity of busy motorways, all suffer from excessive noise by night and day. During the day, other city dwellers can be disturbed by the noise of traffic, especially heavy lorries going past their homes. People who work in heavy industry are subjected to the noise of machines and measures to minimize the effects include the use of noise-abating apparatus and the wearing of ear muffs (see p. 317). As well as affecting sleep, noise is thought to create tension and fatigue, both of which can contribute to accidents and mental ill-health.

One of the most serious consequences of excessive noise exposure is partial deafness which may progress to a substantial hearing loss (see p. 317) and constitute a severe social handicap. Deafness caused by noise at work was reported among metal workers more than 250 years ago, but largely self-inflicted damage to hearing caused by noisy social and leisure activities such as discos and personal stereos, is a 20th century phenomenon (Godlee, 1992).

Preventing pollution is one dimension of maintaining a safe environment which is largely a public rather than a personal responsibility. However, there are many ways in which individuals can protect themselves and others from the potentially dangerous effects of pollutants.

Preventing accidents

Accidents can occur anywhere and at any time. Frequently, though not always, they are avoidable. Preventing accidents — in the home, at work, at play and while travelling — can and should be everyone's concern, both for their own personal safety and for others. The human suffering which results from an accident can be severe and can result in some form of life-long disablement or disfigurement for the victim, not forgetting the stress and guilt which is borne by the person who may have had some responsibility for the accident occurring.

In recent years the problem of accidents and accident prevention has come very much to the fore because the huge scale of the problem is now recognized. In the UK, according to the Royal Society for the Prevention of Accidents (ROSPA) 1994, fatal accidents in 1991 totalled 13 311 and occurred in the following categories:

Road	39.6%
Home	36.5%
Work	4.6%
Sport	2.0%
Other	17.2%

and injuries (hospital and GP treatments) per year are around 9.5 million:

Home	36%
Work	21%
Sport	17%
Road	7%
Other	19%.

Health care professionals have a vital role to play in accident prevention, though the problem needs to be tackled by multidisciplinary effort, organized at national and international levels. Health education is an important aspect of prevention, but that is unlikely to be effective in the absence of increased safety measures and legislation.

Individual effort is also vital. Accident prevention cannot be viewed only in terms of the elimination of hazards. The potential for accidents will always exist, so each individual must become skilled at maintaining safety in the face of hazards inherent in the environment. Some of the ways in which this can be achieved are described in the discussion which follows of preventing accidents *in the home; at work; at play; and while travelling.*

Preventing accidents in the home Most people probably think of their home as a 'safe' place but, in reality, the average home is potentially a very dangerous environment. Even in countries where housing standards have improved immeasurably, and the promotion of safety in the home has been of long-standing concern, the problem of accidents is one of some magnitude.

The ROSPA quotes that there are 5000 deaths each year from home accidents and in addition 2.5 million people will need hospital attention, 150 000 will be admitted, and nearly one million others will go to their general practitioner for treatment.

- *Risks for children.* Young children are particularly at risk (about 200 die each year) and they are dependent on adults to protect them from the potential dangers in their home environment. The type of injury is of import. ROSPA quotes that the most severe injuries are associated with heat-related accidents and falls from a height; that older children are more likely to sustain fractures than younger; and that younger children have a higher percentage of burns and scalds as well as poisoning and ingestion accidents. Children in less advantaged socioeconomic groups are more likely to have fatal accidents.

  The site and time of occurrence are also significant. The most serious accidents occur in the kitchen and on stairs, but the largest number occur in the living/dining room. The most common time of day for accidents to occur is the evening; more happen on Sundays; more during school holidays;

and more in summer. Some happen in times of stress when the usual routine is changed or when in a hurry. Some are caused by lack of familiarity with surroundings, for example when visiting friends or in holiday accommodation.

Not only the injury itself but the aftermath of disability is distressing. It includes brain damage; deformity; loss of mobility; scarring; sensory loss due mainly to eye injuries; and psychological damage.

What then are some of the hazards in the home environment which can cause accidents? Some different groups of hazards are listed in Box 4.5 along with related preventive measures. However, whatever precautions are taken, accidents still happen.

Nevertheless, physical restraint is not a solution to accident prevention and, indeed, excessive over protection will only deny a child the opportunity to explore and learn about the environment. All children have to develop a concept of safety and an ability to cope with the hazards which exist in the environment. Parents and, depending on the circumstances, grandparents and childminders too, have a vital role to play in preventing accidents in the home.

Because they go into homes, health visitors and all community nurses have a unique opportunity to assess levels of safety and to offer appropriate guidance. But others, too, must accept their share of responsibility for safety in the home. They include house designers and manufacturers, especially those concerned with the production of child safety equipment, children's furniture and toys; and household products, especially commonly used chemicals and other potentially dangerous substances and articles.

- *Risks for elderly people.* Apart from children, the other group most vulnerable to accidents in the home are those at the other end of the lifespan, the elderly, particularly those in the over 75 age group and it is estimated that by the year 2023, 4.8 million in the UK will be in this group (Bowling et al, 1992). Falls are of particular concern. There is a high mortality associated with old people who lie undetected for a long time, both related to the injury sustained and to complications; such as hypothermia, dehydration, bronchopneumonia and breakdown of pressure areas. Fear of this happening may cause old people to be admitted to residential homes though, as Bowling et al show, falls are by no means uncommon in that setting either.

In the community, many simple, preventive measures are possible and these range from encouraging elderly people to wear well-fitting shoes rather than slippers, to the use of alarm systems, and the involvement of neighbours and regular callers to an old person's house. Again, as in childhood accidents, prevention of accidents in the home to the elderly requires a variety of approaches. Everything possible needs to be tried

---

Box 4.5 Preventing accidents in the home

Fire hazards
- use fireguards for open fires
- use flame-resistant nightware
- ensure furniture complies with Furniture and Furnishings (Fire) (Safety) Regulations 1988 (it is obligatory to use foam which passes the ignitability test to reduce noxious fumes, and to have match resistant covers, for example).
- instal smoke alarms in strategic areas

Electrical hazards
- keep appliances in good repair
- fit guards on electric sockets to prevent children exploring with a finger or pencil
- ensure that kettle, iron and other flexes are not trailing

Chemical hazards
- store toxic substances in a safe place, out of the reach of children and preferably locked e.g. weed and rodent killer, decorating materials

- use child-proof cupboard fastenings for e.g. dishwasher powder, bleach, hair dye, nail varnish, perfume
- use child-proof medicine containers

Thermal hazards
- fit thermostat valves to hot-water taps
- handle hot liquids with care to prevent scalding accidents
- protect hot cooker surfaces and hot cooking utensils
- ensure that matches are safely stored

Home design
- ensure lighting is adequate especially on stairs
- use a stair-guard for young children
- use a non-slip polish on floors and non-skid pads under rugs
- replace frayed carpets
- instal safety glazing on glass doors and panels, or use shatter-resistant film

if the sought-after goal of independent life at home in the community is to be achieved. The organization, Age Concern, for example, has up-to-date information about many aspects of care for the older person.

- *Risks for people with learning disabilities.* In recent years with the trend to encourage people with learning disabilities to live in a community setting, an important aspect of social skills training is associated with ALs which relate to living in, and running a household. Particular attention is given to measures which prevent accidents in the home although the dangers of overprotection are recognized and the emphasis is on risk management and personal responsibility (Shirtcliffe, 1995).

Preventing accidents at work Even when at work the AL of maintaining a safe environment cannot be forgotten. Mason (1993) reports a recent survey by the Health and Safety Executive (HSE) revealing that some firms could be losing around 37% of their profits dealing with unnecessary accidents. He quotes the director general of the HSE that the total cost of work accidents in Britain is around £10–15 billion a year.

Some groups of health care workers are subject to certain types of injury and accident. For example, back injury is common among nurses and there is growing concern about the need to instruct nurses in proper moving and handling techniques (p. 303). Exposure to radiation is another area of concern affecting radiologists, doctors, dentists and nurses who are involved in the use of X-ray procedures and care of people undergoing treatment with radioactive substances. Female staff of child-bearing age, particularly women who are known to be pregnant, require special protection from radiation hazards and there are codes of practice which apply to radiotherapy and X-ray procedures.

Quite apart from radiation hazards in the health care sector, there is concern about the magnitude of the risk of cancer for workers in the nuclear industry itself. Certainly following the far-flung effects of the disaster at the Chernobyl nuclear power station in 1986, the health hazards associated with nuclear products have been highlighted, not only for employees and people in the immediate environs of a nuclear plant, but also for people and terrain far distant from the scene of the nuclear leak. Considerable public pressure is being put on governments and large companies to utilize energy sources other than nuclear power for industry and commerce, and there are strident demands for stricter supervision to prevent accidents and to monitor the disposal of nuclear waste products.

So important is the subject of a safe work environment that most countries have legislation requiring protective practices at all places of employment. Standards are set also for ventilation, heating, lighting, hygiene, safety features of tools and equipment, care when handling dangerous chemicals or infected materials, fire precautions, first aid facilities; and provision is made for occupational health services. The occupational health nurse can play a vital role in conducting health and safety assessments as well as in counselling, and preventing accidents. In the UK, legislation imposes statutory obligations on employers to set down and implement policy to safeguard the health and safety of their employees. However, the employees also have responsibilities and are required both to exercise reasonable care, and to cooperate with their employers' health and safety policies. More is said about relevant legislation and the subject of safety in the AL of working and playing (p. 317).

At international level, the International Labour Organization (ILO) and the World Health Organization (WHO) collaborate to produce various recommendations which seek to establish worldwide standards of safety with the purpose of preventing avoidable accidents at work.

Preventing accidents at play It seems paradoxical that man must attend to the AL of maintaining a safe environment even during leisure activities. But for those who choose arduous outdoor recreations like climbing, water sports and skiing this is particularly so. Suitable attire is essential; careful attention should be paid to the weather and its forecast; and extra rations and a heat-reflective sheet for warmth must be carried if there is any possibility of encountering adverse environmental conditions.

Those who pursue water-related sports should learn to respect natural events like tides and floods. For safety they should cooperate when local authorities display signs, warning that the seashore is dangerous. Becoming a competent swimmer is obviously sensible and for those who sail a knowledge of seamanship is essential.

Even at festive times like Christmas, extra safety precautions need to be taken with Christmas trees, fairy lights and decorations. Extra precautions are necessary on other occasions when bonfires and fireworks form part of the festivities. An increasing number of countries are moving towards a policy of prohibiting the sale of fireworks to the public and instead, having organized displays operated by experts; ensuring that there is careful segregation of spectators from staff who are igniting the fireworks.

In spite of knowledge of precautions, injuries from accidents during sport and leisure activities are commonplace and account for a significant proportion of emergency admission to hospitals. Tonks (1993) quotes a Sports Council report which reveals there are some 19 million sports injuries costing an estimated £0.5 billion in treatment and days off work. This may reflect the fact that many people today have more leisure and money to spend on such pursuits than in the past. Certainly sports such as motor-cycling, hang-gliding, bungie-jumping, skiing, skating, yachting, diving, skate-boarding, marathon running and squash have become popular among a broad cross-section of the community.

All of these, some more than others, carry the risk of injury from accidents and even the safety of some longstanding sports — notably rugby — has become the focus of attention. It has been roundly criticized because of the risk of cervical spinal cord injury, and there has been a plea for case registers to study the frequency, distribution and nature of rugby injuries; and to monitor the effects on safety when there are changes in the laws of the game (Garraway et al, 1991). Boxing has been the subject of adverse criticism for some time (Dillner, 1993).

In addition to actual physical injury, both rugby and boxing are examples of 'contact' sports and there is increasing concern about the spread of infections while participating in such pastimes, for example, the spread of glandular fever and coxsackievirus B (both are associated with chronic fatigue syndrome, p. 97) and especially the possible risk of HIV contamination when blood is spilt. In rugby union, a player with an open or bleeding wound must leave the field until bleeding is controlled, and in some states of the USA, HIV testing is mandatory for all boxers (Sharp, 1994).

However, not only players of a sport risk injury; spectators may be involved. For example, the problem of football hooliganism has become a matter for concern in several countries and in an attempt to prevent violence and injury, steps have been taken to combat drunkenness at football matches and to improve crowd control. Of course, even in a well-controlled crowd, accidents can occur when many thousands of spectators are gathered together so first aid teams are in attendance, often with a crisis team on call at a local hospital.

In the main, sporting accidents affect young adults; the more challenging and potentially dangerous sports inevitably appeal to people in that age group. However, accidents do happen to school-age children in the course of play, and consistent with the activities of this age group, they suffer fewer accidents in the home (compared with pre-school age children) but more accidents outdoors and in the school playground, some associated with bullying. Some schools have attempted to increase playground safety but here again, as in the home, preventing accidents needs to balance the necessity of supervision and restriction in the interests of safety, against the need for children to enjoy themselves and to develop a sense of personal responsibility for their own safety.

Preventing accidents while travelling Every person has a responsibility for maintaining safety while travelling. Laws and regulations can lay down safety standards, but individuals have to comply with those standards.

Ignorance is no plea in law, so people have to be taught about safety while travelling, and encouraged to develop a positive attitude and strict self-discipline in relation to prevention of accidents.

This is said to be the 'age of travel'. Certainly this century has seen incredible advances in the speed of travel, both inter-city and international, and in the distances people travel — indeed as far as the moon. Holidays and business trips abroad are now commonplace occurrences and an elaborate network of international communication attempts to ensure the safety of travellers by land, sea and air. There are also carefully planned strategies involving multidisciplinary teams to cope with emergencies and the victims of major travel accidents, wherever they may occur in the world.

At national level, the major concern is with preventing accidents on the roads. According to the Department of Transport's Factsheet (1993) the largest number of road casualties coincides with the times of day when traffic is at its heaviest, reaching a peak between 5 and 6 p.m. and with a secondary peak between 8 and 9 a.m. Child casualties peak between 3 and 4 p.m.; are more frequent during the summer months; and for all ages, are more common among boys than girls.

Making comparisons between selected countries (ROSPA, 1993), the number of road deaths in 1991 shows deaths per 100 000 population as follows:

Norway	7.6
UK	8.2
W. Germany	12.0
Japan	12.0
USA	16.0
France	19.0
Portugal	34.0.

Safe road surfaces, adequate street lighting and sign posting, compulsory driving tests, road use regulations, compulsory speed limits and minimum mechanical safety standards for vehicles are all examples of measures taken by national governments to maintain a safe environment on the roads and to prevent accidents. In addition, many governments have extended legislation to other areas, for example, laws which permit police to use a breathalyser test to detect and detain drivers who have been drinking in excess of the alcohol limit (Box 4.6).

In an increasing number of countries, use of seat belts in cars is now obligatory. Since the introduction of seat belt legislation in January 1983 in the UK, there has been a demonstrable reduction in the number of deaths and serious injuries (e.g. internal chest injuries and fractured skull) among front seat car occupants. Now back seat passengers are also obliged to 'belt-up'. Improved baby carriers are constantly being produced and the European Commission proposes to have seat belts in buses and coaches following a series of tragic accidents.

Box 4.6 Drink-drive accidents

In the UK, drink-drive accidents still account for 14% of all road deaths and 7% of all serious casualties, and in 1992, changes to road traffic law created a new offence — 'causing death by careless driving under the influence of drink or drugs'. It carries a maximum of 10 years' imprisonment with a minimum 2 years' disqualification and an unlimited fine (ROSPA 1993). 'Ram-riding' and 'joy-riding' casualties are often associated with drink and/ or drugs usage and frequently involve stolen cars.

It is interesting to see how a law has so rapidly effected a dramatic and important change in people's behaviour concerning safety while travelling where even aggressive publicity campaigns apparently failed to make the necessary impact.

In a number of countries for some years, the wearing of crash helmets by motor cyclists has been obligatory and currently, in an endeavour to reduce serious injury and fatalities, especially among children and teenagers, brightly-coloured helmets for pedal cyclists are popular. Most pedal cycle deaths are caused by severe head injuries and recent studies suggest that head injuries can be substantially reduced by wearing helmets (Thomas et al, 1994; Maimaris et al, 1994). Appleton (1994) describes a head injury rehabilitation unit for children.

Apart from the risks to car drivers, passengers, and cyclists themselves however, *pedestrian* casualty figures are also alarming. Safety campaigns aimed solely at pedestrians are not sufficient in view of the fact that a substantial proportion of pedestrians are struck by vehicles and killed or injured, not on the road but on the pavement.

Preventing accidents while travelling is an enormously complex issue. Legislation has a part to play in maintaining safety, but individuals have a responsibility to control personal behaviour for their own benefit as well as for the survival and well-being of others. Nursing staff in the community setting, in occupational health services and in hospital, have a major role in improving the knowledge, attitudes and behaviour of the road user and a particular responsibility in relation to children, the elderly and those with severe learning difficulties.

Preventing infection

An essential dimension of the AL of maintaining a safe environment is preventing infection. Infection results from the successful invasion of the body by pathogenic microorganisms and, because these are ever-present in the environment, preventing infection is a fundamental issue in disease prevention and health promotion.

Much is now known about the biological characteristics of pathogens and the epidemiology of infection, and successful methods have been developed which can inhibit the growth, the spread, and the harmful effects of these organisms. However, while public health measures at national and international levels can do much to prevent and control infection, the participation of individuals is vital because of the continuing importance of many basic personal and domestic hygiene activities. Therefore, everyone requires to understand about the sources of infection; the modes of transmission of pathogenic microorganisms; the human portals of entry; and the principles basic to the control of infection. These topics are discussed in detail in textbooks dealing with microbiology and will be studied in other parts of the curriculum, but to provide a context for consideration of this AL, some major points related to the first three topics are summarized in Box 4.7, Box 4.8, and Box 4.9, and selected points are made about the control of infection.

Control of infection Several activities are associated with control of infection:

- *Reducing susceptibility.* People will be less susceptible and more resistant to infection if they have an adequate diet and sufficient exercise, sleep and rest. Tired, malnourished people are prone to infection.

  When a person is ill, the body's natural defence mechanisms are already under stress, and therefore, less able than usual to resist the invasion of pathogenic microorganisms. An unfavourable environment may also decrease resistance to infection, for example, prolonged exposure to cold and damp. Resistance to specific infectious diseases can be acquired in several ways (p. 70), and, of course, infants during the first few months of life are relatively unsusceptible to many infections because of transplacentally derived immunity.

- *Destroying pathogens.* Another mode of controlling infection is to destroy the cause. Agents which destroy organisms are called disinfectants or antimicrobial agents, and they are physical or chemical in nature. Physical disinfectants include the natural elements like sunlight and freezing as well as generated heat and cold: chemical disinfectants include liquids and gases. A success story of the 20th century is the discovery of antibiotics, substances which can be introduced into the human body to combat pathogenic microorganisms, although the development of drug resistant strains is causing alarm (Tonks, 1994).

- *Isolation.* Isolating an infected person has long been used as a means of preventing the spread of

Box 4.7 Infection: sources

Human sources

- the source is the site where pathogens grow and multiply
- the natural warmth of the body encourages rapid multiplication, but to establish themselves pathogens must be in the right place, in sufficient numbers, and be sufficiently virulent
- the body defence mechanism — immunity — can usually cope with small numbers and only succumbs when invading numbers are large or when the body's resistance is lowered
- pathogens are usually species specific so common sources in humans are other humans
- *resident flora* (or commensals) are the body's natural flora: the skin and all body orifices are colonized by microorganisms shortly after birth. They only become pathogenic if the body's immune system is not functioning adequately or when transferred to another part of the body, usually by the hands, e.g.

transfer of *E. coli* from the anal area to the entrance of the female urethra causing infection of the urinary tract — autoinfection
- *transient flora* are acquired from other people, e.g. a person incubating an infectious disease; or actually suffering from an infection or recovering; or a carrier who is not personally affected but is harbouring pathogens which can infect others

Animal sources

- animals can harbour and spread pathogens e.g. the house fly can carry several; the mosquito carries malaria and yellow fever; brucellosis can be contracted from milk cows; rabies in man results from a bite by an infected dog

Inanimate sources

- pathogens which cause tetanus are harboured in the soil

Box 4.8 Infection: modes of transmission

In order to understand how infection is spread, it is necessary to know about the main modes of transmission:

- direct contact is most likely to lead to infection of the skin, conjunctiva or mucous membrane. Skin diseases, such as impetigo or scabies, are transmitted by direct contact. The sexually-transmitted diseases (e.g. syphilis, gonorrhoea, AIDS and non-specific urethritis) are so-called because they occur as a result of direct sexual contact with an infected partner. Some oral and respiratory infections follow direct contact: for example, infectious mononucleosis (glandular fever) is frequently described as the 'kissing disease'. Direct hand contact can transmit infection from one person to another or, in the same person, from one location to another. For this reason, *handwashing is the single most important personal activity in preventing infection*, so it is essential that people wash their hands after going to the toilet and before touching food.
- indirect contact involves transmission by fomites (in-animate objects in the environment such as clothing, bedclothes, crockery and cutlery, instruments and furniture) and these can act as reservoirs for infection. Fomites with smooth hard surfaces e.g. glass, are easier

to clean than those made of fabric. Disinfection by physical and chemical means is important in preventing the spread of infection by fomites.
- airborne droplets carry pathogens from infected people when breathing/coughing/sneezing/talking/laughing. Hence the reason for wearing masks e.g. in operating theatres or for wound dressings although there is still controversy about their effectiveness
- floor dust (airborne droplets fall to the floor) and its microbial flora is especially important in steptococcal and staphylococcal infections in hospital
- food and drink can be contaminated by humans, and handwashing before touching food is a basic measure to prevent transmission. People with infected sores (boils, styes) or diarrhoeal conditions should not prepare food. Contaminated food/water/milk can cause an epidemic and infections such as the salmonelloses and bacillary dysentery, are further spread by unwashed hands contaminated with faeces. Milk and food can also be contaminated by infection in the animals which provide them, and preventing transmission of such disease (e.g. brucellosis) involves strict control over the source and supply of animal food products for human consumption. Insects, too (e.g. flies landing on faeces) can then contaminate food and drink and transmit pathogens which cause human ill-health.

Box 4.9 Infection: human portals of entry

- by the placenta — to the fetus from the mother's blood supply, e.g. syphilis, rubella, HIV
- by inhalation — entry of airborne pathogens, e.g. common cold, measles, whooping cough, diphtheria, respiratory tuberculosis
- by ingestion — pathogens in food and drink are ingested and digested, e.g. dysentery, typhoid, gastroenteritis, brucellosis, and bacterial food poisoning
- by the skin — infection of skin and mucous membrane by direct contact, e.g. certain skin diseases, conjunctivitis, infective foot disorders, sexually-transmitted diseases
- by invasion of tissue — via a cut in the skin or surgical wound (e.g. staphylococcal infection, HIV)
  — via the bite of an animal e.g. rabies or insect e.g. malaria

---

infection and has been very effective in campaigns against the more serious and highly infectious diseases, such as smallpox (now eradicated from the world), Lassa fever and tuberculosis. As well as isolating the person suffering from the disease it is, of course, important to locate people who have been in contact with the sufferer and, if necessary, they too must be isolated, treated or kept under surveillance. For this reason, 'contact tracing' has become an integral part of the control of infectious disease.

- *Immunization.* Measures to increase people's resistance to infection are also important in control by means of prevention, and it is in this context that immunization has played such a major role (p. 70). In the United Kingdom, parents are advised to have their children immunized against, for example, diphtheria, tetanus, poliomyelitis, whooping cough, measles, mumps and rubella. Nurses, particularly health visitors, have an important role to play in encouraging parents to take up immunization and there is concern about falling rates of acceptance. This may be partly due to the fact that in the UK, many young parents of today are less aware of the seriousness of some of the above mentioned diseases because they have not had occasion to witness the distress they cause. There is no doubt, too, that parents have become more aware that immunization can carry a risk of adverse reaction and this has been most publicized

in relation to the whooping cough vaccine. On the one hand there have been reports suggesting that the vaccine can cause brain damage, albeit in a tiny minority of children and, on the other, the whooping cough epidemics in recent years have reawakened fears of the damage the disease itself can inflict.

World-wide, the need to raise immunization coverage levels is underscored by the continuing occurrence each year of some 1.6 million preventable deaths from measles, neonatal tetanus and whooping cough; some 120 000 cases of paralytic poliomyelitis; and 1–2 million deaths attributable to hepatitis B infection (WHO, 1993).

A high proportion of the world's children do not even have the opportunity of having protection from some of the major childhood killers, diseases for which vaccines are available — measles for example is a major cause of childhood mortality. Table 4.1 shows the estimated causes of death for the 0–5 age group in developing countries for 1990. However, an increasing number of countries are committing themselves to the WHO disease reduction targets for the decade of the 1990s, for example, the reduction of measles deaths by 95%, and the eradication of poliomyelitis by the year 2000 (WHO, 1993). Of course vaccines alone will not prevent child mortality caused by infectious diseases; better social and economic conditions, and better education about prevention play a major part, as they did in industrialized countries about a century ago.

Table 4.1 Estimated causes of death among children under 5 years of age in developing countries, 1990

Cause of death category	1990	
	Number of deaths (in thousands)	%
1. Acute respiratory infections (ARI) alone (mostly pneumonia)	3560	27.6
2. Diarrhoea alone	3000	23.3
3. Birth asphyxia	860	6.7
4. Malaria	800	6.2
5. Neonatal tetanus	560	4.3
6. ARI — measles	480	3.7
7. Congenital anomalies	450	3.5
8. Birth trauma	430	3.3
9. Prematurity	430	3.3
10. Neonatal sepsis and meningitis	300	2.3
11. Tuberculosis	300	2.3
12. ARI — pertussis	260	2.0
13. Measles alone	220	1.7
14. Accidents	200	1.6
15. Diarrhoea — measles	180	1.4
16. Pertussis alone	100	0.8
17. All other causes	770	6.0
Total	12 900	100.0

(Reproduced with kind permission from World Health Organization (1993).)

Apart from immunization of young children, pregnant women are considered to be a priority group because certain infectious diseases can cause serious damage to the developing fetus. In the UK the rubella vaccine has been offered to all girls in early adolescence and to non-pregnant women of child-bearing age who are found to be serologically negative for this antigen but with the use of the measles/mumps/rubella (MMR) vaccine to small children, started in 1988, and a recently introduced booster injection at secondary school age, this will eventually become unnecessary.

Indications for vaccination against other infectious diseases (e.g. enteric fevers, cholera, typhus, yellow fever and rabies) depend on individual risk of exposure and international travel regulations. The nature of immunization programmes as a means of preventing infection is determined according to the prevailing circumstances of a particular country and readers in countries other than the UK should supplement this section with relevant local information.

Nobody now needs to be, nor should be, vaccinated against smallpox. This disease has been eradicated from the world, an achievement which must rank as one of WHO's greatest successes, although some vaccine is being kept in a limited number of centres in case of resurgence of smallpox.

Control of epidemics   Controlling epidemics is important in preventing infection and, in this age of travel, is a concern which extends beyond the boundaries of any one nation; it requires international collaboration. Incidence of infection in each country is notified to the World Health Organization so that necessary strategies can be implemented to prevent spread to other countries by travellers, cargoes and animals and thus prevent pandemics.

However as one disease is conquered or controlled, others appear, particularly those caused by viruses, and finding cures or methods of immunization is a lengthy exercise. Throughout the world, the virus hepatitis B (Murrell, 1993) has recently become a major health problem. Acute and persistent infection is common and the incidence increasing. The carrier state may lead to chronic liver disease including chronic hepatitis, cirrhosis and hepatocellular carcinoma. High rates of infection have been found in neonates of carrier mothers, sexual contacts of carriers especially among homosexual men, intravenous drug abusers, and health care workers exposed to blood and blood products. WHO recommend that all health care workers receive vaccination against hepatitis B. The spread of the virus causing hepatitis C is also causing concern. It, too, is associated with blood products and intravenous drug abusers.

An even more alarming threat throughout the world is the growth in the incidence, and the accompanying high death rate associated with AIDS (acquired immune deficiency syndrome). Essentially it is a sexually-transmitted disease, but it is also carried in infected blood and blood products so 'at risk' are intravenous drug users; recipients of blood transfusions, for example haemophiliacs; and anyone who is in contact with the blood of infected individuals. The subject of AIDS is discussed in more detail on p. 354.

The risk of infection in a hospital setting is considered later in this chapter.

Preventing fire

Any activity which aims at preventing fire is a component of the AL of maintaining a safe environment. These activities are an essential part of living and in many countries there are educational pamphlets and programmes from several sources to spread knowledge about fire hazards and to encourage self-discipline in carrying out precautions.

Fire in the home   At a domestic level, fire can be prevented by maintaining equipment in a safe working condition, for example repairing frayed flexes, avoiding trailing flexes, ensuring that electrical circuits are not overloaded, having fires adequately guarded, and using self-extinguishing devices for movable articles which can be knocked over with relative ease such as oil lamps and oil-heaters. In the kitchen, a major contribution to safety is care when using fat for cooking purposes; if it ignites, the most effective way of controlling the blaze is to cover the pan with a lid or metal tray and turn off the heat supply to the cooking apparatus. Individuals are responsible for fire safety in their own homes, but most householders insure against the possibility of accidental fire damage to the fabric of their home and to the contents.

Fire in public places   For public buildings — shops, hotels, warehouses — proprietors have the responsibility of taking adequate precautions against fire and there is legislation which permits inspection of premises to ensure that the necessary safety measures are enforced. Despite precautions human carelessness can precipitate the utter devastation caused by fire. Unsafe disposal of lighted cigarette ends has been thought to be the cause of many fires involving buildings used by the public. Similar tragedies can occur even in rather unusual settings and caused by a different train of events, for example the North Sea Piper Alpha episode 1988, where staff died either on the blazing oil installation or drowned in the surrounding sea of fire.

Such disasters with heavy loss of life and the untold misery of injury and scarring for survivors, highlight the need for closer supervision of existing preventive strategies; greater staff awareness of alarm and rescue measures; and increasing vigilance on the part of companies and individuals to reduce human error. It is noteworthy that a British inventor, Maurice Ward, has devised a fire-proof plastic; a ¼ mm-thick piece of this Starlite can survive more than 75 atomic-blast simulations which vaporized ½-inch-thick steel. Among the applications envisioned is the fireproofing of oilrigs (Frankel & Hall, 1993).

Apart from conflagrations in buildings, environmental fires can occur. For example in hot dry weather, carelessly attended picnic fires and inadequate disposal of lighted cigarette ends can start a forest fire, although ignition can occur spontaneously from the heat produced by sun shining through glass carelessly left lying on the ground especially near dry shrubland and trees. Obviously knowledge as well as self-discipline is necessary to prevent accidents and maintain a safe environment.

Strategies for control   When fire does occur, detecting, containing and extinguishing the flames are the main principles of immediate action and the following strategies should be borne in mind:

- detection is often by smell and by seeing smoke and flames, but smoke detectors may give the first alarm and increasingly, these are installed in the home
- smothering the fire with thick material will cut off the atmospheric oxygen supply (combustion requires oxygen) and extinguish the flames, if the fire is limited in extent. Commercially produced fire extinguishers work on this principle
- closed windows and doors help to contain smoke and flames for about 20 minutes and as inhaled smoke can immobilize people who are attempting to escape, these vital minutes may permit an orderly evacuation from other parts of a building and allow time for professional help to arrive
- a paid, professional fire service whose staff are experts in fire-fighting and rescue, is maintained in most countries. They also contribute to fire prevention and play a considerable part in educating the public, especially schoolchildren to become more conscious of fire prevention.

Obviously, the first and foremost purpose in all of the activities discussed — preventing pollution, accidents, fire and infection — is human survival. However, in circumstances when life itself is not threatened, the purpose becomes one of preventing, or at least minimizing, injury and ill-health. An accident can result in some form of disablement or disfigurement and, even if its effects are only temporary, the human suffering involved can be intense. The effects of fire can be devastating: the pain of burned tissue, the stigma of visible scars (p. 364) and the loss of property and personal possessions. Infection too can involve discomfort and absence from work; and it can mean isolation. Pollution, though often more insidious in its effects, can cause ill-health and even permanent intellectual impairment.

To sum up, it seems logical to prevent rather than cure, but of course prevention is also a politicoeconomic consideration.

POLITICOECONOMIC

Both political and economic factors influence the AL of maintaining a safe environment to a very great degree. Although many of the activities involved are carried out by individuals, and there is much scope for personal decision-making and responsibility, the business of maintaining a safe environment is very much a political concern and responsibility — at local, regional, national and international levels.

Government action

As has been described, many aspects of maintaining a safe environment are controlled by legislation. Laws exist which ensure that as far as possible, accidents, fire, infection and pollution are prevented. Governments also accept a responsibility for increasing public awareness of hazards and safety measures and desirable standards of safety through publicity campaigns and education. All such activity is in the interests of both personal and national safety, but also is based on an economic argument.

An unsafe environment will result in accident and ill-health, and both are a burden on a nation's economy. Of course, preventing accidents and promoting safety also cost a great deal of money. Safe houses, roads, vehicles, workplaces and play areas all cost money. So too does the provision of emergency services (such as the fire service) which are sufficiently well-equipped and manned to respond promptly and effectively when required.

The economics of maintaining a safe environment are not just the concern of government, because individuals contribute to the national purse through taxation. For example, a substantial proportion of the road tax levied on vehicle owners goes towards paying for road maintenance and improvements.

Individual action

For individuals, the costs of maintaining a safe environment are, however, by no means all in the category of indirect taxation. Maintaining safety in the home is an expensive business and, for families with children, the purchase of recommended safety equipment — such as car safety seats, stair gates, a playpen and a cooker guard — adds up to a considerable sum. For families of low income such items are almost certainly prohibitively expensive. At other stages of the lifespan, maintaining a safe environment in the home for elderly or disabled people may also be expensive.

People do not need to be politicians to engage in politics. Individuals and pressure groups can exert a considerable influence on government and have indeed done so very effectively in relation to many aspects of the AL of maintaining a safe environment. For example, the introduction of seat belt legislation in the UK was at least in part due to persistent lobbying by sections of the community, including the medical profession. Frequently too, people who live in a particular geographic location combine together to form a pressure group if their neighbourhood has been earmarked by government for the siting of, for example, a new motorway or nuclear power station or the dumping of nuclear waste which is considered to constitute a substantial threat to their safety and health.

All citizens have a responsibility to be involved in the politicoeconomic decisions which influence the AL of maintaining a safe environment — not necessarily for their own safety, but for the safety of others and especially for their children and, indeed, their children's children.

Nuclear threat

It is perhaps that long-term perspective which is at the root of present-day concern over the nuclear arsenal still held by the superpowers and increasingly by lesser powers since the ending of the Cold War or even by smaller fanatical groups. Knowledge of the devastating effect which even a limited nuclear attack would have on the environment and the people in it has motivated increasing numbers to campaign vociferously for nuclear disarmament.

Opinion on the nuclear issue is divided and other arguments are involved too, for example economic considerations. Some people think that the vast amounts of money spent by governments on nuclear weapons and on maintaining existing supplies would be better spent on other needs, such as health care. Protagonists argue that the nation's defence is more important and that the mere possession of nuclear weapons prevents attack by potential users. However, there is no disagreement that preventing the use of nuclear weaponry is vital to maintaining a safe environment for people now, and for future generations.

Individualizing nursing for the AL of maintaining a safe environment

ASSESSING THE INDIVIDUAL IN THE AL

Each day, throughout the day, although not always aware

of it, people are engaged in carrying out numerous activities which have the specific purpose of maintaining a safe environment. As with all of the Activities of Living, there are many similarities in the way different people carry out this AL. However, as the preceding discussion shows, a variety of circumstances determine an individual's vulnerability to certain hazards in the environment, and result in variation in the way necessary preventive activities are carried out. This concept of individuality provides the link between the model of living and the model for nursing.

Individualized nursing is based on knowledge of a person's individuality. Therefore, in relation to the AL of maintaining a safe environment, the nurse needs to know about the patient's individual habits and any actual or potential problems. Such information can be obtained in the course of nursing assessment using as a mental framework, knowledge of the topics outlined in the preceding part of this Chapter (Box 4.10). While observing and discussing relevant topics with the patient, the nurse might bear in mind the following questions:

- what kind of activities does the individual usually engage in with the purpose of maintaining a safe environment?
- what factors influence the way in which the individual carries out the AL of maintaining a safe environment?
- what is the individual's level of knowledge regarding maintaining a safe environment?
- what is the individual's attitude to maintaining a safe environment?
- has the individual experienced any difficulties in the past with maintaining a safe environment and, if so, how have these been coped with?
- does the individual have any actual problems or perceive any potential problems with maintaining a safe environment?

IDENTIFYING ACTUAL AND POTENTIAL PROBLEMS

The objective in collecting this sort of information is to discover the person's usual routines; what can and cannot be done independently; what previous coping mechanisms have been employed; and what problems exist or may develop in relation to this AL. By its very nature it is likely that most will be potential problems relevant to the circumstances (though there may be actual problems too), and, therefore, the goals set and the mutually agreed nursing interventions will be mainly preventive in nature. Accordingly, evaluation will be undertaken to ascertain that the preventive measures implemented have been effective. The goal of individualized nursing for this AL will be achieved if assessing, planning, imple-

Box 4.10 Assessing the individual in the AL of maintaining a safe environment

Lifespan: effect on maintaining a safe environment

- Babies — vulnerable to accidents, infections, excessive heat/cold
- Preschool children — vulnerable to accidents in the home
- Schoolchildren — vulnerable to accidents on the roads and in the playground
- Adolescents — vulnerable to road, bicycle and sporting accidents
- Adults — vulnerable to hazards in the work environment; vulnerable to road traffic accidents; responsible for safety of children
- Elderly people — vulnerable to falls in the home, hazards of infection and fire, pedestrian accidents

Dependence/independence in maintaining a safe environment

- Dependence in infancy/childhood/old age
- Constraints on independence in adulthood (e.g. mental/physical/sensory disability)
- Dependence on others
- Dependence on aids

Factors influencing maintaining a safe environment

- Biological — acuity of the senses
  - physical ability/disability
  - susceptibility to infection
  - state of physical health/ill-health, anatomical and physiological responses to infection and trauma
- Psychological — intellectual ability/impairment
  - attitude to safety (home, work, play, travel)
  - personality and temperament
  - mood and motivation
  - level of confidence
  - level of stress
  - level of knowledge about safety precautions
  - responsiveness to safety legislation/health education
  - non-accidental injury
- Sociocultural — cultural factors (e.g. concept of safety)
  - social factors (e.g. prevalence of infectious diseases)
  - social class (e.g. risk of accident)
  - social unrest and violence
  - deviant cults
- Environmental — housing
  - standard of safety in the home
  - exposure to hazards in work settings
  - hazards in play settings
  - risk of accident on the roads/while travelling
  - exposure to environmental pollution
  - climatic and geographical factors
  - extraterrestrial factors
- Politicoeconomic — knowledge and attitude to safety legislation
  - awareness of local environmental hazards
  - personal spending on safety measures
  - political awareness/involvement (e.g. pollution, nuclear products)
  - legislation
  - government finance

menting and evaluating all take account of the person's individuality in maintaining a safe environment.

That, in the most general of terms, describes how the nursing process method is applied. However, in different circumstances, nursing assessment of the AL of maintaining a safe environment would differ in approach, scope and content. For example, assessment by a health visitor of a mother's knowledge about maintaining a safe environment for her young child in the home would obviously be quite different from an occupational health nurse's assessment of an employee's risk of accident at work or the psychiatric nurse's handling of a person during an acute psychotic attack. Therefore, in different nursing contexts there will be different kinds of problems identified and, accordingly, different types of nursing activities will be implemented.

Teaching is one type of nursing activity which is always relevant in relation to the AL of maintaining a safe environment. Exploiting opportunities for education of people of all ages and in various settings (home, school, workplace, clinic and hospital) is probably the main way in which nurses can contribute to the collective effort to prevent injury and ill-health which is caused by accident, fire, infection and pollution. These subjects were dealt with in detail in Environmental Factors (p. 75) and should be recognized as background knowledge relevant to nursing in relation to the AL of maintaining a safe environment, so are not discussed further.

The remainder of the chapter deals with some circumstances in which nurses are directly involved with assisting people who have actual or potential problems in maintaining a safe environment. There are two sections:

- change of dependence/independence status: considering in very broad terms, the variety of circumstances which can cause a change in status (in a community setting or in a hospital) and which require a nursing input as part of the collective effort
- change of environment and routine: considering nursing in a hospital setting — accidents in hospital; hospital-acquired infection; danger of fire; risks associated with the use of prescribed medications.

CHANGE OF DEPENDENCE/INDEPENDENCE STATUS

The dependence/independence continuum in the model of living serves as a reminder that all people experience change of dependence/independence status for the Activities of Living in the normal course of the lifespan. In the context of nursing, the concept of dependence/independence is an important one. According to the circumstances, nurses either help people to cope with enforced dependence (short- or long-term), or help them to regain the level of independence to which they were accustomed prior to the episode of ill-health. There are many different reasons why people can experience difficulty in achieving or maintaining independence for the AL of maintaining a safe environment and, therefore, may require assistance from nurses or others. The main reasons are briefly described under the following headings: physical problems; mental problems; problems due to sensory impairment/loss.

Physical problems

Physical mobility is essential for many activities aimed at maintaining safety, whether at home, at work, at play or while travelling. Those born with severe deformity of the skeleton, or absence of one or more limbs, usually experience some life-long difficulty in carrying out some of the activities for maintaining a safe environment. Some people, on the other hand, are suddenly rendered immobile, for example certain of the 'emergency' admissions to hospital and those who suddenly collapse or become ill and are nursed at home. For many of them, their inability to maintain a safe environment is only temporary, but for others it may be permanent.

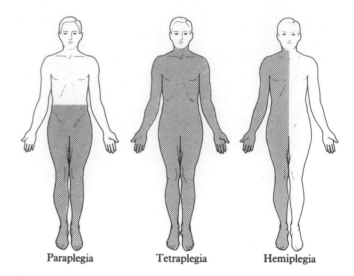

Paraplegia   **Tetraplegia**   **Hemiplegia**

Fig. 4.2 Motor and sensory loss in types of paralysis

Certainly, someone who develops tetraplegia will be permanently and totally dependent for this AL and to some degree, so too with paraplegia and hemiplegia (Fig. 4.2). People who are unconscious are also totally dependent. Severely ill people can experience exhaustion and they simply do not have the energy to carry out the necessary preventive activities; they are dependent on nurses and others for maintaining a safe environment.

Even apparently minor problems, such as any enclosure of the hands or restriction of finger mobility, can render a person less independent for this AL. If there is any restriction on movement, however slight, of the spine, hips and lower limbs, the person may be unable to get out of the way of a dangerous moving object with sufficient speed to prevent mishap. Those who are bedfast or chairfast are similarly unable to take avoiding action.

Physical imbalance of any kind can interfere with independence too, for example, the patient who has had a limb amputated. Recent anaesthesia and certain medications can cause patients to feel dizzy and unable to maintain their balance. People who take sleeping pills can also be at risk of falling, especially if they rise to void during the night, and the 'hang-over' feeling in the morning can create a safety risk.

Most of the physical problems, therefore, are primarily mobilizing problems. These are discussed in more detail in Chapter 11, but for each person the nurse needs to assess what that particular mobilizing problem means in relation to the AL of maintaining a safe environment. She can then identify actual and potential problems and include in the nursing plan whatever precautions are necessary, in order to prevent accidents.

Mental problems

As well as those born with a learning disability, there are people whose intellect is impaired as a result of infection or injury to the brain. They may not recognize when they are in danger, for example when crossing a busy road, or they may not know how to carry out even the most basic safety precautions necessary for the prevention of fire, accidents and infection. In a hospital or home for people with learning disabilities much of the nurse's time is devoted to maintaining a safe environment for the residents and also helping them to understand and take personal responsibility (Shirtcliffe, 1995) for practising essential safety measures when this is realistic.

Certain types of mental illness result in a diminished awareness, so that the sufferers are not able to be completely responsible for carrying out the activities to achieve a safe environment. Depressive illness can result in suicidal thoughts and there may or may not be expression of intent. Such people need help in maintaining their environment in a condition which is safe for them until their mood improves.

If this cannot be assured, then the person may require admission to a psychiatric unit. One important role of such units, is that they provide a safe environment for mentally disturbed people and simultaneously in severe cases, protect members of the community from possible harm as a result of violence to persons (Kay, 1995) or property. Nurses are concerned with the AL of maintaining a safe environment in relation to individual patients but, at the same time, must bear in mind the safety of others. The fact that this AL has a collective dimension in addition to the personal one was mentioned in the early part of this chapter.

Problems due to sensory impairment/loss

All five senses are used in activities carried out with the purpose of maintaining a safe environment and, therefore, impairment or loss of any one can result in problems. Some of the problems can occur so gradually, for example the onset of deafness, that the person adjusts gradually and so is able to maintain independence for this AL. Sudden impairment or loss, however, is likely to cause dependence, at least temporarily.

Visual impairment/loss   It is unusual for a person to lose the sight in both eyes at the same time, but even loss of sight in one can cause several changed perspectives (p. 117). It is important to establish empathy (p. 122) with people who have visual problems in order to discover what they might find helpful, and what is required for independence to be maintained or regained.

Aural impairment/loss   Again it is unusual for a person suddenly to become deaf in both ears, but for example, a loud nearby explosion can cause sudden deafness, perhaps permanently (p. 116). The use of earplugs can simulate the effect, and help one to appreciate the implications for safety if a person does not hear the sound

of a pot of food boiling over, or the noise of approaching traffic.

Sensory impairment/loss   People with sensory loss have a problem in that they cannot feel heat, cold, pain and pressure (p. 118). Sensory loss sometimes occurs in large areas such as the lower limbs and lower trunk; in all four limbs and the whole trunk; in the arm and leg on the same side of the body. Sensory loss frequently occurs with motor loss; the patient is paralysed and it compounds the problem of maintaining a safe environment. The different types of paralysis are illustrated in Figure 4.2.

Smelling and tasting impairment/loss   When cooking, many people check the contents of bottles and packages by smelling or tasting them. When deprived of these sensations they cannot be used as checks when maintaining a safe environment. Nurses can help these people by first observing tactfully whether or not they can read and write. If so, they can be advised to pay special attention to labelling containers and paper bags as to their contents. People who cannot read and write could be advised to use a signing system and could be encouraged to use any available adult literacy programme.

As has been implied from the comments made, the nurse's ability to identify a person's problems with the AL of maintaining a safe environment which result from impairment/loss of the senses, to a great extent depends on an ability to be imaginative and empathetic. Once aware of what the problems are, the nurse can help the person to develop alternative ways of detecting and responding to hazards in the environment, thereby maintaining maximum independence for this AL.

In all of these examples of sensory impairment, the advice of the occupational therapist and other specialists can help in the attainment of maximum independence.

CHANGE OF ENVIRONMENT AND ROUTINE

Most people are conservative and dislike change, particularly the enforced change which occurs when a person is admitted to hospital. The individual can feel insecure and frightened in this new environment and anxiety increases the risk of accident. Someone in an anxious state is more likely to bump into, or trip over objects; shaking or tense hands are more likely to drop or spill objects they are holding. Some patients become disoriented, a more likely reaction if the person is elderly or has already shown signs of mental confusion. Nurses can help all patients by talking with them, keeping in mind the objective of orienting them to the new environment and routine. The sooner this is done the better.

Unfamiliar environment

Familiarity with an environment makes it less hazardous;

for example people adjust spatially to avoid objects in their immediate vicinity. On admission, a patient has not had time to make any necessary spatial adjustments. This could well relate to the design of the hospital bed which may not be at the same height as the one with which the person is familiar. For some people more than others, it is important for the nurses to know that familiar height.

Where mechanically-operated height-adjustment beds are provided and the patient is capable with instruction, of operating the mechanism, independence in this respect can be maintained. When the patient is not capable, then the nurse is responsible for operating the mechanism to maintain the individual's safety.

Patients may have to be nursed on a bed with a ripple mattress or an air bed. While providing greater safety from the pressure hazard, they can create spatial problems for example, the increased height relative to the bedside locker and bed table may require spatial adjustment. Over-reaching for an article on nearby furniture is a frequent cause of accidents. Patients can be helped by nurses who, before leaving the bedside, test whether or not they can comfortably reach articles on the locker.

Sometimes in an attempt to prevent accidents, restraints are used. The use of restraints in the care of elderly people in hospital, especially cot sides, is a topic which nurses have been reluctant to address because of the psychosocial, ethical and legal issues involved, say Ramprogus and Gibson (1991). Nurses face a conflict between the need to maintain a patient's safety and the need to maintain the individual's right to freedom and autonomy. Like everyone else, elderly people have a right to take risks. On the other hand, the person and perhaps other patients have to be protected. In some instances, in fact, it has been demonstrated that restraints exacerbate the very problem they are supposed to avoid, for example, falling out of wheelchairs or beds in an attempt to overcome the restraints. Ramprogus and Gibson carried out a study in an 81-bed elderly care hospital (Box 4.11).

Disabled and older patients who experience difficulty when rising from a chair may like most people, have their 'special' chair at home, out of which they can rise relatively easily, and on which they may hang a walking stick to help with safe rising. These patients can experience many kinds of problems when in a different environment such as increased stiffening of the back and limbs due to lack of exercise because they find it so difficult to get out of the hospital chair; and incontinence for the same reason. Actual shearing injury to the sacral tissues and the heels may even be caused by patients sliding forward on vinyl-covered chairs (p. 246). Nurses can help, within the constraints of the type of chairs provided, by 'matching' the chair to the patient, not just helping the person to any chair.

Box 4.11 Assessing the use of restraints

In an 81-bed 'elderly care' hospital, Ramprogus and Gibson (1991) set out to evaluate:

- the relationship between workload and use of restraints
- the type of restraints used
- the nurse's perception of and justification for the use of restraints
- the use of restraints in practice

The study demonstrated that the main reason for restraining patients would appear to be for safety and the prevention of harm; and the authors quote that this is supported by other studies, indeed is consistent with the most frequent reason given by patients for being restrained. Following the study there were discussions about, and training in the use of non-restraining alternatives, and the use of restraints was reduced by 75%.

Non-restraining alternatives suggested in this study were:

- talk to the patient
- identify the cause of unrest and deal with it
- provide a safe environment
- provide constant observation and supervision
- provide diversional activities
- provide music
- take the patient for a walk if this is appropriate.

Box 4.12 Measuring noise

Noise is measured in decibels (dB). The commonly used A scale (dB(A)) incorporates a weighting to take account of the ear's varying responses to different frequencies—humans are less sensitive to low frequency sounds than to high ones. Noise is measured on a logarithmic scale. This means that a noise of 100 dB(A) has 10 times as much sound energy as one of 90 dB(A). Subjectively, an increase of 10 dB(A) makes the sound twice as loud. (Godlee, 1992)

Noisy environment

Quite justifiably, hospitals have been labelled as noisy environments. Godlee (1992) discussing noise in relation to the human ear's response, uses the dB(A) scale (Box 4.12) and Figure 4.3 gives a comparison of noise levels using this scale.

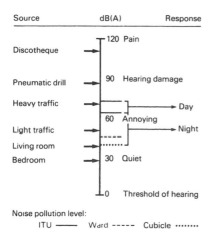

Fig. 4.3 Comparison of noise levels (Reproduced by kind permission of the British Medical Journal.)

Studies about noise levels in hospital in the UK (Soutar & Wilson, 1986) and in the USA (Hilton, 1987) show how disturbing noise can be. Hilton starts by providing references to show how excessive noise can provoke detrimental physiological responses — it can startle; damage hearing; stimulate epinephrine production; induce sensory disturbance; constrict peripheral and coronary arteries; reduce digestive secretions; and slow gastrointestinal motility. Psychological disturbances have also been cited including annoyance and irritation; heightened arousal; impaired judgement; altered perception; interference with thinking; and reduced ability to hear. It is considered, too, that at 50 dB(A), pain perception is enhanced. Hilton's study carried out in four ITUs and two medical/surgical wards showed the noise level above the recommended figure at night. In the recovery room, more than half the talking exceeded 67 dB(A), although considerable noise was also created by oxygen administration equipment, ventilators and alarms on monitors, as well as toilet flushing sounds and telephones ringing. Hilton did a similar study in Canada with similar results.

A more recent study by Dias (1992), although not claiming to be based on the scientific method, was carried out in the UK in a hospital for people who were 'elderly mentally infirm', in an attempt to help them to enjoy a quiet and comfortable sleeping atmosphere. He used observations by staff and patients over a four-week period and classified causes of noise as for example:

- patients — toiletting, coughing, shouting (confused patients)
- staff — talking, handwashing, trolleys, waste-bin lids
- appliances — bedpan-washers, ripple mattress pumps, commodes
- natural phenomena — wind rattling windows/doors
- other factors — vehicles.

Dias made the following observations:

- those who were 'hard of hearing' were less disturbed by noise
- well-oriented patients seemed to be affected most
- those who were depressed or anxious were more sensitive to noise as were those with sleeping difficulties
- certain noises reinforced some patients' delusional systems
- patients receiving higher doses of sedatives were less likely to be affected than those on low doses or none at all.

Improvements are recommended in all of these studies such as shutting doors quietly (and oiling them when necessary); handling equipment carefully to reduce noise; muting the alarm systems and telephones; wearing soft-soled shoes; providing soundproof covers for computer printout machines; reducing conversations between staff and talking quietly; providing earplugs if requested; isolating 'noisy' patients from general wards when practicable so that they create the least possible disturbance to other patients — and, most of these suggestions are simple and inexpensive remedies.

It has been suggested that from time to time, sound engineers should show staff how much they pollute the environment and by means of this simple measurement, educate staff to prevent noise pollution. Of course, noise can mean different things to different people and it is possible to be upset by silence, for example a child in an isolation unit — a salutary reminder of the importance of individualizing nursing according to the circumstances.

Risk of accident

Some mention of accidents has already been made but further, more specific comment is relevant. If nurses are to attempt to prevent avoidable accidents to people who are in care, they need to be aware of what and where the hazards are. For patients who are identified from assessment as being at particular risk, relevant preventive activities should be included in the list of interventions written on the patient's nursing plan.

Sutton et al (1994) carried out research in an attempt to identify predisposition to accidents in a large acute hospital (Box 4.13) and Sweeting (1994) discusses a retrospective audit of falls over a 6-month period in a nine ward 'medical elderly' unit for both acute care and longer-term rehabilitation. As a result of the audit, the Harrogate Trust developed a Patient Fall Assessment Chart which could be scored to indicate fall-proneness according to selected criteria:

- limited mobility

Box 4.13 Patients' accidents in hospital

In 1994, Sutton et al. described a one-year, in-depth study of 728 reported patient accidents (of a non-medical nature) in 10 wards at a large acute hospital, using both primary and secondary data from patients, staff and records. Not surprisingly, higher accident rates coincided with times of increased activity — on rising, at midday, and before settling to sleep in the evening.

Some results confirmed earlier studies, in particular that falls to older patients were the most common type of accident; and that broadly speaking, findings were replicated about distribution of age, sex, diagnosis, mental state, drug treatments and accident location. Among the new findings were the large differences between patients' and staff's accounts of the accidents; that many accidents were poorly recorded; and that lunar cycles may influence accident frequency (this may be, quote the authors, because 'light nights keep patients awake' or could be a manifestation of Leiba's beliefs relating lunar influence and human emotional disturbance).

Two subsequent articles deal with other studies carried out by the authors at the same hospital using the same ward population:

● A comparative study of patients who had accidents and those who did not; investigating further the relationship to accident predisposition of diagnosis, medication, and mental and physical state.
● A study of unreported in-patient accidents — among reported accident patients.

● altered mental state
● unwillingness/inability to call for help
● severely limited vision/speech/hearing
● recent CVA
● known fall before admission
● on medications with potential to induce hypotension
● incontinence/frequency: on diuretics/laxatives.

Subsequently a Fall Prevention Programme was initiated for all staff, and a patient/carer leaflet was also produced to encourage relatives and friends to participate in the preventive measures and become part of the care team.

The Programme generated a high level of awareness of 'at risk' patients among all disciplines, says Sweeting, and in a 6-month trial period, patient falls were reduced by 41%.

Of course, it is the active, more independent elderly person who is most at risk of falling, and it has to be borne in mind that the prevention of all falls is not an appropriate objective in the care of elderly people. Instead the primary aim should be the promotion of patient activity within acceptable limits of safety. This does not, of course, imply that nurses should not be concerned with the prevention of unnecessary accidents. Earlier in this chapter striking a realistic balance between protection and freedom was discussed in the context of preventing accidents in relation to children and in relation to people with learning disabilities. It is equally relevant when providing a nursing service for people who are elderly. One of the themes in developing a mode of thinking about nursing and its practice must surely be preventing the potential problem of accident from becoming an actual one and assessing, planning and implementing appropriate nursing practices for those who are seen to be at risk.

When incidents do occur, an Accident Form must be completed according to the local authority's guidelines; for legal purposes but also to monitor incidence and prevent further accidents.

Of course, injury in hospital may involve one patient assaulting another patient. A pilot scheme to monitor violence was carried out in a psychiatric hospital over a 9-month period (Benson & Den, 1992) and showed that although violent incidents initiated by patients (an average of 12.3 each month) were directed toward staff, property and other patients, the greatest number of incidents occurred between patients — three times more likely to be victims than staff. Box 4.14 outlines the findings, and the authors emphasize the need to continue monitoring changes which are made to reduce aggressive incidents.

Fairlie and Brown (1994) agree with Benson and Den that, in a mental health unit, late afternoon/evening is a high risk period for accidents and incidents among the non-elderly; running on to 22.00 hours for incidents involving aggression and self-harm.

Following some incidents involving injury/death to members of the unsuspecting public which captured media headlines, the UK Health Secretary has emphasized that before discharging inpatients who have a history of violent outbursts, psychiatrists must assess carefully the risk that they might harm themselves or others; and ensure that adequate community care has been set up with named key workers. Ford and Repper (1994) consider how community mental health nurses can comply with guidance issued by the Department of Health and predict that, more than ever, nurses will be accountable for ensuring that people with the most serious mental illness receive the services they require. Ford and Repper suggest an approach pioneered successfully in the USA — assertive outreach (Box 4.15).

Box 4.14 Monitoring violence in a psychiatric unit

Benson and Den (1992) carried out a study to monitor violence in a psychiatric hospital over a 9-month period. From the recording system used, a number of common precursors to violent incidents were identified:

- an overstimulating environment was a clear precursor to violence in a small number of residents
- violence was a method of reducing anxiety:
  — one resident became anxious and stressed in a communal, stimulating environment
  — many used violence as a coping mechanism to combat feelings of helplessness and to control others
  — some violent patients are afraid of their own hostile urges (it is argued they want staff to contain this violence in a safe manner)
- residents who pestered fellow residents for cigarettes often triggered outbursts of fighting or verbal aggression
- incidents increased during evenings and weekends
- some residents displayed certain physical signs before resorting to aggression e.g. agitation
- if compulsorily detained, outbursts were linked to restrictions placed on freedom.

Results from this report enabled staff to recognize that emphasis needed to be consistently placed on:

- the physical environment
- precursors of violence in individuals
- individual management plans to prevent violence
- increasing the amount and range of structured as well as spare-time activities so that residents are encouraged to join in constructive activities for a greater proportion of the time.

Box 4.15 Key factors in 'assertive outreach'

Ford and Repper (1994) suggest the following key tenets of the approach in 'assertive outreach':

- worker accepts responsibility for care provision
- intensity of assertive outreach is balanced against degree of client risk
- long-term persistence is often needed
- long-term aim is a supportive relationship
- client-centred, practical goals should be tackled first
- third-party contact is used where necessary
- accept that limited service provision is better than no service provision.

Risk of infection

When patients come to hospital they are living in close contact with more people than usual. The human body is a reservoir of microorganisms as illustrated in Figure 4.4 and they are easily transferred to other things and people via the hands. A potential problem for patients is the risk of infection because they are in contact with greater numbers of pathogenic microorganisms than at home. Furthermore, this is at a time when resistance is likely to be lowered. A large number of organisms and lowered resistance are two of the necessary conditions for infection to become established.

It was to keep down the population of pathogenic microorganisms in hospital that 'damp dusting' of all laying surfaces used to be considered a nursing activity. Nowadays such activities have been designated 'non-nursing' duties, but nurses liaise with domestic management to achieve a safe environment for patients. Dust invariably contains pathogens which have settled out of the atmosphere.

RESERVOIR	MICROORGANISM	TRANSFERENCE TO HANDS
Nose	Staphylococci	Unprotected sneeze→droplets Protected sneeze→handkerchief Blowing nose→handkerchief Touching nose
Skin	Staphylococci Streptococci	Live and multiply in pores and hair follicles Shed with scales into clothing
Bowel	Salmonella — causing typhoid Bacillus — causing dysentery	From faeces
Mouth and throat	Staphylococci Streptococci	Unprotected sneeze, cough→droplets Protected sneeze, cough→handkerchief

Fig. 4.4 The human body as a reservoir of microorganisms

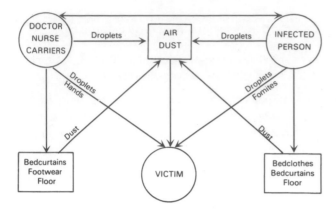

Fig. 4.5 Spread of infection in hospital

In ordinary breathing droplets are projected 150 to 180 cm into the atmosphere and the distance is increased during talking, coughing and sneezing. There is therefore ample opportunity for all surfaces in a ward to be contaminated, particularly bedclothes, bedcurtains, floors and footwear as illustrated in Figure 4.5. It also shows the methods of spread of infection in hospital, an ever present potential problem for the patient. Nurses must be constantly vigilant in every activity so that there is no break in infection control and this is especially necessary because the patient can come into contact with pathogens which have become resistant to one or more of the antibiotics.

From studying Figure 4.5 it will be seen that in hospital there are many potential danger points for contamination by direct contact, for example with infected articles or with hands which have been inadequately washed or not washed at all after dealing with contaminated discharges or materials. Some patients succumb to infection.

Hospital acquired infection Hospital-acquired infection (HAI) or nosocomial infection is notorious for the manner in which it complicates the course of the original illness, delays recovery, and increases the cost of hospital stay. HAI is defined as an infection which is neither present nor incubating before hospital admission, and according to Horton (1993) the level of incidence of HAI has remained unchanged since 1980 — 9.2 per 100 patients. Bowell (1992) provides a chart to help nurses to assess patients who are at risk, and then suggests guidelines for planning protective care.

HAI usually occurs in the urinary and lower respiratory tracts and in surgical wounds. There is evidence that *Staphylococcus aureus* (Beedle, 1993; Siu, 1994) and gram negative bacilli, the main causative agents, reach susceptible patients via contact rather than via airborne routes, predominantly on the hands of staff — and the staff most in contact with patients are nurses.

Handwashing *Handwashing* is undoubtedly the main activity in preventing the spread of infection (Box 4.16).

The bacterial flora of the hands are similar to other skin

Box 4.16 Hand washing

Hand washing is the single most important measure in infection control. Hands should be washed after general patient contact or handling potentially contaminated articles. Hands should be washed:

- before and after aseptic technique or invasive procedures
- before contact with a susceptible patient or site
- after contact with body secretions/excretions
- after handling contaminated laundry/equipment
- prior to administration of drugs
- prior to serving meals and drinks
- after removing articles of protective clothing, for instance masks, gloves, aprons
- at the end of a span of duty
- after any duty which involves close contact with a patient.

Action	Rationale
Remove all rings from your hands	These can harbour microorganisms
Wash with continuous warm running water	Physically removes organisms more efficiently than stagnant water
Wet hands before applying soap	Reduces irritation of hands by soap
Lather all surfaces of hands paying particular attention to fingertips, thumbs and finger webs	
Rinse hands thoroughly	To remove microorganisms. If soap is not removed it can cause dryness and irritation
Turn off taps using elbows on elbow taps, then dry hands thoroughly *or* first dry hands thoroughly, then turn off taps using a dry paper towel	To avoid re-contaminating hands

(Reproduced by kind permission of the Royal College of Nursing from RCN (1994).)

---

sites, but hands are of special significance in the transmission of infectious agents and the most important site of contamination. Most *resident skin flora* (Box 4.7) are not highly virulent and are not normally implicated in infections except when prosthetic surgery or other invasive procedures are performed, or when neonates or immunocompromized patients are involved. In contrast, *transient flora* (Box 4.7) often found on the hands of hospital personnel, can be pathogens acquired from colonized or infected patients and are often involved in cross infection.

Handwashing seems such a simple task. In fact, it is very complex. Discussing its complexity, Gould (1992) identified several critical aspects:

- frequency
- appropriateness e.g. after toiletting, in ICU
- duration
- choice of agent e.g. soap and water, hand disinfectant
- quantity of agent used
- quality of performance (technique) e.g. interdigital surfaces, thumbs, wrists
- drying e.g. roller towels, disposable towels, hot air.

Prefaced by many references to former work, Gould and Ream (1993) report a study to compare hand decontamination in three different clinical settings: ICUs, surgical and medical units. Data were collected from two hospitals, one with comprehensive infection control policies and the other without such facilities. Frequency was highest in the ICU of Hospital 2; technique was superior in ICUs regardless of hospital (and superior to earlier studies); half of all opportunities for essential decontamination were omitted; alcohol handrub was readily available and used more often in the units where the best practice was observed.

Other writers have enumerated several factors which may influence non-compliance with accepted techniques, for example:

- hand paper towels may lead to skin irritation and in turn to skin abrasion and infection
- hot air dryers are noisy, slow and may also lead to irritation and there is some evidence that they may, in fact, spread infection (Journal of Nursing Management, 1994)
- soap may be irritant and therefore not used
- sinks may be inaccessible
- hands may be used to operate faulty foot-operated pedal disposal bins.

Nevertheless, no amount of sterile packs and antiseptic agents will protect a patient from a staff member who has contaminated hands.

Discussing handwashing as a process of judgement and effective decision-making, Elliott (1992) maintains that nurses may not be applying their knowledge in an appropriate manner and are not making informed judgements. He goes on to assert that, apart from the practical considerations, handwashing also has ethical and legal implications: exposing patients and colleagues to the risk of infection is not only unethical, it also contravenes their legal duty as professional practitioners. The UKCC Code of Professional Conduct (1992) reads:

> 'Each registered nurse shall have regard to the environment of care and its physical, psychological and social effects on patients/clients and also to the adequacy of resources, and make known to appropriate persons or authorities any circumstances which could place patients/clients in jeopardy or which militates against safe standards of practice.'

Gloves Quite apart from scrupulous handwashing, hospital staff may wear gloves when undertaking certain activities. The purpose of wearing gloves, quotes Clulow (1994) is either to protect the hands from becoming contaminated with dirt and microorganisms or to prevent the transfer of organisms already present on the hands. Used correctly, appropriate gloves provide an essential added layer of safety for 'hands-on' workers, their colleagues and patients. Taking account of the fact that employees are at great risk of contamination even with small hand-skin blemishes; that more unqualified health care workers are being employed in nursing settings; and that litigation is an ever-increasing risk if employers do not provide PPE (personal protection equipment), Clulow undertook a study to assess the relative benefits of wearing vinyl, latex or plastic gloves during invasive procedures. Her findings agreed with other research, that latex gloves are more effective than vinyl and plastic, and that plastic gloves are only recommended for procedures where there will be no contact with body fluids. However there is concern about health care workers becoming allergic to cheap latex disposable gloves which have flooded the market; latex sensitization seems to make those affected allergic to all rubber products (Nursing Times News, 1994).

Oakley (1994) discusses 'universal precautions' — routine safe working practices to protect staff and patients from infection by blood and body fluids; Gould (1994) reports on a study of the 'uptake' of gloves in two teaching hospitals, and nurses' knowledge of blood/body fluid precautions; and Brookes (1994) presents the results of a study of glove perforation in theatre.

Other issues Other measures to prevent infection related to issues other than handwashing and hand protection by gloves, include subjects as diverse as cleansing hospital mattresses (Viant, 1992); the danger in medicine pots (Thompson, 1993); cleaning dressings trolleys (Lawrence, 1992); the use and abuse of disposal bags (Beaumont, 1992). And the Royal College of Nursing Guidelines on Infection Control (1994) deal with safe handling of for example sharps, specimens, linen, spillages; then discuss methods of decontamination and give examples of recommended methods for various pieces of equipment.

Role of the ICN Infection Control Nurses (ICN) have

a mine of information about the latest research on such topics (Law, 1993) and an interesting article by Murdoch (1992) highlights the particular challenges of the ICN in mental health units when acting as a useful link between hospital and home/hostel in relation to teaching, monitoring and evaluating safe practices. Similarly the control of infection in community and hospital settings for those who have learning difficulties has an added dimension, although the principles are unchanged.

It is salutary that an alarming number of nurses seem unable to countenance some of the basic principles of infection control. So concerned was Horton (1993) that she investigated nurses' perceptions of the subject and deduced that if it is to be improved, nurse education must place a much greater emphasis on microbiology; the current, actual knowledge among nurses falls far short of the level required for informed practice. And once improved, regular monitoring is required to ensure that good practice is maintained in concert with the policies of the local Control of Infection Committee and the work of the Infection Control Nurse (ICN). The importance of assessing each patient's risk factors (potential problems) and planning preventive activities which could be implemented and evaluated is an area which requires much more attention in nursing practice.

Changing patterns of infection   Infection problems faced by hospitals have changed enormously in recent decades. The introduction of antibiotics saved the lives of many who would previously have died, but their use has produced new and complex problems. The widespread use of prophylactic antibiotics has contributed to the development of a dependence on their effectiveness and less emphasis on the importance of surgical principles; a breakdown of isolation procedures; and the establishment of antibiotic-resistant and virulent bacteria in hospital. Moreover, these problems are accentuated by the complexities of modern surgery and the large number of high-risk patients being admitted for hitherto inoperable conditions, particularly the very young; the elderly debilitated patient; diabetic, cancer and transplant patients; the severely injured; the burned; and those undergoing surgery. Other high-risk patients are those undergoing therapy with immunosuppressive agents, anti-cancer medications and steroids.

Infection control is only one element in the care of a patient but it is an indicator of standards and there is no disputing how vital it is when one considers the prevalence of nosocomial or hospital-acquired infection (HAI).

'Source' and 'protective' isolation   The patient, however, rather than succumbing to a nosocomial infection, may have an infectious condition when admitted and probably will be anxious about infecting others. Barrier nursing and isolation will help the patient to feel some security that precautions are being taken. However as Knowles (1993) describes, isolation can have profound emotional effects on the person ranging from anxiety and agitation to severe schizoid behaviour with depression, and one fifth of patients said they felt lonely and insecure. Analysis of her small study indicated that some patients valued the privacy, solitude and control, but expressions of neglect and isolation were common and some perceived themselves to be stigmatized. Therefore it is important for nurses to be aware of the problems of isolation as experienced by the patient, and to attempt to alleviate them. It is essential to explain to them why they are being isolated and the reasons for the various precautions. Information is needed, too, about the part the patient is expected to play in preventing the spread of infection. As always, patient teaching is a vital nursing activity.

Knowles quotes in his study that patients who are isolated because their condition renders them at risk from others (*protective* isolation as opposed to *source* isolation) are significantly involved in the decision to be isolated and seem more able to cope.

Multidisciplinary approach   Just as cooperation between nurse and patient is absolutely essential for infection in hospital to be effectively controlled, so too is cooperation among all members of the multidisciplinary health care team. One profession cannot successfully isolate and combat infection. Only by the cooperation and commitment of all hospital personnel can any infection control programme be really successful; therefore a multidisciplinary approach is logical and must be actively encouraged. A collaborative policy is required, for example, in ensuring that there is safe collection of, and provision of storage for hospital waste prior to incineration; quite apart from installing enough incinerators to deal with the growing amount of disposable equipment now used in hospitals.

Not only hospitals require an infection control policy. As day surgery becomes more common, and as patients are being discharged early from hospital, pressure increases on community nursing services, and Dare and Greenwood (1994) describe the role of the public health nurse — complementing the work of the ICN — who works with Consultants in Communicable Diseases Control (CCDC). In fact HAI may not be detected during a hospital stay. Bell and Fenton (1993) reported on an outbreak of *Staphylococcus aureus* detected by community midwives and GPs through retrospective case finding, which acted as a reminder that infection surveillance does not end in hospital.

Control of infection is a constant challenge, indeed infections which were once thought to have been largely conquered are coming back to plague us. Tuberculosis, malaria and gonorrhoea head the list, fighting a rearguard action against modern drugs; they are mutating rapidly to produce resistant strains. In 1994, pneumonic plague re-surfaced in India. And emerging are apparently comparatively 'new' diseases such as Legionnaire's disease; myalgic encephelomyelitis or postviral fatigue syndrome (Pawlikowska et al, 1994); and acquired immune deficiency syndrome or AIDS (p. 354). In the absence of an infection control policy these infections can become major outbreaks with enormous cost implications, not to mention the suffering, pain and even death of the people involved.

Risk of fire

Fire is a potential problem in all NHS premises. The consequences of fire in hospitals and other health care premises can be especially serious because of the difficulties and dangers associated with the emergency evacuation of patients, many of whom may be highly dependent. The aim therefore is to ensure that outbreaks do not occur; and if they do, that they are rapidly detected, effectively contained and quickly extinguished.

Overall fire safety, depends on physical factors (building design and construction, equipment, furnishings); proper installation and maintenance of detection and alarm systems; local policies for handling emergencies; and staff training in all these matters. Irrespective of specific legislation directly related to fire safety, the Health & Safety at Work Act 1974, places a responsibility on all employers and employees to observe safety in their work premises.

As far as hospital employees are concerned, nurses are the front line operators when fire does occur. It is often the nurse who will have to decide on whether to evacuate or who to move, how and where.

Staff training should cover:

- how to guard against fires
- how to react in case of fire
- how to raise the alarm
- how to help evacuate patients
- how to stop fires spreading
- how to help fight the fire.

The charge nurse of a ward has a special responsibility to know precisely what action should be taken in the event of a fire; to be aware of any special risks, such as oxygen cylinders; and to familiarize all new staff to the ward with the routine and the location of fire alarms, exits and fire-fighting equipment. The professional fire service personnel provide excellent training programmes for health service staff.

Some patients, perhaps especially those who express anxiety about the risk of fire or who are known to have experienced a fire, may welcome being told about the fire precautions in the ward.

The prevention of fire in hospital has had considerable publicity recently via the mass media and patients are more aware of the potential danger, probably partly because in the UK public buildings have been obliged by law to instal smoke doors in public corridors — and they cannot escape one's notice!

Risks associated with medications

At home many people have a personal medication routine such as taking medications orally; inhaling them from a nasal spray; applying them to the skin; putting medicated drops or ointment into the eye; injecting them from a syringe; inserting them in the form of a suppository into the rectum or in the form of a pessary into the vagina. People are responsible in their own homes for maintaining safety in relation to these medications whether they are self-prescribed or doctor-prescribed.

Maintaining safety in relation to medications is a personal responsibility while at home. In hospital, however, the patient usually forfeits this responsibility (it should be noted that in some hospitals, patients are in charge of their own medications; Gaze, 1992) and becomes dependent on nursing, medical and pharmaceutical staff. In these circumstances, in the interests of patient safety, nurses become accountable for giving the correct medicine, at the correct time, in the correct dose, by the correct route to the correct patient.

Due to the potential danger of medications, and in the safety interests of all members of society, most countries legislate to control them. In the UK the Misuse of Drugs Act 1971 and its various amendments are in force. Very strict rules apply to those in the Act called 'controlled drugs'; each dose has to be accounted for in a Controlled Drugs Register, whether it is given in hospital or in the home.

In 1992, the UK Central Council for Nursing, Midwifery and Health Visiting issued guidance about the administration of medicines, whether in a community or a hospital setting. The document makes it quite clear that notwithstanding the expected adherence of registered medical practitioners and pharmacists to specific criteria for prescribing and dispensing medicines, registered nurses, midwives and health visitors are accountable for their own practice — as stated in the Council's Code of Professional Conduct (UKCC, 1992). They are personally responsible for keeping up-to-date with current practices but must also:

> 'acknowledge any limitations in knowledge and competence, and decline any duties or responsibilities unless able to perform them in a safe and skilled manner.'

On rare occasions, medication mistakes are made. The document stresses that the Council's Professional Conduct Committee takes care to distinguish between instances where the error:

- resulted from reckless practice and was concealed

- resulted from serious pressure of work and there was immediate honest disclosure in the patient's interest.

Although recognizing the prerogative of managers to take local disciplinary action, the Council urges that each incident should be considered in its context, along with a thorough investigation of the circumstances which led to the medication error. Nursing staff should not be penalised for making a mistake which might be associated with overwork or poor management.

Compliance with a prescribed medication régime may be a problem. Quite often when a person is discharged from hospital, medications are prescribed as part of their continuing care and this is particularly so with older people. According to Williams (1991) about three-quarters of elderly people in the UK take prescribed medications, often more than one, and a multidrug régime can cause confusion leading to non-compliance or overdosage, both of which carry risks. During a hospital stay, therefore, to minimize the risk of problems, a teaching programme about discharge medications should be discussed by members of the multidisciplinary team, including the pharmacist. It is then the role of the nurse to discuss the régime with the patient and carers before discharge, and to implement a plan prefaced by several assessments including:

- the person's ability to self-medicate: even those who are less able, intellectually or emotionally, can perform satisfactorily if given suitable instruction about the medication, potential side-effects, and mode and time of administration
- the support available at home: carers, community staff
- the need for aids such as suggested by Clarence (1992):
  type of labelling
  diaries, calendars, charts
  compliance packaging, e.g. blister packs
  special containers, caps, systems
  Braille markings for people with visual difficulties
- the form of community monitoring and evaluation and by whom
- the type of help required to ensure attendance at follow-up appointments.

Burns et al (1992) carried out a study to assess compliance among elderly patients, and a study by Williams (1993) highlighted potential solutions for people with ophthalmic difficulties.

Favrod (1993) describes a study involving people with schizophrenia who had been referred to a rehabilitation centre. He worked on the premise that psychosocial treatment with anti-psychotic medication can improve the care of people with schizophrenia, but poor compliance with medication régimes and discontinuation of anti-

psychotic medication are key factors in relapse. He adapted a medication management module developed in USA and concluded it was a useful tool for helping individuals to adopt a more collaborative role which improved their ability to comply; and it also improved the relationships of staff with people who had a long-term mental health problem.

Apart from risks to patients related to medications, nurses themselves may be at risk, for example, when handling cytotoxic medications which are being used in the treatment of cancer. It is, therefore, important for staff to adhere strictly to guidelines regarding the use of protective clothing, especially gloves, when administering them, and also when disposing of any spillages; for their own safety and also for the safety of patients and other staff.

Perhaps the importance of preventing potential problems from becoming actual problems is more obvious in this AL than in some others. And one of the major ways of emphasizing prevention is through health teaching. Health teaching does not necessarily imply an elaborate preplanned programme of instruction; it does involve being alert to cues from the clients and assessing the appropriate time to discuss issues which they and the nurse consider important to the client's circumstances. There may be numerous opportunities for health teaching in the course of a nurse/client relationship; on the other hand, the patient/client may be coping adequately, and therein lies a skilled nursing judgement — knowing when to withdraw.

PLANNING AND IMPLEMENTING NURSING ACTIVITIES AND EVALUATING OUTCOMES

Customarily planning, implementing and evaluating are three phases of the process of nursing and they are entirely dependent on the assessing phase.

When it is appropriate to assess the individual in relation to this AL, we suggest that our conceptualization of nursing is a useful framework. It takes account of:

- the individual's stage on the lifespan
- the individual's dependence/independence status for this AL
- the factors (biological, psychological, sociocultural, environmental and politicoeconomic) which might influence the individual's behaviour in relation to this AL.

Box 4.10 gives a resumé of the type of information which could be used when assessing a client/patient in relation to this AL.

The objective of assessment, of course, is to identify actual and potential problems. It aims to:

- prevent potential problems from becoming actual ones
- solve actual problems
- prevent solved problems from recurring
- alleviate problems which cannot be solved
- help the person to develop positive coping behaviour for problems which cannot be solved or alleviated.

Having identified relevant actual and potential problems, the next step is to devise a nursing plan in collaboration with the person when possible, or with the family/ significant others. This is done in order to set goals (outcomes, objectives) to be achieved; to state how the goals will be evaluated; and to identify the nursing interventions which would be conducive to their achievement (Appendix 1). All nursing staff have to be aware of the plan so that their activities can be coordinated.

For example, a patient might have been admitted to a mental health unit with a psychotic disorder characterized by violent behaviour. In this example, one potential problem is violent behaviour, and a planned goal would be 'no violent episodes' thereby maintaining a safe environment for the person, other patients and the staff. Nursing action to achieve this could, among other things, involve observing the patient for early signs of irritation and restlessness (according to Fairlie and Brown, 1994, research has shown that such people often become more agitated in the late afternoon and evening) and intervening in order to defuse the situation without alienating the patient, thus preventing a potential violent incident. This, along with other goals, would be recorded on the nursing plan so that all staff were aware of the goal; were able to report whether or not the patient had exhibited pre-violent behaviour; and if so, the success or failure of the planned nursing implementation, namely preventive intervention. (Physical contact skills may be necessary but they are techniques of last resort. It is preferable to use the skills of prediction, de-escalation and negotiation.)

To cite another example, a community nurse might discuss with a young mother the care of her 12-month-old child who has been discharged from a paediatric unit following treatment for leg scalding; the mother had tripped on a kitchen rug while carrying a kettle of hot water, which caused the accident. One immediate goal that could be mutually agreed with the mother would be the prevention of infection in the wound area. Initially, the community nurse would do any necessary dressings but might subsequently help the mother to learn to do them safely, including appropriate handwashing procedures. A medium-term goal could be the presence of healed, healthy tissue over the area of the scald; and the eventual goal could be absence of scarring (plastic surgery might be required).

Another immediate goal would be the prevention of similar accidents and the nurse might discuss with the mother any potential accident hazards in the home and suggest appropriate safety measures. A third goal might be the containment of the mother's guilt feelings at causing the accident, and preventing undue stress; it would be important to listen to the mother as she divulged her anxieties. Regarding this third goal, the mother might find it difficult to accept the desirability of maintaining a balance between protecting her daughter from potential accidents yet allowing the freedom of movement so vital to a child's physical, psychological and social development.

As with any goal-setting, of course, it is important to evaluate the outcomes of nursing interventions in relation to the agreed goals. This is a complex matter particularly when, for this AL, goals often involve prevention of, for example, accidents, or incidents, or infections. Prevention is elusive to evaluate in terms of exact measurement. However, throughout the chapter, studies have been cited to indicate the effectiveness of certain measures:

- Box 4.14 suggests monitoring activities which can pre-empt violence in a mental health unit
- Box 4.5 gives several examples of activities which the community health nurse can discuss with a mother to prevent accidents and thus, through an effective teaching programme, help to maintain a safe environment in the home
- On p. 94 the importance of handwashing has been emphasized as one way of preventing wound infection.

It must be recognized, too, that maintaining a safe environment is an obvious example of an AL where the nurse, although identifying problems, does not necessarily work alone in helping to solve them, for example, air pollution or social disorder. Sometimes the main effort comes from government action (e.g. legislation about air pollution or about wearing seat belts), or local authority agencies, or involves a health team effort. Sometimes it is desirable to reinforce verbal discussion with printed material from health education groups or to encourage participation in special interest groups, which are often run by voluntary organizations.

Individualizing nursing has already been discussed in more detail in Chapter 3, and the complexities are overly simplified in Figure 3.9 but the idea is conveyed that feedback, reassessments and adjustments are frequently necessary as the client's problems are solved or changed, or as new problems arise.

Despite the overall importance of this AL in everyday living it is necessary to emphasize, as indicated on p. 37 that there are many instances when it may not be relevant to investigate or to document a client's circumstances in relation to the AL of maintaining a safe environment as such. This is a matter for professional judgement – a subtle mix of knowledge, skills and experience.

When it is necessary to enter this type of information on the nursing plan, it would be combined with information about the person's other relevant ALs. It is only for the purposes of discussion that any AL can be considered on its own; in reality, they are closely related and rarely have distinct boundaries.

REFERENCES

Appleton R 1994 Head injury rehabilitation unit for children. Nursing Times 90(22) June 1: 29–31

Bamber M 1994 Providing support for emergency service staff. Nursing Times 90(22) June 1: 32–33

Beaumont G 1992 Bad riddance to rubbish. Nursing Times 88(14) April 1: 63–64

Beedle D 1993 Beating the bug (methicillin-resistant staphylococcus aureus). Nursing Times (Infection Control) 89(45) November 10: 11–VI

Bell F, Fenton P 1993 Early hospital discharge and cross-infection. The Lancet 342(8863): 120

Benson S, Den A 1992 Monitoring violence (in psychiatric hospitals). Nursing Times 88(41) October 7: 46–48

Bowell B 1992 Infection control: protecting the patient at risk. Nursing Times 88(3) January 15: 32–35

Bowling A, Formby J, Grant K 1992 Accidents in elderly care (Part 1). Nursing Standard 6(29) April 8: 28–30 (Part 2, Part 3 on April 15, April 22)

Brookes A 1994 Surgical glove perforation. Nursing Times 90(21) May 25: 60–62

Burns J, Sneddon I, Lovell M 1992 Age and aging. 21(3): 178–181

Castledine G 1993 First-aid management of psychological emergencies: 2. British Journal of Nursing 2(21): 1079–1083

Clancy J, McVicar A 1993 Subjectivity of stress. British Journal of Nursing 2(8): 410–418

Clarence M 1992 Ensuring compliance with drug regimens. Nursing Standard 7(6) October 28: 24–26

Clulow M 1994 A closer look at disposable gloves: an assessment of the value of vinyl, latex and plastic gloves. Professional Nurse 9(5) February: 324–329

Crewe C 1993 Taking it out on themselves. Sunday Telegraph Review March 28: V

Dare J, Greenwood L 1994 Public outbreak (role of the 'public health nurse'). Nursing Times 90(2) January 12: 38–40

Dawkins J 1995 Bullying in schools; doctors' responsibilities. British Medical Journal 310(6975) February 4: 274–275

Department of Transport 1993 Accident Fact Sheet Series 2(5). DOT, London

Dias B 1992 Things that go bump (noise in hospital). Nursing Times 88(38) September 16: 36–38

Dillner L 1993 Boxing should be counted out say BMA Report. British Medical Journal 306(6892) June 12: 1561–1562

Eaton L 1994 Childhood memories (child abuse). Nursing Times 90(16) April 20: 14–15

Elliott P 1992 Handwashing: a process of judgement and effective decision-making. Professional Nurse 7(5) February: 292–296

Evans-Pritchard A 1993 Foreign news: America. The Sunday Telegraph October 24: 25

Fairlie A, Brown R 1994 Accidents and incidents involving patients in a mental health service. Journal of Advanced Nursing 19(5) May: 864–869

Favrod J 1993 Taking back control (schizophrenia). Nursing Times 89(34) August 25: 68–70

Ferry R 1994 Self-harm: complex causes. Nursing Times 90(3) January 19: 34–35

Ford R, Repper J 1994 Taking responsibility for care (mental health nurses in the Community). Nursing Times 90(31) August 3: 54–57

Frankel M, Hall C 1993 From perms to polymers: British inventor's new plastic baffles scientists. Newsweek CXXI (18) May 3: 19

Garraway W, Macleod D, Sharp J 1991 Rugby injuries. British Medical Journal 303(6810) November 2: 1082–1083

Garrett G 1986 Old age abuse by carers. The Professional Nurse 1(11) August: 304–305

Gaze H 1992 Better late than never. Nursing Times 88(15) April 8: 30–31

Godlee F 1992 Noise: breaking the silence. British Medical Journal 304(6819) January 11: 110–113

Gould D 1992 Hygienic hand decontamination. Nursing Standard 6(32) April 29: 33–36

Gould D 1994 A study of glove use. Nursing Times 90(30) July 27: 57–62

Gould D, Ream E 1993 Assessing nurses' hand decontamination performance. Nursing Times 89(25) June 23: 47–50

Hilton A 1987 The hospital racket: how noisy is your unit? American Journal of Nursing January: 59–61

Hodgkinson P, Stewart M 1991 Coping with catastrophes: a handbook of disaster management. Routledge, London

Horton R 1993 Nurses' knowledge of infection control. Nursing Standard 7(41) June 30: 25–29

Jerram T 1994 Book Review. Recovery from cults: help for victims of psychological and spiritual abuse. British Medical Journal 308(6937) April 30: 1175

Journal of Nursing Management 1994 Hand dryers emit bacteria claims university report. Journal of Nursing Management 2(3) May: 149

Kay B 1995 Challenging behaviours. CE Article 341. Nursing Standard 9 (24) March 8: 31–36

Kingston P, Penhale B 1994 A major problem needing recognition: Assessment and management of elder abuse and neglect. Professional Nurse 9(5) February: 343–347

Knowles H 1993 The experience of infectious patients in isolation. Nursing Times 89(30) July 28: 53–56

Laurent C 1993 Old and at risk. Nursing Times 89(38) September 22: 20–21

Law M 1993 Spearheading the fight against infection: the role of the Infection Control Nurse. Professional Nurse July: 626–631

Lawrence C 1992 Testing alcohol wipes. Nursing Times 88(34) August 19: 63–66

Maimaris C, Summers C, Browning C, Palmer C 1994 Injury patterns in cyclists attending an accident and emergency department: a comparison of helmet-wearers and non-wearers. British Medical Journal 308(6943) June 11: 1537–1540

Mason P 1993 Safety measures. Nursing Times 89(6) February 10: 22–23

Murdoch S 1992 A safe environment for care: infection control nurses' role in mental health units. Professional Nurse 7(8) May: 519–522

Murrell A 1993 Unlocking the virus: providing support and treatment for people with hepatitis. Professional Nurse 8(12) September: 780–783

National Society for Prevention of Cruelty to Children 1993 Annual Report. NSPCC, London

News 1994 Report highlights hidden adult abuse. Nursing Times 90(15) April 13: 5

Nursing Times News 1994 Latex gloves pose hidden health risk. Nursing Times 90(32) August 10: 5

Oakley K 1994 Making sense of universal precautions. Nursing Times 90(27) July 6: 35–36

O'Dwyer F, Dalton A, Pearce J 1991 Adolescent self-harm patients: audit of an assessment in an accident and emergency department. British Medical Journal 303(6803) September 14: 629–630

Pawlikowska T, Chalder T, Hirsch S, Wallace P, Wright D, Wessely S 1994 Population based study of fatigue and psychological distress. British Medical Journal 308(6931) March 19: 763–766

Ralph K, Alexander J 1994 Borne under stress. Nursing Times 90(12) March 23: 28–30

Ramprogus V, Gibson J 1991 Assessing restraints. Nursing Times 87(26) June 26: 45–47

Ravenscroft T 1994 After the crisis (post-traumatic stress disorder). Nursing Times 90(12) March 23: 26–28

Rayner T 1994 Understanding self-harm. Nursing Times 90(3) January 19: 30–31

Royal College of Nursing 1994 Guidelines on Infection Control. RCN, London

Royal Society for the Prevention of Accidents 1994 Home Safety Fact Sheet: the hidden epidemic. ROSPA, Birmingham

Royal Society for the Prevention of Accidents 1993 Road accidents. ROSPA, Birmingham

Sharp J 1994 Infections in sport. British Medical Journal 308(6945) June 25: 1702–1706

Shirtcliffe D 1995 Risk-taking for clients with learning disabilities. Nursing Times 91(5) February 1: 40–42

Siu A 1994 Methicillin-resistant staphylococcus aureus: do we just have to live with it? British Journal of Nursing 3(15): 753–759

Social Services Inspectorate 1993 No longer afraid. HMSO, London

Soutar R, Wilson J 1986 Does hospital noise disturb the patient? British Medical Journal 292(6516) February 1: 305

Sutton J, Standen P, Wallace A 1994 Incidence and documentation of patient accidents in hospital. Nursing Times 90(33) August 17: 29–35

Sweeting H 1994 Patient fall prevention — a structured approach. Journal of Nursing Management 2(4) July: 187–192

Thomas S, Acton C, Nixon J, Battistutta D, Pitt W, Clark R 1994 Effectiveness of bicycle helmets in preventing head injury in children: case-control study. British Medical Journal 308(6922) January 15: 173–176

Thompson L 1993 The danger in medicine pots. Nursing Times 89(29) July 21: 67

Tonks A 1993 Cost of sports injuries may be justified. British Medical Journal 306(6886) May 1: 1148

Tonks A 1994 Drug resistance is a world wide threat. British Medical Journal 309(6962) October 29: 1109

Trevelyan J 1994a Global awareness. Nursing Times 90(10) March 9: 28–30

Trevelyan J 1994b A woman's lot. Nursing Times 90(15) April 13: 48–50

United Kingdom Central Council for Nursing, Midwifery and Health Visiting 1992 Code of Professional Conduct for the Nurse, Midwife and Health Visitor. UKCC, London

United Kingdom Central Council for Nursing, Midwifery and Health Visiting 1992 Standards for the Administration of Medicines. UKCC, London

United Nations 1991 Women: Challenges to the Year 2000. UN, New York

Viant A 1992 Cleaning of hospital mattresses. Nursing Standard 6(21) February 12: 36–37

White C 1992 News: Female sexual abusers are not rare. British Medical Journal 304(6832) April 11: 935–936

White Paper 1990 This common inheritance. HMSO, London

Williams B 1991 Medication education. Nursing Times 87(29) July 17: 50–52

Williams M 1993 Achieving patient compliance. Nursing Times 89(13) March 31: 50–52

World Health Organization 1993 Implementation of the Global Strategy for Health for All by the Year 2000. WHO, Geneva

ADDITIONAL READING

Campbell J 1995 Making sense of clinical features of inflammation. Nursing Times 91(14) April 5: 32–33

Emerson E, McGill P, Mansell J (Ed) 1994 Severe learning disabilities and challenging behaviours. Chapman and Hall, London

Hancock R, Jarvis C 1994 Long term effects of being a carer. HMSO, London

Higgins C 1994 An introduction to the examination of specimens. Nursing Times 90(47) November 23: 29–32

Kingston P, Bennett G 1993 Elder abuse theories, concepts and interventions. Chapman and Hall, London

McLatchie G 1993 Essentials of sports medicine. Churchill Livingstone, Edinburgh

Macmillan Magazines 1994 The carers guide. Macmillan Magazines, Basingstoke

Meadow R 1993 The ABC of child abuse. British Medical Journal Publishing Group, London

Twigg J, Atkin K 1994 Carers perceived: policy and practice in informal care. Open University Press

5 Communicating

The AL of communicating

Man is essentially a social being and spends the major part of each day communicating with other people in one way or another. The activity of communicating is therefore an integral part of all human behaviour.

There is now considerable knowledge from research in the behavioural sciences about body or non-verbal language, use of which can enrich the AL of communicating. And even in the more familiar mode of verbal language, research has uncovered some interesting and illuminating aspects.

An understanding of the complexities of both components of communicating is likely to help people to carry out this AL in a manner which is effective and brings satisfaction to themselves and others. But what does 'communicating' mean?

The process of communicating

The study of cybernetics has contributed considerably to the understanding of the process of communicating. As long ago as 1960, in a classic work, Berlo proposed a model of communication which consists of four distinct components. These are:

(1) Source
(2) Message
(3) Channel
(4) Receiver.

Communication is said to occur when a person (the source) has a message which he sends in a particular medium (channel), so that it is received by a recipient (receiver). This process has been adapted to form a two-way model in which the communication elicits a response in the receiver. The response in turn causes the receiver to become the source of a return message which is sent via a chosen channel, thus providing feedback to the original source (Fig. 5.1).

Broadly speaking, communication generally utilises two main channels. These are 'verbal' and 'non-verbal'. Verbal communication consists of the spoken or written word, whereas non-verbal communication includes paralanguage and kinetics.

Wiggens et al (1994) use the term 'paralanguage' to define the non-semantic

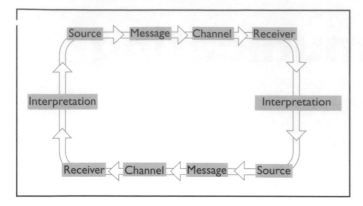

Fig. 5.1 Basic model of communicating (adapted from Berlo, 1960)

aspects of verbal communication which we use to express the meaning that our words convey. Paralanguage concerns *how* we use language, rather than what we say. It includes the tone of voice, the speed with which we speak and our use of 'filler' sounds such as 'um' and 'er'. Such communication can be said to be vocal rather than verbal.

The study of non-verbal communication or body language is now receiving much more attention and the term 'kine' has been adopted for each 'unit' of body movement which transmits a message. The kine is analogous to a letter in the verbal alphabet. Kinetics is still a young science, but it would seem that human ability to exert conscious control over body language is less easy than with verbal communication and most people, at times, are aware of sending contradictory messages. For example, in response to a ring of the doorbell the words 'Do come in, I'm pleased to see you' might be spoken while the facial expression might say 'I'm busy, I wish you hadn't called'.

Non-verbal communication serves a number of purposes depending on the context. The whole body may be conveying a message. Humans use their bodies to express themselves for instance in the way they walk. Walking boldly into a room may be indicative of a feeling of well-being; on the other hand it may be conveying a mood of anger, so analysis of further cues is required to differentiate. In contrast, walking slowly into a room may indicate reticence or apprehension. The stance people take, too, can transmit an impression as varied as boredom, exhaustion, attentiveness and interest.

Facial expression is a rich source of information regarding the emotional state of the individual and some evidence of this can be found in the amount of space and time authors and playwrights give to describing the facial changes in their characters. One can transmit impressions such as disapproval, disgust, anger, irritation, pleasure, love and understanding by facial gesture; indeed its effectiveness is recognized in colloquial expressions such as 'a look enough to kill' or 'a sour look'. The eyes can be par-

ticularly revealing, and people vary in the amount of eye contact they make and maintain while communicating. Eye contact has been shown to be one of the factors which controls the extent to which people participate in a conversation, with 'looking' acting rather as does punctuation in a piece of text (Argyle, 1994). Paralanguage can also provide a similar moderating function.

Hands are particularly important to body language, usually to provide points of emphasis, while shaping with the hands the object being discussed, or an event, or signalling directions. Hands also convey emotion, for example the interviewee attending a selection panel who reflects inner anxiety by restless, wringing movements or fiddling with small objects; or the angry person who shows white knuckles or clenched fists. Feet, too, are used in communicating, for example toe-tapping may express feelings as diverse as a degree of anxiety, or enjoyment of the rhythm of music.

It is apparent that physical appearance and presence are powerful aspects of non-verbal communication, and the amount and variety of make-up products, jewellery, perfume, aftershave, spectacle frames in department stores is an eloquent reflection of the range of taste. Clothes, too, although essentially intended to protect from the elements, provide a great deal of information about the wearer. They can express current mood, state of finance, preparation to take part in sport, or to go to work. Indeed, the term 'language of clothes' is quite commonly used and is discussed in more detail in the chapter dealing with the AL of personal cleansing and dressing (p. 234).

Verbal and non-verbal communication can occur simultaneously. A verbal communication may, for example, take the form of a conversation. At the beginning of the conversation one person (the source) has an idea which becomes the message. The message is encoded in language signals and is sent by speaking (channel). The other person (receiver) hears the signals, decodes and interprets by attaching meaning to them (interpretation). This may be accompanied by a smile or spoken in sarcasm with a mocking expression. The paralanguage will affect the interpretation of the words, as does the associated body language.

Communicating is a highly individual activity. An individual's previous experience can affect, either consciously or unconsciously, how a person interprets interactions which involve communication. Memory therefore has an important influence on the process of communicating. Communicators bring to the conversation their attitudes, beliefs, values and prejudices, these being fashioned by previous experience which must necessarily be affected by social background. The contribution of each person is affected by their current needs: the need to be dominant or submissive; the need to be talkative or silent and so on.

Yet in discussing communicating, it is not the individual who is crucial; it is the interpersonal relationship. To understand the AL of communicating one has to understand how people relate to each other. Although both verbal and non-verbal forms of communication are complementary Argyle (1994) suggests that non-verbal signals are used more effectively than words to convey emotions and attitudes. On the other hand verbal communication is the usual medium for the dissemination of factual information.

Effective communication, of course, is dependent on the communicators' several abilities within the verbal language component, notably those of thinking, speaking, listening, reading and writing (Fig. 5.2). However the necessary skills within the body language component are also of enormous importance.

There are many aspects of the enormous subject of communicating and in this chapter only a sample of topics have been selected to discuss within the concepts of our model — lifespan, dependence/independence, factors influencing the AL, individualizing nursing for the AL of communicating (Fig. 5.3).

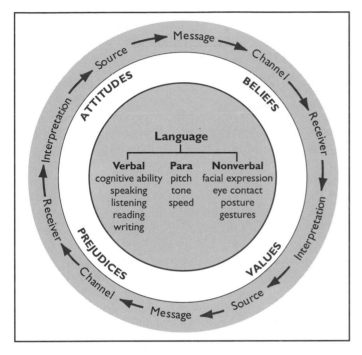

Fig. 5.2 The complexities of communicating

Lifespan: relationship to the AL of communicating

Childhood and adolescence

The lifespan component of the model is particularly

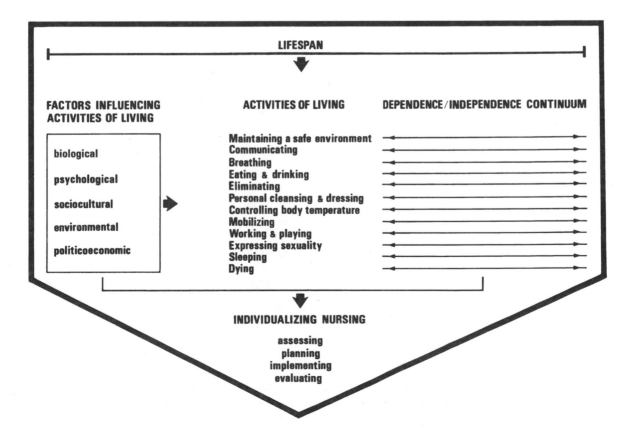

Fig. 5.3 The AL of communicating within the model for nursing

relevant to the AL of communicating. Even in the pre-natal period the fetus is communicating that it is growing in size; and in the later months of pregnancy that it is capable of movement. The baby's first worldly experience of non-verbal communication, however, is usually the touch of the midwife's or obstetrician's hands or sometimes the mother's hands and everyone present at the delivery is relieved to hear the initial cry, the first verbal communication. Thereafter the infant experiments with cooing and babbling and soon can sense the 'meaning' of words and phrases from how they are spoken, and by the volume, intonation and so on. The baby is then ready to associate words with objects or people, and later begins to utter the correct word in response. By a long process the child gradually learns and uses an increasing vocabulary.

A vital aspect of this learning is the stimulation from other people in the environment especially the mother or mother substitute who by speaking and singing to the child, and touching and cuddling, provides the basic experiences for interpersonal communication which are so crucial to further development. Indeed, children deprived of such stimulation may grow up to have difficulty with human relationships.

During adolescence, the teenager may develop special meanings for certain words known only to the peer group and not understood by adults. However as well as this private communication channel, most adolescents extend their vocabulary and modes of expression, verbally and non-verbally, as they move away from the constraints of home and school contacts, and explore new environments with different types of relationship.

Adulthood and old age

It is estimated that the majority of adults have a speaking vocabulary of 3000 to 5000 words although their reading vocabulary may well be more. On the other hand there are those whose speaking vocabulary contains only a few hundred words of not more than three syllables and their reading vocabulary not many more. Often current slang and colloquialisms make up the bulk of such people's language. These factors will naturally have their effect on acquisition of writing skills.

In old age, deterioration of vision and hearing can lessen the ability to communicate effectively by causing distortion of sensory input. Also there is a gradual loss of function of some brain cells which can result in forgetfulness and sometimes confusion. Arthritic finger joints can make writing difficult. Frailty can interfere with body posture and gesture and therefore with body language. All these factors may contribute to problems in the older person's AL of communicating.

Dependence/ independence in the AL of communicating

Communicating is an AL where movement along the dependence/independence continuum has a direct relationship with the lifespan component of the model.

Dependent status

Even when a baby is born with the intact body structures required for communicating, it is necessary to learn to use those structures, to perceive, and to attach meaning to discrete sounds. Stimulation from parents enhances the speed of learning, and great patience is required to perceive and decode the communicating done by babies and children, both verbally and non-verbally.

On the other hand, adults can be curiously lacking in perception. An extreme example would be an instance when there are signs of child abuse and the cues are not picked up by people outside the home setting. Another example is the puzzling situation when an otherwise bright, healthy child has difficulty mastering reading and spelling — a syndrome labelled as dyslexia — and investigation is delayed because cues are overlooked by adults; once recognized, a special educational programme can often compensate.

The young are certainly dependent on others for help with the AL of communicating and likewise, sometimes the elderly, those with learning difficulties, and those with certain mental health problems and physical disabilities.

Coping strategies to enhance independence

Physical body structure, of course, influences the degree of dependence in communicating. Intact physical structures which enable one to see, hear, taste, smell and touch, and those which permit speech and body language are basic to independence, although some degree of impairment can often be compensated for or coped with. However, quite apart from highly specialized surgical techniques, mechanical aids can do much to lessen the disability of impaired body structure, for example:

- the problem of diminished sight can be reduced or corrected by using contact lenses, spectacles or an illuminated magnifying glass; and for those who are severely disabled, the use of specially prepared large-print books or Braille or tape-recordings can help considerably in retaining a measure of independence
- for those who have impaired auditory structure

and function, it is possible now to have quite sophisticated, unobtrusive hearing aids which dramatically improve their quality of living, and there are also amplifiers available for telephone conversations and public meetings

- for those who have difficulties with speech a sign language is useful and especially for mentally disabled people who have speech difficulties, there are symbolic languages such as the Bliss Symbolic Communication System and the Makaton Vocabulary Language Programme which have greatly improved their capacity for communicating

- over a decade ago, it was quite revolutionary to provide an aid, called Possum, for those who were tetraplegic; it enabled the paralysed person, by blowing on a type of keyboard, to manipulate light switches, radio and television sets, telephone and so on. However, more recent technological advances have made possible a robot which can be programmed to carry out a range of services on command. These developments hold great promise for severely disabled people who, although dependent on a machine, can have a feeling of relative independence; their range of control in communicating and getting an appropriate response is increased and they are less dependent on people to carry out a number of everyday living activities.

Factors influencing the AL of communicating

Like all other ALs, communicating is influenced by a variety of factors. In keeping with the relevant component of the model, these are discussed under the following headings — biological, psychological, sociocultural, environmental and politicoeconomic factors.

BIOLOGICAL

Many biological factors influence a person's ability to communicate by means of verbal and non-verbal language, and especially important are adequately functioning body structures in the nervous and endocrine systems.

Functioning body structures

For the acquisition of speech there has to be at least adequate hearing, an adequately functioning speech apparatus and the opportunity to hear others' voices for imitation. The achievement of reading skills requires at least minimal vision, and the accomplishment of writing skills is further dependent on an adequately functioning preferred hand. Communicating by body language is dependent on adequately functioning nervous and musculoskeletal systems and any publicly discernible structural disability may affect, for example, stance, gait, gesture and influence the message received by the onlooker (p. 120).

Hormone production is also related, although less obviously, to communicating. The sex hormones are responsible for the distinguishable difference between the male and female voice. Structurally the male larynx is on average longer anteriorly/posteriorly so that the male voice after puberty is lower in pitch than that of the female. However both males and females differ in the control which they have over the many muscles, including the diaphragm, used in voice production. Thus some people have low, monotonous voices and others can modulate the voice for effective and varied expression.

There are also differences related to patterns of physical contact as a means of communicating between males, between females, and between males/females; and these are mentioned in Chapter 15 when expressing sexuality is discussed.

Physical aspects of language use

Having the physical body structures to make verbal communicating possible, of course, presupposes the existence of language, and use of language involves a number of physical skills mainly speaking and listening; reading and writing.

- *Speaking* involves not only what is said but equally importantly, how it is said. With practice, the clarity, speed, pitch, inflection and tone of voice can all be used to convey exact meaning (paralanguage). In response to a request, the answer 'I don't mind doing it' can be said in a pleasant positive manner, assuring the listener that the task will be done willingly. On the other hand it can be said in a grudging negative manner leaving the listener uncomfortable and possibly guilty at having made the request.

- *Listening* is much more than hearing; it is an active process whereby the listener attends exclusively to the speaker, not only to the words spoken. There are advantages to listening in a face-to-face conversation which communication links such as the telephone and tape recorder do not offer, although being in the presence of the speaker is not an absolute prerequisite for 'effective listening'. For instance a telephone listening service is offered to people in distress by associations such as the

Samaritans. The listeners are trained to hear and interpret silences, sighs, sobs and so on and however mundane the problem may seem, the reception is non-judgemental.

- *Reading* is a skill which many people take for granted. Yet even in developed countries there is concern about the extent of illiteracy among adults, and special classes are offered to cope with this problem. Many readers are hindered by inaudibly 'pronouncing' each word rather than scanning a group of words to get the meaning of a sentence and rapid reading classes can be helpful in correcting this deficiency.
- *Writing* is often taken for granted, yet there are adults who are at a disadvantage because they cannot write their name. Adult literacy campaigns aim to improve writing as well as reading. But even so-called educated people can have difficulty in writing fluently, especially when under stress as, for example, in an examination setting or when emotionally upset.

Even from this brief outline, it can be seen therefore that the apparently physical activities of speaking, listening, reading and writing have other dimensions; according to the circumstances, psychological, social and politicoeconomic factors (as indicated in our model) are often inter-related. Nevertheless, to indicate how human biology relates to our model for nursing the authors suggest that the AL of communicating be particularly associated with the larynx containing the vital vocal cords, and the mouth, tongue and lips; the nervous system including the sense organs; and the endocrine system. This juxtaposition of AL and body system gives guidance for curriculum planning, and also for knowing where to record problems, actual and potential, related to the AL of communicating if our model is used as a guideline for nursing plans (Appendix 1).

PSYCHOLOGICAL

Communicating involves a variety of complex, psychological behaviours which are difficult to slot into specific categories.

Level of intelligence

Level of intelligence undoubtedly affects communicating in that it influences learning ability. It therefore plays an important part in the extent of the vocabulary acquired for use in everyday living. Most written languages have an alphabet, and in English everyone is familiar with the 26 letters from which many thousands of words can be constructed, each having a dictionary definition to help the process of communicating.

A person with a limited vocabulary can usually manage well in familiar surroundings but may experience difficulty, for instance when filling in many of the forms which have become a feature of our modern society. Furthermore, a person with a learning disability who has a slower learning capacity will take longer to achieve their potential in the AL of communicating. However, problems can arise even for 'intelligent' people with an extensive vocabulary, for example, when they are communicating with someone on a subject other than their own specialty.

Communicating, both verbal and non-verbal, and deliberate or non-planned, is the basis of all activities associated with learning and teaching, and there is a considerable literature about the contribution of psychological principles in the approach to information-giving, teaching, and counselling. These psychological principles are used in everyday living related, for example, to child development, all aspects of organized education, the impact of the mass media, and also in a variety of community services including health care services.

Emotions

Emotions are also important when communicating, as people going for an interview know only too well; interviewees may come away feeling annoyed that their ability to respond fluently has been impaired and they have not done themselves justice. For others, in spite of adequate content in their conversation, the non-verbal behaviour of tremulous hands, dilated pupils, perspiration on brow and upper lip, can inform the interviewer of the state of tension.

Current mood also has its effect on communicating. Excitement usually increases the rate of speech, raises the voice pitch and there may be more than usual gesticulation. Anger is usually expressed by raising the voice. Depression flattens the voice almost to monotony; movement is slowed, and a dejected facial expression is characteristic of many people when they are in a low mood. In comparison, cheerfulness lightens the voice, and is likely to be reflected in a smiling expression. Of course communication is two-way, and the mood of the recipients is also important for effective communication. It is not uncommon to refer to a 'hostile audience' or a 'receptive audience'.

Loss of self-respect and faith in self may make communicating a problematic activity. In such circumstances, an event which normally would be considered insignificant might produce a reaction of worthlessness, guilt or shame; or might provoke over-criticism of others, probably a subconscious effort to raise self-esteem. Those who have not experienced some type of long-term, warm, trusting relationship in their early years often lack self-confidence and may find it difficult to communicate effectively with other people.

Some people are aware of their lack of self-confidence. As one of a variety of possible techniques to develop self-confidence, it is sometimes suggested that 'assertiveness training' (AT) is helpful, the idea being that stress is reduced if one knows, in appropriate circumstances, how to be assertive — communicating effectively amid conflict (Williams & Kallmark, 1993) — rather than aggressive, rude or bossy. Fessey (1988) maintains that assertiveness techniques should be used only if a need requires expression or a right is about to be denied. She writes:

'. . . assertiveness skills help to focus the emphasis of the request on the specific problem, and prevent the asserted comment from being aggressive or intensely personal. In this way, the respondent's self-esteem is not severely diminished . . . the technique appears simple but requires an examination of the values and attitudes which shape our responses to others. This process can be painful and revealing but it leads to greater self-awareness — the first step to unambiguous communication.'

The importance of self-awareness is also emphasized by Slater (1990) when describing a group approach to 'enabling' rather than 'teaching' nurses about assertiveness. Enabling assertiveness may be beneficial to patients/clients also and Barker (1990) commends AT for people with severe mental health problems (Box 5.1) Burnard (1992) uses an Open Learning Programme to discuss assertiveness and nursing, a topic he considers to be closely linked to human relationships.

Human relationships

One main purpose of communicating is to establish and maintain human relationships. Most people imagine that they are fairly competent communicators; adults have been doing it all their lives! In fact, it is all too easy to conclude that if one's message is misunderstood, the receiver is at fault; and if the other person's attempt to communicate is not understood, then the other person's mode of expression is deficient in some way. The individual's interpretation of a situation is based on personal beliefs about communication competence — one's own and the other person's — and these beliefs affect how the individual relates to others, and how others relate to the individual.

A lot depends on how individuals view themselves. This self-perception is said to start at birth as the infant begins to develop a feeling of trust. With a feeling of trust comes, among other things, the ability to recognize personal strengths and weaknesses, the development of self-respect and faith in oneself, the development of respect and concern for others; all of which are essential for the establishment and maintenance of human relationships, and are basic to the AL of communicating.

Body image

An important factor in communicating, perhaps especially in non-verbal communicating, is body image. Price (1990) discusses body reality, body ideal and body presentation (an effort to balance reality and ideal) then goes on to suggest a model to assist nurses in assessing patients' body-image needs, thereby improving the nurse's approach to people who might be facing for example, mental or physical rehabilitation, or radical surgery (p. 364). To some degree, body image is linked to physical body structure and the topic is mentioned again on p. 119.

SOCIOCULTURAL

Now more than ever, an increasingly mobile and multiracial society demands that consideration be given to sociocultural factors in communicating.

Verbal language

Foong (1992) discusses potential barriers to communication according to variables such as culture, social class, race, age and gender, and emphasizes that problems arise not only for ethnic groups who have difficulties with a second language; even within one language there can be several local vocabularies. Accent or dialect can communicate place of residence during acquisition of language; and it may take time for the listener to become accustomed to a different dialect. Social status can also be conveyed by language. For example in the UK, the range of vocabulary can be indicative of level of education attained; this can influence the type of job procured which determines economic bracket of income and in turn determines the person's social class according to the Registrar-General's classification (p. 316).

Box 5.1 Assertiveness training for people with mental health problems

The potential of AT to advance the all-round interpersonal effectiveness of people with severe mental health problems is well established quotes Barker (1990). Indeed, he continues, even people with schizophrenia can benefit from being encouraged to look positively, or assertively, at aspects of their psychotic experience. AT can provide a perspective on individuals and their rights as a base for developing holistic care.

Race/ethnicity

Unfortunately, miscommunication is sometimes related to racial differences. When considering mental health, of course, communicating is of paramount importance, and McMillan (1994) describes how one area in England provides psychological support in a community where Asians were not receiving a culturally-sensitive mental health service. He quotes the Department of Health Guidelines on Ethnicity and Health (1993), and Carlisle (1994) describes the Black Mental Health Users and Carers Project. However, there need not always be obstacles. Butrin (1992) considered the cultural diversity between a group of nurses (American-born) and patients (overseas-born) and reported that two-thirds of their encounters during the patients' hospital stay were mutually satisfying experiences.

Technical language

Apart from dialect, accent, social class indicators or racial differences, the specialist vocabulary in certain occupations and professions is almost a 'language culture'. Technical expressions which are in everyday usage within an occupational group, can be totally alien to outsiders. For example, despite the computer revolution, the language of computer users still has to be interpreted to the uninitiated; and for clients in the health care system, the vocabulary of staff is often unintelligible or, when only snatches are over-heard and understood, is open to misinterpretation and can cause the client and family great distress.

It seems ironic that the spoken language can be a barrier to communication! In contrast, people who have no speech and hearing, use a sign language which, in one form or another, has international recognition.

Body language

Sociocultural differences also affect body language, for example, mode of dress can communicate such diverse information as a person's ethnic origin, religious affiliation, occupation or social group.

The acceptability of touching fellow humans also varies. Although communicating by touch is the most primitive mode for the infant, there are culturally determined touching patterns for adults. Some cultures permit a reciprocal hug to signal welcome on arrival, and again on departure to signal appreciation of the visit. The accepted practice in other cultures on these occasions is a kiss on each cheek; yet in others a kiss on the lips; in some it is nose-rubbing; and in others only reciprocal hand-shaking is acceptable.

There are also differences regarding the amount of gesticulation and mobility of the lips when communicating which are culturally determined. There are culturally determined practices related to eye contact, for example certain aborigines, to be polite, do not look into each other's eyes as they talk, whereas in the Western world it is polite to maintain eye contact during conversation.

Values/beliefs

The individual's social and cultural background usually influences the system of values and beliefs which determine behaviour, for example in the expression of spirituality via various ALs, possibly following a formal religion, or in the acquisition of a moral stance on particular issues. In our model, these are subsumed under sociocultural factors and are involved closely with the AL of communicating. Organized religions usually lay considerable stress on group interaction; and the selected places of worship, (sometimes enormously costly to build and maintain and often elaborately decorated), provide the focal point for communication, sometimes in groups or sometimes for personal communion with a god or deity.

A concept which is more encompassing than organized religion is spirituality (Labun, 1988) interpreted as a 'search for meaning' in one's life and encompassing theistic and non-theistic approaches, which applies to agnostics and atheists as well as followers of a recognized religious persuasion. Irrespective of personal interpretation of spirituality it can influence behaviour and the related system of values and beliefs can often bring comfort and reassurance during times of stress or when the individual is faced with moral dilemmas which require resolution.

Dyads and organizations

The simplest form of communication is dyadic, the individual with one other person such as a parent, a spouse, a partner, a friend, a colleague, but there are extensions of the dyad in the form of small group communication, as indeed happens even with children when they go to school and find opportunities for communicating with different children and adults, beyond the home setting. Eventually adults become members of more and more dyadic, small and large group communication systems.

A term often applied to a large group system is an organization and these are usually created to accomplish a specific purpose, for example a hospital is organized for the treatment of people with disease; and it is within a yet larger organization, a national health service, which in addition is responsible for maintenance of health, prevention of disease and rehabilitation.

In an organization such as a hospital, communicating is a means to an end, but in some organizations it is an end in itself. For example in schools and colleges and universities, the purpose is communication in a teaching/learning context. The mass media too are concerned essentially with communicating, usually *giving* information although it may also involve *exchange* in the form of readers' letters to a newspaper or phone-in programmes on radio and television. Of course the mass media are not concerned only with information giving/exchange; they also communicate in order to entertain. And this is true of the theatre, art and music. Music in fact is a universal language of a non-verbal nature which is rich in expression. It can be played, listened to, read and written throughout the world, irrespective of mother tongue and usually brings great satisfaction to sender and receiver.

ENVIRONMENTAL

The appropriateness of the physical environment can certainly contribute to the effectiveness of the AL of communicating. Poor ventilation in a room and extremes of temperature can be conducive to discomfort and interfere with concentration when communicating. Lighting, too, is important. Excessive light and glare can make a person feel too uncomfortable to converse, and poor lighting can mean that important non-verbal cues are missed. Soft lighting is deliberately used by restaurateurs to induce a feeling of relaxation, enhance the enjoyment of the meal, and promote pleasurable conversation.

Environmental noise can have an effect on communicating. Some people find it easier to speak about personal matters if there is background noise, be it music or the hum of conversation, while others find even the slightest noise distracting. Rooms which afford aural privacy usually help when personal matters need to be discussed, for example, an interview or consultation with a member of health care staff. In such a setting, too, conversation is more likely to be encouraged if the furniture is so arranged that the interviewee and the interviewer are not physically separated by a desk; that the chairs are reasonably comfortable and in a position to allow eye contact; and that there are no unplanned interruptions.

Apart from personal interviews, the physical layout of a room is important for any group work; chairs with desks in serried rows for example are not so conducive to discussion as chairs arranged in a circle or round a central table. This type of arrangement allows all members of the group to see who is speaking, to have eye contact, to observe body language and to maximize the impact of non-verbal cues which are so important to the AL of communicating.

POLITICOECONOMIC

The economic status of an individual will almost certainly be communicated to others in a variety of ways, for example by the choice of neighbourhood for a house, the choice of social circle and the type of occupation — at least in Western cultures.

Communicating can also be influenced by the economic status of the Local Government group which serves a neighbourhood. For example it may influence the availability of such services as play-groups and nursery schools when young children have wider opportunities to practice communicating; new types of activities and different relationships can be explored in these settings which add to the child's capacity to communicate and are critical at this stage of development.

Technological advances

Of course, technological advances have greatly enhanced the individual's capacity to communicate. In industrialized societies, even in lower economic echelons, most people have access to and are influenced by mass media communications in the form of newspapers, radio and television.

The availability of telephone, radio and television is often dependent however on services provided by government, so politicoeconomic decisions are involved and some would even maintain that the mass media provide opportunities for political pressure, and for communicating in the form of propaganda.

There is also an elaborate network of rapid, transworld data exchange. In fact, the Information Superhighway has been recognized as having such powerful potential that the world's richest industrial nations (G7) met in 1995 to discuss policy regarding standards and rules of access. They issued a communiqué:

> 'Progress in information technologies and communication is changing the way we live; how we work and do business; how we educate our children, study and do research; train ourselves; and how we are entertained . . . the smooth and effective transition towards the information society is one of the most important tasks that should be undertaken in the last decade of the 20th century.'

Undoubtedly the G7 governments foresee not only the scope for increased global communication but also the economic stakes in the Superhighway's potential.

So politicoeconomic decisions influence several forms of communicating, which inevitably affect the individual, the family, the community and the nation.

Technology and health care

Nowadays all large organizations — including hospitals or indeed a whole health service — are aware of the need for effective communication within and between different levels and grades of staff in order to achieve efficient management. There is widespread use of informal meetings, circulation of reports, notice board announcements, newsletters, fax machines, in addition to the communication associated with committee structures, official correspondence, and videoconferences. Many organizations in fact are overwhelmed by a superabundance of communications and look to computerization to solve some of the problems created by information bombardment.

A vision of the role information technology (IT) will play in health care over the next decade is outlined in Information Management and Technology (IM and T) Strategy for England produced by the NHS Management Executive in 1992 (Willis, 1994). It is envisaged that by the Year 2000:

- all large hospitals will have IT systems networked nationally and locally
- more than 90% of general practices will be computerized and similarly linked to their local hospitals
- family health services authority systems and the purchasers of local health services will have access to good quality IM and T for estimating local health needs and planning services.

To realize this vision, a massive infrastructure is required, says Willis (1994) but meanwhile, the Strategic Advisory Group on Nursing Information Systems (SAGNIS) has drawn up a document which:

'aims to give nurses support and direction as they grapple with the evolution of increasingly sophisticated information systems within their workplace, as well as growing expectations of how such systems can provide useful information for their practice.'

In the process, nurses will have to make some strategic decisions about the nursing input to patient records; records which it is envisaged will be shared by all professional groups (Box 5.2).

In the meantime, Kearsley et al (1994) describe a project using Nursing Information Systems (NIS) which they carried out to demonstrate the value of using a computer database to support quality monitoring of pressure sores; and in so doing they built up a 'care library' to support care planning by having a database of client problems, goals and actions which reflect research-based practice and hospital policies.

The use of technology in health care has enormous potential. The concept of telemedicine which, through computers, cameras and video monitors, enables a far-distant specialist to 'examine' a client in a doctor's office (e.g. in a remote rural area) could be duplicated in a client's home. In fact, advances in robotics and digital communication can give specialists the ability not only to assist with diagnoses but to treat people hundreds of miles away.

Technology and confidentiality

Of course, new technologies bring new problems, and

> **Box 5.2** Patient-based multiprofessional electronic records
>
> To evolve effective electronic records, Willis (1994) suggests, among other things, that:
>
> - nurses must decide what type of information they need to collect and how it will fit with the data of other health workers. It must be capable of being shared with other professional groups, and should not be collected unless it is of value
> - a reconsideration of working relationships among all health workers will be necessary. The use of simple, patient-based electronic records shared by all members of the team ('seamless care' quotes Finnegan, 1994) makes it imperative to recognize the role and contribution of each member of the team
> - health professionals will be forced to look at the language they use to define terms and their practice. Such terms would have to be computer-compatible and nationally agreed.

one cause for anxiety is the ease of retrieval of data. This is especially true of personal data, but also of enormous importance when research data or top secret intelligence are stored in computers. One of the concerns is the use of a password for computer security which, it is now found, can be abused with relative ease.

Other concerns such as theft of computers, hacking, computer viruses, inadvertently sending details to the wrong person or forgetting to log off a terminal (Barber, 1992) apply to computerization in general, but alarm is heightened about confidentiality in the IM and T Project, for example, because of its scale — more information and more people with access to it — and its universal nature.

In the UK, in 1984, the Data Protection Act provided legal safeguards to ensure that computerized personal health data about patients are available only to health professionals and not to groups such as the police, tax authorities, industry, and social services personnel. However, there are doubts about its effective applicability to the huge, ambitious IM and T Project. The British Medical Association, for example, is campaigning for public awareness of the problem and for a code of confidentiality which is legally binding, effectively policed, and the ultimate responsibility of the Secretary of State for Health (Tonks, 1993).

Politicoeconomic and legal factors have enormous potential to influence the AL of communicating in a nursing and health service context.

Individualizing nursing for the AL of communicating

ASSESSING THE INDIVIDUAL IN THE AL

One of the fascinating things about individuality in communicating is that each person develops a distinctive voice, instantly recognizable, for instance, on a telephone. Given the distinctiveness of voice, it is little wonder that people develop individuality in communicating, and this should be taken into account when individualizing nursing. Appropriate information can be obtained in the course of nursing assessment using as a mental framework, a knowledge of the topics outlined in the preceding part of this chapter (Box 5.3). While observing the client, and discussing relevant topics, the nurse could bear in mind the following questions:

- how does the individual usually communicate?
- what factors influence the way the individual carries out the AL of communicating?
- what does the individual understand about communicating?
- what are the individual's attitudes to communicating?
- has the individual any long-standing difficulties with communicating and how have these been coped with?
- what problems, if any, does the person have at present with communicating, or seem likely to develop?

The nurse will find answers to these types of question in the course of conversing with the person and the family and observing their behaviour; and there may also be relevant information in other records such as medical records to which the nurse has access — multiprofessional records are not yet in general use.

Box 5.3 Assessing the individual in the AL of communicating

Lifespan: effect on communicating
- Fetal growth and movement/birth cry
- Infancy and childhood — increasing skills/forming relationships
- Adolescence — extension of skills/relationships
- Adulthood — variety in performance
- Old age — gradual loss of activity/reduction in skills and relationships

Dependence/independence in communicating
- Unimpaired body structure and function
- Visual aids
- Hearing aids
- Speech aids
- Electronic aids

Factors influencing communicating
- Biological — intact body structure and function
  - speaking/voice pitch
  - hearing
  - seeing
  - reading
  - writing
  - gesticulating
- Psychological — intelligence/range of vocabulary/learning
  - self-confidence
  - self-respect, perception of self, and effect on perception of others
  - body image
  - prevailing mood
  - information giving, teaching and counselling
  - assertiveness
  - human relationships
- Sociocultural — mother tongue
  - dialect/accent
  - vocabulary
  - ethnicity and discrimination
  - personal appearance/dress
  - patterns of touching
  - eye contact/gesticulation
  - attitudes, values and beliefs
  - dyads and groups
- Environmental — temperature/ventilation
  - light
  - noise
  - type/size of room
  - arrangement of furniture
- Politicoeconomic — income
  - occupation
  - communication channels/mass media
  - computers
  - legislation to protect data/individual

IDENTIFYING ACTUAL AND POTENTIAL PROBLEMS

The collected information can then be examined, in collaboration with the individual when relevant, to identify any problems being experienced with the AL. The nurse may recognize potential problems and it may be appropriate to discuss them with the person so that mutual, realistic goals can be set to prevent potential problems from becoming actual ones; to alleviate or solve the actual problems; or to help the person cope with those which cannot be alleviated or solved.

Bearing in mind what the person can and cannot do independently the nursing interventions to achieve the set goals can then be selected according to local circumstances and available resources. These interventions should be recorded on the nursing plan along with the date on which evaluation will be carried out in order to decide whether or not the stated goals have been, or are being, achieved. All these actions, reactions and interactions are necessary in order to provide individualized nursing.

These same activities are used whatever the setting — home, clinic or hospital — and communicating is even more important (if that is possible), when a child is involved, or when the person has a learning disability or when the contact is made for mental health problems.

Particularly in hospital, communicating is the only means people have of acquiring information about their progress, telling staff of problems, keeping in contact with relatives and relating to other patients.

Many consumers have the highest praise for the effectiveness of communication with nursing staff but there is also, undoubtedly, a lot of criticism, and it is useful to outline some of the problems which can arise. Against the background of the general discussion in the first part of this chapter, the remainder of this section highlights some types of consumer problems related to communicating and the relevant nursing activities. They are grouped under headings which indicate how the problem can arise:

- Change of dependence/independence status
- Change of environment and routine
- Experience of pain.

CHANGE OF DEPENDENCE/INDEPENDENCE STATUS

It is understandable that with an Activity of Living which has so many dimensions, a number of variables can affect the individual's capacity to be independent. Any change in status can be influenced by the age of onset, perhaps congenital; the type of onset, sudden or gradual; the degree of difficulty, ranging from partial to complete; and whether or not the problem is reversible. Some of the main problems which people can encounter in relation to the AL of communicating are outlined below and often, the nurse works in collaboration with other professionals to assist the patient to achieve their potential.

Problems related to cognition

Children who are born with a learning disability frequently do not possess the necessary intellectual ability to communicate verbally so start life with a severe impediment as far as independence in communicating is concerned. However with painstaking teaching, many can learn to respond to verbal messages such as greetings and simple instructions, and many are able to learn to speak. For children who have a learning disability, non-verbal communication can assume greater importance than usual. Through play, physical contact, hand language and body language, these people can be encouraged to achieve their optimal level for communicating, and several studies are reported by Hunter (1987) where they, as well as brain-damaged people and those with mental health problems have been helped to learn, using computers.

Another problem related to cognition, called autism, involves a trio of impairments affecting communication, social interaction and imagination (Martell, 1994). The autistic child may develop only a limited, repetitive pattern of activities, and the social world and communication with others can be 'unpredictable, confusing and frightening'. Learning activities which can help such children to achieve their potential are described by Wimpory, 1991.

Impaired cognition can also follow an illness or an accident. Prior to the event, communication had not been a problem, and this loss of mental acuity may involve drastic changes in lifestyle related to employment and loss of earning capacity, as well as loss of self-respect and hardship to the family. The nurse needs to know how aware such patients are of the impairment, how they experience the impairment, and what they feel about it. They need to talk about what the change means in their lives; whether or not they will be able to communicate sufficiently to continue at work and carry out their leisure time activities. If they do not recognize their assets, it is important that they are helped to do so, and positive comment on whatever they accomplish will help them to regain self-respect.

Cognitive impairment — and memory deficit — is also a feature of Alzheimer's disease. It affects 400 000 people in the UK, usually in the older age groups, and is the commonest cause of dementia (Rossor, 1993; Allison & Marshall, 1994). Alzheimer's disease can pose gradually increasing problems not only with the AL of communicating but with all ALs, for the person and the carers. Early access to community support, including the community mental health nurse, is valuable, and the Alzheimer's Disease Society provides excellent information leaflets for the use of carers.

Quite apart from Alzheimer's disease, some people in their declining years show signs of diminishing skills in thinking and remembering, and McCourt (1994) describes how she used reminiscence as part of her work with elderly people. Reminiscing can occur spontaneously, but can be used in a more planned manner for therapeutic purposes, either individually or in groups. It can help older people to retain self-esteem and a sense of individual identity, but it can also evoke powerful and painful emotions. Not everyone wishes to reminisce. As a therapeutic practice it has to be carefully planned, and McCourt scrupulously outlines the potential disasters as well as the benefits to the older person and the carer.

Problems related to speech

Independence in verbal communication may be impaired by distortion of the voice caused by a variety of physical dysfunctions. Dryness of the mouth interferes with speech. It may be due to a variety of causes such as reduced fluid intake; or associated with excitement or anxiety; or infection; or it may be caused by the use of medications, for example certain anti-emetics and anti-depressants. Dryness of the mouth, of course, is deliberately caused preoperatively when a drug such as atropine is given to dry up secretions prior to general anaesthesia. Mouth dryness is frequently a feature, too, when parenteral feeding has been prescribed (p. 191) and among other things, can inhibit verbal communication at a time when the patient particularly requires interpersonal contact. Unless contraindicated, a drink will relieve dryness of the mouth, a mouthwash may prove helpful, and something as simple as sucking a sweet or medicated lozenge may stimulate salivation sufficiently to relieve discomfort.

Specific local infections such as laryngitis and swelling such as enlarged tonsils will also cause speaking problems but these conditions are usually temporary in nature and reversible. A distortion of longer duration occurs when a child is born with congenital hare lip or cleft palate. These can be corrected by surgery, but a considerable amount of speech therapy is required in the post-surgery period to ensure that such children can communicate in a way which is understandable to others.

A stammer, too, can deter communication and Fewster (1990) describes a useful approach by speech therapists which considers not just the stammer but the whole person.

There are occasions when one is at a loss for words, but most people find it difficult to imagine what it would be like to be unable to speak. Certainly one could still see, listen, read, write and communicate non-verbally. So these are the modes which have to be exploited when someone suddenly loses the ability to speak, whether it be temporary or permanent in nature.

Sudden impairment A temporary inability to speak — mutism — may be a manifestation of a mental health problem. Hysterical psychoneurosis consists of a reproduction of symptoms or signs of an illness for some personal purpose without the person being aware of the motive, for example to evade a particularly painful or embarrassing occurrence. The loss does not obey any anatomical or physiological laws and the process of treatment involves discovering what situation the person subconsciously seeks to avoid. It is necessary to convey to the person that their condition is recognized as genuine, and in need of exploration and resolution.

Temporary loss can also be produced when, for instance it is necessary to make a surgical incision into the trachea and insert a tracheostomy tube to maintain patency (p. 160). Where possible it is important that the patient understands the nature of the operation, but sometimes it has to be performed in an emergency. The person will almost certainly be conscious and needs considerable support which the nurse can supply by the manner in which activities are carried out. A pad and pencil is an alternative means of communicating, and it is important that some means, such as a bell, is within the patient's reach in order to attract the nurse's attention when help is required.

Permanent impairment Permanent loss occurs when there is surgical removal of the larynx, a laryngectomy (Harding, 1994). In such circumstances the patient needs to understand the permanency of the loss of natural voice production. Usually every encouragement is given to develop oesophageal speech (Box 5.4), and effective collaboration between nurse and speech therapist will do much to assist the patient and family during the early stages of learning. The nursing contribution involves encouraging the patient to carry out the speech therapist's instructions; not showing impatience as the person practises; and not showing embarrassment at the changed voice. Such people can be advised to join one of the self-help groups — Laryngectomee Clubs — which exist to give support and encouragement to those with similar problems and assist them to regain independence in verbal communication.

Dysphasia and aphasia For other reasons, of course,

Box 5.4 Oesophageal speech

Air is swallowed and forced into the oesophagus by locking the tongue to the roof of the mouth.

When air is expelled the walls of the oesophagus and pharynx vibrate, causing the column of air in the oesophagus to vibrate and produce a low-pitched sound.

The sound is formed into words by the patient's tongue, lips, teeth and palate to form intelligible speech.

there can be dysphasia (speech difficulties) or aphasia (loss of ability to speak) for example, these problems may arise when someone has a cerebrovascular accident (CVA) – a stroke. Depending on the exact location of the CVA in the brain, so the person's problems are different. A variety of terms is used to indicate varying degrees and forms of difficulty with speech and comprehension (Smith, 1991; Stewart & Creed, 1994) and it is important for the nurse to work in conjunction with the speech therapist. Two broad categories are often used — expressive aphasia and receptive aphasia (Box 5.5).

Ireland (1990) gives a graphic account of her personal difficulties with communicating when she had a CVA just before her 38th birthday and MacIsaac (1993) describes how she found a way to communicate with an elderly, woman who had dysphasia and was admitted to a unit for people who were mentally ill.

Of crucial importance is the continuation of encouragement and support in the community once the person is discharged from hospital. Family, friends and home helps can collaborate effectively even when progress seems slow, and groups such as Action for the Dysphasic Adult Group (ADA) produce leaflets containing helpful exercises and useful ideas to assist communicating. Local groups, too, organize social activities where people with a dysphasia can meet others with speaking difficulties, and with whom they can empathise with less embarrassment.

Problems related to hearing

The congenitally deaf or hearing-impaired baby has difficulty in acquiring vocal communication skills because of the inability to hear. One of the early assessments of all babies is a simple hearing test so that, should any impairment be identified, specialist advice can be sought early (Davies, 1993).

Recurrent middle ear infections can produce a problem for young children who are still acquiring basic communication skills and the resulting reduction in hearing capacity can retard the learning process. Of course at any stage on the lifespan an ear infection or even the presence of excessive wax may interfere with hearing. However these are usually transient impediments.

Sudden impairment It is a different matter when there is a sudden loss of hearing; the person is now in a silent world; and even in the midst of people, there is intense loneliness. Nevertheless visual cues are still received and sometimes when others glance in the deaf person's direction while talking, the reaction varies. There may be signs of paranoid behaviour; there may be loss of self-respect; the person may become more easily cross and irritable; indeed, these people may feel so uncomfortable in the company of others that there is physical withdrawal which may well increase the feeling of loneliness.

A discomfort which sometimes accompanies hearing

Box 5.5 Aphasia

Two broad categories are often used in the discussion of aphasia:

- *Expressive aphasia* is a term used when people know what they want to say, yet although able to move the mouth, simply cannot speak. It is the right-handed person's problem when there is a CVA in the left motor speech area, because the speech area is best developed in the left cerebral hemisphere. It is frustrating because intelligence is unimpaired. Also hearing has not changed, although CVAs tend to occur in the older age group who may already have some impairment, so it is important in these circumstances to collect information about hearing ability.

  It is also important for the nurse to note whether the patient does manage to speak any word or words. With the objective of the patient speaking an increasing number of words, the nurse puts into practice advice given by the speech therapist. This usually consists of encouraging the person to say particular words, separately at first to ensure success, then short sentences and so on. Nursing time is much better spent on these exercises than on long one-sided conversations, which may only produce frustration when the person cannot talk. Indeed great distress can be caused when nurses and relatives do not appear to understand the disability and talk as if to a child.

- *Receptive aphasia* is a term used when there is impaired comprehension of spoken and written words, although the patient can still say the words aloud. According to the person's previous reading ability and hearing acuity, (and this information must be collected) the words can still be seen and heard but there is difficulty understanding and remembering. The right-handed person can have receptive aphasia when there is a CVA in the left sensory speech area, again because it is best developed on the left side and the fibres cross over. The ability to think and vocalise words is retained, but the words spoken may be out of context. The person requires to re-learn association of words with things — the things needed in everyday living such as toothbrush, toothpaste and so on, and it is useful to keep these articles on a tray nearby so that the nurse can encourage extra repetition whenever opportunities are available to spend time with the patient.

impairments is tinnitus (Luxon, 1993). Hearing therapists are trained to counsel people who suffer from it, and the British Tinnitus Association provides support and help (Box 5.6).

Permanent impairment When permanent impairment is inevitable, everything possible must be done by the nurse to convey to the person that, although hearing-impaired, he/she is still valued as a person. Nurses can use non-verbal language as much as possible. The patient has no loss in cognitive ability and speech and usually will begin to lip-read. To help lip-reading, the nurse's face should be at the same level as the patient's, at a comfortable distance to accommodate the patient's vision, and in a good light.

Patients and members of their families may decide that use of a hand language would solve their communicating problem. With practice it can be quicker for the other members than writing the input part of conversation with the hearing-impaired person who can still speak in reply! With tolerance and good humour the problem of communicating can at least be reduced, if not overcome. Within a group of hearing-impaired people, the British Sign Language (BSL) may be used and Wright (1993) carried out an interesting study investigating BSL-users' perceptions of communication with nurses. It has its own rules and grammar and uses finger-spelling instead of words, but is not suitable for deaf people who have a learning difficulty — Makaton (Tompkins, 1988) may be helpful for them. Makaton uses selected words and signs graded in complexity from basic needs to more complex concepts and can be taught to individuals or groups without the need for any sophisticated equipment.

It is interesting to contemplate whether or not a deaf person who has a psychosis can 'hear' voices and

---

Box 5.6 Tinnitus

The perception of sound originates from within the head rather than from the external world and the pathophysiology remains obscure (Luxon, 1993).

Almost everyone can hear noises in the ear if in quiet enough surroundings but environmental noise usually masks this. However, the tinnitus which accompanies impairment of hearing is said by sufferers to be worse than hearing loss and the monotonous buzzing or ringing sounds can cause insomnia, depression, and total distortion of their living pattern.

Drugs, surgery, electrical stimulation of the cochlea, and biofeedback techniques have been tried with varying success. Portable masking devices such as an ear-level hearing aid which delivers a continuous masking sound — often closely imitating the distressing tinnitus sound — can be helpful.

McGough (1990) examines the challenge, emphasizing that communicating is one of the prime skills of a mental health nurse.

Hearing aids If there is even minimal hearing, it may be possible to augment it with a hearing aid. However the aid magnifies every sound and at first some sounds can be startling until the patient learns to filter them out. It needs a lot of encouragement and support during the learning period to use the aid to best advantage and nurses should speak slowly and clearly, and encourage lip-reading. With technological developments, it is now possible to have small, unobtrusive aids which are effective as well as being more aesthetically acceptable than the older body-worn models.

Various home aids have also been devised for the use of people with impaired hearing, for example, a flashing light when the doorbell or telephone rings; and there are special adaptors for radio, television and telephones (British Telecom supply excellent advice, and some services free of charge). Special reception facilities in selected areas of some theatres and concert halls are helpful and these are available in some churches, too, so that people with hearing impairments can enjoy spiritual enrichment in the company of like-minded worshippers. There is also a scheme to provide 'Hearing Dogs'. Guide dogs for people who are visually impaired have been used in the UK since 1931 and this is an extension of the same idea.

Problems related to sight

In contrast to hearing problems, it is usually possible to notice quite readily that someone has a visual problem. It may be congenital and as soon as it is detected, the parents require careful, specialist advice so that other communication channels are exploited to the optimum. At the other end of the lifespan, gradual visual impairment is a frequent problem which is age-related, and Kelly (1993) discusses the key role of nurses — in the community as well as in hospital — in identifying and intervening to suggest solutions. Sight can be crucial to independence and so often, nowadays, older people live alone.

Sudden impairment People who lose the sense of sight suddenly face a different problem; there is a change from a world of light and colour to a world of perpetual darkness. They cannot see their environment or the person to whom they are speaking, so miss all the visual communication cues. They cannot write letters although they may be able to use a computer and they may still be able to write a signature if the hand is placed exactly where it is required. They cannot read letters and the friendships maintained in this way are no longer 'private' because a nurse or volunteer has to read them to the patient. Of course there are tape recordings, but again they are less 'private'. A phone at home can be modified, but it may be less easy to use the hospital telephone.

When there is a sudden loss of sight the nurse can give more effective help if she understands that people, suffering any form of loss go through similar psychological stages to those of dying (p. 405). The nurse therefore needs to help them to deal with, and not deny, the feelings of anger and frustration, and must convey the intended message by voice alone since it is not complemented by visual cues. However such people still have visual memory of colour, shape, size and so on and can be helped to develop mental images if the nurse describes the environment and what is going on, emphasizes landmarks, and encourages others to do likewise. Description is particularly important if any treatment is going to be carried out so that the patient knows what to expect but it is also helpful to have ordinary activities such as a food tray described. For anyone whose sight has been suddenly impaired, it is important that nurses indicate their approach before touching the person and that they speak in a normal voice; sudden loud speech merely serves to startle.

For those who have undergone certain types of ophthalmic surgery the covering of both eyes in the immediate postoperative period, although transient, can be alarming. If such patients are in the older age group, they are usually less adaptable and inability to see can add to the confusion at being in the strange environment of a hospital; in fact, some can become disoriented. Waterman and Webb (1992) describe a study to investigate the visually-impaired patients' perceptions of their needs while in hospital.

Permanent impairment   If the impairment is permanent, the transition from hospital to the community can be traumatic as the person attempts to adjust to living in the everyday world without the advantage of sight. Donnelly (1987) carried out a study of 71 people who had recently been registered as blind. Major concerns were the loss of independence; loss of finance and work opportunities; anxiety about being a burden on others; in fact, some were doubly concerned as they themselves were carers of a disabled spouse.

In a more positive vein, special parentcraft provision is discussed by Nolan (1994) for women who have a permanent visual impairment and become pregnant. Tactile teaching aids; handling a model of the pelvis; visiting the labour room in advance to accustom them to the sounds and smells of the unit; and arranging a visit with another mother who has a visual impairment to share the experience can all be valuable. By working in partnership, says Nolan, the midwife can play a vital role in helping these women to achieve fulfilling motherhood.

Visual aids   Visually impaired people have to cope with many disadvantages, one being the impediment to learning at the same speed as sighted people; they rely on large-print books, talking books, tapes, and Braille (invented 1824). However, the computer revolution pro-

vides considerable extensions to their options. As well as a learning aid, computers can be used to increase the potential for work opportunities as well as for pleasure activities.

The Royal National Institute for the Blind (RNIB) produces a number of sensitive booklets which suggest ways of helping people who are visually impaired, indeed they provide nearly 60 different services, for example, they offer advice and support; design and sell special equipment; and supply information in print, Braille, Moon and on tape.

In the community, a number of visually-impaired people use specially trained dogs as an aid to their everyday activities, but as well as increasing their capacity for independence, the dog provides them with faithful companionship in a world where social contacts may be diminishing.

Problems related to body sensation

Sensation via the skin is a topic which people do not readily discuss. Only when deprived of skin sensation does the individual realise what an important, and indeed pleasurable, part of communicating it can be. Research has suggested, however, that as well as being a potent medium for communication, it is essential to physical and mental health (Carter, 1995).

Touch is the earliest and most primitive form of communication in the infant and continues to be an important form of non-verbal communication throughout life; it can convey a myriad of positive and negative messages between people. However the use and acceptance of touch depends on numerous cultural norms and personal characteristics; each culture has rules about how, when, and where to touch another human, and this is related to gender, age, and maturity.

Use of conscious touch   Carruthers (1992) quotes various research studies where intentional, 'therapeutic touch' (a concept first used by Krieger in 1960) had a beneficial effect in reducing anxiety; alleviating acute and chronic pain; and reducing labour delivery times and complications during childbirth.

Although the use of conscious touch is usually beneficial, it can, however, produce problems. In a small study carried out by McCann and McKenna (1993) they discuss situational and personal factors associated with conscious, therapeutic touch and factors impinging on touch perception. They enlarge on two main categories which are identified in the literature:

- instrumental touch (procedural or task-oriented e.g. washing a patient, or dressing a wound)
- expressive touch (comforting or non-necessary or affective e.g. holding a patient's hand to convey concern, or during a painful procedure).

Nurses hold a licence to touch that is sanctioned by the client, they quote, and outside this context few, except intimate, significant others, would be allowed such complete access to a person's body. Following their study, they caution that patients (in this instance, elderly people) may misinterpret the goal or the motivation behind touch initiated by the nurse, and react negatively. In fact, in certain circumstances, perhaps in a psychiatric setting, touch can be interpreted to the point of precipitating aggressive behaviour. Skill is required to detect any reservations by the recipient, especially in circumstances where the person has reduced personal independence.

Loss of touch perception Different problems arise when there is loss of the sensation of touch via the skin. Protective cues cannot be communicated and for example, it is not possible to detect excessive heat so the skin area may be burned; or the person may bump into sharp objects without realizing the damage to the skin and underlying tissues. Impaired sensation is often a feature following a CVA and certain spinal injuries, occurring along with impaired movement.

Problems related to body movement

When people lose the ability to move, the affected area of the body can no longer be used to convey non-verbal messages. According to the extent of the paralysis (Fig. 4.2, p. 88), so the change in mode of communicating is different as are the compensatory needs to maximize the remaining components of verbal language.

Hemiplegia People who have a hemiplegia can be deprived of up to 50% of their ability to communicate non-verbally. Hemiplegia is most commonly associated with a cerebrovascular accident (CVA). When it occurs in the right cerebral hemisphere there is a left hemiplegia because the nerve fibres cross at the base of the brain. A left CVA results in a right hemiplegia, and since the majority of the population is right handed, many people with a left CVA are also deprived of the writing component of communicating.

Furthermore hemiplegia can be accompanied by facial paralysis. The lip lies limp and down-drawn on one side but it may not be conveying the sadness and depression which body language experts associate with down-drawn lips. Facial paralysis may include a drooping eyelid which minimizes the eye contact component of body language and the visual input component of verbal language. A left hemiplegia can also interfere with speaking.

Again it is a case of the nurse helping the patient to work through the various emotional stages of coming to terms with lost abilities in the several components of communicating. Nurses need to become skilled at recognizing cues (other than down-drawn lips) of sadness and depression and dealing with these as seems appropriate. The nurse when communicating with the patient should be on the same side as the unaffected eye both for the patient's comfort and to maximize visual input.

Whatever the extent of the hemiplegia, nursing activities include provision of emotional support, and encouragement to relearn control of the paralysed muscles — as advised by the physiotherapist — so that there will be improvement in the person's AL of communicating non-verbally and by writing.

Paraplegia People who have a paraplegia can also be deprived of up to 50% of the ability to communicate non-verbally, but it is a different distribution from the hemiplegic patient, so the problems are different. The most common cause of the condition is an accident and a preponderance of the victims are young males. They cannot move from the waist downwards so they are deprived of their characteristic walk and the other information conveyed by this portion of the body, one of the greatest anxieties usually being related to the communicating elements of expressing sexuality.

Helping the patient with the AL of communicating includes several of the nursing activities given for the hemiplegic patient. However as soon as possible the person with paraplegia is rehabilitated to a wheelchair life, which in itself can present communicating problems. Just as a small child's eye level when standing is at the adult's leg level, so the wheelchair person's eye level is at most people's waist level. Nurses can help by offering same level eye contact to prevent a feeling of being talked down to — physically, of course!

Tetraplegia Tetraplegia deprives people of most of the ability to communicate non-verbally; only facial expression and the ability to make eye contact remain intact. It is not possible to use a hand to write but the function for communicating by verbal language is intact and indeed, some learn to write holding a pen in their mouths, or even paint. However, the computer revolution has provided enormous opportunities for extending communicating capacity; a rod held in the mouth can tap computer keys to print, or to activate switches for lighting, television, telephones and so on. And verbal instructions can now motivate a robot to perform a range of activities.

Problems related to body language

Much of present-day knowledge about body language is the result of research on 'normal' subjects. However, there are people who do not have a 'normal' body either in structure or function, with which to transmit such a language.

For example:

- When there is impaired structure and function not only is there a problem in transmission of body language, but there is a problem in interpreting the body language transmitted by these people (Box 5.7).

- Patients in intensive care units (ICUs) also have problems with communicating. Some distressing event has led to their admission; they are surrounded by strange equipment and unusual sights and sounds, including other critically ill patients; and staff carry out frequent investigations and treatments. They may feel too ill or too drained of energy to ask appropriate questions or may get the impression that the staff are much too busy to

listen, or may have an injury which impedes conversation or makes it difficult to receive a communication. When patients have difficulty in responding, research has shown that they often receive limited deliberate communication. Turnock (1991) explores the reasons for poor nurse/patient verbal and non-verbal communication in ICUs and maintains that appropriate communication skills must be learned by the nurse in order to identify priorities between the patient's physical/technical needs and the psychological needs, so that the person's coping strategies can be enhanced. It is a subtle balance.

- For a patient in coma (p. 389) there is no communication by any mode. However any gradual return to consciousness is often observed as a response to touch. The manner in which a nurse communicates her concern while for instance bathing an unconscious patient, is obviously important. The stimulus of a constant familiar voice or repetition of a familiar tune — and nowadays these may be utilized in the form of tape-recordings — may also eventually produce a response and help to re-establish the AL of communicating.

Changes in various modes of communicating have been discussed separately in order to give each its importance but in reality, the patient may be adapting to change in several modes simultaneously. For example someone with a left hemiplegia may have both a sensory and a motor loss; and may have either a receptive or expressive aphasia, or a mixture of both. Because such a person is likely to be in an older age group, there may also be lessened visual and auditory input, so helping with the AL of communicating is an enormous challenge to the nurse.

Of course, a number of patients who are admitted to hospital may have been visually or hearing impaired, or have impaired speech, or have been partially paralysed for a period of time. It is particularly important that the nurse discovers what the individuals' usual coping mechanisms have been so that as far as possible, they can continue these practices and use their limited capacities for communicating to the optimum level.

Obviously communicating is not easy. Patients need and enjoy the human interest of social conversation and this is usually an effective way of establishing the basis of a relationship. But planned purposeful communication is also required. Observing and listening, as well as asking appropriate questions, can help the nurse to assess the timing of planned communication and the level at which information is given. Although effective communicating is not easy, it is possible for the student nurse to learn the skills.

Box 5.7 Body language: examples of problems

- *Impaired posture and gait*
Structural or functional defects can affect body language, for example, a curvature of the spine is usually associated with a drooping shoulder or shoulders. One of the person's problems is an inability to assume the 'upright' posture with braced shoulders which is characteristic of a confident, cheerful and optimistic mood. They therefore have to express these emotions and reactions in other ways.

- *Generalized overactivity*
This is often an expression of anger. However, there are people who, while not being angry or frustrated, simply cannot relax and sit still; it is characteristic of hyperactive children and some mental illnesses, and can be a problem to the individual and to others in the family. It is usually inadvisable to restrain forcibly such individuals as this can make them angry or even violent. Special attention therefore needs to be paid to the environment so that they do not harm themselves or others, as they pace restlessly back and forth or indulge in meaningless movement which distorts the usual cues of body language.

- *Localized overactivity*
This can be observed as an inability to control one or more muscle groups. For example, the arms may swing in purposeless movement, so the person is unable to communicate by pointing to something that is wanted. Localized overactivity is sometimes associated with a reduced level of intelligence which precludes effective acquisition of verbal skills, so nurses need to observe body movements carefully to discover whether or not a message is being transmitted.

- *Enforced posture*
Confinement to bed or sitting in a wheelchair can produce body language problems, particularly in relation to eye contact. Nurses can help by being seated when talking with people whose movement is restricted in this way.

CHANGE OF ENVIRONMENT AND ROUTINE

Once people are admitted to hospital, several dimensions of communicating have changed, for example, the social dimensions. Members of the group with whom they live, usually the family, are no longer present; the people with whom they communicate at work are absent; and likewise, the people with whom they choose to spend the leisure part of each day.

Unfamiliar people

The person's problem is that he has joined a group of unfamiliar people, some of whom, the patients, are present all the time; others, the nurses, are in his vicinity for some of the time; and a whole variety of others appear 'to come and go'. It is little wonder that even the most confident individuals experience some difficulty in trying to make sense of such an environment, one which is alien to most people.

Admission In some instances the patient is very ill on admission and in these circumstances explanations and introductions have a lower priority than life-sustaining treatment and nursing. So what can the nurse do to help the patient with the AL of communicating? Initially only essential information need be communicated — that they are in hospital, that relatives have been informed, how to summon the nurse and so on. As the condition improves there can be gradual and fuller exchange of information between nurse and patient.

For people admitted from the waiting list, the nurse who 'admits' them should help with the inevitable quandary of meeting new people in somewhat unusual circumstances. It should be remembered that an anxious person, even an intelligent one, does not retain as much new information as normally. The nurse should therefore attempt to communicate only the information necessary for the patient to manage say, the next 24 hours. Throughout a hospital stay, communicating is important for all patients but in mental health nursing, communicating is the major therapeutic tool and the patient's initial relationship can particularly influence the effectiveness of the subsequent therapy.

Communicating with children (and their parents) requires special skills and Glasper et al (1989) discuss this, as well as the importance of the communication links between hospital and community services when children are ill (see also p. 335).

Introduction of nurse and patient/client The first nursing activity is introduction of the nurse, by name, to the patient. When name badges are worn, nurses need to remember that people who wear bifocal spectacles have difficulty in reading at that level, and any cues regarding inadequate vision should be noted. The patient should be told of the mode of address used in that particular

hospital for professional staff. It is important to remember that patients need some information about the different members of the health care team so that they can relate satisfactorily to them. If uniforms distinguish the different grades of nursing and domestic staff, then this is useful information for the nurse to communicate.

It is of crucial importance that the nurse addresses adults as Mr, Mrs, Ms. or other appropriate title unless they request otherwise. Older people in particular may object strongly to being addressed by their first name, in fact Leach (1994) maintains it can show lack of insight into how a person feels on entering hospital, with all the loss of power which this change of status threatens. Williams (1991) suggests some guidelines for effective communication with elderly people, but they have general relevance.

Introduction to other patients/clients For all but the very ill or those admitted as an emergency the nurse can help the patient with his problem of being among unfamiliar people by introducing him to the other patients in his immediate vicinity. These are the people who will be present throughout each day and they help to give the new patient a feeling of 'belonging', indeed other patients can be a great support and source of information. It is important for the nurse to remember the professional responsibility of maintaining confidentiality so the medical diagnosis and any personal details about the other patients must not be divulged.

Communicating staffing patterns The nurse who admits new patients needs to explain whether or not they have been allocated to a named nurse as part of a patient allocation scheme; if so, for how long the nurse will be on duty; and the staffing arrangements that will be made for other shifts. They should be encouraged to express any particular anxieties and queries until the nurse assesses from verbal and non-verbal interaction that they have a reasonable grasp of the staffing pattern as it applies to them and know from whom they can seek any further help. Patients cannot be expected to feel safe and secure without this information.

Nurse-patient/client relationship The relationship between nurse and patient is essentially a human one. However each patient is in the health care system for a purpose, seeking help with health problems, actual or potential. The nurse is there to make the nursing contribution to the solution; amelioration or prevention of the patients' actual or potential problems. Nurses therefore are not in the individual patient/nurse relationship from choice, but in the capacity of making a professional contribution. A consideration of what the nurse brings to the relationship is therefore necessary. Of course, it is not only in the hospital that this relationship is crucial; it is of paramount importance in any health care setting.

Nurses bring to the relationship themselves as unique human beings, the culmination of their particular life experiences. They also bring compassion for people and a commitment to nursing, together with nursing knowledge and skills. Their emotional maturity should be such that they do not have to gratify personal needs at the patient's expense. For example a need to be dominant and make decisions may deprive patients of practice which they require in order to deal with, for example, their problem of indecision, common in some mental illnesses. Or again, a strong parenting need may motivate a nurse to dress patients when it would be in their best interest to re-learn dressing skills.

The nurse brings to the relationship a maturity which permits toleration of frustration if, for example, the person presents challenging behaviour (Kay, 1995). The trigger points are innumerable, but the nurse should have the maturity to deal with the resultant feelings in a constructive way that avoids reflecting any annoyance on to the patient. Nobody expects a paragon of virtue but the nurse is meant to be realistic, is meant to have self-knowledge because the 'self' must be used in the relationship. The nurse's personal needs have to be met by other supporting staff, by counsellors or by the significant others in the nurse's life.

The patient/client is also a unique human being who has been fashioned by life experiences. Something is wrong, so already the image of self has changed. Change is uncomfortable at the best of times and the patient is discomforted. If there is a mental health problem, the person may be apprehensive about stigma at home or at work — stigma still exists. If the diagnosis is uncertain and an array of diagnostic tests is required, then the patient is bound to be anxious both about the tests and the potential results, and inevitably, is worried if surgery is prescribed. Worried people do not concentrate, hear or understand so well as usual. However, if the nurse takes the time to give information to the patient, it has been shown in various studies to be beneficial, although Teasdale (1993), reviewing a number of studies dealing with this topic, emphasizes that human communication depends less on interpretation (Fig. 5.1) of semantic information than on inferences which recipients draw from the context.

Anthonypillai (quoted in the Nursing Times 1994) highlights communication skills which can be effective when nursing non-English speaking patients in an ICU; Dodds (1993) identifies ways of using communicating skills to help relieve perioperative anxiety; and Hunt (1991) describes a study he carried out in a psychiatric hospital emphasizing the language skills involved during admission of new clients when information-giving and -seeking is so crucial to the nurse-patient relationship.

Psychological comfort is inextricably linked to physical comfort and some interactions can be planned, deliberately, by staff to contribute to psychological comfort. It may be as fleeting as a look of acknowledgement when passing the patient's bed; or using expressive touch (p. 118) to convey empathy, trust, reassurance, security or the proximity of another person; or it may be less transient, for example, helping someone through the stages of accepting and coping with chronic illness; or when someone has a mental health problem, it can be the major emphasis for most interactions.

Many activities carried out in the vicinity of the patient offer the nurse an opportunity to show empathy. Empathy is described in various ways — Gould (1990) provides a review of literature — and Burnard (1987a) discussing its use in psychiatric nursing quotes Carl Rogers' definition as 'a process of entering into the perceptual world of another person'. Burnard goes on to mention some of the skills involved: the ability to listen (to the words but also noting volume, pitch, eye movements and related body language); ability to offer free attention (to note and accept, not analyse and interpret); to suspend judgement (to refrain from categorizing as good/bad, right/wrong); and to control what is said in reply and how it is said, with a facial expression which is genuine, not mechanical. By behaving in this way, the nurse shows respect for the person's individuality, a point reinforced in our model for nursing.

In another article, Burnard (1988) compares empathy and sympathy:

'To empathize is to set aside our own perception of things and attempt to think the way the other person thinks, or feel the way he feels . . . a very different quality to sympathy. Sympathy involves 'feeling sorry' for the other person — or perhaps, it involves our imagining how we would feel if we were experiencing what is happening to him. With empathy, we try to imagine what it is like being the other person and experiencing things as he does.'

Empathy of course does have limits. It is not possible to completely enter someone else's frame of reference because other people live different lives and Jones (1990) considers the difficulties of 'walking into the world of another' when counselling someone with a life-threatening illness, in this instance AIDS. Speaking in general, he cautions that there are occasions when an empathetic response could be inappropriate; clients may be unable to tolerate the anxiety which can be aroused. This intuitive aspect of empathy arising from cues picked up from the client, is just as important as a repertoire of communication techniques.

In all community and hospital settings, the nurse needs to develop psychological and social skills as well as manual skills in order to maintain an effective nurse/patient relationship while the patient requires it; and these skills are also required to relinquish the relationship when appropriate.

Of course it is not only the nurse-patient relationship which contributes to the patient's care and well-being.

Inter-professional communication is required between nurses and other members of the health team. When deficient, there are omissions or repetitions of activities; uncoordinated interruptions to the patient's rest and comfort; failure to meet the patient's psychological needs — in essence poor communication causing a breakdown in the continuity of care.

Too often, breakdown occurs in relation to transfer back into the community.

Discharge Providing patients with information on admission to hospital and throughout their stay may be acknowledged as an important part of nursing but frequently, discharge is a very rushed affair.

Information about planning the convalescent period, about continued medication and treatments, about potential complications, expected rate of progress, return to employment are all important to patients and their families; and is highlighted as one of the national charter standards in The Patient's Charter (1992). Even during the admission procedure, the nurse should be alerted to consider what the person requires to know on discharge in order to resume the usual Activities of Living.

Staff-to-staff communicating between hospital and community services is another important aspect when considering discharge and this is even more crucial for short-stay admissions. Markanday and Platzer (1994) describe a framework for communicating with, and assessing the suitability of, people who are potential day-surgery clients. And Stephenson (1990) discusses discharge criteria; the seven categories she chose arose from a literature search combined with data from a descriptive research study about the recovery and welfare of patients following day surgery. Quite apart from the negative effect of patient's emotions on learning, it has been demonstrated, she quotes, that simple anaesthetic techniques can produce considerable impairment to the ability for retaining new information in the immediate postoperative period. Instruction sheets, verbal conversation, cassettes and telephone calls have all been used to give and receive information before, as well as following, surgery.

Norris (1992) discusses the need for perioperative communication related to the child and parents in a paediatric day-surgery programme, and at the other end of the lifespan, King and Macmillan (1994) report the findings of their research based on data from 326 elderly patients. King and Macmillan considered that the assessment of the patients' needs, and social and home circumstances were inadequate for the purposes of discharge planning and decision-making. There was also concern about the tendency to assume that relatives or carers were willing to give increased support following a person's discharge home; sometimes carers were also old and frail, or had family and work commitments, or had recently been discharged from hospital themselves. The authors maintain that information about social circumstances and about carers should be an intrinsic part of admission assessment and should be documented to assist with discharge arrangements. Williams (1994) discusses the rehabilitation process for older people and their carers and stresses assessment, planning, implementing and evaluating.

With the trend to close hospitals for people who have mental health problems or who have learning difficulties, the need for pre-discharge communication with the client, the potential carers and the multidisciplinary teams is crucial. Unfortunately there is some alarm about apparent breaks in the communication chain with community support systems, and a number of vulnerable ex-hospital patients seem to be more isolated than ever, while their health and their coping strategies deteriorate.

Certainly, recorded information must be available to the multidisciplinary team in the community; the attitude should be transfer-back-to-the-community rather than discharge planning, says Ryan (1994). Perhaps combined records for all professional staff will help to ameliorate communicating problems.

Unfamiliar place

Lack of usual contacts People newly admitted to the hospital environment will naturally be anxious about keeping in touch with family, friends and work associates. Anxiety may be lessened by information about such things as a mobile shop where stationery and newspapers can be bought; ward arrangements for collection and delivery of mail; for making and receiving telephone calls, and for visiting. Gradually the patients' new environment seems less strange and threatening as they become aware of the possibilities for communication between hospital and their familiar environment.

Disorientation Information is also needed by the patient to permit the continuance of other everyday activities. It can be communicated by adequate labelling of, for example, toilets and bathrooms. The letters should be sufficiently large and should be placed so as to cater for those with poor vision. This is especially helpful to older people who may have difficulty in learning and remembering, and who may require to visit the toilet during the night.

As the days pass in this unfamiliar environment, some patients (particularly those with deficient vision and hearing, and those who for one reason or another do not read a daily newspaper) can lose track of the time of day, the day of the week and the day of the month. The provision of a large calendar and clock in each ward can be useful in preventing this apparent disorientation.

The problem of disorientation has been studied particularly in relation to elderly people and the techniques of reality orientation (RO) seem a promising area for development. It is really a psychological approach to the confused elderly person which aims to improve and maintain their level of functioning by stimulating them and their environment. Ratcliffe (1988) describes it as a technique used in rehabilitating people with memory loss, confusion and time-place-person disorientation which adds a humanistic element to care, and discusses in some detail how it affects communicating.

Unfamiliar language

Lack of understanding The new patient who probably has the biggest problem with communication is the one who does not speak the national language. With increasing multiracial societies in most countries and the speed of modern-day travel such patients are found in health service settings throughout the world. This is recognized as an international problem and voluntary organizations such as the League of Red Cross Societies have produced helpful translations in many languages. At a local level, voluntary help is usually available; there is often a list of people speaking other languages who are willing to act as interpreters. Failing this, nurses can help by using empathy, ingenuity and miming.

Even when the same national language is spoken by client and nurse, both can experience problems in aural perception when their attention has to be directed to listening because of accent or dialect. The nurse can help to avoid this problem by speaking clearly and slowly, stopping for clarification of interpretation when this seems necessary.

A problem can also be experienced when there is a difference in the vocabulary used by client and nurse. This can operate in both ways — the client might use words which the nurse does not readily understand and vice versa. Take the words used for the place for eliminating: bathroom, convenience, lavatory, loo, toilet, water closet (WC). There are countless other examples but the above should serve to alert nurses so that they can prevent problems in this area. This is accomplished by becoming expert at observing and interpreting nonverbal cues indicating incomprehension, and by exploring the cause of the break in the chain of communication and correcting it.

Technical terms Further differences in vocabulary can produce problems for patients when words with a medical definition are used in the process of communicating: insomnia, migraine, obstruction or 'hospital speak' such as 'ivee' and where an 'engee' tube goes (Lynn, 1993). She states that 'patient empowerment has a long way to go', in her study involving communicating with people who have cancer.

Nurses should therefore discover from clients what meaning these words have for them, so that they can be sure that they are talking about the same conditions. This naturally applies also to specific medical words, and when they are used, the nurse may find it necessary to correct inaccuracies and add explanations.

Embarrassing topics Some patients experience difficulty when talking with nurses about activities such as eliminating and expressing sexuality. They may fear that they are not using the 'right' words. It is therefore helpful if nurses start by saying that people use different words, and asking patients to give the information in their own words. Yet another type of vocabulary can have difference in meaning for patient and nurse and thereby give rise to difficulties — words describing parts of the body, though having a particular anatomical reference, do not necessarily have that reference for lay people, even intelligent lay people. Where appropriate, pointing to the area on one's own body is helpful or using visual aids, which can be as simple as drawing a diagram while explaining the location of the part; this, and using a model doll can be useful when communicating with children and with people who have learning difficulties.

Unfamiliar activities

Giving information to patients/clients The activities which occur inside hospital and are taken so much for granted by staff can be bewilderingly strange to the patients. Not surprisingly they feel anxious and Dodds (1993) discusses anxiety as a response to stress. It is now recognized by staff that much of the apprehension and anxiety can be traced back to lack of communication and Wilson-Barnett (1988) discusses the development of different approaches to rectify the situation, drawing distinctions between information-giving, patient teaching or education, and counselling. The provision of factual information seems to alleviate some of the initial anxiety on immediate arrival at the ward and many hospitals send to those who are being admitted from the waiting list, some type of preparatory material ranging from a leaflet to an illustrated brochure, the latter in particular for children. But this type of information presupposes that the recipients have the necessary vision and can read, and that they are sufficiently orientated to understand what they are reading. When this is not so, they are deprived of this initial preparation as are all those who are admitted as 'emergencies'. Of course, the written word is enhanced when given in conjunction with verbal information; it is possible to assess interpretation.

The value of giving information about specific nursing interventions, too, has been studied and in a review of literature, Radcliffe (1993) quotes studies which indicate that information-giving can reduce anxiety to the extent that patients, for example, require less anaesthesia; less analgesia; have less postoperative complications; and recover more quickly.

These studies are examples which illustrate the results

of effective staff communication, but there is also evidence from patients of breakdown. On investigation, a recurring point seems to be a lack of communication skills teaching for nursing staff, or inability to use it in practice, and this is borne out by Radcliffe (1993), Zylinski (1993) and Dodds (1993). Even in a psychiatric hospital Dunn (1991) found that taught communication skills were not effective in practice.

Giving information to relatives Relatives, too, seem concerned about lack of communication and the 'unavailability of the nurses'. Dodds (1993) and Radcliffe (1993) extol the value of including families (or significant others) in perioperative education for example to reduce their fears and anxieties, and enable them to become a source of support to the patient thereby enhancing recovery. However in all health care settings the giving of information to families is usually appropriate and is one of the national charter standards in the Patient's Charter, 1992, outlined by Cohen (1994a).

Of course, information-giving may be in the form of breaking bad news and the role of the nurse in undertaking this aspect of nursing is discussed in the Professional Development Series of the Nursing Times (1994). The Series seeks to promote the skills involved in understanding the effect such information may have on the recipients.

Teaching and counselling v. information-giving Having commented on the perceived need for information-giving experienced by staff, patients and relatives, it is interesting to note work which shows that facilitating certain strategies for *coping* during stressful procedures is more effective than information per se for reducing signs of distress. Wilson-Barnett (1988) indicates how information-giving is gravitating towards 'teaching' individuals how to cope. Wilson-Barnett differentiates between teaching (involving a change in behaviour) and information-giving (a process, and having less concern with how it is received . . . and not necessarily involving interaction or assessment of individual need). The didactic emphasis, she continues, is now shifting towards a more patient-centred involvement. And as patients have become more involved in identifying and negotiating areas for learning and behavioural change, the field of investigation has come to borrow from the theories and practice of counselling.

Burnard (1991) recommends that all nurses should be taught how to use what he calls 'minimal' counselling skills (Box 5.8). In an earlier article (1987b) he writes that central to patient-centred counselling is that individuals are the best arbiters of what is and is not right for them. They may listen to others, but decide on their own course of action. People are free to choose their own future, so the patient knows what is best. Listening is the basis of counselling. In the process of counselling, he goes on, the nurse does not offer interpretations laced with 'oughts'

Box 5.8 Counselling skills

Formal counselling requires lengthy training but, says Burnard (1991) all nurses should be taught 'minimal' counselling skills to enable them to help clients with their problems in a positive, therapeutic way. He suggests:

- *listening and attending:* giving the person one's full attention, and avoiding thinking about the 'rightness' or 'wrongness' of what is being said — listening without being judgmental
- *using open questions:* they usually begin with 'what', 'how', 'when', or 'where' enabling the person to expand on their problems i.e. questions which avoid single word or 'yes', 'no' answers
- *reflecting:*
  (a) reflection of thoughts e.g. echoing the last few words the person has used
  (b) reflection of feelings i.e. echoing to the person, the feelings or unstated thoughts which underline a statement just made
  Both need to be used judiciously, not over-used
- *summarizing:*
  (a) to pull together disparate strands of conversation and help the person to organize their thoughts
  (b) to end a therapeutic conversation while still focusing on the other person's concerns
- *checking for understanding:* seeking clarification by asking e.g. 'Can I just check what you are saying?' or 'You seem to be saying that .....'

---

and 'shoulds' — or the exercise degenerates into advice which may not fit the patient's beliefs and value systems. Vanderslott (1992) for example advocates counselling skills as one form of preventing ward violence without alienating the individual.

Essentially counselling is non-directive and without censure. The objective is that the patient gains the insight to make a personal decision from the options available. This approach, Burnard maintains, is different from other aspects of nursing when the nurse uses knowledge and expertise to advise and educate. Counselling is concerned with coping mechanisms which may be related to physical health problems, or may be personal and linked to relationships, or sociocultural issues including spiritual beliefs, or may be linked to economic difficulties.

McLeod Clark et al (1991) discuss the role of communicating skills, counselling skills and counselling, and to clear the confusion, they suggest a hierarchy of activities (Fig. 5.4).

Nowadays nurses are faced with complex situations, not only to take account of psychological and sociocultural factors during illness but also as promoters of

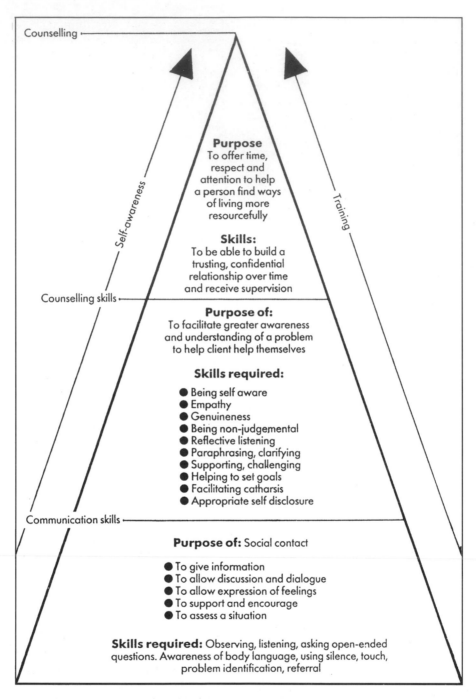

Counselling

Self-awareness

Training

Purpose
To offer time, respect and attention to help a person find ways of living more resourcefully

Skills:
To be able to build a trusting, confidential relationship over time and receive supervision

Counselling skills

Purpose of:
To facilitate greater awareness and understanding of a problem to help client help themselves

Skills required:
● Being self aware
● Empathy
● Genuineness
● Being non-judgemental
● Reflective listening
● Paraphrasing, clarifying
● Supporting, challenging
● Helping to set goals
● Facilitating catharsis
● Appropriate self disclosure

Communication skills

Purpose of: Social contact

● To give information
● To allow discussion and dialogue
● To allow expression of feelings
● To support and encourage
● To assess a situation

Skills required: Observing, listening, asking open-ended questions. Awareness of body language, using silence, touch, problem identification, referral

Fig. 5.4 From communication skills to counselling (Reproduced by kind permission of Nursing Times where this Figure first appeared with the article 'Progression to counselling' on February 20 1991.)

health, and in helping patients and families to become involved in their own health care. Appropriate knowledge and communication skills (information-giving, teaching, counselling skills) are required for these activities and skill is needed also to decide which communication approach is relevant to the circumstances.

Nurses must be able to function in this way or complaints will continue to be made by patients and relatives about poor communication. The freedom to complain

about communication failures, as well as other problems, and the ability of an organization to handle complaints effectively is part of the idea that a public service should be accountable and the DoH report 'Being Heard', discussed by Downey (1994), covers both community and hospital problems.

However, legitimate concern about improvements in communicating must be tempered by the countless instances when it certainly is effective.

Change of role

In the familiar world of the adult individual many parts are played and there is communication with many people: spouse, partner, offspring, other family, friend, acquaintance, co-worker, employer and club-member. There is control over when, how and where they communicate. Now, on admission to hospital, the AL of communicating has to continue while assuming the sick role or patient role discussed on p. 46.

Family relationships In hospital, the spouse's communication with the patient, in a setting that includes nightclothes, bed, single or multiple room/ward, is essentially different. When the visiting spouse or partner is accompanied by offspring or other family members, further modification of the partners' behaviour may be perceived to be necessary. At this sensitive period in these people's lives, such modification can be misinterpreted by any one or more members of this group and may have repercussions in family relationships. Nursing includes 'caring' about the family and what they mean to the individual. Indeed family disruption may have contributed to the illness. After visitors have departed, nurses should pay attention to a patient's non-verbal behaviour as well as to what is said. Nurses should not pry but they need to be sensitive to any cues which indicate a desire to discuss anxieties.

Reversal of roles The reversal of roles can cause the patient anxiety. Should the patient be the person who had attended to the business and financial side of family life, then there will have to be a reversal of roles; these items will have to be attended to by a responsible other person, usually the spouse or partner. And the previous level of frankness in communication about these matters can narrow or widen the possibility of stress between them during these communications in a hospital ward.

Visitors The reaction of friends to the change of role can be a sensitive matter. Patients may find it difficult to come to terms with which of their friends, co-workers and employers did, or did not, communicate with them during hospitalization. Some of these people may have phoned; and it is important that the patients' lines of communication are kept open by relaying these enquiries to them — they are easily jotted on a memo pad and delivered at a convenient moment. More is said about the importance of visiting on p. 337.

Information-giver and confidentiality Another potential problem for patients is that they find themselves in the role of information-giver, and it is often information of a very personal nature. They may not see the relevance of giving information about their social history when their problem is a physical one — and it may not be. When it is relevant, great sensitivity is required in eliciting such information and telling them how it helps in planning their nursing. For example, when an elderly, confused person is admitted, it is important for discharge planning, to know about social circumstances and about the potential carers. It is therefore important to understand at the outset that anything communicated to members of the professional staff will be treated as confidential.

The knowledge that confidence will be respected is an important feature of effective nurse/patient communication, and is incorporated in professional codes of practice in a number of countries. The UKCC Code of Professional Conduct (1992) states that registered nurses, midwives and health visitors shall:

'respect confidential information obtained in the course of professional practice and refrain from disclosing such information without the consent of the patient/client or a person entitled to act on his/her behalf except where disclosure is required by law or by order of a court, or is necessary in the public interest.'

This sounds reasonable but application of the principle may contain inherent conflicts of interest as Korgaonkar and Tribe (1994) describe in an AIDS-related circumstance where private rights and public interest were at variance. In certain instances, of course, reporting is required by law, for example, reporting of infectious diseases (Public Health Regulations, 1988), reporting for statistical purposes (Abortion Regulations, 1968), reporting deaths (Coroners Act, 1988) but nurses who breach patients' confidentiality with no good reason could face disciplinary procedures or even removal from the Register.

Related to confidentiality is the collection, storage and retrieval of written or computerized records (p. 112) a permanent form of communication (Box 5.9).

Box 5.9 Confidentiality and records

Information imparted by, and collected about the patient is given in confidence, so the information gatherer has a responsibility to be familiar with the records system in use, know who has access, and be aware of risks associated with the legitimate use of records (Barber, 1992). Do all health professionals have access? Do students have access? Do research workers have access? Is the system supervised? With the advent of computer storage of records, the topic of confidentiality has received considerable coverage and some aspects of the Data Protection Act, 1984, are considered to be insufficiently stringent (GMC, 1992).

Members of the public are concerned also and where health information is stored in computers, it is important that the public understand the safeguards against unauthorized people gaining access.

Information-receiver and informed consent As already mentioned, an increasing number of research reports show that a frequent complaint made by patients is lack of information. Sometimes the required information is about what tests are going to be performed and why; the results of tests; the medical diagnosis, particularly if, for example, a mental illness is confirmed, or heart disease or cancer are suspected; how long to expect to be away from work and so on. Whatever the nurse staffing arrangements, each one needs to know what the patient has been told and what currently appears to be understood. Adequacy of communication is an essential part of nursing, not only to reduce patients' complaints but to permit nurses to comply with their professional duty to be accountable. The UKCC Code of Professional Conduct (1992) states:

'Each registered nurse, midwife or health visitor is accountable for his or her practice, and in the exercise of professional accountability shall: act always in such a way as to promote and safeguard the well-being and interests of patients/clients.'

Pyne (1992) examines accountability in principle and in practice, and how it relates not only to the revised Code but also to another UKCC document 'The Scope of Professional Practice'.

Apart from receiving and understanding information, has the patient consented to the various tests and treatments – what has come to be termed 'informed consent'. The nurse/patient and doctor/patient relationship used to be founded on trust but now the accent is on mutual partnership, patient involvement, patient empowerment, and patient autonomy (McCormack, 1993). The nub of informed consent quote Korgaonkar and Tribe (1993) is that every human of adult years and sound mind has a right to determine what will be done with his or her own body, and, adds Robson (1994) to accept or reject treatment, even when the outcome may be immediate death.

For all surgical procedures, informed consent is a legal requirement but despite this, say Lavelle-Jones et al (1993) a substantial number of patients seem unaware of important details concerning their surgery (Box 5.10).

The legal rights of children (Box 5.11) in giving or withholding consent to medical treatment now receive much more attention (for young children, the parent or guardian will give consent on the child's behalf). However certain issues are unresolved, say Korgaonkar and Tribe (1994), for example the law makes no reference to the right to withhold treatment, or to non-therapeutic procedures such as organ donation.

Franklin (1994) discussing the speciality of organ transplantation reports that in decisions which may involve a child's life or death, the child is often excluded from the discussion. And Peace (1994) working in the area of palliative care maintains that adults frequently underestimate a child's understanding and awareness of the situation. Focusing on the child's rights does not exclude parental views, and those of siblings and professionals of course but, they say, children should be given a voice — and listened to.

Informed consent is also relevant when considering research which necessitates patient participation (Box 5.12), and in the UK, nursing research involving patients must be scrutinized by the local ethics committee.

In psychiatric nursing where the importance of acting on behalf of the client can be a daily ethical dilemma, Hackney (1993) discusses informed consent. He uses as an example the administration of neuroleptic drugs and raises the issues of accountability and advocacy. Fox (1995) too, emphasises the ethical dilemma when nursing an elderly man who had a chronic organic brain syndrome and who refused medication.

Advocacy Related to informed consent is the concept

Box 5.10 Informed consent: communication and recall about a surgical procedure

Lavelle-Jones et al (1993) studied, prospectively, the effects of certain variables on recall of medical information related to selected elective surgery procedures:

- information about the procedures and common complications was given to patients verbally; with permission the session was taped; questions were answered
- a random allocation of written 'operation information cards' containing the same content was given to half of these patients; they were left to read them for 30 minutes; another opportunity was given to ask questions
- recall was checked at sequential intervals:
  * within one hour of signing the consent form
  * on the day of discharge from hospital
  * 4–6 weeks after discharge
  * 6 months after discharge

The authors found that patients were best informed immediately after signing the consent form. From then on, recall deteriorated with time to reach the lowest level at the six-month review.

They concluded that elderly people and those with below average IQ (psychological and psychometric tests were conducted independent of the surgical team), with impaired cognitive function, and with an external locus of control (an internal locus = believed their health to be within their own control) have poor information recall; and that written information may be more useful if given before admission to hospital.

Box 5.11 Informed consent: the rights of children

Children do have some rights from international and national charters, quote Shield and Baum (1994):

- the UN Convention on the Rights of the Child advocates the right of every child to self-determination, dignity, respect, non-interference, and the right to make informed decisions
- the European Charter for children in hospital states that children and parents have the right to informed participation in all decisions involving their health care. Every child should be protected from unnecessary medical treatment and investigation
- in the UK, the Children Act 1989 states that children's wishes and feelings should be incorporated into the decision-making concerning them.

Box 5.12 Informed consent: communication and recall regarding participation in a research trial

Susman et al (1992) studied the consent process related to participation in research as viewed by children, adolescents, young adults and physicians.

Verbal and written explanations about the study were given to patients and parents. Written consent was given by the patient or parent, depending on age.

Standardized tests and taped interviews were used with the 44 patients, aged 7–21 years, to examine their knowledge of the research process and their own involvement.

In their conclusions, the authors found that more than half of the subjects knew, for example, the benefits to themselves of participating in the study; the duration of the research; their role as a participant; and understood that participation was voluntary.

However, fewer than half knew, for example, the purpose of the research; the potential benefits to others; alternative treatments; and that they were free to withdraw.

of patient advocacy. Graham (1992) quotes various sources to indicate that, in recent times, the emphasis has moved away from 'doing things for' the patient and evolved towards an approach which has more respect for the autonomy, self-determination and empowerment of the client.

But can the nurse really be an advocate? The nurse certainly has more contact with clients than most other health professionals and, says Sutor (1993) could be seen as in a strong position to 'advocate'. She considers the nurse's role using a four-model framework posited by Fowler:

- guardian of patient rights
- preserver of patient values
- champion of social justice in the provision of health care
- conservator of the patient's best interests.

In making a case for the nurse as an advocate she considers the UKCC Code of Practice (1992) which states:

'Each registered nurse, midwife and health visitor shall act at all times in such a manner as to justify public trust and confidence . . . . . . and above all to safeguard the interests of individual patients and clients.'

The implication from such a statement, suggests Sutor, is that nurses should act as advocates for their clients, representing their points of view when they are unable to represent themselves.

The role of a nurse as advocate is discussed by others in relation to specific groups of clients, for example, people who have a mental health problem (Sines, 1993); older people (Cohen, 1994b; Evans, 1994); and in relation to children (Chambers, 1992). But nurses are not the only people who understand patients' problems, and it should not be assumed that the nurse would always be the best advocate; indeed, other health professionals could see this stance as pretentious and offensive (Allmark & Klarzynski, 1992), conducive to interprofessional tension, and detrimental to teamwork.

Some authors, in fact, attack the notion that nurses can, or should, be advocates. An advocate, say Allmark and Klarzynski (1992) should plead a person's cause as the person sees it, not as the advocate sees it, and they give examples. Would the nurse provide the alcoholic with a drink (what the person wishes); or plead for someone *not* to be treated, who has been admitted because of a drug overdose; or plead that a 'sectioned' person be allowed to leave a psychiatric hospital? The nurse as health promotor and health care provider cannot plead the client's cause, only their best interests; and a patient's cause and best interests may not coincide. They maintain that what is often described as advocacy is no more, and no less, than nurses trying to act in the best interests of their patients, a role which has always been theirs.

Patient advocacy, obviously, is a broad and controversial issue and an interesting development is the initiation and funding by local councils of Citizen Advocacy Schemes. The advocates are lay people from the community and include representatives of many ethnic groups, which can also help when there are language problems (Hubert, 1993). Their role is seen as that of a friend, supporting and communicating the views and wishes of the patient to the health professionals when requested to do so by the person.

The idea was initiated in the USA as long ago as 1966. In the UK, the Advocacy Alliance was launched in 1982 by five major charities including MIND and the Spastics Society and although initially, the movement concentrated on people with learning difficulties, it has grown to include other groups including older people and those with mental health problems, says Cohen (1994b). The issue of independence from health providers is central to all the advocacy groups and he quotes the Wertheimer Report that although there can be pitfalls in citizen advocacy — it too can promote client dependency and threaten autonomy — the conclusions about its effectiveness were positive.

EXPERIENCE OF PAIN

Of all the features of illness, pain is probably the most common. It is a peculiarly individual phenomenon. Because of its subjective nature (discussed by Clancy & McVicar, 1992), it is difficult to measure and only people afflicted can communicate their perception of its presence and intensity. Hence the reason for allocating the main discussion of pain to the AL of communicating. The relevance of the link with communicating is corroborated by McCaffery (1983) who considers that 'pain is what the patient says it is, existing where he says it does'.

Most people who know what it feels like to be in pain regard it as an unpleasant sensation and something to be avoided if at all possible. In fact, in some circumstances it can be a protective mechanism, a warning signal; it is the body's response to any number of stressors ranging from the invasion of pathogens to physical injury to mental trauma.

People bereft of the ability to feel pain are therefore constantly in danger of accidentally being burned, bruised or cut, and of failing to recognize the onset of disease. At the opposite pole are people who experience pain even in the absence of any apparently painful stimulus. These two extremes are part of the phenomenon of pain.

For over 2000 years, work has gone on, unceasingly, to unravel the mystery of pain and provide relief — and Astley (1990) traces historical trends — but even now, some pains have defied all efforts made to resolve them. The challenge continues.

Physical aspects of pain

Pain is manifested by the nervous system, one of the biological systems aligned with the AL of communicating in our model, and research carried out in recent years has greatly increased our understanding of the phenomenon. In brief, at the site of pain certain chemicals are released; they sensitise the nerve endings and help trans-

mit the impulse to the spinal cord, from where it is relayed to the brain. Primitive sensations of pain can occur in the mid-brain, with more refined sensations occurring in the thalamus. However the most refined are at the level of the cerebral cortex where the type, intensity and location of pain are recognized. Notwithstanding, the painful stimulus can be so intense that the impulse is not transmitted to the brain and an immediate response is initiated by a reflex action, which is processed in the spinal cord. The classic example of this is the reflex withdrawal of the hand on touching something very hot.

For a long time it was thought that painful stimuli were received by special pain receptors in the tissue and transmitted along special pain pathways to a pain centre in the brain. However, this theory, called the *specificity theory*, does not account for the complexities of pain perception. A more acceptable explanation was provided by *pattern theory* which assumes that the pathways in the central nervous system are not narrowly specific but deal with patterns of impulses, pain therefore being transmitted along pathways which convey other sensations too. But this theory is said to be physiologically flawed (Hollinworth, 1994).

One of the widely accepted theories of pain is the *gate theory* put forward as long ago as 1965 by Wall and Melzack (their 1994 publication is *Textbook of Pain*). As the name suggests, gate theory proposes the idea that there is a mechanism at spinal cord level which acts as a gate. It can decrease or increase the number and intensity of pain signals which reach the brain from the peripheral sensory receptors. Also, impulses from the higher centres of the brain (for example, anxiety or suggestion) can descend and modulate the ascending pain impulses. The gate-control theory helps to explain some of the strange features of the pain experienced, such as why the amount of pain perceived does not necessarily correlate with the intensity of the painful stimulus, and why the emotional status of the person appears to influence the process of pain perception.

In fact the role of the brain itself in suppressing pain sensations is now accepted as an area of knowledge crucial to understand. In 1975, a powerful pain-blocking chemical called endorphin was found to be present, naturally, in the human brain and spinal cord. Since then, several such substances have been identified, as well as enkephalins (they have an action similar to morphine) which are also produced in the body; and they all have a complicated part to play in closing the gate to pain. Such discoveries add an important dimension to understanding the physiology of pain (overviewed by Jacques, 1994) but it is recognized that there is still much to learn.

Perception of pain

This aspect of the pain experience is one of the most fascinating. It concerns the individual's interpretation of the meaning of the signals received in the brain — the perception of the pain. It can be influenced by, for example:

- *Past experience.* Children respond to parental attitudes e.g. some parents fuss about a child's minor injury whereas others reserve attention for more severe pain and as a result, the children concerned adopt different ways of responding to pain. And Davis (1993) quotes studies to show how past experiences of pain influence perception e.g. premedication with anaesthetic blockage and/or opiates reduce postoperative pain
- *Personality.* Kitson (1994) quotes studies where introverts were found to have more intense pain but complained less than extroverts. Of course, Freud regarded pain as a common conversion syndrome representing the transformation of a repressed drive into physical symptoms; the pain need not be created, but selected from a background of possible pain that best fulfils a symbolic function. Reflecting on this, East (1992) suggests that although the health care professional is taught to relieve pain, this may not be welcomed by the client
- *Anxiety.* In a review of literature, Baillie (1994) concludes that anxiety, fear and depression can increase pain sensation and if the level is reduced, less pain is reported
- *Suggestion.* Pain control can be affected by e.g. placebo drugs (Hollinworth, 1994). Placebos are often innocuous confections of sugar and can, in selected instances relieve pain because of the implicit suggestion that medications relieve pain, although an effective receiver-giver relationship is usually a prerequisite. However, other mechanisms may also be involved
- *Cultural beliefs and attitudes.* These can affect the way people grow up to perceive and react to pain, e.g. in Western cultures childbirth is generally considered to be a painful experience (Mander 1992 reviews the literature and discusses pharmacological and non-pharmacological methods of relief) but in other parts of the world, women appear to have minimal pain in labour. In certain societies, ritualistic ceremonies involving piercing the lips or cheeks with stakes are carried out with little apparent pain and the resulting wounds heal quickly. Also, a study quoted in Hollinworth (1994) suggests that despite a high degree of assimilation of ethnic groups into American culture, individual expressions of pain are still conditioned by the patient's ethnic background
- *Religion.* Attitudes to pain may be influenced by

beliefs which can provide a rationale for pain. For example, says East (1992) Hindus may associate pain with Karma (a burden from a past incarnation).

It is often said that these variations in the perception of pain are the result of people's different 'pain thresholds' — some people having a low threshold and feeling only slightly painful stimuli, and others having a high threshold and being immune to everything except the most intensely painful stimuli. In fact, all people have the same 'sensation threshold' (that is, the point at which sensation of any kind is experienced): it is the '*pain perception threshold*' — the point at which the sensation of pain is experienced — which varies between individuals.

Of course, the ability to perceive pain requires a fully functioning nervous system and any damage to the sensory nerve endings, sensory tracts in the spinal cord or the involved areas of the cerebral cortex of the brain will interfere with pain perception. For example, there may be no perception of pain affecting the lower limbs in a person paralysed because of paraplegia. Sometimes, on the other hand, there is an increased sensitivity to pain and this often occurs in neuritis, an inflammatory condition affecting nerve tissue. Level of consciousness is also relevant; as the level lowers, the pain perception threshold is correspondingly depressed.

It should be remembered, however, that even when able to perceive pain, the person may not be able to communicate the perception effectively because of, for example, a speech impediment; lack of fluency in the language; age (a child, an elderly person); a learning disability; certain mental health problems. Such people are even more dependent on the nurse's communication skills to help them convey their feelings.

Reaction to pain

Like the perception of pain, the reaction to pain is highly individual and again, is partly determined by upbringing, personality and sociocultural factors, for example, the renowned (though highly generalized) British reaction of 'keeping a stiff upper lip'.

The major differences between reactions to acute and chronic pain are outlined in Box 5.13 and Doverty (1994) reminds us that the expectation of the person with chronic pain is attainment of day-to-day symptom control rather than pain resolution (as in, for example, trauma) so specific nursing interventions must be suited to each pain experience.

Many people who have chronic pain are at home in the community and Snelling (1990) reviews some research and examines the family's aetiological role in chronic pain; the ways in which the family can influence and maintain pain; and the impact chronic pain has on the family unit.

Box 5.13 Features of acute and chronic pain

ACUTE	CHRONIC
relatively short duration	lasts > 6 months although an initial episode may be identifiable
usually localized	less localized
well-defined pattern of onset with subjective symptoms and objective physical signs	insidious onset lacking the objective signs commonly associated with acute pain
rapid pulse raised blood pressure raised respiratory rate skin pale and sweaty muscle tension in affected part anxious expression anorexia nausea } may occur if restlessness } unrelieved irritability insomnia	personality changes anxiety depression irritability helplessness/ powerlessness weariness alteration in ability for ALs alteration in lifestyle

At home, the social, psychological, environmental and economic circumstances are perhaps more obvious to the nurse and Walker (1992) emphasizes how essential it is to consider the reactions and needs of the carers:

'some sufferers cope well at the expense of someone else; others fail to do well because their carer is doing too good a job, and has unwittingly denied them their role in self-care.'

Types of pain

Pain manifests itself in different ways according to the location, cause, intensity and duration. There is no one definition, but it is possible to categorize pain into various types. For example:

- *superficial pain* is felt in the skin and subcutaneous tissue often with an obvious cause such as heat, pressure or mechanical trauma;
- *deep pain* usually involving muscles and joints may be described as 'aching' or gnawing';
- *visceral pain* often is associated with a specific organ, for example the 'tight' pain of angina when there is a reduction in oxygenated blood reaching the myocardium;

- *neuralgic pain* arises from damage to peripheral nerves and is often caused by infection, inflammation or poor circulation;
- *referred pain*, for example angina, may be experienced as shoulder pain;
- *phantom limb pain*, a tingling pins-and-needles pain experienced in an amputated limb, may continue for months although eventually it does disappear. Davis (1993) refers to the influence of past experience on pain perception and quotes a study where it was shown that phantom limb pain is reduced if patients are rendered pain-free by epidural blockade prior to amputation;
- *psychogenic pain* occurs in the absence of apparent physical stimuli. Increasingly it is being recognized that psychological factors can cause pain and it is not imaginary; to the person experiencing the pain, it is real.

Assessment of pain

Because pain is a subjective experience and such a complex phenomenon (including neurological, physiological, behavioural and affective aspects) it is not easy to assess. There are three main methods of assessment:

(1) obtaining the person's own description; this allows them to feel involved in the management of the pain
(2) obtaining a history
(3) observing the individual's reactions to pain.

The following aspects can be explored:

- *The location of the pain* is one of the first facts to ascertain. The person may be able to point to or describe the gross area involved, such as in the arm or may need help to locate it more specifically.
- *The temporal pattern of the pain* may be important in diagnosis, for example, whether stomach pain occurs before, during or after a meal. The time of the onset of the pain, the duration and the time at which it gets worse or less or better can be established from questioning.
- *The intensity of pain* must be assessed as the patient's own perception and is not necessarily reflected by the pain reaction. An effective way of finding out how intense the patient's pain is, and how the intensity varies, is to use a pain rating scale. They can be Visual Analogue Scales or VAS (a line marked with no pain at one end and unbearable pain at the other; clients mark the line with a cross at the point which best represents their level of pain) with variations on that theme which include numbers or colours or words or descriptions (Fig. 5.5 and Fig. 5.6). There are also

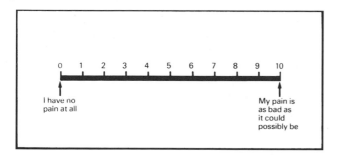

Fig. 5.5 A painometer — an example of a pain rating scale

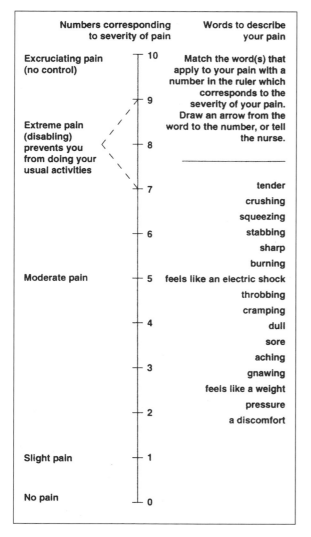

Fig. 5.6 The pain ruler — an example of a pain-rating scale (Source: Baillie (1993))

graphic rating scales to measure pain relief. Several are described by Kitson (1994) in her literature review of postoperative pain management.

Using a rating scale is more informative than spontaneous verbal statements such as 'I can't bear it' or 'Its terrible'. Doverty (1994) reviews the literature, mentions several rating scales and quotes that different tools can be combined such as

a VAS, a linear scale and the McGill Pain Questionnaire (it contains sensory, affective and evaluative aspects and is used in a study by Fortin et al 1992).

For children, Van Cleeve and Savedra (1993) adapted a body outline model to assess pain in 4–7 year olds and Nethercott (1994) conducted an exploratory study related to the assessment and management of postoperative pain in children as viewed by the children, parents and nurses.

- *The reaction to pain*, if observed carefully, may provide important information particularly when the person has difficulty in communicating verbally or has a depressed level of consciousness. Pallor, rapid breathing, a raised blood pressure and excessive sweating may accompany intense pain. Nonverbal cues may assist with assessment. Facial gestures such as screwing up the face or gritting the teeth are common reactions to pain. Body posture may also be relevant; for instance with stomach pain people often curl up, whereas with chest pain they may want to lean forward or lie on the affected side. Crying and groaning may occur and if the pain is intermittent yet intense, the person may shout aloud or shriek.

  As long ago as 1984 Sofaer was reminding us that some patients need nurses to tell them that their pain behaviour is acceptable and normal, and other people also react in a similar way.

- *The character of the pain* is the way it is described. Some of the ways in which pain can be described have already been mentioned; 'aching', 'gnawing', 'tightness', 'tingling' are a few of the words commonly used. Some others are 'stabbing', 'burning', 'twisting' and 'shooting'. Sometimes the description is a comprehensive statement of the pain being experienced; for example, the person may say 'I have a sharp pain in my chest when I breathe in' or 'I have a burning pain when I pass water' or 'I get cramp-like stomach pains with my periods' or 'I have a throbbing or stabbing migraine' (Reilly, 1994).

- *Factors precipitating the pain* are important elements for identification in assessment. Pain is often related to everyday activities of living such as eating and drinking, eliminating, breathing, working and playing, to name a few. Whether pain is associated with mobility or whether it occurs even at rest is of crucial importance. Environmental factors such as noise, and psychological factors such as anxiety or fear may also precipitate pain. The person may describe without difficulty what precipitates the pain: 'The pain in my chest comes on when I get short of breath, for instance after climbing a flight of stairs'.

- *Past experience of pain* is relevant in assessment because it may affect subsequent pain experiences (Davis, 1993). Discussion can also provide information about measures which have been effective in alleviating pain, or it may indicate sources of anxiety which could be reduced by adequate understanding of what to expect, for instance regarding an operation (Hiscock, 1993; Walding, 1991), and so reduce pain in the postoperative period.

Having gathered all the information about the person's experience of pain, including their normal coping strategies, the assessment must be documented. This is conducive to continuity of care by the health team; it allows re-assessments to be compared; and permits evaluation of pain relief.

Of all the health care staff, nurses are probably the most involved with ongoing assessment of pain yet various studies indicate that nursing inferences were made by observing appearance and behaviour rather than asking the sufferer to describe and assess the pain; and there seems to be lack of correspondence between observer inferences and patient self-reported pain. Many studies expose the inadequacy of pain documentation and by inference, the inadequacy of pain assessment.

Despite the considerable research, and related recommendations for solving some of the problems, patients/clients are still suffering unnecessary pain (Closs et al, 1993; Davis, 1993; MacKintosh, 1994) and the plea continues that nurses (and doctors) must equip themselves with the necessary knowledge and skills to minimize and alleviate pain. In a comparative study of an ICU and a hospice Fothergill-Bourbonnais and Wilson-Barnet (1992) found that 88% of nurses thought they needed more knowledge and skills to care for patients in pain. And in a survey of neonatal ICUs reported by Lyall (1990) 70% of the units thought analgesia was commonly under-prescribed by doctors, and 33% thought it was under-administered by nurses; a finding echoed in other paediatric settings (Nursing Standard Supplement, 1993).

Control of pain

The relief of pain and suffering is one of the most important objectives in health care and in many instances, some form of medication is used — by the oral, sublingual, subcutaneous, rectal, intramuscular, spinal or parenteral routes. Nurses do not prescribe medications, but they do have a considerable role in relation to their administration and even when the medical practitioner physically administers the medication, for example a local anaesthetic block, nurses still have responsibilities in preparing and supporting the patient before, during and after the treatment. This is especially so with children. May (1992)

discusses pain control in a children's neurosurgery unit, and a series of articles in the Nursing Standard Supplement (1993) feature pain management in the infant and child.

Patients primarily look to the nurse for pain relief and the nurse, along with the individual concerned (and/or the parents if the patient is a child), assesses the individual's current experience of pain before administering the prescribed medication and evaluating the effect. It is important therefore that nurses understand how analgesics work and this subject is studied in other parts of the student curriculum.

Exploring the provision of postoperative analgesic medications Closs (1990) quotes that many researchers have commented on the under-use of narcotic analgesics in hospital, with adverse effects on the patient, physical and psychological. The reasons for underprovision appear to fall into two main areas:

- exaggerated beliefs about the addiction properties of opiates and their side effect on respiratory depression
- difficulties in assessing pain compounded by the reluctance of many patients to ask for analgesics.

She went on to investigate the relationship between pain and sleep, and in her retrospective study concerned with 200 patients in surgical wards, it was found that 179 had sleep disturbance by pain at some point in their hospital stay. Although there was no difference in analgesic provision related to time of day, it was found that analgesics were given approximately half as frequently during the night. This lack of pain relief plus the effects of sleep deprivation (p. 375) can produce undesirable physiological and psychological reactions.

Duggleby and Lander (1994), in a postoperative study of older patients, included (among several measures) the assessment of night pain intensity and sleep disturbance. One of their important findings was that poor pain management may be a precursor of acute decline in cognitive status.

As well as the individually-administered medications given by nursing staff, there is a new generation of medication delivery systems which offer the patient a large measure of personal control, and the possibility of staying at home, or even at work, because efficacious control techniques are available.

The technique of patient-controlled analgesia or PCA (Box 5.14) is described by Warwick (1992); and Thomas and Rose (1993) discuss some of the criteria for allocating PCA, emphasizing the nurse's responsibilities. It requires careful planning. Staff must be trained to use it and the patient should be carefully selected, effectively instructed about the technique, and willing to use it. Thomas and Rose quote studies where it has been effective for postoperative pain, myocardial pain, for burns, for bone

---

Box 5.14 Patient-controlled analgesia

The purpose built equipment has a previously programmed medication injection which is connected to a venous cannula in the patient's arm or hand. A preset dose can be delivered over a predetermined time by the patient activating a press-button switch. This is done when the patient feels the need for pain relief, but there is a built-in mechanism to prevent overdosage.

It helps the patient to feel 'in control' and this is considered to be psychologically desirable as well as having positive physical effects e.g. in relation to early ambulation, therefore lessening the risk of respiratory infection, embolus and pressure area problems.

---

marrow transplant, and for cancer. It can also be successfully used for older children.

However, acute pain is not only a hospital concern. Although historically, postoperative pain control has been the domain of the hospital, Hollinworth (1994) reminds us that the use of day surgery and shorter hospital stays draws community nurses into the arena of postoperative pain control.

Community nurses are certainly involved with the management of chronic pain. Jones (1993) discusses the evolution of acute to chronic pain and outlines the stages of adaptation the individual goes through. She refers to the coping strategies used in the attempt to return to a 'normal' life, the success of which determines whether or not they enter the chronic phase. An important determinant, she says, is the person's attributional style i.e. the way the person explains and controls events:

- the internal locus governs the way individuals see themselves as being in control of their progress
- the external locus governs the belief that outside factors or other people (e.g. nurses, doctors) control their progress

and she maintains that as pain becomes more chronic, the locus of control moves from internal to external.

In the community, many elderly people suffer from ailments which cause chronic pain and Walker (1991) carried out a study to investigate coping strategies and pain control among elderly people visited by district nurses. Latham (1993), too, discusses pain management in later life, sometimes the result of diseases associated with the ageing process. She particularly mentions problems of communication, and discusses the use not only of medications, but other therapies which are effective in pain control. Closs (1994) reminds readers that older people frequently have more than one source of pain, and she, too, stresses the problems of assessment when the person has communication difficulties and/or dementia.

She quotes Ferrell's ten principles of pain management for elderly people as a basis for minimizing suffering and improving their quality of life.

Quite apart from pharmacological remedies prescribed by the medical practitioner, there are other pain therapies, some of which lie directly within the province of the nurse. Any sensory distraction or diversion such as change of position, application of heat or cold and relaxation techniques may provide competition to stimuli which prevent them getting through the 'gate' and therefore reduce the pain signals. Also rubbing or lightly slapping an injured part can reduce the pain.

Transcutaneous nerve stimulations or TENS (mentioned by Hollinworth, 1994) is another 'competitive' measure as are acupuncture and biofeedback; many are described in a special issue of the Nursing Times called Complementary Therapy (1993) and in subsequent issues during 1993 and 1994. Several require special training if used by the nurse; and others require collaboration with recognized health therapists. A Nursing Times Leader (1994) however, reminds nurses that a number of complementary therapies have not yet been adequately researched.

In several countries, multidisciplinary pain control clinics have been established as a focus of specialized knowledge and expertise for chronic pain. Patients come with a variety of problems including pain associated with arthritis, cancer, orthopaedic disabilities and back pain. Different treatments are offered including medications and psychiatric assessment, and those who need inpatient treatment are admitted. Chronic pain affects the person's lifestyle. The emphasis may be on how to cope with pain and how to live with it rather than 'curing' the pain; and measuring the person's increase in activity level may be more relevant than diminishing the pain level.

It is now recognized that the skills and expertise of various health therapists can be used to manage pain and these clinics (Box 5.15) offer diverse methods of pain control which can be summarized under three headings — physical, psychological and pharmacological:

physical methods of pain control	change of position applications of heat/cold massage and vibration electrical stimulation techniques neurosurgical techniques acupuncture
psychological methods of pain control	communicating sensory distraction and diversion music therapy relaxation techniques desensitization hypnosis biofeedback behaviour modification

Box 5.15 A pain unit for somatoform pain

Wilson (1991) describes a pain unit where most people referred had a diagnosis of somatoform pain whose essential feature, he quotes, is:

'a preoccupation with pain in the absence of adequate physical findings to account for the pain or its severity'.

The Unit (based in a psychiatric wing) offers individually tailored packages following an assessment carried out by members of the multidisciplinary pain team. The rehabilitation programme of five-weeks duration is behaviourally based. This approach, he says, can help sufferers to gain control over their lives and movements, achieving a measure of independence which they may have assumed they had lost forever.

pharmacological
methods
of
pain control
{
analgesics (local and general), medication to treat the cause of the pain, tranquillizers to reduce anxiety, anaesthetic blocking agents (for example, epidural anaesthesia), inhalations

The search for new and more effective techniques of pain control goes on year by year. However as far as medications are concerned, their availability is not universal so politicoeconomic factors can influence methods of pain relief. In developing countries, for example, where it is difficult to procure or to afford oral narcotics, pain relief by other than pharmacological means assumes enormous importance. Any discussion of pain illustrates yet again the relatedness of biological, psychological, sociocultural, environmental and politicoeconomic factors.

Patients may complain of pain in any part of the body and in many instances it is not possible to see the cause, so for our model for nursing, McCaffery's (1983) definition is used 'Pain is what the patient says it is, existing where he says it does'. Consequently, the problem of pain in our model, is associated with the AL of communicating.

It is suggested therefore that, in any proforma based on our model which is used for documenting a Nursing Plan, the nurse would normally assess and chart the incidence of pain under the AL of communicating unless it were AL-specific, that is, if someone with a respiratory infection had a pain in the chest, the pain would be recorded under the AL of breathing. Examples of pain related to specific ALs are mentioned in the appropriate AL chapter in Section 2.

PLANNING AND IMPLEMENTING NURSING ACTIVITIES AND EVALUATING OUTCOMES

In the preceding section, some examples of clients' pro-

blems in the AL of communicating have been outlined and it will be apparent that the causes and effects of problems are varied and often complex. In fact, the entire chapter provides a background of *general* information about the AL of communicating which can be used by the beginning student as a mental framework to assess the individual (Box 5.3) and then identify some *specific* problems which any one client might experience.

Having identified the individual's problems, actual and potential, it is possible in conjunction with the person and/or carers, to agree on goals to cope with or solve them; or to prevent potential problems from becoming actual problems. Goal-setting is the first part of planning and goals should be stated in terms of how they will be evaluated.

For example, for a man who has early stages of dementia with reduced short-term memory, one goal (in an attempt to retain his optimum independence at home) might be to teach his wife and/or carers — or rather, help them to learn — about communicating effectively. Emphasis could be on how to give clear verbal messages, and how to use memory and orientation jogs at regular intervals throughout the day while ascertaining his response.

This goal, along with others, would be recorded on the nursing plan, and over a period of weeks or months the community nurse would evaluate, at predetermined dates, the degree of independence retained by the client and the response of the wife/carers in terms of their capacity to cope with the client's deteriorating ability to communicate.

Another example might be of an adolescent girl who has limited intellectual capacity and severe speech difficulties, and who has been admitted as an emergency, having sustained a fractured leg in a car accident. One immediate goal would be 'effective communication' with this girl, and if her family were available, one nursing activity related to this goal would involve collaborating with them in order to learn about her usual repertoire of communicative techniques. This information would be recorded on the nursing plan as soon as an assessment could be made, so that all staff were aware of her abilities to communicate as well as her limitations.

On return from the recovery room, ward nursing staff might deduce — by means of careful observation and continuing assessment — that restlessness and discernibly different grunting sounds were used by the girl when she appeared to be in pain, and when she wished to eliminate. To meet the goal of 'effective communication' would involve interpreting her unique methods of 'speaking' and responding, and adapting to them in order to anticipate her needs; not only to increase her comfort but also as a means of helping to reduce her level of anxiety in a strange environment among strange people.

When appropriate, goals would be geared to the girl's

pending discharge from hospital, and it would be important to give the community nurse well documented information about the girl's modes of communicating in order to effect a smooth handover of nursing responsibilities until such time as her pre-accident level of independence in ALs had been achieved.

These are two examples but throughout this Chapter, in the course of discussing individuals' problems with the AL of communicating, nursing interventions have been mentioned along with possible outcomes.

Finding exact measures to evaluate outcomes is recognized as a field where more research is required but meantime, attempts are made to use measures which reduce subjectivity to a minimum, for example a pain-rating scale for the assessment of pain and an evaluation of the effectiveness of nursing interventions.

It must be recognized, too, that in achieving a stated goal, the nurse may not be the only person who makes a contribution to the achievement. Other members of the health team may be involved, and in the home setting, the contribution of family and carers may be virtually inestimable, not to mention the client's own personal contribution. However a statement of goals; the agreed actions for achieving them; and the method of evaluating whether or not they are achieved (even with tools which are not proven to be exact measurements) assists all those involved to unite in concentrating their efforts towards a common end.

Figure 3.9 attempts to emphasize that the four phases of individualizing nursing (using the process of nursing) which have been discussed are not linear; there is frequent feedback, re-assessment and adjustment as the person's problems are resolved or change, or as new problems arise. The whole topic of individualizing nursing has already been discussed in more detail in Chapter 3.

It is necessary to emphasize, however, that there are many instances when it may not be relevant to investigate or document a client's circumstances in relation to the AL of communicating. This is a matter for professional judgement. When it is necessary, the information would be combined with information about the person's other relevant ALs. It is only for the purposes of discussion that any AL can be considered on its own; in reality they are closely related and frequently overlap.

ACKNOWLEDGEMENT

Thanks are extended to Dr Hazel Watson, Assistant Head, Department of Nursing and Community Health, Glasgow Caledonian University, for preparing the section, 'Process of Communicating'.

REFERENCES RELEVANT TO COMMUNICATING (except PAIN)

Allison A, Marshall M 1994 Dementia in acute units: the issues. Nursing Standard 8(52) September 21: 28–30

Allmark P, Klarzynski R 1992 The case against nurse advocacy. British Journal of Nursing 2(1): 33–36

Anthonypillai F 1994 Overcoming language barriers in ICU. Nursing Times 90(8) February 23: 12

Argyle M 1994 The psychology of interpersonal behaviour 5th edition. Penguin, London

Barber B 1992 Security screening. Nursing Times 88(49) December 2: 50–52

Barker P 1990 Breaking the shell. Nursing Times 86(46) November 14: 36–38

Berlo D 1960 The process of communication: an introduction of theory and practice. Henry Holt, New York

Burnard P 1987a Sharing a viewpoint. Senior Nurse 7(3) September: 38–39

Burnard P 1987b Counselling — basic principles in nursing. Professional Nurse 3(10) July: 388–391

Burnard P 1988 Empathy: the key to understanding. Professional Nurse 3(10) July: 388–391

Burnard P 1991 Acquiring minimal counselling skills. Nursing Standard 5(46) August 7: 37–39

Burnard P 1992 Assertiveness. Part 1. Nursing Times Management Module 88(22) May 27: i–viii

Butrin J 1992 Cultural diversity in the nurse-client encounter. Clinical Nursing Research 1(3) August: 238–251

Carlisle D 1994 Facing up to race. Nursing Times 90(26) June 29: 14–15

Carruthers A 1992 A force to promote bonding and well-being: therapeutic touch and massage. Professional Nurse 7(5) February: 297–300

Carter A 1995 The use of touch in nursing practice. Nursing Standard 9(16) January 11: 31–35

Chambers M 1992 Who speaks for children? Journal of Clinical Nursing 1: 73–76

Cohen P 1994a Passing the buck? Nursing Times 90(13) March 30: 28–30

Cohen P 1994b Advocates of independence. Nursing Times 90(9) March 2: 67–69

Davies P 1993 Diagnosing hearing loss in children. Nursing Standard 7(35) May 19: 33–36

Department of Health 1993 Ethnicity and health; a guide for the NHS. DOH, London

Department of Health 1994 Being Heard. DOH, London

Dodds F 1993 Access to the coping strategies: managing anxiety in elective surgical patients. Professional Nurse October: 45–52

Donnelly D 1987 Focus on disability: registered hopeless? Nursing Times 83(24) June 17: 49–51

Downey R 1994 A listening ear. Nursing Times 90(24) June 15: 14–15

Dunn B 1991 Communication interaction skills. Senior Nurse 11(4) July/August: 4–8

Evans G 1994 Supporting role. Nursing Times 90(9) March 2: 70–71

Fessey C 1988 Communication difficulties and assertiveness/negotiation skills. The Add-on Journal of Clinical Nursing 3(27) March/April: 1002–1005

Fewster C 1990 Trapped in a stammer. Nursing Times 86(7) February 14: 40–41

Finnegan L 1994 Lives at a glance. Nursing Times 90(16) April 20: 52–54

Foong A 1992 Challenging the tower of Babel. Nursing 5(5) March 12–25: 8–10

Fox G 1995 Guiding principles. Nursing Times 91(4) January 25: 62–63

Franklin P 1994 Straight talking. Nursing Times 90(8) February 23: 33–34

General Medical Council 1992 News review. GMC, London (2): 1

Glasper A, Gow M, Yerrell P 1989 A family friend. Nursing Times 85(4) January 25: 63–65

Gould D 1990 Empathy: a review of the literature with suggestions for an alternative research strategy. Journal of Advanced Nursing 15(10) October: 1167–1174

Graham A 1992 Advocacy: what the future holds. British Journal of Nursing 1(3): 148–150

Hackney A 1993 Truth about drugs. Nursing Times 89(8) February 24: 66–68

Harding E 1994 Preparing patients for the effects of laryngectomy. Nursing Times 90(32) August 10: 36–37

Her Majesty's Stationery Office 1992 The Patient's Charter. HMSO, Edinburgh

Hubert J 1993 Speaking up. Nursing Times 89(44) November 3: 59–61

Hunt A 1991 The admission process. Nursing Times 87(20) May 15: 30–32

Hunter L 1987 Keyboard rehabilitation. Nursing Times 83(32) August 12: 45–47

Ireland C 1990 I'm not mad — I'm angry. Nursing Times 86(20) May 16: 45–47

Jones A 1990 Empathy in the counselling process. Nursing Standard 4(44) July 25: 53–55

Kay B 1995 Challenging behaviours. Nursing Standard 9(24) March 8: 31–36

Kearsley N, Little T, Wiseman C 1994 Realised potential. Nursing Times 90(24) June 15: 44–45

Kelly J 1993 Visual impairment among older people. British Journal of Nursing 2(2): 110–116

King C, Macmillan M 1994 Documentation and discharge planning for elderly patients. Nursing Times 90(20) May 18: 31–33

Korgaonkar G, Tribe D 1993 Children and consent to medical treatment. British Journal of Nursing 2(7): 383–384

Korgaonkar G, Tribe D 1994 Confidentiality, patients and the law. British Journal of Nursing 3(2): 91–93

Lavelle-Jones C, Byrne D, Rice P, Cuschieri A 1993 Factors affecting quality of informed consent. British Medical Journal 306(6882) April 3: 885–890

Leach V 1994 More on familiarity and contempt. Nursing Standard 8(25) March 16: 41

Luxon L 1993 Tinnitus: its causes, diagnosis and treatment. British Medical Journal 306 June 5: 1490–1491

Lynn J 1993 Don't tell the patient. Nursing Standard 7(27) March 24: 50–51

McCann K, McKenna H 1993 An examination of touch between nurses and elderly patients in a continuing care setting in Northern Ireland. Journal of Advanced Nursing 18: 838–846

McCormack B 1993 How to promote quality of care and preserve patient autonomy. British Journal of Nursing 2(6): 338–341

McCourt V 1994 Cherish the memory (Reminiscence Groups). Nursing Times 90(29) July 20: 63–64

McGough S 1990 An extraordinary skill. Nursing Times 86(20) May 16: 35–37

MacIsaac E 1993 Answer that soon. Nursing Times 89(1) January 6: 43

Macleod Clark J, Hopper L, Jesson A 1991 Progression to counselling. Nursing Times 87(8) February 20: 41–43

McMillan I 1994 Minority interest. Nursing Times 90(10) March 9: 20–21

Markanday L, Platzer H 1994 Brief encounters. Nursing Times 90(7) February 16: 38–42

Martell R 1994 The enigma of autism. Nursing Standard 8(15) January 5: 20–21

Nolan M 1994 Maternity care for the visually impaired. Modern Midwife May: 18–20

Norris E 1992 Care of the paediatric day-surgery patient. British Journal of Nursing 1(11): 547–551

Peace G 1994 Sensitive choices. Nursing Times 90(8) February 23: 35–36

Price B 1990 A model for body-image care. Journal of Advanced Nursing 15(5): 585–593

Professional Development 1994 Breaking bad news: the role of the nurse. Unit 2 Part 2 Nursing Times 90(11) March 16: 5–8

Pyne R 1992 Accountability in principle and in practice. British Journal of Nursing 1 (6): 301–305

Radcliffe S 1993 Preoperative information: the role of the ward nurse. British Journal of Nursing 2(16): 305–309

Ratcliffe J 1988 Worth a try. Nursing Times 84(6) February 10: 29–30

Robson R 1994 Refusing treatment. Nursing Standard 8(29) April 13: 23

Rossor M 1993 Alzheimer's disease. British Medical Journal 307(6907) September 25: 779–782

Royal College of Nursing 1993 Advocacy: the nurse's responsibilities. Nursing Standard 8(2) September 29: 29–30

Ryan A 1994 Improving discharge planning. Nursing Times 90(20) May 18: 33–34

Shield J, Baum J 1994 Children's consent to treatment. British Medical Journal 308(6938) May 7: 1182–1183

Sines D 1993 Balance of power. Nursing Times 89(46) November 17: 52–55

Slater J 1990 Effecting personal effectiveness: assertiveness training for nurses. Journal of Advanced Nursing 15(3) March: 337–356

Smith M 1991 Understanding speech disorders. Nursing Standard 5(48) August 21: 30–33

Stephenson M 1990 Discharge criteria in day surgery. Journal of Advanced Nursing 15(5) May: 601–613

Stewart J, Creed J 1994 Aphasia: a care study. British Journal of Nursing 3(5): 226–229

Susman E, Dorn L, Fletcher J 1992 Children and the question of consent. The Journal of Paediatrics 121(4): 547–552

Sutor J 1993 Can nurses be effective advocates? Nursing Standard 7(22) February 17: 30–32

Teasdale K 1993 Information and anxiety: a critical reappraisal. Journal of Advanced Nursing 18: 1125–1132

Tompkins J 1988 A good sign (Makaton). Nursing Standard 32(2) May 14: 31

Tonks A 1993 Information management and patient privacy in the NHS. British Medical Journal 307(6914) November 13: 1227–1228

Turnock C 1991 Communicating with patients in ICU. Nursing Standard 5(15) January 9: 38–40

United Kingdom Central Council 1992 Code of Professional Conduct for the Nurse, Midwife and Health Visitor. UKCC, London

Vanderslott J 1992 A supportive therapy that undermines violence: counselling to prevent ward violence. Professional Nurse 7(7) April: 427–430

Waterman H, Webb C 1992 Visually impaired patients' perceptions of their needs in hospital. Nursing Practice 5(3): 6–9

Wiggens J, Wiggens B, Sanden J 1994 Social psychology. 5th edition. McGraw-Hill, New York

Williams J 1991 Meaningful dialogue. Nursing Times 87(4) January 23: 52–53

Williams J 1994 The rehabilitation process. Nursing Times 90(29) July 20: 33–34

Williams K, Kallmark A 1993 Confidence trick. Nursing Times 89(24) June 16: 31–33

Willis J 1994 Strategic decisions. Nursing Times 90(7) February 16: 52–53

Wilson-Barnett J 1988 Patient teaching or patient counselling? Journal of Advanced Nursing 13 (March): 215–222

Wimpory D 1991 Breaking through the barriers. Nursing Times 87(34) August 21: 58–61

Wright D 1993 Deaf people's perceptions of communication with nurses. British Journal of Nursing 2(11): 567–571

Zylinski J 1993 Patient education: postoperative needs. Nursing Standard 8(6) October 27: 31–35

ADDITIONAL READING

Baillie L 1995 Empathy in the nurse-patient relationship. Nursing Standard 9(20) February 8: 29–32

Burnard P 1992 A communication skills guide for health care workers. Edward Arnold, London

McNally S 1995 The experience of advocacy. British Journal of Nursing 4(2): 87–89

REFERENCES RELEVANT TO COMMUNICATING AND PAIN

Astley A 1990 A history of pain. Nursing 4(17) August 23 – Sept 12: 33–35

Baillie L 1993 A review of pain assessment tools. Nursing Standard 7(23) February 24: 25–29

Clancy J, McVicar A 1992 Subjectivity of pain. British Journal of Nursing 1(1): 8–12

Closs S 1990 An exploratory analysis of nurses' provision of postoperative analgesic drugs. Journal of Advanced Nursing 15(1) January: 42–49

Closs J 1994 Pain in elderly patients: a neglected phenomenon? Journal of Advanced Nursing 19(6) June: 1072–1081

Closs S, Fairtlough H, Tierney A, Currie C 1993 Pain in elderly orthopaedic patients. Journal of Clinical Nursing 2: 41–45

Davis P 1993 Opening up the gate control theory. Nursing Standard 7(45) July 28: 25–27

Doverty N 1994 Make pain assessment your priority. Professional Nurse 9(4) January: 230–237

Duggleby W, Lander J 1994 Cognitive status and postoperative pain. Journal of Pain and Symptom Management 9(1): 19–27

East E 1992 How much does it hurt? Nursing Times 88(40) September 30: 48–49

Fortin J, Schwartz-Barcott D, Rossi S 1992 The postoperative pain experience: a description based on the McGill Pain Questionnaire. Clinical Nursing Research 1(3) August: 292–304

Fothergill-Bourbonnais F, Wilson-Barnett J 1992 A comparative study of intensive therapy unit and hospice nurses' knowledge on pain management. Journal of Advanced Nursing 17: 362–372

Hiscock M 1993 Complex reactions requiring empathy and knowledge. Professional Nurse 9(3) December: 158–160

Hollinworth H 1994 No gain? — postoperative pain. Nursing Times 90(1) January 5: 24–27

Jacques A 1992 Do you believe I'm in pain? Nurses' assessment of patients' pain. Professional Nurse 7(4) January: 249–251

Jacques A 1994 Physiology of pain. British Journal of Nursing 3(12): 607–610

Jones S 1993 Effect of psychological processes on chronic pain. British Journal of Nursing 2(9): 463–467

Kitson A 1994 Postoperative pain management: a literature review. Journal of Clinical Nursing 3: 7–18

Latham J 1993 Treatment we can all believe in: pain and its management in later life. Professional Nurse 8(4) January: 212–220

Lyall J 1990 Painful admission. Nursing Times 86(43) October 24: 16–17

McCaffery M 1983 Nursing the patient in pain (Adapted for the UK by B Sofaer). Harper & Row, London

MacKintosh C 1994 Do nurses provide adequate postoperative pain relief? British Journal of Nursing 3(7): 342–347

Mander R 1992 The control of pain in labour. Journal of Clinical Nursing 1: 219–223

May L 1992 Reducing pain and anxiety in children. Nursing Standard 6(44) July 22: 25–28

Nethercott S 1994 The assessment and management of postoperative pain in children by registered sick children's nurses: an exploratory study. Journal of Clinical Nursing 3: 109–114

Nursing Standard Special Supplement 1993 Managing pain in children. Nursing Standard 7(25) March 10

Nursing Times Leader 1994 Dire need for data. Nursing Times 90(30) July 27: 3

Nursing Times Special Issue 1993 Complementary therapy. Nursing Times, London

Reilly R 1994 Acute and prophylactic treatment of migraine. Nursing Times 90(29) July 20: 35–36

Snelling J 1990 The role of the family in relation to chronic pain: review of the literature. Journal of Advanced Nursing 15: 771–776

Thomas V, Rose F 1993 Patient-controlled analgesia: a new method for old. Journal of Advanced Nursing 18: 1719–1726

Van Cleeve L, Savedra M 1993 Pain location: validity and reliability of body outline markings by four-to-seven-year-old children who are hospitalised. Pediatric Nursing 19(3): 217–220

Walding M 1991 Pain anxiety and powerlessness. Journal of Advanced Nursing 16: 388–397

Walker J 1991 Living with pain: elderly people in the community. Nursing Times 87(43) October 23: 28–32

Walker J 1992 Taking pains. Nursing Times 88(29) July 15: 38–40

Wall P, Melzack R 1994 Textbook of pain. Churchill Livingstone, Edinburgh

Warwick P 1992 Making sense of the principles of patient controlled analgesia. Nursing Times 88(41) October 7: 38–40

Wilson P 1991 Breaking the barrier: behavioural management of chronic pain. Professional Nurse 6(11) August: 639–643

Breathing

The AL of breathing

The AL of breathing was introduced albeit briefly in the model of living (p. 21). It was mentioned in the model for nursing in the context of priorities among ALs (p. 36). Here we consider that 'taking the first breath' is of crucial importance at the birth of every baby and determines whether or not the infant will have a viable existence as a human being. From then on breathing seems effortless and people are not usually consciously aware of the AL of breathing until some abnormal circumstance forces it to their attention.

The purpose of this chapter is to focus the four concepts of our model to the particular AL of breathing as illustrated in Figure 6.1.

Lifespan: relationship to the AL of breathing

At birth it may be necessary to suction the baby's upper respiratory tract to remove any debris collected during the birth process, but for most people, the AL of breathing is an independent activity throughout the lifespan. A newborn infant can be cyanosed because of a heart malformation which diminishes the volume of blood reaching the lungs for oxygenation. Early corrective surgery is usually successful. There can be minor congenital malformations which may not be detected until a school medical examination reveals a 'murmur' on auscultation of the heart. Often such minor malformations are only discovered at a postmortem examination. They may produce symptoms in adulthood, but people may reach their later years before symptoms occur.

The earlier the indulgence in smoking the greater the likelihood of succumbing to cancer of the lung, or narrowing of the arteries supplying the heart muscle resulting in a myocardial infarction, both conditions occurring most commonly in the adult and late phase of life. However, the fact that there is a direct relationship between age and the rate of breathing (and also pulse rate and blood pressure) is relevant knowledge in the present context (Box 6.1).

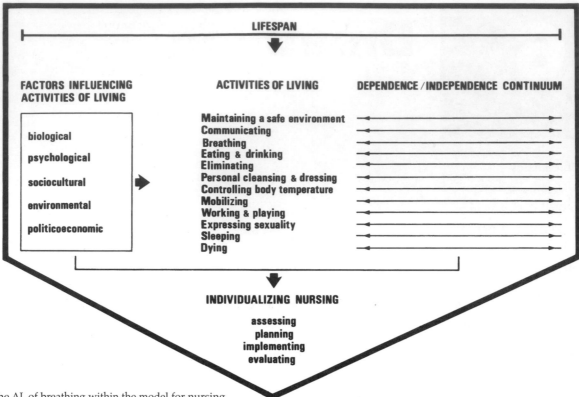

Fig. 6.1 The AL of breathing within the model for nursing

Dependence/independence in the AL of breathing

For most of the ALs, the dependence/independence continuum is closely related to the lifespan, during which a state of dependence in the early years is the norm. Breathing is the exception; it is the only AL which the majority of people perform independently right from birth throughout the entire lifespan, until the moment of death. In health, changes in dependence/independence status for breathing do not occur.

However, there are people who are dependent on smoking and this subject is considered more fully on p. 143. Some people are dependent on the local 'pollen count' for organizing their outdoor activities, thereby achieving their optimal independent status despite their allergy to these substances — a condition known as hay fever. Asthmatic people are dependent on medications which dilate the bronchi, most of these being inhaled. Many such people learn to manage their medication regime and achieve their optimal independence status in their AL of breathing.

Because we juxtaposed the cardiopulmonary system with the AL of breathing, it has to be considered that people with high blood pressure may be dependent on

prescribed anti-hypertensive medications for maintenance of medication-assisted positive health status in the interest of preventing stroke and heart attack. Similarly many people with atrial fibrillation and early congestive heart failure can achieve 'independence' in their AL of breathing despite their dependence on such medications as digoxin.

There are certain illnesses which cause people to be dependent on more sophisticated medical investigation, and subsequent treatment, either temporarily or permanently, with the goal of adequate functioning of the cardiopulmonary system, thereafter achieving optimal independence in the AL of breathing.

Enough has been said about the concept of 'dependence/independence in breathing' to alert the beginning student to its complexity.

Factors influencing the AL of breathing

Commonly occurring activities such as speaking, laughing and eating cause minor alterations in the breathing pattern, though rarely is the individual really aware of these adjustments. Even in the healthy person, however, a number of factors can in a more obvious way influence the rate, depth and regularity of breathing, pulse rate and

Box 6.1 Rate of breathing, pulse rate, and blood pressure: related to lifespan

- *Rate of breathing* is measured by counting the number of times the chest wall rises and falls over a given period. An infant's rate of breathing may be up to 44 per minute but in children it is about 20 per minute and the range of normal for adults is 12 to 18 breaths per minute. In the older person, however, the breathing rate increases and respirations are shallower. These changes are due to the decreasing elasticity of the lungs and less efficient gaseous exchange between the alveoli and the pulmonary capillaries.

- *The pulse rate* also varies in relation to age, the average of 140 beats per minute in the young baby decreasing gradually to around 70 beats per minute in adulthood. Males tend to have a slightly lower rate than females. The pulse rate tends to remain stable at the adult level for the rest of a person's life, unless altered by disease processes.

- *Blood pressure* increases with age. In infancy the blood pressure is around 90/60 whereas in adulthood the average is 120/80, with little change in the later years unless due to the effects of disease. Adults with pressures above 140 mmHg systolic and/or 100 mmHg diastolic are referred to as hypertensive; adults with pressures below 100 systolic are considered to be hypotensive.

blood pressure. These are: the degree of physical activity, and the body's physiological response to stressors (biological factors); changes in mood and emotion (psychological factors); and, of course, the composition of inhaled air and the presence of abnormal constituents in the atmosphere (environmental factors). The fourth group of factors included in this component of the model — sociocultural factors — is only tangentially relevant in the West, but deserves mention under its own heading. Under the fifth heading, politicoeconomic factors, control of pollution is mentioned, and the problem of smoking is discussed from this particular point of view.

BIOLOGICAL

The biological factors most directly influencing the AL of breathing are of course the body structures and functions required for this AL. In biological terms these are the organs which collectively form the respiratory system, the function of which is to provide every cell in the body with oxygen by the processes known as external and internal respiration (Box 6.2). To accomplish this, the blood, together with the vessels and organs comprising the circulatory and lymphatic systems are also relevant biological factors which influence the AL of breathing. In human biology terms, therefore, in the model for nursing the AL of breathing is not only juxtaposed with the respiratory system but also with the cardiovascular system. The purpose of this juxtaposition is to provide guidance when devising a nursing plan which takes account of nurse-initiated interventions. It also enables understanding of the nursing interventions which result from medical prescription and the suggested documents in Appendix 1 accommodate this.

During vigorous exercise in the healthy adult there is a normal physiological increase in respiratory rate, because the muscles require more oxygen. To transport the oxygen more quickly, the heart beats faster so the pulse rate is simultaneously increased; in fact, respiration and pulse rates are related in a ratio of 1:4, and an alteration in one is usually accompanied by an alteration in the other. Conversely when the body is resting, particularly when sleeping, the respiratory rate and pulse rate are usually decreased.

Not only rate but the rhythm of breathing can be affected during such physical activities as talking, laughing, eating, singing, yet seldom are these variations given conscious thought. Even sneezing and coughing, if transient, are rarely pondered over as a deviation in the normal pattern of breathing. But the tissues of both the respiratory and cardiovascular system can be damaged by such activities as smoking.

The effects of smoking

Many people are now aware that cigarette smoking is a factor which can influence the respiratory system, but fewer people know that it can also affect the cardiovascular system. Disturbance in one or other, or both of these systems can affect the AL of breathing. Cancer in other organs of the body can be associated with inhalation of tobacco smoke, for example, the mouth, throat, oesophagus and pancreas. Expressing sexuality is the AL associated with fetal damage from tobacco smoke causing low birth weight and even stillbirth. The AL of eliminating is affected when there is cancer of the bladder and kidney and smoking predisposes to these conditions (Burgess, 1994).

The effects of passive smoking

Current interest is focused on passive smoking. There is now considerable evidence of risks to health among non-smokers who are exposed to environmental tobacco smoke (Hill, 1993). They have a 10 to 30 per cent higher risk of developing lung cancer than non-smokers who have not been so exposed (Burgess, 1994).

Children are also affected by sidestream smoke and in

Box 6.2 External and internal respiration

Biologically speaking, breathing in is called inspiration, breathing out is expiration and the whole process is referred to as respiration. Inspiration is concerned mainly with the intake of oxygen from the atmosphere, and expiration with the expulsion of carbon dioxide and because of the site at which this occurs, it is called 'external respiration'. The whole point of breathing is to convey oxygen (O_2) from the atmosphere to each cell in the body so that it can create the energy to engage in its various activities. The cell is the basic unit of all life and respiration is the most fundamental of its processes; respiration is needed for all cellular activities and in the process carbon dioxide (CO_2) is formed as a waste product of metabolism. Because of the site at which this occurs, it is referred to as 'internal respiration'. The CO_2 is absorbed into the blood, in which it is transported along the cardiovascular system and arrives in the lungs to be breathed out as expired air. In very broad functional terms the requisites to achieve both external and internal respiration are:

- adequate oxygen in the atmosphere
- a functioning respiratory system
- a large moist surface in the lungs where the oxygen and blood are in close proximity to allow exchange of O_2 and CO_2.
- a physical 'bellows' arrangement (the thoracic cage) with muscles to operate it and nerves to control the muscles
- a 'transport' system, the blood
- a 'carrier' in the transport system, the haemoglobin
- thin-walled capillaries in close proximity to the cells where O_2 and CO_2 can be exchanged
- healthy cells which are capable of using the O_2 and releasing CO_2.

This complex integrated activity is in constant use to collect O_2 from the atmosphere; transport it in the blood to the cells; collect the cells' CO_2; and transport it to the lungs where it is released to the atmosphere. It is evident that the action of the heart and blood vessels are complementary to breathing. It is therefore logical to expect that impairment at any point in this complex sequence of the cardiopulmonary system is going to affect the exchange of gases and the individual's ability to 'breathe'.

It is not the intention in this book to describe these complex biological processes in detail, but to alert the student to the need for integration of knowledge from other disciplines into nursing.

smoking households are more prone to chest problems and upper respiratory tract infections.

Tobacco smoke contains carbon monoxide (CO) which binds with haemoglobin in the red blood cells to form carboxyhaemoglobin which does not easily exchange oxygen. Consequently there is a reduction in the blood's oxygen-carrying capacity of between 10 and 15%, so it is understandable that there can be such widespread effects throughout the body. CO increases the permeability of arterial walls to cholesterol and this predisposes to atherosclerosis which increases blood pressure. The nicotine increases the heart rate and is another factor which raises blood pressure. The combination of nicotine and CO also seems to have the effect of increasing the viscosity of blood by making the platelets more sticky, predisposing to thrombosis. The condensate from tobacco smoke is deposited in the smoker's lungs and causes local tissue damage including cancer.

Smoking and respiratory changes

Most people associate the ill effects of smoking with lung cancer. It is the world's most common cancer, accounting for 12 per cent of all cancers (Parkin, 1993). But it also causes many chronic chest conditions.

'Smokers' cough' is an explanation given frequently for a cough with expectoration of phlegm. Increasingly frequent incidents of bronchitis may occur and there is usually difficulty in breathing caused by narrowing of the small bronchial tubes. There are changes in the minute air sacs in the lungs which decrease the area of membrane available for gaseous exchange; the condition is called chronic obstructive pulmonary disease. The impaired microcirculation in the lungs causes backlog problems in the pulmonary arteries and veins which is the beginning of chronic heart failure.

Smoking and cardiovascular changes

Men are still more likely than women to experience problems related to cardiovascular changes and in general the risk increases with age, and in association with smoking, high blood pressure, lack of exercise, high blood cholesterol and diabetes. There is a risk of coronary heart disease in the presence of more than one of these factors, together with a predisposing family history (p. 153).

Smokers

It is not only adults who risk physical pathology by smoking. The Office of Population Census and Surveys (OPCS) has carried out surveys among secondary school children of 11 to 15 years old on a two yearly basis since 1982. An extra survey was carried out in 1993 for two reasons. Firstly in 1989 the Health Education Authority introduced a five year teenage smoking programme in England aimed at reducing smoking prevalence among teenagers, especially girls because of the known adverse effects should they become pregnant. Secondly the target set by the Department of Health (1991) in The Health of the Nation was a reduction in smoking prevalence among 11 to 15 year olds of at least 33% by 1994 (from the 1988 baseline).

The two year statistics plus the extra 1993 statistics show little change. Ten per cent of the sampled pupils were regular smokers (defined as usually smoking one or more cigarettes a week). However the average number of cigarettes recorded in the previous week by regular smokers was 47. Smoking was more prevalent among girls than boys, but the difference was not statistically significant.

The teenagers are risking pathological changes in their respiratory and cardiovascular systems in the future. The younger people are when they start smoking the greater the risk.

Shock: circulatory/respiratory failure

It is pertinent here to re-state that in the model for nursing, the respiratory, circulatory and lymphatic systems were juxtaposed to the AL of breathing. Consequently another biological factor influencing both internal and external respiration is the condition of shock which is basically a manifestation of circulatory failure. With decreased venous blood reaching the respiratory surface membrane, there is decreased exchange of O_2 and CO_2 so that there is a concomitant respiratory failure with a change in the body's electrolyte balance. First-aiders are taught to recognize 'collapse' and render help by using the mnemonic ABC:

- Airway — ensure that it is clear
- Breathing — mouth to mouth
- Circulation — external cardiac compression.

The objective is to keep the collapsed person alive until more sophisticated equipment to maintain these bodily functions is available in a hospital setting; 'cardiopulmonary resuscitation' is the term used. More will be said about this later.

'Fight or flight' syndrome

As well as the biological processes related to smoking and the phenomenon of shock, there are others which become active in response to perceived danger — sometimes called environmental stressors. The response increases the rate and depth of respiration, as well as the heart rate, blood pressure and flow of blood to the muscles. In extreme form, these increases are part of the 'fight or flight' syndrome facilitating man's survival. However for most of the time most people's reaction to fear is much less intense. Physiologically the body reacts to anxiety in a similar way, but frequently the reaction is of much longer duration.

PSYCHOLOGICAL

In very general terms the AL of breathing can be seen to be influenced by a variety of psychological factors. Certain emotional events in life can affect the individual's breathing. Sadness and grieving, for example, may affect the rate and depth of respirations resulting in audible and visible activities such as sighing and sobbing.

And at some time or another, everyone has had the experience of being suddenly startled; fright is often accompanied by an indrawn, gasping respiration followed by an increase in breathing and pulse rates. The two quite different emotions of anxiety and pleasurable excitement may also cause an increase in breathing and pulse rates and even minor, fairly transient pain can have a similar effect.

Anxiety

Anxiety can be troublesome and most people can be helped to overcome its effects by learning simple relaxation techniques, many of which involve controlled breathing as practised in chanting, transcendental meditation and yoga. Currently there is great interest in helping tense people to relax and lower their blood pressure and pulse rate by constant visual technological monitoring of these functions called biofeedback.

As the feeling of anxiety is so unpleasant, everyone, sometimes consciously but mostly subconsciously, attempts to avoid it. To do so, everyone indulges in an enormous diversity of coping mechanisms in an attempt to reduce stressful anxiety to a tolerable level. For those who are employed it may involve going home to family, and learning to leave work worries behind; for others, who perhaps live alone, it may mean the discipline of organizing non-work time in a recreational way, and many local authorities are offering those who are unemployed the means to minimize stress by reduction of entrance fees to sports facilities and so on. In all these examples, the goal is to achieve relaxation and thereby prevent increased blood pressure which can predispose to conditions such as coronary heart disease and stroke.

However, the part played by temperament and emotional factors is difficult to assess. There is no doubt that worry about high blood pressure is only likely to exacerbate the problem.

Smoking was discussed as one of the biological factors which can affect the AL of breathing, but there is also a psychological dimension. One of the problems about smoking is that it produces a state of dependence.

Dependence on tobacco is a form of addiction. In an attempt to help people to recognize the complex set of circumstances which precede the state of absolute dependence on any chemical substance be it tobacco, alcohol or drugs, the World Health Organization (1980) has defined three types of dependence:

- *social dependence:* the person depends on a chemical in order to conform to the behaviour patterns of his particular community
- *psychological dependence:* the person depends on a chemical to provide enjoyment and/or suppress or come to terms with mental or emotional conflicts
- *physical dependence:* the person becomes dependent on a chemical for normal functioning.

It seems that dependence on tobacco grows insidiously over the years. In many instances it starts as social dependence perhaps even at an early age while at school, as already mentioned. It may be that there is oral gratification in having a cigarette between the lips; or the act of inhaling gives a special pleasure; or the feeling of relaxation may be associated with exhaling; or perhaps the greatest attraction lies in having something to do with the hands which would otherwise fidget. Sooner or later there is physical dependence, and some people in spite of determined effort to give up smoking find it impossible.

Those who do manage to give up smoking may suffer from unpleasant psychological symptoms for several weeks: for example, depression, irritability, anxiety, restlessness and lack of concentration. These are symptoms which result from the withdrawal of nicotine. More will be said about this later.

SOCIOCULTURAL

There is also a sociocultural dimension to smoking. Formal adherence to some religions does not permit smoking. There are also other social groups of people who work together to promote anti-smoking activities, and others who equally fervently extol the rights of smokers.

Quite apart from the spitting associated with 'smokers' cough, there is a normal secretion of phlegm from the upper respiratory tract, most of which is swallowed, and in many cultures children are socialized into disposing of any excess phlegm by using a tissue. However, when people are outdoors, they sometimes spit this secretion onto the street, which can be offensive to onlookers. And when there is secretion from the lower respiratory tract, usually caused by chronic infection, coughing expels it into the upper respiratory tract. If it is expelled onto the street it can be dangerous, because, for instance, any microorganisms dry, are wafted in the dust and can be inhaled by other people, thereby influencing the AL of breathing by causing chest infection. During the process of dessication the microorganisms have acquired an 'environmental dimension' and this is an example of the relatedness of the factors influencing breathing.

It is interesting that currently in some Third World countries, there are notices on public transport and in public places exhorting people to refrain from spitting, along with reminders that spitting spreads disease — notices which were common, certainly in the UK, about four decades ago but are now no longer in use. It is also interesting that currently in discussions on the radio and television about litter in the streets, spitting is being mentioned more frequently and is offensive to many citizens. It is also relevant to note that policemen in the UK report spitting as one of the assaults perpetrated against them and they were recently concerned that it might transmit AIDS, although this fear is unsupported by currently available knowledge.

ENVIRONMENTAL

Some environmental factors were discussed in general in the model of living (p. 28) and in the model for nursing (p. 47); here they are focused to the AL of breathing. The aspect of the environment which is obviously most relevant to consider in relation to this AL is the atmosphere. It is logical to expect that the composition of inspired air will affect the rate, depth and rhythm of breathing. Atmospheric air is a mixture of gases; it has a variable humidity as shown in Box 6.3. It can also contain microorganisms and pollutants.

Microorganisms

Dispersed throughout the atmosphere are many millions of microorganisms; most are non-pathogenic but some, when inhaled, can cause infection in the respiratory tract, for example the common cold. Microorganisms fall to the floor or settle on objects in a room by force of gravity, and convection currents can recirculate them in the atmosphere and perpetuate the possibility of inhalation by man.

Pollutants

While out-of-doors in and around an *urban area*, man is frequently exposed to possible abrasion of the tissue in the respiratory tract by inhalation of smoke, containing minute particles which are the products of combustion in domestic heating systems, industrial furnaces and transport vehicles. The latter currently causes the greatest pollution and the four major pollutants affecting the AL of breathing are sulphur dioxide, oxides of nitrogen, ozone and particulates (Monkley-Poole, 1992).

In many large cities, attempts have been made to

Box 6.3 Composition of the atmosphere

- *Oxygen.* Every cell in the human body requires oxygen and each time a person breathes, 4% of the oxygen content of inspired air is retained for cell metabolism.

  At high altitudes, the air has a lower oxygen content than at sea level and even at moderate heights, the human respiration rate will increase in an attempt to compensate. On the other hand, too high a concentration of oxygen would support combustion too readily and be incompatible with life.

- *Nitrogen.* Although present in atmospheric air, it cannot be used by the human body; it is in the form of an inert gas and acts as a diluent to the oxygen.

- *Carbon dioxide.* Exhaled air contains 4% more carbon dioxide than inhaled air. In the process of preserving the ecological balance, plants and other vegetation, during photosynthesis, utilise carbon dioxide by retaining the carbon as a form of food and releasing the oxygen into the atmosphere and so the cycle of gas exchange between humans/animals and the plant world goes on.

- *Water vapour.* The air breathed by humans is moistened by the water vapour in the atmosphere, thus preventing irritation of the respiratory mucous membrane. On the other hand, expired air has picked up some of the body's water so has a higher water content than inspired air, and saturation is reached when the water vapour begins to condense, visible on the breath when atmospheric temperature is low.

  If the atmospheric humidity is very high, perspiration lies on the skin and the body cannot cool itself by the process of evaporation. For this reason, living in a very hot climate where there is high humidity can cause discomfort and in extreme cases heat exhaustion, one of the features being respiratory distress.

- *Environmental temperature.* In a temperate climate, at sea level, the environmental temperature is usually lower than body temperature and consequently, some heat is lost from the body with each breath. Most people find this a reasonably comfortable environment for living, working and playing. When the environmental temperature is considerably higher, it is more difficult to maintain a comfortable balance between the human body and the atmosphere and, in extreme cases, heat exhaustion will result. Conversely, when the environmental temperature is low, the loss of body heat may cause chilling of the whole body and hypothermia will result.

reduce this health hazard by encouraging the use of smokeless fuels for household purposes. Some governments have passed legislation making it obligatory that grit is extracted before furnace smoke is released into the atmosphere: condensation around the solid particles produces fog, often referred to as smog, a reminder that the smoke is the real hazard.

Other measures to mimimize pollutants are street-cleaning machines which spray water on the dust before sweeping; garbage collection vehicles which have mechanisms to prevent dust from dispersing into the atmosphere.

At an international level, the World Health Organization is studying and monitoring the problem of atmospheric pollution and assisting with the exchange of information about prevention on a worldwide scale so that the air, so necessary to human life, will be less of a health hazard.

Work environment

In the *work environment*, there may be exposure to respiratory abrasion from industrial waste particles, organic and inorganic, for example from linen, hemp, wool, metal, stone and coal. The coal-mining industry has a long history of protective practices to prevent the onset of the dreaded disease, pneumoconiosis, which develops when coal-dust particles become embedded in the lung tissue and eventually cause gross impairment in the capacity to breathe. Inhalation of minute particles of asbestos can cause cancer of the lung and a detailed Code of Practice has been designed in the UK to help workers protect themselves from the hazard. In this instance, even more widespread education is necessary because some householders continue to use asbestos for lagging pipes and insulating roofs.

Workers who are at risk in these types of industries are encouraged to use the appropriate preventive measures provided and to have regular chest X-rays so that any adverse effects will be promptly detected and treated. At international level, the International Labour Organization (ILO) has taken measures to encourage governments to provide employees with protection from several types of respiratory health hazards.

Another hazardous environmental factor has been identified in the last two decades. Water droplets from infected humidifier cooling towers, and stagnant water in cisterns and shower heads, are now known to transmit Legionnaires' disease. It is primarily a type of pneumonia and undoubtedly influences the AL of breathing.

Home environment

At *home*, householders can pollute the air by failing to provide good ventilation, thus increasing the concentration of products from expired air. The oxygen and carbon dioxide content does not reach dangerous levels but the increased temperature and humidity is conducive to rapid multiplication of microorganisms. If poorly ventilated, the household atmosphere may also be permeated with unpleasant odours from the kitchen or toilet accommodation. Inhalation of gases leaking from appliances and from paraffin stoves can cause headaches, drowsiness or indeed, in large quantity, may render the occupants unconscious.

POLITICOECONOMIC

Many of the topics discussed in the preceding section have an obvious politicoeconomic dimension: for example, the problem of atmospheric pollution. That problem is primarily a responsibility of government and in many industrialized countries legislation exists to control and reduce the hazards associated with atmospheric pollution for city dwellers and workers at risk. However, individuals have responsibilities too; for example, to comply with the requirement to burn smokeless fuel or to wear a protective breathing mask when engaged in certain types of work. In such ways individuals minimize risks to others and avoid hazards which might affect their own breathing.

There are many other ways in which politicoeconomic factors can influence the implementation of preventive activities to reduce, for example, the risk of coronary heart disease and stroke in those people who have a symptomless raised blood pressure. Before setting up 'well persons' clinics' or in some areas imaginatively called 'MOT clinics' (an abbreviation for the UK's Ministry of Transport's road-worthiness certificate required annually for vehicles which are 3 years old or more), extensive advertising (which is expensive) is necessary to inform members of the local community of the desirability of using this facility. Setting up the clinic costs money; it has to be available at times convenient to members of the local community, which may involve overtime payment of staff. It will involve the cost of medication for those found to be 'at risk'. Some health authorities, when allocating their financial budget, do not give priority to these preventive activities. This introduces an ethical dimension to the debate, namely, should the decision of a health authority deprive members of the local community who have a 'silent' raised blood pressure, of the facilities which might help to prevent it causing coronary heart disease or stroke?

And with regard to cigarette smoking, the debate continues about the politicoeconomic factors related to it. Mention has already been made of this problem in terms of its physical effects on the body, and in relation to the development of dependence, a psychological state. Con-

sideration of smoking as a politicoeconomic issue is yet another perspective. Most governments are concerned that smoking is a recognized and serious threat to health and are aware of the fact that treatment of smoking-related disease is a drain on the finances available for health care. However, at the same time, the government obtains revenue from the tax on cigarettes and so there are two sides to the economics of the problem.

Many other groups with health interests engage in education and mount vigorous campaigns against smoking: for example, ASH (Action on Smoking and Health) which was set up by the Royal College of Physicians, and the National Society of Non-smokers which was founded in 1926 and may be best known for its instigation of an annual National 'No Smoking' Day.

However, the money spent on prevention by the government and all the various organizations is infinitesimal compared to the millions of pounds spent on sales promotion by the cigarette companies. Anti-smoking advertising campaigns play a part in bringing about changes in smoking behaviour but a variety of approaches is needed, aimed at both the individual and at society as a whole. Programmes in schools have a crucial role in attempting to stop people ever starting to smoke; advice and information by doctors and other health professionals remain important, for healthy people as well as those suffering from smoking-related disease; improved methods to help people to give up smoking are being developed, for example the use of nicotine gum and skin patches and behavioural techniques; and, for the protection of non-smokers from sidestream smoke, there has been a gradual increase in restriction on smoking.

Over the past few years such protection has been most noticeable on public transport, particularly on planes and trains, where a majority of seats are designated 'No smoking', indeed on some short and long distance flights smoking is prohibited. Many restaurants have followed suit. Some work places have always had a 'No smoking' rule, necessary because of the work undertaken, and employees are aware of this before being employed there. However, at other work places, there is governmental encouragement to separate smokers from non-smokers. Another method is to have a 'No smoking' rule while working, but to provide a smoking room which can be visited in the rest periods.

So far in this chapter, the AL of breathing has been discussed in relation to the other three components of the model — lifespan, the dependence/independence continuum and the five factors influencing the ALs: biological, psychological, sociocultural, environmental and politicoeconomic factors. From the interaction of all these components, individuality in breathing develops, which is the base from which individualized nursing is developed.

Individualizing nursing for the AL of breathing

The four cyclical phases of the process — assessing, planning, implementing and evaluating — are the means by which individualizing nursing for the AL of breathing is accomplished. Assessing is the method by which nurses discover the person's individuality related to this AL, and it is from this individuality that the nursing plan (Appendix 1) develops. Because the three concepts already discussed contribute to individuality, we have prepared an aide-memoire (Box 6.4) which can be bourne in mind during an initial assessment.

Box 6.4 Assessing the individual in the AL of breathing

Lifespan: effect on breathing
- Age vis à vis rate of breathing
- pulse rate
  blood pressure

Dependence/independence in breathing
Independence normal in health
Dependence associated with ill-health

Factors influencing breathing

Biological	— characteristics of breathing (rate, depth, rhythm, sound)
	— level of activity
	— cough (if any)
	— smoking (habits if smokers; exposure to tobacco smoke if non-smoker)
	— evidence of peripheral circulatory deficiency
Psychological	— dependence on tobacco ⎫
	— motivation to ⎬ smokers
	stop smoking ⎭
	— knowledge of and attitudes to smoking
	— effects of emotional status on breathing
Sociocultural	— safe expectoration
Environmental	— exposure to air pollution; at home, at work
	— knowledge of and attitudes to air pollution
Politicoeconomic	— knowledge of and attitudes to air pollution
	— prevention of smoking-related disease

ASSESSING THE INDIVIDUAL IN THE AL

At the initial nursing assessment, people, if they are given the opportunity, can tell how they perceive any problem they may have with this AL, and nurses can bear in mind the various topics noted in the preceding part of this chapter. If coughing is mentioned, the nurse can enquire when it occurs; whether or not it is productive of sputum; characteristics of the sputum (p. 151); whether or not there is breathlessness; the relationship of breathlessness to exercise and so on. Certainly in all instances the person's age has an important bearing on the characteristics of breathing. For example mouth breathing in children can be indicative of enlarged adenoids which should alert the nurse to the possibility of impaired hearing when assessing the AL of communicating, thus again demonstrating the relatedness of the ALs. If the person is a smoker, then detailed information about smoking habits should be collected (Department of Health, 1991). This may be relevant in the context of understanding the person's disease; and would be utilized in the context of health education concerning smoking.

While assessing the AL of breathing the nurse would have some other questions in mind:

- does the individual breathe normally?
- what factors influence the individual's breathing?
- what knowledge does the individual have about breathing?
- has the individual experienced any difficulties with breathing in the past (or a longstanding breathing problem) and, if so, how have these been coped with?
- does the individual appear to have any problems (actual and/or potential) with breathing at present and are any likely to develop?

Other questions may be pertinent because in the model for nursing the AL of breathing is concerned not only with the respiratory system, but also with the cardiovascular system.

- has the individual ever been unduly conscious of the heart beating, probably faster, without an obvious cause such as circumstances causing fear or excitement?
- has the individual ever experienced more than transient cold in the extremities?
- has the individual experienced pain in the chest or legs on walking?

The objective in collecting this information is to discover the person's usual habits in relation to the AL of breathing; whether there is any impediment to independence in breathing, remembering that cardiovascular problems can impede breathing; previous coping mechanisms in relation to breathing or circulatory difficulties; and any current or incipient problems with breathing and/or circulation.

Of course, for people admitted specifically for investigation or treatment (medical or surgical) of an actual breathing problem, in other words, when there is dysfunction of either of the body systems required for breathing (respiratory system and circulatory system), nursing assessment would require to be much more detailed and specific as will become evident at appropriate places in the ensuing text.

IDENTIFYING ACTUAL AND POTENTIAL PROBLEMS

Before students can begin to think comprehensively about individualizing a nursing plan for a person who is experiencing a problem with this AL, it is pertinent that they have a generalized idea of the sort of actual and potential problems which can arise in relation to the AL of breathing. They are numerous and complex, but in this introductory discussion they will be grouped according to a broad classification of causes:

- change of dependence/independence status
- change in habit
- change in heart, pulse rate and blood pressure
- change in mode
- change of environment and routine.

CHANGE OF DEPENDENCE/INDEPENDENCE STATUS

Various discomforts in varying degrees of intensity can cause change in a person's dependence/independence status and some of these will now be discussed.

Coughing

Coughing is a frequently encountered respiratory problem and is really a reflex protective mechanism used by the body to expel foreign material from the respiratory tract. There are various assessments/observations which nurses should make (Box 6.5).

Coughing can cause considerable distress to the person, may interfere with many daily activities and may even prevent sleeping. If sputum is produced the person should be helped to cough in order to remove the excess secretions and reduce the possibility of superimposed infection. It is for this reason that postoperatively, especially after thoracic and abdominal surgery, patients are dependent on the physiotherapist and nurse to teach and supervise deep breathing and coughing. They usually find it reassuring, if nurses 'splint' the surgical incision with their hands as patients often fear that the sutures will give way because of the muscular effort involved.

Box 6.5 Assessment/observation of coughing

- *Character*
  — a 'dry' cough has little expectoration
  — a 'loose' cough is associated with the production of sputum
  — a short restrained, suppressed cough accompanies pleurisy and pneumonia
  — there is a short, frequent, dry cough in early tuberculosis
  — a breathless, distressing cough is associated with cardiac conditions.

- *Duration and frequency*
  — a cough is described as continuous in untreated pneumonia for example, and as spasmodic in asthma. It can accompany an acute episode of infection such as bronchitis, or a chronic condition such as cardiac insufficiency.

- *Time*
  — with many disease conditions coughing is worse in the morning when the person awakens and changes body position.

- *Effect on the person*
  — a cough can be irritating but shallow, or it may involve strenuous effort and leave the person exhausted.

Expectorant medications may be prescribed when a cough is productive of sputum, but when it is unproductive, irritating and preventing sleep, soothing cough syrup can be given to reduce discomfort and permit longer periods of rest.

Sputum   Sputum is usually the outcome of coughing. It is a secretion poured out from the irritated lining of the respiratory tract and consists mainly of mucus but if associated with an infection, pathogens will also be present.

People can be very distressed by the appearance of sputum and by having to spit in front of others. If the amount is small, they may prefer to spit into a tissue which is folded and placed immediately into a disposal bag at the bedside. Otherwise they may use a disposable sputum mug which has the lid replaced when not in use.

There are several assessments/observations of the sputum which the nurse should make (Box 6.6).

Blood (haemoptysis)   Coughing up blood is called haemoptysis and may vary in severity from mere streaking of the sputum, a common symptom in bronchitis, to a massive haemorrhage. Coughing up frank blood is alarming to the patient and to those in the vicinity, so the bed should be screened. The nurse should remain with

---

Box 6.6 Assessments/observations of sputum

- *Quantity.* The daily amount may have to be measured.
- *Consistency.* In acute conditions sputum is sticky and tenacious; in long-term conditions it can be fluid; if associated with infection it is purulent.
- *Colour.* Sputum is usually greenish-yellow in the presence of pus; blood stained in mild tuberculosis and pneumonia.
- *Odour.* Malodorous sputum is usually associated with infectious conditions such as abscess of the lung, bronchiectasis or pulmonary gangrene and large quantities of foul-smelling sputum are expectorated (it is this type of condition which often requires postural drainage (p. 161)). It is sometimes necessary to send a specimen of sputum to the laboratory for bacteriological culture of microorganisms. It is therefore necessary for nurses to realize that sputum can contain pathogenic bacteria, and meticulous handwashing is essential to remove any transient flora which can include the opportunistic *Pneumocystis carinii*. Pneumonia caused by this organism is the main presenting disease seen in AIDS, and is by far the most frequent cause of death in persons with AIDS.

---

patients and they should be helped into a comfortable position, which usually by choice will be sitting up supported by pillows. Unless massive and resulting in sudden death, the bleeding will stop provided the patient can rest quietly. Usually a sedative is ordered immediately, and the calming effect of the medication enables the patient to control the cough and to use it effectively instead of dissipating energies in useless coughing bouts which merely aggravate the bleeding. 'Universal precautions' should be taken whenever nurses are exposed to possible contamination from blood because it may contain the hepatitis B virus (Trevelyan, 1991) or the AIDS virus (Royal College of Nursing, 1994).

Linen soiled with blood must be placed in a water soluble plastic bag labelled with a hazard warning and then double bagged in accordance with local practice for the processing of infected linen. Blood may spill onto the floor or furniture and should be dealt with immediately using an appropriate chemical disinfectant for example, sodium hypochlorite (10 000 parts per million available chlorine) and disposable towels. Nurses should wear disposable plastic aprons and gloves during these procedures.

The patient's face and hands should be sponged and a mouthwash offered. Careful observation is subsequently

required and restlessness may be an indication that a further episode will occur.

However small in amount, haemoptysis should be considered as potentially serious and should be reported to the nurse in charge or the doctor. Carcinoma of the lung and pulmonary tuberculosis are often causes of haemoptysis.

Palpitation

While collecting information about the AL of breathing, the patient may report being conscious of a rapid, forceful beating of the heart. Listening carefully to the patient, the nurse may discover that it only occurs after exercise, or when lying down. If it occurs in other conditions, ascertainment of whether or not it is regular or irregular has relevance to the medical diagnosis and the information should be shared with the doctor. In the first two instances mentioned, though it is disconcerting, it is not usually indicative of disease.

Choking

It is very discomforting when food 'goes the wrong way'. Most people experience this phenomenon at some time in their lifespan. It usually results in a bout of coughing accompanied by excessive watering of the eyes. Should the face become livid, immediate action is necessary to dislodge the foreign body. The choking person will probably be standing to maximize contraction of the abdominal muscles in order to produce effective coughing. The helper stands behind the person; puts one hand as a clenched fist on the person's abdomen so that the midline of its lower border is just above the umbilicus; covers the 'fist' with the other hand; applies pressure with both these positioned hands and directs it upwards to dislodge the obstruction (Heimlich manoeuvre). It is a frightening experience and the person may be best comforted by touch such as holding the hand until the breath has been regained and the person can talk comfortably.

In the case of choking in small children, a finger sweep of the mouth may cause sufficient retching to dislodge the 'foreign object'. If this fails, the adult should sit on a chair, put the knees lower than the hips, place the child face down on the downward sloping thighs. The child's upper chest and lower neck should be supported by one hand while the other hand should apply back blows (Fig. 6.2).

Pain

The main discussion about pain is in the chapter on communicating (p. 130). In this chapter it will be discussed as a manifestation in the cardiopulmonary system required for the AL of breathing.

Respiratory pain Given that pain in any part of the

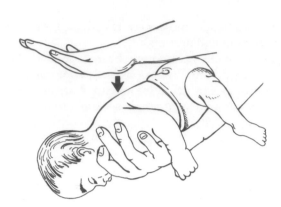

Fig. 6.2 Back blows for removal of foreign body in small children

body may cause alterations in the normal breathing pattern, pain in relation to the respiratory tract itself is of two main types:

- pain made worse by coughing and experienced behind the sternum — the type of pain associated with inflammation of the trachea
- sharp, stabbing pain made worse by deep breathing and coughing and caused by inflammation of the pleura.

Note should be made of the site, onset, duration, and intensity and any precipitation factors. The person's perception of the intensity can be assessed, and response to treatment evaluated by using a painometer (p. 133). As with pain of any kind every attempt should be made to remove the cause or minimize the effect and if these measures are unsuccessful, to help the person to cope with pain. In many instances, assisting the person into a comfortable position will help and someone with pleuritic pain will usually lie on the affected side. If an unproductive cough is the cause, soothing cough syrup may alleviate the discomfort and if antibiotics are prescribed for an inflammatory condition they will counteract the infection and thereby relieve the pain-producing inflammation.

Deep vein thrombosis pain   Deep vein thrombosis usually produces pain in the calf muscles, although it can also be a painless condition. It is a potential problem which can become an actual one in women who take oral contraceptives for a prolonged period. Deep vein thrombosis is also a potential problem postoperatively; almost all postoperative thromboses begin during, or within 72 hours of operation. Different preventive routines are used such as compression stockings, calf compression during operation, and injections of low-dose heparin (Evans, 1991; Smith, 1992). As a routine preventive measure, all patients who are having less exercise than usual should be encouraged to breathe deeply and exercise the feet several times daily. It is customary in some hospitals for the physiotherapist to initiate this preventive activity, but

it is necessary for nurses to encourage its continuance at intervals during the day. The potential problem of pulmonary embolism exists when there is a deep vein thrombosis.

Ischaemic pain in lower limb   The calf muscles can also be the site of ischaemic pain because atheromatous plaques in the arteries supplying the lower limbs are preventing the flow of an adequate blood supply. However, if the person is mobilizing and experiences such pain, pausing for a minute or so permits the person to walk a little further. Smoking should be discouraged because the chemicals in smoke are considered to reduce the efficiency of blood supply to the calf muscles. After examination of the blood there may be a prescription for medication to lower the blood cholesterol; and there may also be dietary modification to assist in lowering the blood cholesterol. Encouragement is usually necessary to help these people to persevere with walking as it helps in the development of collateral circulation. Obese people will be advised to reduce their intake of calories (Kilojoules).

Such people can be encouraged to keep a pain diary to note what they were doing when pain was experienced; at what level they graded the pain; duration of each episode; what coping mechanisms were found to be effective, for example warming or cooling the limb, raising or lowering it, exercising it and so on. If a pattern is manifest, this can be checked with the time medications such as vasodilators or pain controllers were taken. Adjustment of the drug programme may give relief (Janman, 1993). Complementary therapies may be useful.

Lower leg pain from ulcers   Local pain arising in the medial aspect of the lower legs can also be caused by superficial ulcers which are a manifestation of impairment in the cardiovascular system. Severe pain is more frequent in arterial ulcers — those secondary to arterial insufficiency — in one study they were responsible for 22% of leg ulcers (Roe et al, 1994): they have a less favourable prognosis than venous ulcers which are estimated to comprise 75% of leg ulcers. The new types of wound dressings have improved the healing of all types of leg ulcer (Smith, 1994).

Pain from lymphoedema   Lymphoedema occurs mainly in the upper limbs, sometimes in the lower limbs and occasionally in the tissues of the trunk. Most of the literature deals with the condition in upper limbs developing after radiotherapy for breast cancer. Pain occurs in 50% of people with cancer-related lymphoedema (Carroll & Rose, 1992). The subject is under-researched, but epidemiological data are improving as clarification of definition of the condition is agreed. One research project revealed that the greatest reduction of arm lymphoedema occurred in the first four days of treatments. This was implemented and resulted in financial savings (Rose, Taylor & Twycross, 1993).

Treatment of lymphoedema is an area where nursing initiatives from which patients benefit are paramount (Carroll & Rose, 1992; Jeffs, 1992; Sneddon, 1992; Dickson, 1993).

The majority of people with lymphoedema are in the community and are dependent on the knowledge of the professional staff at primary level. The number of nurses with a special interest in this distressing condition is increasing as well as specialist clinics which the person visits every 6 to 12 weeks (Williams, 1992, 1993).

Pain from intravenous infusions Intravenous infusions and blood transfusions are frequent forms of treatment and they may cause problems which manifest in pain. The most common problems are extravasation of fluid into the tissues and phlebitis (Jamieson et al, 1992; Lamb, 1993; Wilson, 1994). When phlebitis develops there is a potential problem of thrombus formation; the thrombus can become an embolus which commonly lodges in the lungs when the condition is called pulmonary embolism (Smith, 1992). The pain from pulmonary embolism is of the pleuritic type.

Cardiac pain There are instances when chest pain which affects the activity of breathing is really cardiac pain sometimes referred to as angina; the site is characteristically behind the sternum or across the chest. It is usually described as being crushing in character and there may be radiation down one or both arms or even into the neck and shoulders or through to the back. The person can become profoundly shocked and cardiac arrest may occur and it requires immediate treatment. This type of pain is also a feature of myocardial infarction and it must be relieved so that the shocked state may be reversed. A number of people with this condition are admitted to intensive coronary care units which have highly specialized health teams skilled in emergency treatment. However there are patients in these units, who for a variety of reasons do not report their pain as Mackintosh (1994) discovered. She recommended that this should be recognized as a potential problem when assessing, prior to formulating an individualized nursing plan. Such 'under reporting' of pain was discovered as long ago as 1989 by Willetts.

Cardiac rehabilitation

Rehabilitation of patients with heart disease, particularly myocardial infarction and cardiac surgery, is crucial if patients are to regain their confidence and return to optimal functioning in the community (Evans, 1993; McCrissican, 1991). A research-based multidisciplinary approach is reported by Doughty (1991). It is now well recognized that the physical effects of heart disease are influenced by both psychological and social well-being. Consequently education and emotional support for both patient and family increase the chance of a full recovery. They need

information about, and sometimes practice at, such activities as exercise, relaxation, stress management, safe taking of medicines, a healthy diet, alcohol intake and of course help with stopping smoking and losing weight if appropriate (Campbell, 1993a). It is entirely appropriate to offer sexual counselling before discharging these people from hospital (Piper, 1992; Jones, 1992; Briggs, 1994). Piper provides a handout which can be photocopied.

Prevention of coronary heart disease

Prevention of coronary heart disease is indeed better than cure. Clinical specialists have developed a computer-based health education programme for primary school children 7 to 11 years old. It deals with prevention and healthy lifestyles (Lindsay et al, 1994).

There is a 'heart chart' to assess a person's risk of developing coronary heart disease. For each of the following criteria — family history, blood pressure, lung expansion, smoking, fat in diet, weight, alcohol, stress, exercise, aerobic fitness (step test) — there is a numerical allocation of 0 to 4. The higher the score the greater the risk (Deans & Hoskins, 1987). Permission is given for photocopying the chart and it is suggested that health visitors, occupational health nurses and practice nurses are particularly well placed to use the chart. However, all nurses should bear it in mind when assessing patients.

There is room for improvement of strategy if the Health of the Nations target of reducing death's from coronary heart disease by 30% by the year 2000 is to be achieved. A survey of the various projects which have been carried out revealed an uncoordinated approach to the subject with regard to government spending, the work of the Health Education Authority, as well as that done by voluntary organizations at both national and local level. Projects carried out by health professionals at local level were similarly fragmented related to intended outcome, method and design, and a lack of collaboration and coordination among the professional groups (Twinn, 1990).

Anxiety about investigations

Sometimes investigations which are carried out to assess dysfunction in the respiratory and/or circulatory system cause discomfort or pain. Probably the most commonly used investigative technique is X-ray which is not in itself painful, although it may cause discomfort if performed in conjunction with the introduction of an opaque dye to outline the bronchi and bronchioles, a bronchogram; or to outline the inner surfaces of arteries (aortogram); or the heart (cardiogram). The structure and motion of the heart can be viewed on a screen by using ultrasound-echocardiography. An electrocardiogram (ECG) records the various phases of the heart's action on a moving strip of paper. The last two are non-invasive techniques.

Respiratory function tests are sometimes prescribed and they may cause discomfort. A bronchoscopy on the other hand, may be painful and can be alarming; a tube is passed into the upper respiratory tract and the tissue lining can be viewed by means of a lens in the eyepiece. In all these procedures, people will have some anxiety about what they will be expected to do, how they will react and what the result will be.

The nurse must take time to explain any preparation involved prior to the procedure, and what to expect during and after. Any relevant instructions about the person's expected behaviour should be stated clearly and simply. Factual information about the preparation and technique will be found in the ward procedure book but the nurse must interpret it to patients according to perceived preparedness of each patient to receive the information; and on the basis of assessed level of comprehension; and perhaps most important of all, in response to the patient's own expressed fears and anxieties.

It is evident that a large number of conditions can change a person's dependence/independence status, and the conditions themselves can vary from being a nuisance (hay fever) to life threatening (choking). Some other conditions can also change the dependence/independence status, but in this text they are allocated to change of habit, as well as to change in mode and they will now be discussed in that order.

CHANGE IN HABIT

Change in habit is the second broad classification for discussion of people's actual and potential problems with the AL of breathing. Many people erroneously believe that problems associated with breathing indicate only disorders of the lungs or upper airways. As mentioned earlier in the chapter, any alteration to the cardiopulmonary sequence of events will have an effect on the individual's respiration, pulse and blood pressure. With regard to respiration, the person may experience problems related to change in rate, rhythm and character of breathing.

Rate of breathing

Apart from atmospheric changes, the rate of respiration may be increased if there is:

- obstruction in any part of the respiratory tract such as a foreign body or a swelling which narrows the lumen of respiratory passages
- loss of functioning tissue in the respiratory tract because of injury or disease
- defect in the intercostal muscles or diaphragm

perhaps because of injury, or disease of the nerves serving those muscles as in poliomyelitis
- defect in the circulatory system such as impaired cardiac action which impedes circulation, or reduction in the size of the blood vessel lumen because of the deposit of fatty plaques as in atherosclerosis
- decrease in the volume of blood as in haemorrhage, or reduced haemoglobin in the red blood corpuscles which occurs in iron deficiency anaemia.

Usually these defects cause an increase in respiration rate as the body tries to make up for the O_2 deficit by breathing faster but in some instances such as head injury, brain tumours, or meningitis when the respiratory centre is depressed, the respiration rate is slower. A decrease is also associated with toxic conditions or with the intake of certain medications (such as morphine) which depress the respiratory centre; indeed overdosage of morphine will cause respiratory arrest.

Rhythm of breathing

The *rhythm* involves the time interval between each respiration (which should be equal) and the depth of respiration. Usually deep slow breathing occurs when a patient is in coma, and shallow restrained breathing occurs in for example pleurisy when the patient is attempting to diminish the sharp stabbing pain caused by inflammation of the pleura. In a type of breathing known as Cheyne-Stokes breathing there is a marked and somewhat eerie change of rhythm found in a variety of conditions where the patient is critically ill. It begins slow, shallow and quiet, becomes deeper and noisier then dies away; and may be followed by a short period of apnoea (cessation of breathing), then the cycle recommences.

Character of breathing

The *character* of the patient's breathing may also be altered. Loud snoring or stertorous breathing is associated with brain injuries and alcoholism; a harsh grating sound called stridor occurs when there is obstruction of the larynx; a grunting note on expiration may occur in pneumonia; and wheezing is associated with asthma.

These are all subjective assessments and can be detected by the ear unaided, but by using a stethoscope various sounds can be identified which are indicative of the state of the lung tissue such as constriction, consolidation and the presence of excess mucus and fluid.

Moderate change in breathing habit

There are many viruses which cause the common cold resulting in discomfort when breathing because of congestion in the upper respiratory tract. There are many over the counter remedies and the acute signs and symptoms usually subside in 72 hours. All people should be advised to cover the nose and mouth with a tissue when sneezing and dispose of it immediately in a hygienic manner.

A traditional remedy which can be used at home to relieve upper respiratory infection is the steam inhalation to which menthol crystals may be added; it helps to loosen abnormal secretions in the respiratory tract and thereby eases breathing. A Nelson's inhaler may be used but an ordinary spouted domestic jug and towel serves the same purpose. Whether in home or hospital, care must be taken to ensure that steam inhalation equipment is handled carefully to prevent spillage and scalding, and to prevent irritation to the eyes (Jamieson et al, 1992).

When use of steam is dangerous, specially designed apparatus such as a croupette (with canopy) or a croupaire (without canopy) may be used to humidify the atmosphere; they can be used continuously without the exertion of holding equipment and without the anxiety of scalding so are particularly useful for children who have respiratory problems, or for confused people.

Hay fever (seasonal rhinitis) Seasonal rhinitis which is commonly called 'hay fever' is an allergic reaction to such things as pollen, moulds and the common dust mite. People can be tested to discover the specific antigen to help them develop a lifestyle which will avoid it, even when on holiday! (Brydon, 1993). She provides a two page handout 'Managing your hay fever on holiday' with permission to photocopy it. The media help by publicizing daily 'pollen counts' so that when these are high, allergic people may be able to stay indoors.

Asthma Distress may be more marked in those who have asthma, and knowledge about its aetiology, treatment and control has increased in the last few years. There are 3 million sufferers in the UK (Partridge, 1994). The person's problems are principally intermittent dyspnoea, wheezing and coughing. Many asthmatic people can learn to manage their condition and nurses working in asthma clinics enable them to do so (Reynolds & Ward, 1994). Treatment has to be set in a social context, for example where children are concerned, other members of the family need to understand what triggers increased sensitivity of the airways, narrowing the lumen and resulting in wheezing, coughing and dyspnoea with increased mucus production. The medicament is introduced directly into the tract from an inhaler or nebulizer (Smith & Kendrick, 1993).

Children do not have to be deprived of exercise and sport; they can inhale a preventive medicament before such activity. Should an attack occur at school, inhalation of a bronchodilator will curtail it (Strudley, 1990). However, a survey carried out by the National Asthma Campaign found that one in four secondary schools restricted the children's access to their inhalers by keeping them in locked desks or the staffroom (Nursing Standard, 1994). A nurse devised and tested an educational programme for hospitalized children with asthma (Collins, 1994). People who have asthma need to understand that it is a chronic condition, and that even during a trouble-free period they should take the prescribed maintenance medications (Tettersell, 1993).

Asthma is one of the dyspnoeic conditions in which a flow meter can be used to assess the expiratory flow rate, and again at intervals to evaluate response to treatment. Indeed the National Asthma Campaign recommends them for those asthmatic people who can benefit from a self-management plan (Sharp, 1993; Leach, 1994).

Marked change in breathing habit

Dyspnoea is the noun used for difficult breathing and the adjective dyspnoeic was used in the previous paragraph in the context of asthmatic people. However, there are other medical diagnoses which cause the distressing condition of chronic continuous dyspnoea.

For the person, it is a distressing symptom but it does in fact indicate that a compensatory body mechanism is attempting to convey more O_2 to the cells. Every movement of the body uses up O_2 and produces CO_2 so it is obvious that everything should be done to spare the patient unnecessary activity. Lying flat, normally the most restful position, is however contraindicated as it further embarrasses breathing; when flat the abdominal organs slide against the inferior aspect of the diaphragm and inhibit its movement, and the rib cage also has limited expansion.

The patient usually prefers to sit up in a well-ventilated room and indeed often requests to be near an open window. Special beds may be available which help to maintain the sitting position and are often more comfortable for the patient, but if these are not available, the nurse should be skilful in helping the patient to find a comfortable sitting position well supported by pillows. A bedtable with a pillow on which the patient may lean forward supported on the arms sometimes gives considerable relief and is restful. Many patients find it more comfortable however to sit well supported in an armchair and, at home, a person with chronic breathlessness usually prefers to do so. The inability to breathe except when in the sitting position is called orthopnoea.

Breathing is such a vital activity of living and marked difficulty causes patients great anxiety and distress so the nurse must adopt a quiet, calm manner when carrying out procedures and should anticipate their needs as much as possible.

Because dyspnoeic people are gasping for air, they are breathing through the mouth as well as the nose, and the mouth can become very dry so a drink in a covered container should be at hand. Should a reduced fluid intake be prescribed, a pleasantly flavoured mouthwash can be comforting. Milky drinks may have to be followed by oral hygiene if the mouth is to be kept clean and comfortable and cracked lips require an application of vaseline (p. 245).

Apart from the change in rate, rhythm and character of breathing associated with chronic dyspnoea other effects on total body functioning may cause the person distress. Nervous tissue is particularly sensitive to oxygen deficit and such people may show signs of impaired brain function: headache, dizziness, drowsiness, restlessness, faulty judgement and disorientation. Nurses must therefore be on the alert for indications of abnormal behaviour and remember that such symptoms are often reversible if the O_2 supply is improved.

The patient's colour may also be altered. Cyanosis, a bluish tinge in the skin, the lips, the nail beds and in mucous membrane is indicative of lack of oxygen. The muscular system too reacts to oxygen deficit and the person tires easily and feels exhausted on very slight exertion. People who are breathless require skilful nursing. Activities and relatively minor anxieties with which they would normally cope unaided assume abnormal importance when they are fighting for breath, and nurses must not be irritated by their frequent attempts to seek attention, and to seek reassurance of the presence of a nurse.

For dyspnoeic people, malnutrition is always a potential problem. If an oxygen mask is being used it can usually be replaced by oxygen spectacles at mealtimes. Because of early tiring, small meals of soft but tasty food should be given. Sips of nutritious fluid between meals are helpful (Poole, 1993).

There is a greater awareness of the nurse's role as a health educator to enable dyspnoeic people to take control of their chronic condition (Brown & Mann, 1990). Their article provides a handout with permission to photocopy.

Hyperventilation   Another marked change in breathing habit is hyperventilation; it is characterized by rapid shallow breathing, chest pain, anxiety and a tingling sensation in the fingers and toes. It is associated with high anxiety and arousal states and the faulty breathing can change the blood pH to a level of alkalinity which can produce tetany. Early recognition and treatment is necessary to prevent this happening. Once diagnosed, a paper bag into which the person breathes and re-breathes expired air usually relieves the symptoms. This simple method works because the inhaled air has a higher than normal level of carbon dioxide, and thus corrects the low level in the blood.

Change in heart and pulse rate

The origin of the pulse beat arises in the heart and it is responsible for supplying an adequate amount of venous blood to the diffusing surface of the pulmonary alveoli. As has already been described, inhaled air exchanges 4% of its oxygen to this circulating blood, while at the same time 4% of the blood's carbonic acid which changes to carbon dioxide is diffused into it, to be exhaled. This is essential for maintenance of the blood pH within the normal range of 7.45 to 7.55. Some heart diseases can lessen the amount of blood reaching the pulmonary alveoli and can therefore interfere with this aspect of the blood pH regulating mechanism. Also the disadvantageous change in blood pH can occur at the 'internal breathing' sites in the body which involves the metabolic activity of each cell. It is not the objective of this text to deal with these complex phenomena, but the foregoing facts are merely mentioned to help the beginning student who is learning about the Roper, Logan and Tierney model for nursing to appreciate that the AL of breathing includes 'biological factors'.

Everyone's heart beats at a characteristic rate and this is transmitted via the arteries as the pulse. The pulse rate can be counted by gentle compression of an artery as it passes over a bone, the most usual site being the radial artery. Various medical conditions can lower the pulse rate to less than 60 beats per minute (bradycardia), although it has to be remembered that healthy athletes can achieve this lower rate after a period of intensive training. A decreasing pulse rate can be indicative of an increasing intracranial pressure and it is for this reason that people suffering from cerebral conditions, including head injuries, require to have the pulse counted hourly or even half hourly. Medicines, however, may be prescribed to deliberately reduce the heart rate; digitalis preparations are taken to slow and strengthen the heart beat, but in order to prevent the drug reducing the rate too drastically, the pulse is checked regularly to ensure that it does not drop below 60 beats per minute in an adult.

Various medical conditions can raise the pulse rate and if it is over 100 beats per minute, the term tachycardia is used. It characterizes such diverse conditions as cardiac failure, fever, haemorrhage, shock and thyrotoxicosis, when accurate pulse counting is essential to monitor the patients' response to treatment (Jamieson et al, 1992).

Change in blood pressure

The blood exerts pressure on the walls of the vessels in which it flows. In the living body, arteries are full of blood which causes a continuous stretch in their elastic walls. When the left ventricle contracts and discharges blood into an already full aorta, the increased pressure produced is known as systole. In the adult the systolic blood pressure is around 120 millimeters (mm) of mercury (Hg) that is, it supports a column of mercury in a sphygmomanometer 120 mm high.

When the heart is resting with no discharge of blood

from the aorta the pressure within the blood vessels is termed diastolic pressure and is around 80 mmHg. Blood pressure is expressed therefore as 120/80 mmHg.

A sphygmomanometer and stethoscope are required to assess the blood pressure, if the procedure is performed manually. The sphygmomanometer's inflatable cuff, acting as a tourniquet is used to compress the brachial artery until no pulse is discernible. As the inflated cuff gradually deflates, a stethoscope is placed over the brachial artery below the antecubital fossa to detect the returning pulse.

The sounds were first described by Korotkoff and take his name. They consist of:

- phase 1 a clear tapping recorded as the systolic pressure
- phase 2 a softening of the sound
- phase 3 return of sharper sound
- phase 4 abrupt muffling — diastolic 4
- phase 5 disappearance of sound — diastolic 5.

In the USA it is customary to record diastolic 5 as the diastolic pressure, and although traditionally in the UK, diastolic 4 was recorded, the current recommendation is to record diastolic 5 for adults, only retaining diastolic 4 for children and pregnant women (Kemp, Foster & McKinlay, 1994).

There are no agreed numbers for the upper limits of a 'normal' blood pressure, but it has to include a systolic and a diastolic pressure. For diagnostic purposes the diastolic pressure is used and Feher et al (1992) considered this as:

- mild hypertension   95 to 104   mmHg
- moderate hypertension   105 to 114   mmHg
- severe hypertension   115   mmHg.

In many areas a nursing custom/ritual of measuring the blood pressure of people newly admitted to the health service persists. Yet there are so many acknowledged variables regarding assessment of blood pressure that such a once-only measurement provides an unreliable datum. It is possible that considerable nursing time is spent collecting blood pressure data which are of questionable use (O'Brien & Davison, 1994).

In the 1970s and 80s a number of research projects identified various deficiencies in health staff's knowledge about the technique of measuring blood pressure using a mercurial sphygmomanometer and stethoscope. Data were collected by questionnaires.

In the early 1990s researchers found similar deficiencies and were concerned that 'assessing blood pressure' had not included recommendations from the earlier studies. Considering that it is the main assessing/evaluating tool when identifying hypertensive people and stabilizing them on an antihypertensive medication regime this is worrying.

From the literature, particularly the project carried out by Nolan and Nolan (1993) we have prepared a résumé of the many pertinent points which have been made regarding assessing/evaluating blood pressure (Box 6.7). However each health authority devises its own protocol, with which students need to be familiar.

There is a range of difference when the blood pressure is estimated in the right and left arm. This was found in some young people but in more of the elderly people in one study (Fotherby et al, 1993). With an ageing population, estimation in both arms, at least once may become part of blood pressure protocols.

Box 6.7 Taking blood pressure

- Use accurate equipment (sphygmomonometers and stethoscopes should be serviced annually)
- There are three different cuff sizes — leg, arm and paediatric
- Size should be stated on the nursing plan or blood pressure chart
- Too small a 'bladder' can result in over-estimation of blood pressure
- Person so placed that antecubital fossa and heart are at the same level
- Place sphygmomonometer so that meniscus of mercury is at your eye level
- Place cuff around upper arm so that there is a gap of 2 to 3 cm between it and the antecubital fossa with centre of cuff bladder over upper arm brachial artery
- Place oneself no more than 0.914 m (3 ft) from the person
- Palpate radial pulse, rapidly inflate cuff until radial pulse cannot be felt (palpated systolic pressure)
- Inflate cuff for a further 30 mmHg
- Place stethoscope on brachial artery just below antecubital fossa
- Deflate cuff at 2 to 3 mmHg per second
- Record systolic to the nearest 2 mmHg at which a clear tapping sound is heard (Korotkoff phase 1)
- Continue slow deflation (2 to 3 mmHg) and recognize Korotkoff phases 2, 3, 4 and 5
- Current recommendation is to document Korotkoff/ diastolic 5 for adults. However some centres require documentation of Korotkoff/ diastolic 4 only, or as well as 5, for example 120/80/75
- After use apply an alcoholic wipe to the ear pieces and the sphygmomonometer diaphragm
- Document the pressures
- Five minutes is the estimated time for efficient assessment/evaluation of blood pressure
- A rushed procedure underestimates systolic/ overestimates diastolic pressure

Students should be aware that 24 hour ambulatory blood pressure monitoring is becoming more frequent and has obvious advantages over single assessments carried out at primary level and in outpatient departments (Foster, McKinlay & Kemp, 1993). And lastly, some centres are teaching hypertensive pregnant women to monitor their blood pressure at home (Kennedy, 1991). A handout is provided in the article with permission to photocopy.

Change in pulse and blood pressure in shock

Changes in both pulse and blood pressure are manifested in the condition of shock.

Basically shock is a state of circulatory failure. The average adult body contains about 6 litres of blood and if all the innumerable blood vessels were widely open simultaneously, there would be insufficient blood to fill them. The body functions with this relatively small volume of blood by controlling the muscle tissue in the walls of the small arteries (arterioles), thereby narrowing (vasoconstricting) or widening (vasodilating) the lumen. The control is very exact and normally it is a state of vasoconstriction. However, when the control is disturbed and the lumen of many arterioles are simultaneously vasodilated, the volume of blood is insufficient to maintain effective circulation and there is some degree of shock.

The most common causes of shock are the inhibition of vasoconstriction due to:

- loss of blood, as in haemorrhage
- loss of plasma, as in severe burns
- loss of electrolytes, as in continued vomiting and/ or diarrhoea, and heat exhaustion
- alteration in permeability of blood vessel walls, as in injured tissue
- severe pain
- severe fright.

When there is, for example, loss of blood or plasma, (sometimes called hypovolaemic shock) the reason for circulatory failure is more readily understood and expected because there is actual loss of circulatory volume and the treatment is intravenous infusion to replace the lost fluid (Buckley, 1992; Campbell, 1993b; Adomat, 1992). But in instances of severe pain or severe fright there is no loss of fluid; shock (sometimes called neurogenic shock) is due to reduced vasoconstriction. It is just as important to expect and recognize the body's warning signals of neurogenic shock so that it can be effectively treated.

In shock, the body defences immediately try to compensate by permitting the vessels supplying blood to vital organs such as the brain, heart and kidneys to continue to do so, while the supply to muscles, skin and intestines is severely restricted. In a severe state of shock,

the body temperature falls; the blood pressure falls; the pulse increases; the person complains of feeling cold; the skin is grey, cold and moist; and there is generalized prostration. If the cause of shock is treated satisfactorily, these adverse changes will be reversed but if not, the blood pressure falls further and death will ensue.

Cardiac arrest

There is another type of shock produced by cardiopulmonary failure, sometimes called cardiogenic shock or cardiac arrest which requires special mention (Williams, 1993). Immediate treatment is essential as the brain is damaged when deprived of oxygen for as short a time as 3–5 minutes. It is estimated that every year in Britain 60 000, i.e., 60% of deaths from myocardial infarction (one cause of cardiogenic shock) occur before the patients reach hospital.

Cardiopulmonary resuscitation Resuscitation techniques are continually undergoing re-evaluation as more research knowledge becomes available. The current guidelines were prepared by the European Resuscitation Council to ensure that the same techniques were taught throughout Europe (Wynne, 1993; Bruce-Jones, 1993; Gee, 1993; Coady & Calne, 1994; Alton, 1994; Gardiner & Halliday, 1994).

The ABC sequence is now accepted as the best method. The mnemonic stands for Airway, Breathing and Compression. A flaccid tongue obstructing the airway is illustrated in Figure 6.3 and it is prevented by using the jaw

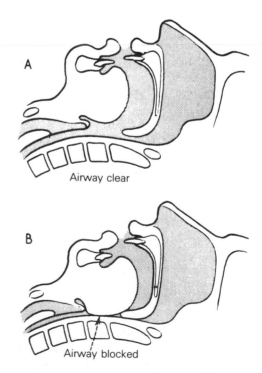

Fig. 6.3 Flaccid tongue and jaw muscles interfering with breathing

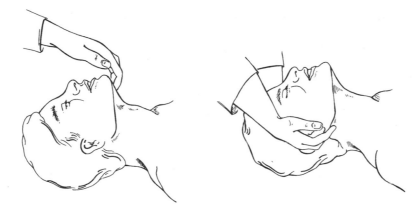

Fig. 6.4 Jaw lift, jaw thrust: the recommended method for maximizing airway

lift or jaw thrust illustrated in Figure 6.4. For breathing, it is recommended that two ventilations (usually mouth-to-mouth) of 1–1½ seconds allowing for deflation between them, should be carried out initially, and then repeated after 15 external chest compressions, there being at least 80 compressions per minute. The Royal College of Nursing AIDS Working Party (1994) recommends that devices for cardiopulmonary resuscitation should be readily available to enable this procedure to be carried out without direct mouth-to-mouth contact. Advanced Life Support is usually carried out by a medical member of the 'crash team' and consists of tracheal intubation and attempts to restart the arrested heart (Toulson, 1993).

The same principles apply when children require cardiopulmonary resuscitation, but of course modification of practice is required (Simpson, 1994; Williams, 1994).

It is worrying that various surveys testing nurses' knowledge and skills re cardiac arrest and cardiopulmonary resuscitation continue to reveal deficiences. The new guidelines suggest that the subject should be in the student curriculum and that all students should acquire proficient skills on an electronic manikin and that knowledge and skills should be updated six monthly.

To finish this section about 'Change in habit' it is important to raise some of the ethical issues which may need to be considered in relation to resuscitation. When cardiac arrest occurs in a person who is frail, ill and in the older age group, the case for resuscitation is sometimes questioned and thought to be inappropriate. In hospital, resuscitation is most often initiated by nurses (Godkin & Toth, 1994) and they worry about the consequences of withholding resuscitation (Pottle, 1992; Rundell & Rundell, 1992; Speck, 1992; Gibson, 1991). These dilemmas have resulted in the concept 'Do not resuscitate'.

A joint formulation by the Royal College of Nursing and the British Medical Association (BMA/RCN, 1993) states that the consultant concerned should finalize the decision, and document it in the patient's records, and effectively communicate it to other members of staff. It should be recorded in the nursing notes by the primary nurse (or most senior nurse) and it is her responsibility to inform other members of the nursing team (Nursing Standard, 1993). However Schutz (1994) writes that the joint statement is not exempt from criticism on moral and ethical grounds. A further joint statement (British Medical Association, 1995) deals with 'advance statements about medical treatment'. The terms 'living wills' and 'advance directives' are in more common usage.

Student nurses have considerable doubts and problems related to the concept 'Do not resuscitate'. Some of these were revealed in Candy's project (1991). Nurses need to be aware of the statistics related to the outcome of resuscitation (Chellel, 1993b) from which she states that they show 'a remarkably poor success rate'.

There is no doubt that for students and registered nurses cardiopulmonary resuscitation remains a source of fear and anxiety. It is no less so for nearby patients who 'witness' the drama, and who miss the 'resuscitated' patient who will be removed to intensive care. When the 'event' has been unsuccessful they naturally feel sad and need special support from nursing staff (Chellel, 1993a).

CHANGE IN MODE OF BREATHING

Change of mode in both body systems is undoubtedly problematic and can render a person totally dependent for the AL of breathing, which is a frightening experience. To maintain independence in the crucial activity of breathing, the most obvious need is the maintenance of a clear airway in the upper respiratory tract.

Obstructed air passages

Obstruction of the airway was mentioned on p. 151 in relation to choking. Upper airway obstruction can occur in many situations outside hospital and requires first aid (Innes, 1992) to dislodge it. Some newborn babies need to have mucus, blood and amniotic fluid removed from the respiratory tract (Nursing Times, 1991). Conscious

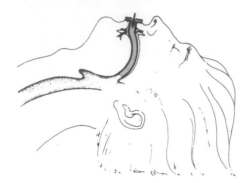

Fig. 6.5 An airway in position

patients will cough to remove obstructions but those in an altered state of consciousness (p. 389) must be carefully observed as the cough reflex is depressed and it may be necessary to clear their air passages mechanically. In emergency situations nurses may have to do this with a finger, suitably protected against clenching of the teeth, by for instance, wrapping with a wad of tissues.

In a hospital setting, clearance may be achieved by using a catheter and suction to the mouth or nose (Ashurst, 1992), or by inserting an artificial airway into the throat in order to keep the tongue forward and the airway patent (Fig. 6.5; McGarvey, 1990). Laryngeal masks are increasingly being used instead of endotracheal tubes (Green, 1991). Patients in an altered state of consciousness (coma) should be kept in the semiprone position to facilitate drainage from the mouth and prevent accumulation in the pharynx (Fig. 6.6).

Tracheostomy Obstruction due to excessive secretion or sputum retention may however be beyond the reach of an artificial airway or a catheter inserted via the mouth/nose (Hough, 1992). A *tracheostomy* may be required. An incision is made into the trachea, and a tube inserted and secured in position by tapes tied at the back of the neck (Fig. 6.7). The air entering a tracheostomy is not warmed, moistened and filtered as normally occurs in the nose and upper respiratory tract so the person is more liable to infection. The removal of secretions by suction is therefore performed using a sterile catheter and gloved hands and the inner cannula of the tube can be removed for cleansing and replaced by a sterile substitute cannula (Jamieson et al, 1992). There is always a risk of mucosal damage; to minimize this the suction catheter should be less than half the diameter of the tracheostomy

tube. The suction apparatus pressure gauge should be between 100 and 120 mmHg.

To conscious people, tracheostomy suctioning can be a most alarming procedure and must be carefully explained, although when the use of a tracheostomy is a long-term measure, people may eventually learn to carry out the suction themselves. When they are in control of the situation they usually feel less dependent.

In the initial stages the person may develop an irritation of the skin around the tracheostomy but a soothing keyhole dressing under the flange of the tube usually brings relief. The tapes holding the tube in position may cause distress and should be checked to ensure that they are sufficiently tightly tied to hold the tube securely without causing skin irritation. When soiled, the tapes should be changed not only for comfort but for prevention of infection, and the person may be concerned about the appearance.

It is not common but there are occasions when air gets into the tissues around the tube and it causes a rapidly spreading puffiness in the surrounding tissue which crackles when touched. The surgeon must be informed so that the obstruction can be relieved to ease the patient's discomfort and distress.

Reflecting the relatedness of the ALs, communicating is a problem when people have a tracheostomy because they are unable to talk, so a pad and pencil should be provided to lessen the frustration which comes with this type of dependence and a handbell must be within hand reach so that they can summon help. Sometimes a light gauze dressing is placed over the opening of the tube and when people are shown how to place a finger over the dressing, it is possible though difficult to speak.

Initially there may be difficulty with feeding and sometimes thickened fluids are easier to manage than thin liquids. Mouthwashes and mouth care are comforting and also help to prevent infection.

Some children developed iatrogenic subglottic stenosis from tissue damage when passing tubes when they were pre-term neonates. Their mothers learned to apply suction and change the inner tube.

In Britain in 1990 there were 225 children under 12 years of age with a long-term tracheostomy. A nurse researcher worked with 10 of these children and their families to gain an understanding of how all of them are affected (Jennings, 1990).

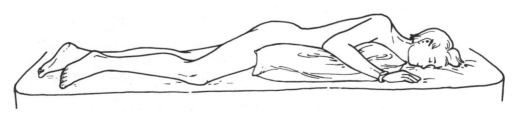

Fig. 6.6 Patient in semiprone position

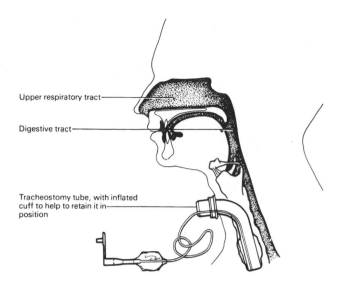

Upper respiratory tract

Digestive tract

Tracheostomy tube, with inflated cuff to help to retain it in position

Fig. 6.7 A tracheostomy tube in position

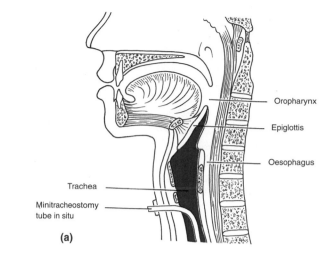

Oropharynx

Epiglottis

Oesophagus

Trachea

Minitracheostomy tube in situ

(a)

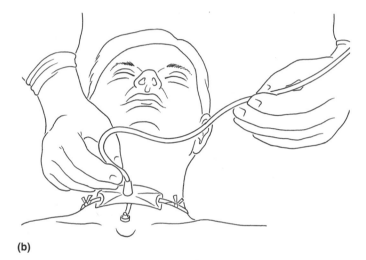

(b)

Minitracheostomy In some instances of sputum retention, minitracheostomy is being used more frequently. It avoids speech impairment. A special tube (Fig. 6.8) is inserted under local anaesthetic and secured round the neck. The small plastic bung is only removed during suctioning to enable the person to cough and evacuate sputum. Suctioning is an aseptic procedure and suction is only applied during withdrawal of catheter (Nelson, 1992).

Postural drainage Some lung conditions produce excessive sputum which obstructs the airway and interferes with oxygenation of the blood. Its removal by postural drainage is frequently necessary (Hough, 1992).

It is important in the first instance to teach deep breathing exercises. The person is then helped into a position, depending on the site from which secretions must be drained, which will encourage the excess mucus and pus to move by gravity into contact with healthy tissue and initiate coughing. Postural drainage usually involves leaning over the side of the bed then coughing and spitting into a large receptacle placed on the floor which is suitably protected by a disposable paper sheet so the nurse must ensure privacy as this is a somewhat undignified position to adopt, and most people dislike coughing and spitting in public. The physiotherapist in these circumstances can be an important member of the health team and may assist with vibration and percussion movements over the affected lung area. When children with fibrocystic disease are involved, parents learn to help with this treatment at home. The appearance and odour from the sputum may cause distress and the receptacle should be removed as soon as possible.

The exertion involved in this technique of postural drainage usually leaves people exhausted and they may benefit from a rest on the bed to recover, before sponging

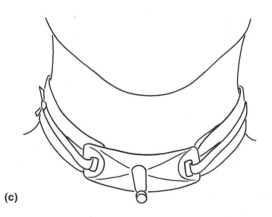

(c)

Fig. 6.8 a. Position of minitracheostomy tube. b. Suctioning by catheter. c. Bung in position between episodes of suction

the face and hands and rinsing the mouth. Despite the unpleasantness, postural drainage can bring quite dramatic relief especially in the morning after wakening: secretions gather during sleeping hours when there is relatively little change in body position.

Oxygen insufficiency

Oxygen insufficiency renders people dependent, not only on the apparatus via which oxygen will be administered, but also on the medical staff for safe prescription and the laboratory staff for monitoring the blood gases and acid/base status. Patients depend on nurses having adequate knowledge and skills to use the apparatus so that maximum benefit is achieved without risk. They depend on nurses' sensitivity to their anxiety and nurses should offer patients every opportunity to retain as much independence and decision making as possible.

Oxygen apparatus The apparatus via which oxygen can be administered is usually selected from a variety of facemasks, nasal cannulae, T-pieces which are used in conjunction with an endotracheal tube or a tracheostomy tube, and oxygen tents. Oxygen tents are now rarely used for adults, but in modified form such as incubators and head tents they are useful for babies and young children. An introduction to the types of apparatus follows.

Facemask Modern facemasks are usually transparent and are made of plastic. Many of them are disposable which is a considerable contribution to prevention of infection. They fit over the nose and under the jaw and are anchored in this position by a strap attached to either side, passing along the cheeks and round the back of the head, so all these areas should be inspected for signs of any response to friction and/or pressure. Some air is breathed in (entrained) around these masks but with well fitting masks and a high flow of oxygen, an inspiratory concentration of 60% or more can be achieved.

Masks are prescribed when oxygen is needed for a relatively short time and the lungs are not diseased. They are not suitable for people with chronic chest conditions because the respiratory centre has become less sensitive to carbon dioxide (Foss, 1990), but there are masks which have a small adjustable valve facilitating a more reliable percentage, and some masks can have several different valves fitted so that percentages of inspired oxygen from 24 to 60 can be achieved (Bell, 1995; Ashurt, 1995).

The placing of a mask on the face of a person who is already breathless can be frightening and the nurse should remain until anxiety is at least diminished if not completely allayed. Patients need to be encouraged to control the rate and depth of respiration because, as noted in the previous paragraph, this contributes to the decreasing or increasing of the percentage of oxygen reaching the lungs for diffusion into the blood.

While the mask is in position, it is not possible for the patient to talk and this barrier to communication increases anxiety, so a bell or buzzer within reach with which to summon assistance is a physical nursing intervention allied to the goal of decreasing anxiety. Understandably, the mask must be removed for eating and drinking; however, in some instances oxygen has to be given via nasal cannulae during the meal. The mask should be dried and the patient provided with facilities to sponge the face before it is replaced. Because of the drying effects of increased oxygen intake, oral hygiene is necessary and nursing interventions for the prevention and treatment of cracked lips.

Nasal cannulae Nasal cannulae are less restricting than a face mask as, while in situ, they permit speech, eating and drinking. Also there is less facial perspiration but this type of apparatus can be just as frightening to the patient. The central part has two light plastic tubes which are inserted into each nostril. A tube on each side passes along the cheek and is supported on the top of each ear lobe and descends to form a Y-junction with the tube leading to the oxygen supply. But a unilateral nasal cannula is now available. The catheter is passed along the floor of one nasal cavity to deliver oxygen into the nasopharynx. The outer end is enveloped within a sponge which rests in the anterior nostril (Fig. 6.9).

Nasal administration of oxygen has gained in popularity as several research projects have compared this method with that of face masks. Most of these comparative surveys have been in the area of postoperative oxygen therapy (Bambridge, 1993; English & Brown, 1994). One set of comparisons is given in Box 6.8. Having established the efficacy of nasal administration current interest is in financial audit and nasal catheter administration is cheaper than mask administration.

However efficacy of the monitoring of administration by nurses has been challenged. Oxygen was prescribed at 4 litres per minute by Hudson face mask, and data were collected during the first postoperative night (Baxter et al, 1993). They recommended:

- improvement in nurse education related to oxygen therapy

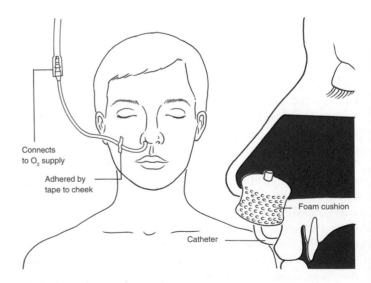

Fig. 6.9 Unilateral nasal catheter (attached)

Box 6.8 Advantages and disadvantages of masks and nasal catheters

Hudson masks		Nasal catheters	
Advantages	**Disadvantages**	**Advantages**	**Disadvantages**
Versatile in that, during an emergency, high oxygen concentrations can be achieved quite easily	Patients cannot eat and drink, take oral drugs, expectorate, vomit, have oral temperatures taken or have oral hygiene without discontinuing oxygen therapy	Patients can eat and drink, take oral drugs, expectorate, vomit and have oral temperatures taken without discontinuing oxygen therapy	Less versatile than masks in an emergency. Less able to produce high oxygen concentrations without risk of damaging the nasal passages. Less able to accommodate patients with high minute volume requirements
More suitable for patients with high minute volume requirements	Patients often feel as if the mask is suffocating them. Some hate having anything on their face or dislike the mask's smell	Permits patients to communicate easily with staff and visitors	Catheters can fall out and need to be taped to the side of the face to stay in place; may be dislodged by sneezing
	Mask can be hot and uncomfortable, and may cause pressure sores on the nose and behind the ears	Cheaper than masks	Catheters may become disconnected from oxygen tubing without nurses noticing
	Masks can cause spectacles to steam up		
	Masks impair communication with staff and visitors	Patients can have oral hygiene and be 'sucked out' without discontinuing therapy	Staff may mistake a nasal catheter for a NG tube and inadvertently discontinue oxygen therapy
	Few patients wear masks correctly, so oxygen concentrations can be variable		Can be uncomfortable for patients with small nostrils

NB. Neither masks nor nasal catheters have been found to reliably produce set oxygen concentrations at specific flow rates but, when worn correctly, masks are slightly more accurate (Fairfield *et al*, 1991).
(Reproduced by kind permission of Professional Nurse, Fairfield et al and Macmillan Magazines Ltd.)

- more emphasis on the use of nasal administration
- assessment of improved staff education on the compliance of supplementary postoperative oxygen therapy (Study in progress).

Oxygen administration in hospital The oxygen supply may be piped to the ward or it may be stored in cylinders which stand at the bedside and cylinder changes should be effected outside the ward as the noise involved in changing a cylinder head can be acutely distressing to an already anxious patient.

Emergency O_2 equipment in the ward should be checked daily to be ready for use, and empty cylinders must be clearly marked and removed from the ward precinct as quickly as possible.

Any supply of oxygen presents a fire hazard. It is the nurse's responsibility to ensure that when oxygen is in use, a warning notice is placed on the cylinder and the dangers explained to the patient, to visitors and to fellow patients. Smoking is forbidden; mechanical toys, electric bells and heating pads are removed; bedmaking and hair combing should be done with care to avoid creating static electricity; and every member of staff should know how to use the nearest fire extinguisher and raise the fire alarm.

Oxygen level in the blood Lack of oxygen in the blood (hypoxaemia) is obviously the reason for administering oxygen to prevent lack of oxygen in the tissues (hypoxia). This can be a preventive measure as in the postoperative studies mentioned, or a therapeutic measure when there is lack of perfusion in the lungs. Whatever the rationale for giving oxygen, a non-invasive tool to measure the oxygen level in the blood when assessing and evaluating is to be welcomed (Coull, 1992; Jones, 1995). A pulse oximeter is such a tool and one version is illustrated in Figure 6.10. It is a portable one with a digital display. The probe is opened to enclose a finger. Another type is illustrated in Nursing Times (1995).

Oxygen administration in the community People who have chronic obstructive pulmonary disease can be

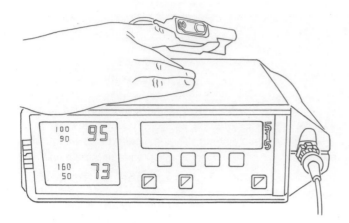

Fig. 6.10 A pulse oximeter

helped to live in their own homes and surroundings by the use of a 'domiciliary oxygen policy'. It is predicted that the number of people requiring this service will increase as the population ages (Williams & Nicholl, 1992). Cylinders are provided and it seems that they are mostly used intermittently for symptom relief. However, concentrators can be installed in the home, maintained and removed when no longer necessary. This may have both administrative and financial advantages but data about the therapeutic response needs to be collected before guidelines are issued (Williams & Nicholl, 1992).

Pre-term infants can develop bronchopulmonary dysplasia and this prolongs the period during which oxygen therapy is required via the nasal route. There are now schemes in some areas whereby two involved adults participate in a teaching/learning programme, the outcome of which is that they become proficient at:

- changing the nasal catheter
- changing the oxygen cylinder head
- using an apnoea monitor
- using a mucus extractor
- recognizing clinical signs of hypoxia
- taking relevant action
- carrying out cardiopulmonary resuscitation.

It has to be remembered that the adults will have witnessed the nurses in the neonatal intensive care unit doing these procedures. Gradually as they gain confidence they carry out the procedures under supervision (Sadler, 1989; Robinson, 1994) before taking their baby home.

Mechanical defects

Anything which interferes with the mechanics of breathing is going to cause problems for the person. A defect in the respiratory muscles or the nerves supplying them means that the person cannot breathe without mechanical assistance. Artificial ventilators can be divided into two groups; firstly, those operating on the principle of

negative pressure on the outside of the chest (the traditional 'iron lung') which was used in the polio epidemic in the 1950s. A cuirass is an updated version working on the same principles. It encloses the chest, and an accompanying pump produces the negative pressure for inspiration, and elastic recoil causes expiration. Secondly there are ventilators which operate on the principle of positive pressure which forces air from a power-driven source into the lungs by means of a tracheostomy tube causing the chest and lungs to expand. The technical aspects of artificial ventilation are often bewildering, and caring for patients can appear daunting (CE Article 337, 1994; CE Article 338, 1994).

Assisted ventilation in hospital The nursing of ventilated people follows the same principles as care of the totally dependent person. Prevention of sensory monotony, orientation to time and place, maintenance of nutritional status, and prevention of pressure sores assume a high priority. Even if such patients cannot talk, nurses should continue to explain procedures, and to inform them of what is going on around them. After a period on the ventilator, full return to spontaneous breathing may take several days or weeks. Weaning from the respirator is usually determined by the patient, but for a few patients this is not possible. All such people need psychological help to come to terms with the many changes involving self-image and self-esteem.

Assisted ventilation in the community Some of the people who require to be ventilated for life may be able to live at home, but many wide-ranging issues need consideration to make this possible. There are also some ventilation-dependent children; they suffer not only from lack of exercise, but they also experience frustration and boredom stemming from their total dependence on a machine. With some ingenuity, swimming and sunbathing have been used as effective therapies (Carter, 1988).

People who require assisted ventilation are highly dependent for the AL of breathing and they and their families require considerable emotional support.

As long ago as 1979, Ashworth's research indicated that of all types of respiratory problems, the greatest difficulties were experienced by the patient whose breathing was being maintained artificially via a tracheal tube and who was also paralysed by medications or the pathological condition which caused the respiratory failure. She wrote:

'Speech and other forms of communication may be impossible except perhaps blinking of the eyelids and other small movements. It can be very frightening to be unable to indicate needs or feelings, and also very frustrating. To add to the problem, even experienced nurses may find it very difficult to go on talking to someone who appears unresponsive, who cannot talk, move, smile or perhaps open their eyes.'

In a small study in five intensive care units it was found that there was a correlation between the amount of communication by the patient and by the nurse: the less the patient communicated, the less intentional communication there was by the nurse. An awareness of this should encourage nurses to seek to maintain communication (and to encourage relatives to do so too) even with apparently unresponsive patients, for the reason Ashworth gave:

> 'To someone who is aware yet totally helpless and unable to control even his own breathing, it is essential to have people to talk to him by name about things which interest and concern him, if he is not to lose his sense of identity and to feel like 'just another body in a bed'.'

Artificial pacing of the heart beat   There are various conditions which interfere with the mechanics of the heart, rendering it less effective as a pump. When the pulse rate and rhythm can no longer be controlled by oral medications, some people require surgical insertion of an electronic pacemaker under the skin of the left chest. Those who are dependent on a pacemaker are usually satisfied with their consequent improved health status.

CHANGE OF ENVIRONMENT AND ROUTINE

When people who have problems with the AL of breathing are to be nursed at home, there may have to be changes in the environment, for example, if possible it is better for all concerned if a single bed is used which is easily accessible from both sides. There may also have to be modification of the daily routine to accommodate for instance learning about inhaling from nebulizers.

However, the person may have to be admitted to hospital. Irrespective of the individual's diagnosis, merely coming into hospital can alter normal breathing activity and circulation. The ward temperature may be so warm that it produces a feeling of 'suffocating'; or the central heating may reduce the atmospheric water content causing irritation to the nose and mouth; or the odours peculiar to hospital may be unpleasant; or the strangeness of the surroundings may be so overwhelming as to produce the rapid, shallow breathing which often accompanies anxiety. And of course, the accompanying emotional upset can increase the pulse rate.

Health services are moving towards a total non-smoking policy, and smokers may feel restricted and irritated by rules about limitations on indulging in this activity. Non-smokers may abhor even a whiff of stale smoke or may be apprehensive about the fire hazards when fellow patients seem careless about extinguishing cigarettes.

Nurses must be alert to these circumstances and within the constraints of communal living attempt to accommodate the requirements of both smokers and non-smokers, as far as it is possible. The risk of fire in buildings on account of smoking was mentioned in the context of maintaining a safe environment (p. 84), and nurses should be ever vigilant on this account.

Change of environment and routine which results in reduced exercise can contribute to the potential problems of deep vein thrombosis with possible consequent pulmonary embolism. It is relevant to mention them here, because these conditions pertain to the cardiopulmonary system, but there is further discussion on p. 305 in the context of decreased mobilizing related to possible nursing interventions.

Summarizing, some of the actual and potential problems with the AL of breathing have been discussed using four broad classifications. It is possible to discuss them from a general point of view, but in reality they are experienced uniquely by the individual person. Identification of problems is the prelude to planning and implementing nursing activities and evaluating outcomes.

Planning and implementing nursing activities and evaluating outcomes

From the preceeding section it can be seen that the possible actual and potential problems are not only numerous but some of them are also of a complex biological/pathological nature. Congruent with our model we believe that the expected outcomes when planning and implementing nursing practices for the AL of breathing are that people will be helped:

- to prevent potential problems from becoming actual problems, smoking related diseases having high priority
- to solve or alleviate actual problems in the respiratory system, lymphatic system, cardiovascular system or any combination of these
- to prevent solved problems from recurring
- to develop positive coping mechanisms for those problems which cannot be solved.

So far, individualizing nursing for the AL of breathing has been discussed under the headings of 'Assessing the individual in the AL of breathing' and 'Identifying actual and potential problems' but the reality is that two other phases of the process of nursing — planning and implementing have been mentioned many times. This is indicative of the fact that the phases of the process are not linear, sequential or separate but all phases can be part of a single nursing event because of their interactive nature.

The nurse's role as health educator is acowledged in The Health of the Nation (Department of Health, 1991) in relation to reaching the target of reducing the number of smokers by the year 2000. In many health centres there are 'Stop smoking' clinics planned and staffed by the practice nurses. They have at their disposal leaflets and booklets produced by the Health Education Authority. Each client will select a preferred route/plan to achieve the stated expected outcome 'cessation of smoking'. Nursing help and advice will probably be needed for the person to 'implement' the plan at home, at work and during leisure activities. There will be evaluation and re-evaluation at follow up visits, which may well strengthen motivation to persevere. An annual visit may reinforce this as well as helping to improve the data bank about permanent cessation.

Nurses are being encouraged to take a 'smoking history' at the initial assessment of people entering the health service. When the contact is going to be short, ward nurses for instance could refer people who smoke (and want to stop) to their local 'Stop smoking clinic'. Midwives and nursing staff in contact with intending mothers in what is now being referred to as the pre-conceptual period, as well as the antenatal period, plan and implement similar programmes emphasising the risk of smoking in pregnancy.

Another example of using the process flexibly might be practice nurses can plan to offer information to, for instance chronically breathless people to help them understand their condition. The plan might include advice to keep a diary so that activities which increase their breathlessness can be identified. From the diaries the plan would be to help these people to plan their daily activities in such a way as to minimize incidents of increased breathlessness, or the information might guide the time at which medications are taken. Planning for these people is an ongoing cooperative activity, and it is the breathless person who 'implements' the plan. Planning includes stating expected outcomes and these might be — decrease in the incidents of increased breathlessness: managing their daily lives to their satisfaction. On evaluation the first is a recordable datum which can be compared with the previous one, but the second is subjective and individual to each chronically breathless person.

A similar pattern of the nurse's role is required in helping people to cope with such chronic conditions as asthma. They need information/education about what happens in their body during an attack; they need help to identify the allergen which precipitates an attack; and they need information about their medications. However, they have an additional need — demonstration and practice in the effective use of a nebulizer. Ineffective use of nebulizers is a frequent finding reported by Smith and Kendrick (1993). People do not learn at the same rate and some are more dexterous than others and this has to be remembered when setting the date for evaluation of the expected outcome which might be — understands function of medications; less frequent attacks; nebulizer used effectively. The expected outcomes do not end here; these people have to incorporate into their body image a change which eventually can be very restricting of many ALs and finally can mean severe breathlessness, even at rest, so that there is dependence on others for most of the ALs.

This chapter has been concerned with focusing the concepts of our model to the AL of breathing with the objective of individualizing nursing by using flexibly the phases of the process of nursing as illustrated in Figure 3.9, p. 60. Breathing is essential for living, and any impediment in this AL can affect all the others. Indeed cessation of breathing and circulation is the end point of the AL of dying.

REFERENCES

Adomat R 1992 Understanding shock. British Journal of Nursing 1 (3): 124–128

Alton R 1994 Arrhythmias associated with cardiopulmonary arrest. Nursing Times 90 (19) May 11: 42–44

Ashworth P 1979 Psychological and social aspects of respiratory care. Nursing 1st Series (7) November: 295–299

Ashurt S 1992 Suction therapy in the critically ill patient. British Journal of Nursing 1 (10): 485–489

Bambridge A D 1993 Comparison of oxygen mask and nasal catheter in the provision of postoperative oxygen therapy. Professional Nurse 8 (8) May: 513, 515–518

Barnes K, Clifford R, Holgate S T 1987 Bacterial contamination of home nebulisers. British Medical Journal 295: 812

Baxter K, Nolan K M, Winyard J A, Roulson C J, Goldhill D R 1993 Are they getting enough? Meeting the oxygen needs of postoperative patients. Professional Nurse 8 (5) February: 310–312

Bell C 1995 Is this what the doctor ordered? Accuracy of oxygen therapy prescribed and delivered in hospital. Professional Nurse 10 (5) February: 297–300

Briggs L M 1994 Sexual healing: caring for patients recovering from myocardial infarction. British Journal of Nursing 3 (16): 837–842

BMA/RCN 1993 Statement on cardiopulmonary resuscitation. BMA/RCN, London

British Medical Association 1995 Advance statements about medical treatment. BMJ Publishing Group, London

Brown S, Mann R 1990 Breaking the cycle: control of breathlessness in chronic lung disease. Professional Nurse 5 (6) March: 325–328

Bruce-Jones R 1993 Resuscitation update. Nursing Standard 7 (44) July 21: 48–50

Brydon M J 1993 Understanding is the means to control. Seasonal rhinitis. Professional Nurse 8 (10) July: 662–666

Buckley R 1992 The management of hypovolaemic shock. Nursing Standard 6 (41) July 1: 25–28

Burgess L 1994 An epidemic of massive proportions. Smoking and the health of the nation. Professional Nurse 9 (8) May: 566, 568, 570, 572

Campbell J 1993b Making sense of shock. Nursing Times 89 (15) February 3: 34–36

Campbell J 1993a How necessary is cardiac rehabilitation? Professional Nurse 8 (5) February: 279–283

Candy C E 1991 'Not for resuscitation': the student nurses' viewpoint. Journal of Advanced Nursing 16: 138–146

Carroll D, Rose K 1992 Treatment leads to significant improvement. Professional Nursing 8 (1) October: 32, 33, 35, 36

Carter B 1988 Simple! (Chronically ventilated children) Nursing Times 84 (13) March 30: 38

CE (Continuing Education) 1994 Article 337. Assisted ventilation: methods and observation. Nursing Standard 9 (6) November 2: 43–47

CE (Continuing Education) 1994 Article 338. Assisted ventilation: psychological and physical care. Nursing Standard 9 (8) November 16: 51–56

Chellel A 1993a CPR: the problems and solutions. Nursing Standard 7 (21) February 10: 33–36

Chellel A 1993b Outcomes, ethics and accountability. Nursing Standard 7 (22) February 17: 37–39

Coady E, Calne S 1994 Artificial ventilation and chest compression. Nursing Times 90 (17) April 27: 36–38

Deans W, Hoskins R 1987 Preventing coronary heart disease. Professional Nurse 2 (10) July: 328–329

Dickson D 1993 Lower limb lymphoedema. Wound Management 3(1): 15

Department of Health 1991 The Health of the Nation. A consultative document for health in England. HMSO, London CM 1523

Department of Health 1988 National Breastfeeding Initiative. HMSO, London

Doughty C 1991 A multidisciplinary approach to cardiac rehabilitation. Nursing Standard 5 (45) July 31: 13–15

English I, Brown C 1994 Oxygen mask or nasal catheter — an analysis. (Postoperative patients) Nursing Standard 8 (26) March 23: 27–31

Evans A 1991 Sensible stockings. Nursing Times 87 (51) December 18: 40–41

Evans P 1993 Back to basics. Cardiac rehabilitation. Nursing Times 89 (48) December 1: 48–50

Fairfield J E, Goroszeniuk T, Tully A M, Adams A P 1991 Oxygen delivery systems: a comparison of two devices. Anaesthesia 46(2): 135–138

Feher M, Harris-St John K, Lant A 1992 Blood pressure measurement by junior hospital doctors — a gap in medical education. Health Trends 24 (2): 59–61

Foss M A 1990 Oxygen therapy. Professional Nurse 5 (4) January: 188–190

Foster C, McKinlay S, Kemp F 1993 Ambulatory blood pressure monitoring. Nursing Times 89 (1) January 6: 23–24

Fotherby M D, Panayiotou B, Potter J F 1993 Age-related differences in simultaneous blood pressure measurements. Postgraduate Medical Journal 69 (809): 194–196

Gardiner J, Halliday A 1994 Resuscitation in special circumstances. Nursing Times 90 (20) May 18: 35–37

Gee K 1993 Cardiopulmonary resuscitation. British Journal of Nursing 2 (2): 138–141

Gibson P 1991 The ethical dilemma. Resuscitation. Nursing 4 (26) January: 16–18

Godkin M D, Toth E L 1994 Cardiopulmonary resuscitation decision making in long-term care: a role for the nurse? Journal of Advanced Nursing 19: 1 January 97–104

Green A 1991 Laryngeal masks. Nursing Times 87 (10) March 6: 36–37

Hill S C 1993 Health warning. Passive smoking. Nursing Times 89 (24) June 16: 40–49

Hough A 1992 Sputum retention. Nursing Times 88 (36) September 2: 33–35

Innes M H 1992 Managing upper airway obstruction. British Journal of Nursing 1 (14): 732–735

Jamieson E M, McCall J M, Blythe R 1992 Guidelines for Clinical Nursing Practice. Churchill Livingstone, Edinburgh

Janman L 1993 Assessment brings its own relief. Ischaemic leg pain. Professional Nurse 8 (8) May: 524, 526–529

Jeffs E 1992 Management of lymphoedema. Journal of Tissue Viability 2 (4): 127–131

Jennings P 1990 Caring for a child with a tracheostomy. Nursing Standard 4 (30) April 18: 24–26

Jennings P 1990 Caring for a child with a tracheostomy. Nursing Standard 4 (32) May 2: 38–40

Jones C 1992 Sexual activity after myocardial infarction. Nursing Standard 6 (48) August 19: 25–28

Jones S E 1995 Getting the balance right: pulse oximetry and inspired oxygen concentration. Professional Nurse 10 (6) March: 368–373

Kemp F, Foster C, McKinlay S 1994 How effective is training for

blood pressure measurement? Professional Nurse 9 (8) May: 521–524

Kennedy S 1991 A measure of independence. Teaching home blood pressure monitoring. Professional Nurse 6 (12) September: 730–731

Lamb J 1993 Peripheral IV therapy. Nursing Standard 7 (36) May 26: 31–34 (Continuing Education Series)

Leach A 1994 Making sense of peak-flow recordings of lung function. Nursing Times 90 (44) November 2: 34–35

Lindsay G M, Christie J, Gaw A, Packard C J, Shepherd J 1994 Educating children (7 to 11) about heart disease. Nursing Standard 8 (45) August 3: 32–35 (Computer programme)

Lyall J 1993 Off target (in reducing smoking among young teenagers). Nursing Times 89 (29) July 21: 19

Mackintosh C 1994 Non-reporting of cardiac pain. Nursing Times 90 (13) March 30: 36–39

Monkley-Poole S 1992 Vehicle pollutants: effects on the lung. Nursing Standard 7 (5) October 21: 35–38

McCrissican D 1991 Patient education in coronary care. Nursing Standard 5 (40) June 26: 37–39

McGarvey H 1990 Endotracheal intubation. Nursing Times 86 (42) October 17: 35–37

Nelson A 1992 Minitracheostomy: the benefits for patient care. British Journal of Nursing 1 (10): 492, 493, 495

Nolan J, Nolan M 1993 Can nurses take an accurate blood pressure? British Journal of Nursing 2 (14): 724–729

Nursing Standard 1994 Children suffer over school asthma ignorance. Nursing Standard 8 (17) January 19: 14

Nursing Standard 1993 Making the decision on resuscitation. Nursing Standard 7 (48) August 18: 39 (A statement jointly prepared by the Royal College of Nursing and the British Medical Association)

Nursing Times 1991 Comparing endotracheal suction regimes (Babies). Nursing Times 87 (50) December 11: 44

Nursing Times 1995 Staff confusion in the use of pulse oximetry. Nursing Times 91 (12) March 22: 11

O'Brien D, Davison M 1994 Blood pressure measurement: rational and ritual actions. British Journal of Nursing 3 (8): 393–396

Office of Population Censuses and Surveys. OPCS 1993 Smoking among secondary school children in England in 1993. HMSO, London

Oliver E 1994 Maintaining nutritional support in the community. Journal of Tissue Viability 4 (1): 28–32

Parkin M 1993 The avoidability of cancer: world-wide totals and world-wide variation. Paper presented to Conference on strategies for chronic disease control. Royal Society, London, 15 February 1993

Partridge M R 1994 Asthma: guided self management. British Medical Journal 308 (6928) February 26: 547–548

Piper K M 1992 When can I do 'it' again nurse? Sexual counselling after a heart attack. Professional Nurse 8 (3) December: 168–171

Poole S 1993 Nutritional aspects of respiratory disease. Professional Nurse 8 (4) January: 252, 254–256

Purtell M 1994 Teenage girls' attitudes to breastfeeding. Health Visitor 67 (5): 156–157

Pottle A 1992 Tough decisions. Nursing Times 88 (42) October 14: 32–33

Reynolds D, Ward C 1994 Intensive training. Asthma education. Nursing Times 90 (27) July 6: 46–47

Robinson J 1994 Settling David. Paediatric long-term oxygen therapy at home. Nursing Times 90 (1) January 5: 30

Roe B, Griffiths J, Kenrick M, Cullum N, Hutton J 1993 Nursing treatment of patients with chronic leg ulcers in the community. Journal of Clinical Nursing 3 (3) May: 159–168

Roper N 1988 Churchill Livingstone Nurses' Dictionary. Churchill Livingstone, Edinburgh

Rose K, Taylor H, Twycross R 1993 Volume reduction in arm lymphoedema. Nursing Standard 7 (35) May 19: 29–32

Royal College of Nursing 1994 2E AIDS nursing guidelines. Royal College of Nursing, London

Rundell S, Rundell L 1992 The nursing contribution to the resuscitation debate. Journal of Clinical Nursing 1: 195–198

Sadler C 1989 And baby came too. Training mothers prior to discharge of their premature babies. Nursing Times 85 (23) June 7: 16–17

Schutz S E 1994 Patient involvement in resuscitation decisions. British Journal of Nursing 3 (20) November 10–23: 1075, 1077–1079

Sharp J 1993 Which peak flow meter? Nursing Times 89 (3) January 20: 61–63

Simpson S M 1994 Paediatric advanced life support — an update. Nursing Times 90 (27) July 6: 37–39

Smith B 1994 The dressing makes the difference. Venous ulcers. Professional Nurse 9 (5) February: 350–352

Smith E C, Kendrick A H 1993 How do inhaled bronchodilators work? Professional Nurse 8 (8) May: 531–535

Smith P 1992 Compression hosiery in a surgical unit. Nursing Standard 6 (49) August 26: 25–28

Sneddon M 1992 Management of the oedematous limb. Professional Nurse 7 (12) September: 818, 820–822

Speck P 1992 Who draws the line? Resuscitation. Nursing Times 88 (39) September 23: 22

Strudley M 1990 Asthma in the classroom. Nursing Standard 5 (7) November 7: 49–50

Tettersell M J 1993 Asthma patients' knowledge in relation to compliance with drug therapy. Journal of Advanced Nursing 18: 103–113

Toulson S 1993 A guide to advanced trauma life support. Professional Nurse 8 (2) November: 95–97

Trevelyan J 1991 Hepatitis B. Who is at risk? Nursing Times 87 (5) January 30: 26–29

Twinn S 1990 The heart of the matter. Community Outlook. August: 11, 12, 14

While A 1990 Getting it right. Weaning. Community Outlook. October: 14, 18

Willetts K 1989 Assessing cardiac pain. Nursing Times 85 (47) November 22: 52–54

Williams A 1993 Management of cardiogenic shock. Professional Nurse 8 (8) May: 520–523

Williams A 1993 Management of lymphoedema: a community-based approach. British Journal of Nursing 2 (13): 678–681

Williams A 1992 Management of lymphoedema: a community-based approach. British Journal of Nursing 1 (8): 385–387

Williams B, Nicholl J 1992 Recent trends in the use of domiciliary oxygen in England and Wales. Health Trends 23 (45): 166–167

Williams C 1994 Paediatric cardiopulmonary resuscitation. British Journal of Nursing 3 (15) August 11 — September 7: 760–764

Wilson J A 1994 Preventing infection during IV therapy. Professional Nurse 9 (6) March: 388–390, 392

World Health Organization 1980 International classification of impairments, disabilities and handicaps: a manual classification relating to the consequences of disease. WHO, Geneva

Wynne G 1993 Revival techniques. Nursing Times 89 (11) March 17: 26–31

ADDITIONAL READING

Ball S 1994 Breath of life: adult respiratory distress syndrome. Nursing Times 90 (37) September 14: 60

Benington G 1991 Nursing management of lymphoedema. Nursing Standard 6 (7) November 6: 24–27

Blackler P, Sinclair D 1993 Audit of inhaled asthma therapy. Nursing Standard 7 (33) May 5: 28–30

Brewin A M, Hughes J A 1995 Effect of patient education on asthma management. British Journal of Nursing 4 (2) January 26–February 8: 81, 82, 99, 101

Campbell J 1993 Underwater sealed drainage. Nursing Times 89 (9) March 3: 34–36

CE (Continuing Education) 1995 Article 342 Venous and arterial leg ulcers. Nursing Standard 9 (26) March 22: 25–30

de Belder A 1993 Understanding atherosclerosis. Nursing Standard 7 (30) April 14: 48–49

Drago S S 1992 Banking on your own blood (autologous blood transfusion). American Journal of Nursing 82 (3): 61–65

Ferns T 1994 Home mechanical ventilation in a changing health service. Nursing Times 90 (40) October 5: 43–45

Flynn M 1993 Management of chronic obstructive airways disease. British Journal of Nursing 2 (14): 717, 718, 720–723

Gee C F, Noble W 1990 Transparent film dressings in preventing infection in intravenous cannula sites. Nursing 4 (21) November 7: 39–41

Gee K 1993 Cardiopulmonary resuscitation: basic life support skills. British Journal of Nursing 2 (1): 87–89

Heath M 1993 Management of obstructive sleep apnoea. British Journal of Nursing 2 (16): 802–804

Higgins C 1994 Blood transfusion: risks and benefits. British Journal of Nursing 3 (19) October 27–November 9: 986–991

McKenzie S 1994 Drugs used to control asthma. British Journal of Nursing 3 (17) September 22–October 12: 872, 873, 875–877, 879, 880

Midence K, Graham V, Acheampong C, Okuyiga E 1994 Measuring knowledge of sickle cell disease in adult patients. Professional Nurse 9 (4) January: 255, 256, 258

Mitchell E, Scragg R, Stewart A W et al 1991 Cot death supplement. Results from the first year of the New Zealand cot death study. New Zealand Medical Journal 104 (906): 71–76

Moffatt C J, Oldroyd M I 1994 A pioneering service to the community. The Riverside Community leg ulcer project. Professional Nurse 8 (7) April: 486, 488, 490, 492, 494, 497

Nursing Times 1995 Professional Development Unit 15, Part 1. Blood pressure. Nursing Times 91 (14) April 5: 1–4

Oldham P 1991 A sticky situation? Microbiological study of adhesive tape used to secure IV cannulae. Professional Nurse 6 (5) February: 265, 266, 268, 269

Rowland R 1991 Venepuncture. Nursing Times 87 (32) August 7: 41–43

Shemwell A, Wilson P A 1994 Rest and respiration during obstructive sleep apnoea. Nursing Times 90 (19) May 11: 30–32

Sutcliffe L 1992 Heart health. Nursing Times 85 (24) June 14: RCN Nursing Update: 3–8

Wilkinson R 1991 The challenge of intravenous therapy. Nursing Standard 5 (28) April 3: 24–27

Williams T 1992 To clamp or not to clamp? Chest drainage tubes. Nursing Times 88 (18) April 29: 33

Willis J 1995 Infusion therapy: principles and practice. Nursing Times 91 (12) March 22: 67–68

Woods M 1991 Developing a service for the management of lymphoedema. Nursing Standard 5 (445) July 31: 10–11

Woods M 1994 An audit of swollen limb measurements. Nursing Standard 9 (5) October 26: 24–26

7

Eating and drinking

The AL of eating and drinking

Human life cannot exist without eating and drinking, such is the essential nature of this activity. It takes up a considerable part of each day since apart from the time involved in eating, food has to be procured and prepared; indeed in some instances it has to be grown by the individual family. In most cultures it is the women who select, buy and cook the family's food. However in many industrialized societies, with the movement towards a greater sharing of parental and domestic activities, this is beginning to change and men are playing a much more active part in matters related to food and feeding. And in the world of chefs there are more men than women!

In keeping with our models, the four concepts — lifespan; dependence/independence; factors influencing; and individuality in living and individualizing nursing — will in this chapter be focused to the fifth concept, the ALs, emphasizing the particular AL of eating and drinking as illustrated in Figure 7.1.

Lifespan: relationship to the AL of eating and drinking

It is not difficult to appreciate that the activity of eating and drinking will vary according to the individual's stage on the lifespan. The close relationship of the lifespan and the dependence/independence component is integral to the model, and this is certainly so for the AL of eating and drinking particularly for the very young, and in some instances at the other end of the age spectrum for the elderly.

The physical growth and development of the fetus are dependent on nutrition received from the mother via the umbilical cord, so the quality and quantity of the maternal diet is important throughout pregnancy and features highly in health education during the prenatal period. Indeed in the preconceptual period, women are being encouraged to maximize their health status by attending to their diet (Anderson, 1994) and minimizing alcohol intake.

Up-to-date research reveals that ethnic minority pregnant women need help

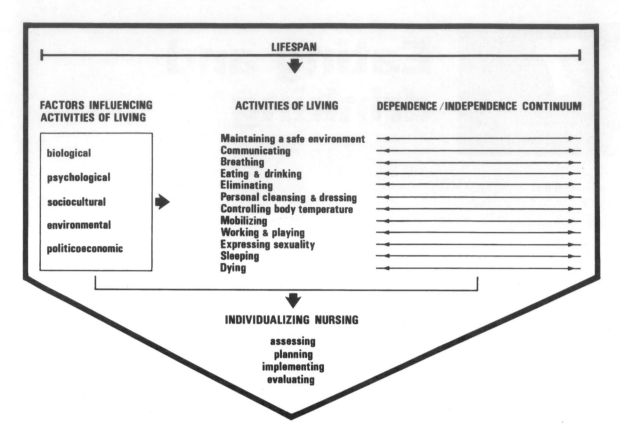

Fig. 7.1 The AL of eating and drinking within the model for nursing

to adjust their diet according to their cultural and spiritual beliefs about food (Way, 1991).

The goal of health education is to enable pregnant women to make the best choices under the circumstances, particularly if they are adverse, and these may be as varied as inadequate food supply to the geographical area, or an inadequate financial income to buy the recommended diet.

Infancy

Newborn babies are incapable of choosing and it would seem that most mothers have a straightforward personal choice (influenced by knowledge, attitude and beliefs) either to breast feed or bottle feed their baby. However, due to a variety of circumstances, some mothers may not be able to be in contact with their baby (who may be in a neonatal intensive care unit), but they may be able to express their breast milk by using a pump, so that although such babies are not being breastfed in the accepted sense, they are receiving breast milk.

Breast feeding Currently, if the mother has decided to breast feed, it is customary to put the newborn infant to the breast almost immediately after delivery (Box 7.1), as advocated by UNICEF and WHO.

In the infant stage of the lifespan, breast milk provides protection against infection and allergy, as well as nutri-

tion for the baby in the form most suited to human infants. Provided the mother is taking a reasonable diet, the constituents of breast milk are present in the correct ratio for the human infant's digestive system; at the correct temperature; available without elaborate preparation; and is cheaper than formula milk (Black, 1993). The intimacy of breast feeding is known to induce a special relationship between mother and baby, called 'bonding'.

Despite the acknowledged superiority of breast milk, including its protective effect against cot death (Mitchell, Scragg, Stewart et al, 1991) and more controversially, protection against breast cancer in young women (Chilvers, 1993; Schwarz, 1990), the practice of breast feeding is declining in the UK.

The Infant Feeding Survey (Social Survey Division, 1992) shows that in 1990 63% of parturient women began breast feeding compared to 64% in 1985. Fifty per cent were still breast feeding at two weeks compared to 51% in 1985. The DHSS backed a National Breastfeeding Initiative (1988) with the objective of increasing the number of breast feeding mothers, as well as the duration, (and there are local groups throughout the country). The survey also showed that 45% of babies were given formula milk while in the maternity unit, and that at six weeks more mothers were combining breast with formula feeds. And the mother's social class was also signifi-

Box 7.1 Ten steps to successful breast feeding

UNICEF and WHO have drawn up a code of practice for all maternity units. All hospitals following the 'Ten Steps to Successful Breast feeding' will be designated as 'baby-friendly'. The ten steps?

1. Have a written breast feeding policy — routinely communicated to all health staff.
2. Train all health staff to implement this policy.
3. Inform all pregnant women about the benefits and management of breast feeding.
4. Help mothers initiate breast feeding within half an hour of birth.
5. Show mothers how to breast feed, and how to maintain lactation even if they are separated from their infants.
6. Give newborn infants no food or drink other than breast milk, unless *medically* indicated.
7. Practise rooming-in (mothers and children to remain together) 24 hours a day.
8. Encourage breast feeding on demand.
9. Give no artificial teats or pacifiers (also called dummies or soothers) to breast feeding infants.
10. Foster the establishment of breast feeding support groups and refer mothers to them on discharge from the hospital or clinic.

cant – 86% in class one initiated breast feeding compared with 41% in class five.

Some mothers who are HIV seropositive have given birth to a seropositive baby. If the baby is negative, mothers in this country are being discouraged from breast feeding in favour of a safe feeding alternative (World Health Organization, 1992; Curtis, 1992; Morley, 1994).

The decreasing number of breast feeding women already mentioned is not confined to the UK; it is prevalent in many countries throughout the world, and is accompanied by an increase in the number of babies who are bottle fed. Intensive marketing and advertising of 'breast milk substitutes' are known to be a contributing factor to the undesirable changes. The World Health Organization's International Code of Practice on the marketing of 'breast milk substitutes' was mainly for commercial firms. However, it also recommended that health professionals should refrain from offering samples of these formulae (provided by sales representatives) to new mothers, or advertising them in any way, for example in maternity hospitals and clinics. This was reinforced by the UK responding to a European Union Directive which concerns the composition, labelling and marketing of formula milk. It restricts the advertisement of formula milk and follow-on formulae to professional journals and for-

bids health professionals from promoting sales of such products (Briggs, 1992; Nursing Times, 1993).

If the number of infants who are breast fed at birth is to reach the target set by the government, then teenage girls need to be educated about the benefits of breast feeding (Purtell, 1994). The subjects in the study said they would prefer to be educated by health professionals, but if so, it may encourage the notion that breast feeding is a medical issue rather than a natural one.

In the early 1990s the UK national press discussed the subject of men objecting to mothers breast feeding their babies in public places such as restaurants. In response, The National Opinion Poll surveyed 924 men and half of them objected to breast feeding 'in any place they chose', while 14% found breast feeding in parks and shopping centres 'unacceptable' or 'very unacceptable'. They said it was embarrassing, unnecessary, a form of exhibitionism, attracted attention or was 'disgusting behaviour' (Laurent, 1993). There are suggestions that in school, health/sex education should emphasize that the primary function of the female breast is nurturing and that their sexual erotic function is secondary. There is also a suggestion that breast feeding is put on a par with immunization; the public as well as prospective parents need to be informed that both are for the well-being of the child. The role that the public can play in helping breast feeding mothers to feel at ease also needs to be stressed (Thomson, 1991; Clarke, 1991).

There is greater emphasis in the literature about helping first time mothers to breast feed. Although babies root instinctively they usually need help to take the areola as well as the nipple into their mouths (Reid, 1992). She emphasizes that time has to be spent with mothers while they gain confidence as well as knowledge. She also says that despite progress, we are still imprisoned by a task-oriented view of work. And finally a teaching package has been prepared for midwives. It is a research-based approach to show how professionals can best pass on their expertise (Jamieson, 1994).

Bottle feeding For a variety of reasons, however, bottle feeding may be the method of choice. In these circumstances, dried milk preparations are frequently used. It is most important that the amount is carefully calculated using the measuring spoon provided in the packet, and the prescribed measure of liquid. Otherwise the baby may develop an electrolyte imbalance which can lead to a dramatic disruption of physiological processes. If a bottle fed baby appears to be hungry, the volume of the feed can be increased, but not the concentration (DHSS, 1988). To prevent infection the bottle and teat are scrupulously cleaned and then sterilized between feeds, usually by immersion in a hypochlorite solution, which is discarded and replaced daily. Close bodily contact between mother and baby during feeding enhances the 'togetherness' part of bonding.

Weaning As the infant grows, milk is no longer adequate for nutritional requirements and the process of weaning from breast or bottle feeding begins. Many young mothers, including members of minority groups, believe that the commercial weaning foods are 'superior', but this multimillion financial market is being challenged. Not only are they relatively expensive, but the nutritional information on the labels is increasingly difficult to interpret (Todd, 1992). Pureed family food, gradually thickened, exposes the infant's palate to different textures as well as tastes (Holmes, 1991).

Another word about weaning in ethnic minority groups. National research (DHSS, 1988) had shown iron deficiency anaemia. A Nursing Development Unit is participating in an action research project exploring users' health and dietary beliefs, and their feelings about weaning (Buxton, 1993).

Infants have to develop a different eating skill; instead of sucking they have to cope with food on a spoon and manipulate the semisolid in the mouth before swallowing. Not surprisingly there is initial awkwardness and time must be given for experimentation.

Eventually infants begin to handle the spoon themselves and lift the food to the mouth. They experiment with gripping and controlling the spoon and tracing the spatial pathway from plate to mouth. The resultant 'messiness' is inevitable, but patience and the presence of a warm supporting mother or mother substitute permit acquisition of the necessary dexterity. Gradually, solid foods are introduced into the diet and eventually the majority of children become independent in the necessary skills for eating and drinking. However, a minority of people have physical disabilities which prevent them from acquiring independence as they progress along the lifespan. More will be said about this later.

In the interest of health education, to prevent the potential problems of dental caries, periodontal disease, and obesity from becoming actual problems in later life, it is important to wean all infants on to foods which have a savoury rather than a sweet taste (Todd, 1992).

The Department of Health's report on weaning (1994) advises that solid food should not be given before the age of four months; from four to six months, spoon-feeding should complement breast or bottle milk, progressing to 'finger feeding', puréed and minced food until nine months. Until 12 months, minced and cubed 'family' food can gradually be managed using a small knife and fork. Mathieson (1995) discusses the report in more detail.

Children

But what should children be eating? In the last 20 years several research reports have associated a high fat intake, particularly saturated (animal) fats, with coronary heart disease. Consequently some nutritionists recommended that from an early age, children should be given a diet low in animal (saturated) fat; others believed that this is inappropriate as milk fat makes an important contribution to a child's available energy as well as supplying vitamins and trace elements. Recommendations from the DHSS report (1988) are still valid. Skimmed milk should not be given to children under 2 years, but 2-year-olds can be given semi-skimmed milk, and 5-year-olds may be given skimmed milk.

Other general recommendations were for decreased salt and sugar, and increased fibre in the diet (of adults). There was concern that this dietary advice could be inappropriately applied to the under-5-year-olds. However at whatever age, energy requirements are dependent on age, gender, weight, height and physical activity and must be met for each individual to promote optimal growth (Department of Health, 1991).

Adolescents

Throughout adolescence many people are physically active, expending a great deal of energy. Consequently the appetites of adolescents tend to be large and in the Western world seem to be satiated by high energy snacks rather than traditional meals. Many young people live away from home for the first time, and they become independent for providing their own diet. Some experiment with changing to, for example, a vegetarian diet. But in the interests of health, all should try to follow the main recommendations from the Committee on Medical Aspects of Food Policy (COMA) (Department of Health, 1991). These are to eat sufficient food to maintain optimal weight for height, and to take adequate exercise. A decrease in salt and sugar intake is recommended. Dietary fat should provide a maximum of one-third of the total daily energy intake; and only one-third of this should be saturated (animal) fat and the rest should be made up of polyunsaturated fat. Alcohol should comprise no more than 4% of daily energy intake. And, of course, dietary fibre should be increased by eating wholegrain cereals, pulses, fruit and vegetables (Department of Health, 1991).

Adults

The variation in food and drink preferred by adults is legion and the variety becomes more obvious when there is a multicultural society. The report previously mentioned in the context of adolescents, was originally recommended to promote healthier eating practices in the adult population, and they should be continued throughout life. The prime objective of the reports was to prevent coronary heart disease (p. 153) but there are other diet-related diseases — diverticulosis, obesity, dental caries and periodontal disease. It is important in adult years to take sufficient exercise, because the increased metabolism is beneficial to the cardiovascular system in particular.

Elderly people

Going to the other end of the lifespan the elderly person often has less appetite for food; there is usually less physical activity so there is not the same requirement for the energy-giving foodstuffs. There may also be less interest in cooking and preparing a meal for one, if the person is living alone, and hastily prepared snacks often do not provide the necessary vitamins or minerals. Being housebound may be due to apathy or dementia, but a physical disability can also make it difficult or impossible to go out for shopping. There is usually an increasing dependence on others as the old person moves to the end of the lifespan and this will probably influence the choice of food and drink, and perhaps reduce the pleasure usually associated with this AL.

Dependence/ independence in the AL of eating and drinking

Independence in eating and drinking obviously is associated with the individual's stage on the lifespan. There is the obvious dependence of the young and the potential dependence of the elderly. At any stage of the lifespan, persons previously independent for this AL can become dependent, temporarily or permanently, from either physical or psychological disability. Behaviourally disturbed people may not be able to leave home and go shopping for food; or decision-making may be difficult and so on. There are others who may have a hand or arm defect or who have diminished sight yet can still be independent for eating and drinking, provided they have the use of mechanical aids as recommended by the occupational therapist. These aids may be in the kitchen for preparing food, or used when cooking and eating food and allow the individual to retain the maximum self-esteem and dignity despite a physical disability. For a quite different reason people who have a learning disability will often have eating and drinking problems and the importance of good positioning with a suitable size of chair and table, in a relaxed atmosphere, are basic to progressive independence.

Some hospitals have equipped a special unit organized by occupational therapists. Here they assess patients who are experiencing problems related to the AL of eating and drinking, including cooking and kitchen skills. Occupational therapists may also visit the patient's home prior to discharge, to advise on possible adaptations so that the increased independence learned in the unit can be maintained or even improved after discharge from hospital.

And some local health authorities provide a demonstration unit with an occupational therapist in charge. It can be visited, not only by those in need of advice and equipment, but also by other professionals, and indeed any 'non-professional carers', so that people in need of help can achieve their optimal independence in the AL of eating and drinking.

Factors influencing the AL of eating and drinking

Eating and drinking play a significant part in the everyday living pattern of all age groups and for most people they are pleasurable activities. However, there are many factors which can influence this AL and affect the individual's reaction to food and drink. The various factors are described, using the categories which appear in the model under the headings of biological, psychological, sociocultural, environmental and politicoeconomic factors.

BIOLOGICAL

The human body is a highly complex collection of millions of cells. The cycle of each cell's growth and development as well as the constant cell activity requires an energy source, and the source of all energy used by the body is obtained from eating and drinking. At subsistence level, human beings will eat almost any available food, often in its raw state, in order to meet the basic need for sustenance.

Human milk of course is the natural food for infants, and the sucking reflex is present at birth. As the baby grows, milk on its own does not supply enough nutrients to satisfy appetite so semisolid and solid foods are introduced to the diet; and the child becomes proficient in chewing as the teeth appear. The sense of taste is developed too: milk is somewhat bland in flavour and as solids are added, the child learns to experiment with a variety of tastes.

In our model, the biological factors related to the AL of eating and drinking are the ones required for three functions — ingestion, digestion and absorption; namely the mouth, oropharynx, oesophagus, stomach and small intestine, together with the salivary glands, pancreas, liver and gallbladder which provide juices and enzymes to facilitate these three functions. For the purpose of the model, in human biology terms, the upper alimentary tract and the accessory organs of digestion are juxtaposed with the AL of eating and drinking. The purpose of this juxtaposition is to help students to integrate their increasing knowledge of biology into our AL framework for application in clinical practice.

To provide understanding of the problems faced by people who have feeding difficulties, the body structure and function required for swallowing are described in Box 7.2.

Body size is a visible physical dimension resulting from eating and drinking, and height and weight are measurable physical aspects. Also included in the concept of biological factors influencing this AL are the basic constituents of food. The study of food and the associated biological processes of growth, maintenance and repair are known as the science of nutrition and a brief outline of this subject follows.

Nutrition

From every country in the world comes an enormous variety of foodstuffs and they are classified first as macronutrients and micronutrients. The macronutrients are the energy providers and, according to the Department of Health, COMA Report (1991) consist of:

- protein
- carbohydrates
  — starches
  — sugars
- fats
- alcohol.

Inclusion of alcohol acknowledges a changed style of living in the 1990s.

The micronutrients include the vitamins and minerals which do not provide energy, but may release energy from the other food groups. To function effectively each cell in the body requires these substances, and to maintain health and efficiency the individual must have a balanced daily intake of all these constituents. Carbohydrates, proteins and fats are oxidized in the body to provide it with energy and the amount of energy produced by these different nutrients can be measured in the laboratory for research purposes, or to assist medical diagnosis, for example thyrotoxicosis which causes a raised basal metabolic rate.

In many countries, it is assessed in heat units called Calories — weight-watchers frequently maintain that they are 'watching their Calories'. Since 1975 however, the United Kingdom has adopted the kilojoule (kJ), and SI (Système International) unit for dietetic calculations. The kilojoule requirement for an individual varies with height, weight, age, gender, climate and occupation. In other words, each individual has a particular daily kilojoule requirement which naturally changes along the different stages of the lifespan. Consequently the 1991 COMA Report gives a range (dietary reference values),

---

Box 7.2 Swallowing

It is customary to describe swallowing in three stages:

- **Preparatory stage** The preparatory stage includes appreciation of what, for that person, is a 'manageable mouthful' on a fork or spoon; then tracing the visuospatial pathway without spillage from vessel to mouth, so that food is brought to the mouth at an appropriately sequenced time interval. As the food arrives, the lips part, the mouth opens and food is deposited on the tongue, the lips close around the cutlery helping to remove the food from it; the fork or spoon is then withdrawn and the lip seal completed. The concept of biological factors has therefore to widen to include at least one functioning upper limb, or some other way of conveying food from a plate to the mouth, and this may mean the assistance of another person.

- **Voluntary/pre-swallow/oral stage** The next stage is variously called the voluntary, pre-swallow or oral stage. It starts when the lip seal is formed around the food. Although the tongue is the sensory organ for taste, texture and temperature; it is also the motor organ for moving food in the mouth, to enable biting, chewing and grinding by the teeth on the preferred side. Correct apposition of teeth in the upper and lower jaws is necessary to accomplish this and the service of an orthodontist may be necessary to facilitate this. Correct apposition is equally important when fitting dentures. Saliva and mucus both help to soften the food and bind it into a bolus, which is rolled to the back of the tongue which is the lowest part of the ring of swallow receptors, the ring being completed by the pillars of the fauces at the sides, and the soft palate at the top.

- **Involuntary/swallow/pharyngeal stage** The final stage of swallowing is involuntary; called the swallow or pharyngeal stage. Stimulation of the sensory ring is the beginning of a complicated reflex action; the soft palate moves upwards and backwards to prevent food rising into the nasopharynx with possible nasal regurgitation. The tongue rises to occlude food returning to the mouth which may cause dribbling or drooling. The glottis closes and the epiglottal folds close over the entrance to the larynx to prevent aspiration of food into the respiratory tract. Further assistance in this is provided by momentary cessation of breathing as the oropharyngeal constrictor muscles push the food into the oesophagus, along which it travels by peristalsis to the stomach and small intestine for subsequent digestion and absorption.

rather than the previous specific quantity which was called 'recommended daily amount'. This affirms the fact that assessing and planning a person's diet must be an 'individualized' activity.

Vitamins, mineral salts, dietary fibre and water are essential to health, but do not provide kilojoules of energy.

Carbohydrates The starches and sugars are composed of carbon, hydrogen and oxygen and are found in foods such as sugar, potatoes, cereals, fruit and vegetables. Before they can be used by the body they must be reduced to glucose.

1 gram of carbohydrate yields 16 kJ (roughly 4 C).

Carbohydrates provide heat and energy and can be stored in the liver as glucogen but when eaten in excess are incorporated into the fat depots of the body as adipose tissue.

Proteins The body relies on proteins for its supply of nitrogen, but they also contain carbon, hydrogen, oxygen, sulphur and phosphorous; they are broken down to amino acids prior to absorption. Protein foods are, for example, meat, fish, eggs, milk products, soya beans, peas, beans and lentils.

1 gram of protein yields 17 kJ (roughly 4 C).

These foods supply the essential amino acids for building and repairing body tissue. For this reason, children require a higher proportion of protein foods than adults, and people who have been ill may be prescribed a high-protein diet to replace damaged tissue and to replace weight loss.

Fats Carbon, hydrogen and oxygen are present in fats but in different proportions to carbohydrates and before they can be absorbed they must be broken down to fatty acids and glycerol. The terms 'animal fats' and 'vegetable fats' have been superseded by 'saturated fats' and 'polyunsaturated fats' respectively. The latter terms not only designate content, but they are less restrictive regarding source; for example, some saturated fats are of vegetable origin — coconut and palm oil; and some polyunsaturated fats found in fowl and fish are obviously of animal origin. A decreased fat intake was recommended in the first COMA report. Over the last decade nutritionists, health educationists as well as nurses working in many different clinical areas have helped to disseminate this information. Yet several surveys published in the 1990s found that many of the population were still eating a diet which was not conducive to health.

However the debate continues as to whether or not a low fat intake prevents coronary heart disease. The second COMA report (Department of Health, 1991) states that scientists have extensively researched the number and structure of dietary fatty substances, as well as their metabolism and role within the human body. Words like low and high density lipoproteins have filtered into the medical vocabulary because of their involvement in cholesterol metabolism.

1 gram of fat yields 37 kJ (roughly 9 C).

In the body, fatty deposits are found around delicate organs like the eye or kidney to protect and maintain their position, and fats also have an important function in transporting fat-soluble vitamins, but the general functions of fatty foods, as with carbohydrates, is to provide heat and energy.

Vitamins Good health is dependent on vitamins and most cannot be manufactured in the body so they must be obtained from food. Vitamins are chemical compounds which are classified into two main groups:

- fat-soluble vitamins: A D E K
- water-soluble vitamins: B C P.

Vitamins are required in only small amounts. In many instances their function is catalytic, as components of enzyme systems involved in essential metabolic reactions. Although not supplying energy to the body, some are needed for the regulation of energy; and some are needed for the regulation of tissue synthesis. They are required therefore for the general health of tissues and gross deficiency can lead to specific disease conditions for example rickets (lack of vitamin D); scurvy (lack of vitamin C); beri-beri and pellagra (lack of vitamin B). Vitamins are found in many foods; the fat-soluble are mostly in dairy products, fat meat and fish oils; and the water-soluble in fresh fruit and vegetables, nuts and the germ of cereals.

Antioxidants Vitamins A, C and E are 'anti-oxidants' and are currently thought to reduce the risk of coronary heart disease and some cancers, although their role in this reduction is imperfectly understood (Hunt, 1992).

Trace elements Although required only in small quantities, these inorganic elements have many essential roles. They are components of body tissues and fluids, and of many specialized substances such as hormones, transport molecules and enzymes. For example, calcium and phosphorus are required for teeth and bone production; iron is required for red blood corpuscles; iodine is needed for the hormone secreted by the thyroid, an endocrine gland; sodium is important in the maintenance of the fluid volume in the body.

Sodium is an example of an electrolyte and the balance of the various electrolytes in the body is of critical importance. An electrolyte is formed when an inorganic compound such as salt (sodium chloride) is dissolved in water and dissociates into two or more electrically charged particles. For example, in the body, sodium chloride (NaCl is the chemical symbol) is present in solution as sodium (Na^+) and chlorine (Cl^-). The desired range of the different electrolytes in the cell fluid and in the extracellular fluid is known. When, because of disease or loss of fluid from the body this electrolyte balance is upset, the function of body cells may be grossly impaired. Mineral salts are widely dispersed in foods, including meat, fish, dairy products, and vegetables.

Dietary fibre   The cellulose part of food which passes through the digestive tract and is excreted as part of the faeces is called dietary fibre. It does not at any time become part of the body structure but its bulk helps to stimulate muscular movement in the large intestine and promotes defaecation thus preventing constipation (Bennett, 1988). There is also evidence that the breaking down of fibre by colonic bacteria makes the stool more acid and this is one of the reasons why fibre is believed to reduce the amount of possible carcinogens (Burkitt, 1983).

Water   The chemical symbol H_2O represents water and signifies that each molecule is composed of two parts hydrogen to one part oxygen. Water is essential to life and makes up about two-thirds of the body weight. Death will follow if there is water deprivation for more than a few days as many body processes are dependent on its presence: water is the main constituent of all body fluids; many physiochemical changes take place in the environment of the body fluids; most nutrients and cellular waste products are soluble in water.

A review of a variety of physiology texts revealed a range of 'normal' daily intakes from 2500 to 1000 ml with a mean of 1500 ml (Burns, 1992). If the intake is inadequate or if the loss of water is excessive most people will experience the sensation of thirst.

Normally, provided that an adequate well balanced diet is available, food and fluid intake is controlled by complex biochemical processes. There are centres in the brain which are sensitive to changes in the levels of nutrients and trace elements in the blood thereby controlling appetite and thirst.

A National Food Guide called The Balance of Good Health has been prepared by the Health Education Authority (1994). It is colourful and attractive and uses the food groups with which the majority of people are familiar. It is illustrated in Figure 7.2.

PSYCHOLOGICAL

Most people are aware that 'eating' and 'drinking' have a psychological dimension. They experience pleasure on seeing food arranged attractively; displeasure when what should be a hot course, is almost cold when it arrives; and loss of appetite when they are worried. But few people realise the wide implications of level of intelligence for the AL of eating and drinking.

Level of intelligence

A minimal level of intelligence is necessary to master the skills used in the process of eating and drinking. This is apparent when observing a young child as he experiments intellectually as well as physically with the development of mealtime skills, and likewise it is apparent when observing children whose intellectual development

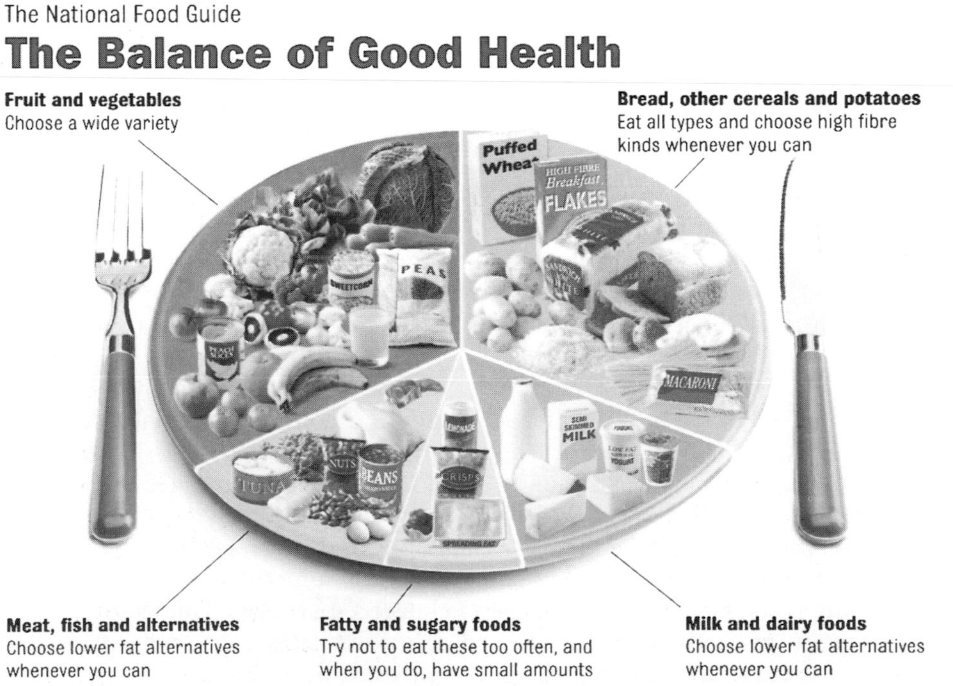

The National Food Guide
The Balance of Good Health

Fruit and vegetables
Choose a wide variety

Bread, other cereals and potatoes
Eat all types and choose high fibre kinds whenever you can

Meat, fish and alternatives
Choose lower fat alternatives whenever you can

Fatty and sugary foods
Try not to eat these too often, and when you do, have small amounts

Milk and dairy foods
Choose lower fat alternatives whenever you can

Fig. 7.2 The National Food Guide: The Balance of Good Health. (Reproduced with kind permission from the Health Education Authority.)

is impaired; they often have great difficulty in acquiring eating and drinking skills.

A certain intellectual level is also required for the acquisition and application of the knowledge needed to select and prepare a diet which will maintain health, and a great deal of time and effort are expended by the government, the health professions and the media in health education to interest the general public in desirable eating practices. The acquisition of knowledge is required also to apply appropriate hygiene practices when handling food; and to dispose of food waste in such a manner that it will not attract vermin and flies which have the potential to harbour and spread pathogenic microorganisms to humans.

Emotional state: undereating

The individual's emotional state may sometimes affect food intake. The child's excitement prior to a holiday, the anxiety associated with examinations, the stress of a change of job may well reduce the accustomed intake for that individual. These however are usually transient. Loss of appetite or lack of desire for food over a prolonged period can be indicative of a more serious disturbance in emotional states.

Anorexia nervosa Appetite disturbance over a prolonged period is called anorexia nervosa. It has a peak incidence in adolescence especially among young women, although the number of men is increasing. In the UK, one per cent, that is 10 000 secondary schoolgirls suffer from anorexia (Lyall, 1991). Despite evidence to the contrary, the individual views herself as fat (distorted body image) and will refuse to eat or will deliberately vomit following food intake. Anorexia nervosa is usually considered to be a disturbance in personality development, often in the relationship with one parent. However, research has shown that when people with a 'normal' appetite are starved, the higher mental functions are impaired; there is selfishness, withdrawal from social activities and a decreased interest in sex, together with increasing self-centredness and rigid thinking, so that compromise cannot be considered. All these manifestations have been seen in people with anorexia nervosa (Fretwell, 1991; Kenny, 1991).

Emotional state: overeating

Most people, at particular times in their lives indulge in overeating. Such events are of a periodic nature and are usually associated with some sort of special social occasion.

Obesity In contradistinction some people use food as a source of comfort and security. Overeating in the majority of people leads to obesity (p. 183), and those who are comfortable with their body image will not be motivated to lose weight. However the doctor may advise a reduction in weight, for example, if surgery becomes necessary, or if arthritis develops in the joints of the lower limbs.

Bulimia nervosa Compulsive overeating means that the person no longer has control over what is eaten although aware of the enormous quantity being eaten. There is usually a morbid fear of becoming fat, but this is avoided by self-induced vomiting or laxative abuse or both. 'Binge eating' has long been recognized as a feature in some people with anorexia nervosa or obesity. It is only in more recent years that it has been identified in people who are not suffering from either of these psychological problems influencing eating, and it is called bulimia nervosa (Jones and Stone, 1992). A Nursing Development (nurse-led) Unit is functioning to help people overcome eating disorders such as anorexia and bulimia (McMillan, 1994).

Alcohol dependence/abuse

Currently alcohol dependence/abuse is a major problem in many countries of the world. Usually the onset of dependence on alcohol is insidious, starting with social drinking but when out of control, the habit can lead to irresponsible behaviour, petty crime or even assault, and bring distress not only to the individual but to family and friends. It is discussed in more detail on p. 183.

SOCIOCULTURAL

Providing nutrients is the biological reason for eating and drinking, but they also serve several other purposes in everyday living. During family mealtimes, for example, eating plays an important part in learning about the culture. The meal provides an opportunity for the young child to learn about the rituals of serving food, about the vessels from which different foods are eaten, and about the utensils used for certain items in the diet.

As children explore relationships with people both within and outside the family circle, they began to appreciate that food can have considerable social significance concerned with interpersonal relationships. In almost all cultures, eating and drinking are considered social occasions and offering a meal to visitors is one overt way of expressing friendship and hospitality. Eating and drinking in most societies are also an integral part of such diverse family ceremonies as birth, marriage and death; and of some national holiday festivities and religious festivals.

In certain cultures it is customary to take meals in the home in a special room set aside for the purpose but there are many variations, and it may be accepted practice to eat under a tree, round a camp fire or in a tent. Not only the setting but the style of eating may vary considerably.

Some societies make use of fingers, others use chopsticks, and yet others use knives, forks and spoons; some eat food from a communal bowl, others from individual plates or bowls; some sit cross-legged on the floor, others customarily use a chair.

In a few cultures there may even be segregation of the sexes at mealtimes with adult males eating together but separately from adult females eating together. More commonly, however, the meal is an occasion when all members of the family are sharing news about the day's activities although in some industrialized countries, the increasing use of 'fast' foods and the consuming dominance of TV-viewing are altering the pattern of mealtime socializing.

Certain religious groups have definite rules about the choice and preparation of specific items on the menu. For example orthodox Jews must prepare and serve dairy products and meat dishes separately, while the Koran forbids Muslims to touch pork and alcohol, and the devout Hindu will not eat animal products. There are however other groups who, not for religious reasons, are vegetarians and will not eat animal products.

With the interaction of these many variables, and remembering the interaction of the other four groups of factors influencing the AL of eating and drinking, it is not surprising that each person develops deep-rooted beliefs and attitudes as well as an individual pattern related to this AL.

Even in the same family, there are individual differences related to food and drink; there may be large appetites and some small, some may be quick eaters, some may be slow. Even at a young age, each individual is consciously aware of this essential AL of eating and drinking; indeed throughout life, the waking day is punctuated by meals — breakfast, lunch, supper or some variation of these words — and many other Activities of Living are arranged around them.

ENVIRONMENTAL

Physical environmental factors can affect the choice of food. Obviously geographical position, soil fertility, climate and rainfall will determine the type of food which can be grown locally, and will also influence the meat, fish and poultry content of the diet. Nowadays, for industrial nations with their extensive import/export networks, reliance on local food is not such a dominant feature of everyday living but it is crucial for about two-thirds of the world who are dependent on local produce.

Availability of fuel is also a consideration. Although certain groups such as Eskimos eat raw fish and seal, it is customary in most countries to improve the palatability of food by cooking many of the vegetables and fruit fibres, and the flesh of fish, fowl and animals. Also some

form of fuel is needed for preservation of food for example in bottling, canning or deep freezing, and making storage possible.

However, careful planning for storage of new food, whether scarce or abundant, may be negated if the environment is plagued by vectors such as cockroaches, flies, mice and rats. Not only can they deplete the supply; they may 'spoil' food by contamination with excreta and make it unfit for human consumption, or they may even transfer pathogens which can lead to food poisoning.

Food is imperative for human existence but an adequate supply of water is even more important. Three-quarters of the world's surface is water but getting an adequate supply of fresh, clean water which is safe to use for drinking and cooking is one of the world's pressing problems. Most of the world's water is salt and in the oceans; only 3% is fresh and only a small amount of that is accessible as a public water supply. Many of the world's women and children have to walk miles to draw water from a stream or well which may be inadequate for all the Activities of Living; when a safe supply is available on tap, water is so much taken for granted. Accessibility and distribution of food and water in the local environment certainly contributes to the ease of eating and drinking.

In a slightly different sense, the environment is obviously taken into account by restaurateurs who consider that the ambience of the environment can contribute to food and drink enjoyment. Noise, hustle and bustle are not thought to be good for digestion and many hoteliers give considerable thought to the provision of carpeting, lowered lights and soft background music as an environmental aid to both the physiological and psychological enjoyment of eating and drinking.

POLITICOECONOMIC

Any consideration of eating and drinking presupposes that food and drink are available. This is not always the case, indeed, about half of the world's population is hungry. In certain areas even now, hundreds of people die every day due to starvation, and many thousands of others are undernourished because they have insufficient food to eat. There are many complex reasons for this maldistribution of food throughout the world, such as infertile soil, inferior seed, inadequate crop rotation, overgrazing, soil erosion, lack of irrigation, lack of knowledge and lack of finance, all of which contribute to a poor yield. Some parts of the world, too, are more liable to suffer from natural disasters such as drought, floods or pestilence which result in crop failure or even large-scale famine. When this occurs, scarcity creates an increase in the price of food which often takes it beyond the financial reach of lower income groups so the people are undernourished or may in fact 'starve to death'. Considerable attempts have been made at national and international levels to redress these gross inequalities but still the problem remains, much of it due to economic and political constraints highlighted in the Brandt Report as long ago as 1980.

Preventing protein-calorie malnutrition

Protein is the most expensive food nutrient to process and protein-calorie malnutrition is a widespread and serious problem especially in the first years of life. Very young children are highly susceptible to lack of adequate nutrients, and in developing countries babies who have initially been breast-fed may suffer severe nutritional deficiencies, especially of protein, when they are weaned. One of the gross manifestations of protein deficiency in young children is kwashiorkor.

The WHO (World Health Organization) collaborates with the FAO (Food and Agricultural Organization) and UNICEF (United Nations Children's Fund) in the Protein-Calorie Advisory Group set up by the UN and it is paying particular attention to the development of low-cost, protein-rich weaning foods suitable for local production in developing countries. Enhancing self-help is a much more enduring policy than encouraging import of foreign-produced foodstuffs to an undernourished or malnourished nation.

Helping people in the poverty/health trap

The reasons are legion for many people having to exist on a minimal income even in those countries where there is governmental financial assistance. It is estimated that over eight million people in England and Wales are on income support. Various cities are providing initiatives whereby these people can purchase 'healthy' food at a price they can afford at such places as 'food co-operatives' (George, 1993).

Elderly people

To help to prevent malnutrition in the older person, some countries have instituted a 'meals-on-wheels' service. At a small cost or free of charge in cases of financial hardship, a cooked meal is delivered in the middle of the day to the home of those who, because of physical disability or frailty, are unable to go shopping for food or are disinclined to cook for themselves. For those elderly people who are still ambulant, voluntarily organized local luncheon clubs are becoming popular. They provide a cooked nutritious meal and have the advantage of being a social event.

Food hygiene

There is no point in exhorting the nation to eat a healthy diet if the food and water provided are not free from the potential of causing illness in the consumers. Most countries have government Food Laws about the standard of hygiene to be maintained in, for example food retail outlets and restaurants, and the food additives and colourings that may be used, and the pesticides to be used for spraying crops. Because of the tremendous advances in food technology in the last few decades, many of these laws are now inadequate, and the UK government is having to respond to public pressure about the increasing incidence of illness arising from microbial contamination of food. From one decade to another, the pathogens present in food are not necessarily the same ones, and this applies to the foods transmitting the pathogens.

It is recommended that after purchase, many foods should be put in the fridge or freezer as soon as possible. Domestic refrigeration of precooked foods should be at 2°C and such foods should be heated to 70°C before eating; any food left over should not be reheated.

Irradiation of food

It is claimed that irradiation of food would remove *all* pathogens thereby rendering food safe to eat and drink. But would it also kill the microorganisms, multiplication of which warns that food is no longer fit for consumption? There are still members of the public who have reservations about this food technology. However, if further research answers many of the queries, and the public gain confidence in it, it may well be that the government in the future will change the Food Laws in order to provide the safest possible food and drink. These are examples of the necessity for nurses to continually update their knowledge.

Alcohol

The drinking of alcohol can be influenced by several politicoeconomic factors. For example there are usually laws about where and under what circumstances alcohol can be sold. In some countries it can only be sold from government controlled premises, and from licensed social institutions such as public bars, restaurants and hotels. In others, it is more readily available, for instance in superstores, along with groceries and other household commodities. This means that drinking alcohol is not confined to the hours set by some governments for drinking in licensed premises. There may be a minimum age at which people can buy alcohol, or drink it in a licensed place, and there is usually imposition of a fine for selling alcohol to under-age drinkers. Also there is usually a maximum permitted level of alcohol in the blood when driving a vehicle.

Individualizing nursing for the AL of eating and drinking

Individuality is the base from which individualized nursing is developed. From the preceding discussion it is evident that there are many dimensions of the other components of the model which contribute to the development of individuality in the AL of eating and drinking. Box 7.3 contains the main points in the discussion, and it can be used during the initial assessment as an aide memoire.

ASSESSING THE INDIVIDUAL IN THE AL

'Assessing' this AL is not the prerogative of nurses and other health workers. For example, many mothers can give details about the kind and quantity of food taken by each of their children. They assess the outcome of their children attending to this AL by noting when the child has outgrown various garments.

The nursing literature is emphasizing that nutritional assessments should be carried out by nurses working at primary level. According to the King's Fund Report (Lennard-Jones, 1992) 50% of surgical and 44% of medical patients are malnourished on admission to hospital. People on a waiting list for admission could therefore be helped by primary level staff to avoid this. A pre-admission dietary diary could alert nurses to the potential need for discreet health education (Mairis, 1992).

Assessing involves observing the person; acquiring information about eating and drinking habits by asking appropriate questions, and by listening to the comments and questions raised by the person and family; and using relevant material from available records such as medical ones. The nurse would be seeking answers to the following questions:

- how often does the individual usually eat and drink?
- what does the individual usually eat and drink?

Box 7.3 Assessing the individual in the AL of eating and drinking

Lifespan: effect on eating and drinking
- Nutrition in utero
- Breast/bottle-feeding and weaning in infancy
- Increasing skills in eating and drinking during childhood
- Prudent diet during adolescence and adulthood
- Reduced appetite/potential nutritional deficiency in old age

Dependence/independence in eating and drinking
- Special utensils
- Mechanical aids
- Kitchen gadgets
- Special transport for shopping

Factors influencing eating and drinking
- Biological
  - state of mouth and teeth
  - swallowing
  - intact digestive system
  - nutrition
  - physical proficiency in shopping for/preparing food
  - physical proficiency in taking food and drink
  - appetite/thirst regulation
- Psychological
  - intellectual capacity to procure and prepare food and drink
  - knowledge about diet and health
  - weight control
  - distorted body image
  - alcohol dependence/abuse
  - food hygiene
  - disposal of food waste
  - attitude to eating and drinking
  - emotional status
  - likes and dislikes
- Sociocultural
  - family traditions
  - cultural idiocyncrasies
  - religious commendations/ restrictions
- Environmental
  - climate and geographical position
  - facilities for procuring/growing food
  - distance from home to shopping area
  - availability of transport
  - means of cooking
  - means of storage
  - vectors and food spoilage
- Politicoeconomic
  - malnutrition/finance
  - choice of food and drink
  - quantity and quality of food and drink
  - published national reports about healthy diet
  - safe food

- when does the individual eat and drink?
- where does the individual eat and drink?
- what factors influence the way the individual carries out the AL of eating and drinking?
- has the individual any long-standing difficulties with eating and drinking and how have these been coped with?
- what problems, if any, does the individual have at present with eating and drinking and are any likely to develop?

Of course the nurse does not necessarily ask these actual questions because much of the information can be acquired in the course of conversation with the person and by observation. For example, if there has been recent weight loss, the clothes may hang loosely, or if the change has been weight gain the clothes will probably be tight.

Dietitians and nurse specialists in nutrition have published their suggestions about what is important to assess (Wallace, 1993; Mairis, 1992; Charalambous, 1993). Height and weight are the two obvious objective measurements. However, machines may not weigh accurately as Harrison (1991) discovered. It is therefore important to write down which scales were used, to maximize efficiency of ongoing evaluation. There are two non-invasive assessment/evaluating tools which nurses are being encouraged to use. Fat is stored in subcutaneous tissue and it can be metabolized in periods of deficient intake of nutrients; evidence of this happening can be provided by grasping a portion of skin with calibrated calipers. The body does not have a protein store, but protein is a structural part of muscle tissue and evidence of it being used for metabolism is provided by measuring the circumference of the upper arm.

The outcome of the initial assessment is identification of any actual problems which the person is experiencing with the AL of eating and drinking. And indeed, potential problems may be recognized.

In the early days when a person is experiencing difficulty in swallowing (dysphagia), whether being cared for at home, or in hospital, the speech therapist will carry out a 'swallowing assessment' and prescribe the texture of food and fluid which can be swallowed safely, thus avoiding the potential problem of aspiration pneumonia (Oliver, 1994).

But there may not be any problems! Nevertheless it is important to 'assess' this AL because the information about the person's individuality in eating and drinking will be useful to nurses on each succeeding shift.

IDENTIFYING ACTUAL AND POTENTIAL PROBLEMS

However before nurses can begin to think in terms of individualized nursing, they require a general idea of the sort of problems which people can experience in relation

to our concept of the AL of eating and drinking. For example, the domestic activities re buying, washing, storing, cooking and serving food may become progressively problematic because of increasingly painful and deformed hands.

There follows a general discussion of the types of patients' problems related to eating and drinking. They are grouped under headings which indicate how they can arise:

- Change of dependence/independence status
- Change in eating and drinking habit
- Change in mode of eating and drinking
- Change of environment and routine.

CHANGE OF DEPENDENCE/INDEPENDENCE STATUS

The ability to help oneself to food and drink is usually taken so much for granted until circumstances occur which interfere with this activity of living and result in problems of dependence, either temporarily or permanently.

For a variety of reasons people may require assistance with the actual activity of eating and drinking, and this should be given graciously and with dexterity so that they will be protected from needless embarrassment resulting from their lack of independence in this AL.

People can, in a general sense, be dependent for help, often from a multidisciplinary team, for keeping their bodies as well nourished as possible under the circumstances. Examples are people with cancer (Holmes, 1991a), people who are terminally ill (Williams, 1990), and people who are resident in an institution for those with learning disabilities; but as Sines (1992) writes, such people are 'characterized by a combination of physical, emotional, psychological, sensory and intellectual disabilities'.

However, beginning students can be helped to acquire knowledge in this complex area by thinking of these different kinds of dependencies separately.

Problems associated with physical dependence

Posture Even something apparently simple such as a change of physical posture may create ingestion and swallowing problems, for example when people are forced to lie flat when eating. The distress, difficulty and even indignity suffered in such circumstances should be appreciated by nurses and dealt with sensitively.

Such people may have to be fed by a nurse, and it is almost impossible for them to feel relaxed if the nurse is standing over them. Nurses should therefore be seated when feeding patients. Obviously food on the plate will have been prepared so that it can be lifted to the mouth by one piece of cutlery, a fork or spoon, whichever the person prefers. The question arises, should the nurse sit at one side, facing the same way as the patient, so that the nurse's hand can mimic the movement of the patient's preferred hand when lifting food from plate to mouth? Or should the nurse sit facing the patient? Perhaps patients can be asked about their preference which should be written on the nursing plan, so that nurses on each shift offer the same sort of help. Greenhorn (1992) offers some advice from his experience of having to be fed.

Liquids may be interspersed throughout the meal or offered at the end according to the person's wishes. Liquids can be given from a spouted feeding cup, but a drinking straw usually allows better control of the flow and nowadays, angled straws made from materials which can withstand warm fluids make mealtimes less difficult for people who require help with feeding.

Oral hygiene is often required before and after the meal and it is a cardinal rule that, unless contraindicated (for example when a patient is unconscious, or is on restricted fluids) anyone who needs special oral hygiene, needs also to be helped to take oral fluids in order to keep the mouth tissues in a healthy, comfortable state.

Physical disability The majority of people who become physically disabled live at home. When assessing their dependence/independence status for eating and drinking one has to start with the early preparations. Can they go shopping for food? Can they prepare food in the kitchen? Can they cook it? If they cannot be helped to go shopping themselves, usually the social services can make arrangements for their shopping to be done by another person. In the UK there are some centres where gadgets which can help with preparing and cooking food are displayed and demonstrated, together with advice from an occupational therapist.

There are several devices available for 'stabilizing' food or containers, which is the key problem for a one-handed person, for example vegetables can be mobilized on a spiked board to accomplish peeling and chopping. There are 'tip-up' stands to enable pouring from teapots and kettles, as well as non-spill cups, plate guards, unbreakable crockery and several types of modified cutlery.

In hospital the occupational therapist can often make useful suggestions which will help the person to retain independence and dignity at mealtimes. Spilling of food and soiling of clothes are distasteful to most people, especially when eating in the company of others who are not at a physical disadvantage.

However, there are some people whose physical disability precludes them from achieving independence and they remain dependent for feeding throughout the lifespan. Non-progressive brain damage (usually at birth) can result in spasticity of muscles, and/or inability to control muscular movement so that the limbs, and perhaps the head and neck, are never still; there is continuous purposeless movement.

Speech therapists have highlighted the complexities of feeding such people, and Anderson (1991) wrote a book, *Feeding — a guide to assessment and intervention with handicapped children*, to help parents and professionals working with children who have profound learning difficulties, including learning to eat and drink. Though described in clear language there is no doubt about the complexity of eating and drinking. Such disabled people may be admitted to a general hospital for a reason other than the disability. If the usual 'feeder' cannot attend all mealtimes, nurses should observe the technique so that they can provide 'continuity of feeding' when necessary.

Respiratory distress Many breathless people live in the community and may indeed manage to go to work. They and their family where appropriate need information to help them cope, so that the person remains well nourished. Unnecessary effort in chewing has to be avoided, so meat can be flaked and served to look like meat on the plate. It is tempting to puree all food, but the result can be visually displeasing and devastating to the appetite. Dry foods such as biscuits are to be avoided or accompanied with fluid to moisten them. It may be helpful if smaller meals can be arranged more frequently, especially when the breathless person eventually becomes housebound. Naturally eating takes longer and nurses can help to forestall family tension by explaining this.

Impaired vision Occasionally blind people are admitted to hospital and they are usually able to tell the nurse what sort of help they need to minimize increasing their dependence. For a variety of reasons other people may have both eyes bandaged for a shorter or longer time, and certainly become dependent for feeding. In these circumstances the food should be cut into mouth-size pieces and the type of food described when served.

Problems associated with emotional/psychological dependence

Stress At some time or other in their lives, most people have experienced emotional stress and one of the manifestations of anxiety can be loss of appetite. The stress and the accompanying upset of the AL of eating and drinking are usually transient. When a person persistently refuses food and fluid, however, skill, tact and perseverence are required by the nurse to discover the motive. Disruption of eating and drinking activities may be due to neurotic or psychotic disorders.

Psychiatric illness Many depressed people are too apathetic and listless to eat. They are not hungry, have no desire for food, and do not want to be bothered with eating and drinking activities. In some instances, they may be merely passive and uninterested and may respond to spoon-feeding, when it is relatively easy to ensure an adequate food and fluid intake. On the other hand, people in a manic phase of a depressive illness are often much too active to eat. Frequently attempts to persuade them to remain at a set table for a meal are only marginally successful, and a sandwich in the hand may be a more effective way of introducing nourishment.

People who are medically diagnosed as suffering from dementia exhibit a wide range of unusual behaviour. They cannot remember the time at which they last had a meal, or what has been eaten in the 24 h. Watson (1990) gives some suggestions for feeding people who are demented.

Some disturbed people, however, refuse to eat. They suffer from delusions and although they seem bizarre the delusions are very real to such people — they have no money to pay for food; they are unworthy; their 'bowels are blocked'; the food has been poisoned; a voice is telling them not to eat. At every mealtime, therefore, they require persuasion to eat and having done so, may vomit in order to avert the awful consequences they think will ensue if they retain the food in their body.

Other problems with eating which have an emotional connotation may be exacerbated by advertisements in the media in Western countries which propagate the message that to be slim is to be attractive. But most people make dietary choices which (together with the exercise they take) enable them to feel reasonably comfortable with their psychological body image regarding its physical shape and size.

However, as mentioned on p. 177, for a minority of people, mainly young women (usually adolescents), their eating programme gets beyond their control, and they experience feelings such as shame, and guilt at their behaviour which can include undereating, overeating, self-induced vomiting achieved by drinking large amounts of water; over-use of laxatives, diuretics, and even self-administered enemas. Three names are given to the conditions which may include one or more of these behaviours:

- compulsive eating
- anorexia nervosa
- bulimia nervosa.

They are not mutually exclusive and people can have periods when any one of the three predominates.

Meades (1993) gives an account of the role of the community psychiatric nurse in helping people who are experiencing these conditions. And Waller (1991) discusses sexual abuse as a factor in such eating disorders.

Learning disability More and more attention is being paid to helping people who have a learning disability to acquire the functional skills required in everyday living (Richardson, 1993; Perry, 1992). As a rule pre-school places are not available for this group of children, so it is usually the parents and other siblings who need to be involved and supported in a behaviour development programme to achieve the actions necessary for independent eating and drinking. Achievement is a great boon for all concerned and will be one of the criteria used for admission to primary and then secondary school.

Alcohol abuse Alcohol has been mentioned in the context of psychological factors (p. 177) and politico-economic factors (p. 179). It is relevant to consider 'alcoholism' here, as not only is it associated with the AL of drinking, but it inevitably changes individuals' dependence/independence status. Factual information about the volume and frequency of alcohol intake required to produce the state of dependence is difficult to obtain, because only individual drinkers know this, and both volume and frequency may be minimized or maximized when giving information for a 'drinking history'.

Surveys in the last two decades have revealed that one in five adults admitted to a general hospital have a problem triggered by excessive alcohol consumption. But what is an acceptable and what is an excessive alcohol intake?

The health education experts have for years provided the information that an acceptable weekly intake is 21 units for men and 14 for women. A 'unit' is illustrated in Figure 7.3. The health educationists advise people to plan their drinking for the week ahead according to their social programme. Some people's lifestyle might accommodate three units for men, two for women on each of the seven days. A lifestyle which is not conducive to healthy drinking is one where the units are saved for two weekend parties.

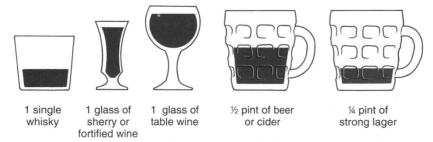

| 1 single whisky | 1 glass of sherry or fortified wine | 1 glass of table wine | ½ pint of beer or cider | ¼ pint of strong lager |

Fig. 7.3 1 unit = 7.9 g of alcohol

Two other ways of measuring the outcome from excessive alcohol are cited by Cooper (1994); one is estimating the number of deaths which in 1988 was 28 000 in England and Wales; the other is counting the annual financial cost to the health service which in 1989 was £120 million.

In 'The Health of the Nation' nurses were recognized as being able to play a key role in identifying people who have alcohol related problems and in intervening therapeutically. In 1993, the Department of Health's publication encourages nurses to contribute to changing behaviour in relation to specific risk factors and identifies the active role nurses must play in improving awareness of the dangers of alcohol, often in conjunction with lifestyle assessments (Cooper, 1994; Campbell, 1995). However, a survey revealed that 'a major health education opportunity is being wasted because nurses know too little about alcohol-related problems' (Friend, 1992a): the survey referred to was carried out by Watson (1992) at the University of Strathclyde, Glasgow. Of 168 ward-based nurses, half did not know the safe limits for drinking alcohol.

Leslie and Learmonth (1994) offer information to overcome this. They report a service which evolved to increase the awareness of staff in a general hospital about alcohol intake and possible problems when this is excessive. As well as including a 'drinking history' as part of the initial assessment, staff are encouraged to explain a 'unit of alcohol' whereby one can assess safe drinking levels, and a 'drinking diary' whereby a weekly pattern of drinking can be traced. Midwives are also being encouraged to take a drinking history as part of the routine booking process (Plant, 1990).

Now that people with learning disabilities are being transferred from hospital to the community, some of them are risking becoming dependent on alcohol. They are drinking considerably more than the accepted safe level and training programmes are being devised and implemented in some areas (Lindsay & Allen, 1992).

Several research groups found that advising teenagers about alcohol abuse can be too late! They pooled their information and prepared an 'Alcohol information package' for children aged between eight and eleven years (Nursing Standard, 1994). The development of alcohol dependence is usually insidious. In some countries, wine drinking may be a normal part of mealtimes and in many societies, people can enjoy a drink socially without experiencing any compulsion to take more. Some people, however, come to be dependent on alcohol and this may manifest itself in behaviour which is atypical for that person such as disregard for personal appearance, unpunctuality, irritability or absence from work. Excessive drinking may also lead to irresponsible behaviour, petty crime, casual sexual activity which can be sexual abuse, and even disorderly behaviour amounting to assault, per-

haps involving police custody. All these deviations bring attendant distress to family and friends.

Sometimes the problem is less easy to detect because the person appears to function adequately in everyday activities yet needs to imbibe at increasingly frequent intervals during the day in order to cope with commitments. As might be expected, the affected individual begins to suffer from malnutrition because the appetite for food decreases; weight is then lost and health deteriorates. Eventually there are economic overtones as more and more money is spent on procuring alcohol to the detriment of the family budget, and work capacity may become impaired, often to the point of loss of employment.

In the UK, various voluntary associations work in conjunction with the National Council for Alcoholism. One is for ex-alcoholics and is called Alcoholics Anonymous (AA), a world-wide association. Members of local branches meet frequently to give each other moral support in the long and continuous process of refraining from drinking alcohol. Another is called the Al-Anon Family Group which is for the spouse, friends and relatives of the alcoholic person, and they help one another to cope with the many problems of alcoholism which impinge on family life and cause untold upset (A worker from Al-Anon, 1993). A newly formed group is SCAD — Support for Children of Adult Drinkers (Friend, 1992b).

There are physical discomforts which are problematic and can change a person's status on the dependence/ independence continuum for the AL of eating and drinking. Some of them will now be discussed.

Problems associated with physical discomforts

Sore mouth A sore mouth is always a potential problem in dehydrated patients and those with an insufficient flow of saliva; febrile and ill patients are at risk of developing an actual problem. A sore mouth can be an actual problem of which patients are all too aware. When one considers the many structures forming the mouth — the tongue, teeth, gums, inner cheeks, upper palate, tonsils and the salivary glands which pour their secretion into the mouth — one realizes that there has to be location of the 'soreness' before appropriate nurse-initiated intervention can be planned.

Causes A sore tongue for example can be due to something as straightforward as the sharp edge of a damaged natural tooth, or friction from dentures. The nurse-initiated intervention will be vigilant oral hygiene described on p. 244. Application of a local anaesthetic gel will produce temporary relief to facilitate eating and drinking, but an appointment with a dental member of the health team will be necessary. On the other hand, a sore tongue can result from insufficient intake or poor absorption of vitamins B and C and dietary iron, contributing to different types of anaemia. If investigations confirm these causes, there will be a medical prescription to remedy them.

'Toothache' is applied to several phenomena — the constant dull ache from dental caries, and the throbbing ache from a root abscess, as well as the jagging pain when an exposed nerve is in contact with hot or cold fluid or food. Obviously dental treatment is required for these conditions and a dental appointment has to be made for long stay patients. In an emergency, to provide relief, the usual household remedies can be used, for example the application of oil of cloves and use of a local anaesthetic gel to facilitate toothbrushing so that the healthy teeth are not compromised. Soft food can be offered when chewing triggers toothache, and food and fluids at body temperature will be appreciated when there is an exposed nerve.

Inflammation of the gums (gingivitis), the tongue (glossitis) and the whole mouth (stomatitis) can occur when the natural oral flora (non-pathogenic commensals) are compromised, that is the state of colonisation ends and infection begins. The subject is important because the change can be caused by treatments such as antibiotics, chemotherapy and radiotherapy: it can also be changed by a specific infection such as AIDS. For example, the fungus *Candida albicans*, a normal commensal in the mouth, can become pathogenic causing thrush.

Treatment Some patients have found Redoxon mouth washes refreshing, and half a Redoxon tablet left on the tongue effervesces and cleans, and helps the person to feel more comfortable. Gentian violet mouthwashes three times a day, for 4 days, may also be recommended. Or antifungal tablets may be medically prescribed to be retained in the mouth for as long as possible four times daily for at least 4 days. Part of the resultant nursing intervention is helping patients to understand the prescription and to resist resorting to chewing the tablets, as well as continuing the full course even if they think that the condition has been 'cured' after only 2 or 3 days.

Swallowing/dysphagia Knowledge about the complex activities related to swallowing (p. 174) is essential to facilitate understanding of the problems which can be experienced with this part of the AL of eating and drinking. Much of the recent knowledge about feeding patients has been contributed by speech and language therapists who realised that treatment for the motor and sensory neuromuscular dysfunctions involved in speech impediments, whether congenital, or acquired as a result of disease, were in fact related in many instances to swallowing.

Multidisciplinary approach With the increased multidisciplinary interest in people who have feeding and swallowing problems, 'Feeding aids resource centres' are being developed in various parts of the UK. In some areas a specialist 'feeding team' has been established comprising a nurse, dietition, occupational therapist, physiotherapist, speech therapist and sometimes a technical aids officer. The team carries out a full assessment and, in conjunction with nurses, plans suitable individual programmes so that people with these problems can achieve their optimal independence, according to their circumstances, to achieve the goal of optimal nourishment without loss of social or psychological dignity. It is important that nurses record the amount of food and fluid taken, as well as the rate of progress towards optimal independence.

Re-learning feeding mechanism After a stroke, many people have feeding and swallowing difficulties. Re-educating the feeding mechanism is a necessary nursing contribution which requires guidance from the dietitian and speech therapist (Cabell, 1990, includes a swallowing assessment; Beadle, Townsend & Palmer, 1995). Frequent practice at biting a Bikkipeg strengthens the relevant muscles. As does protruding the tongue, then moving it up, down, and from side to side; as well as making specific sounds for example the five vowels. A syringe may be used to place a small quantity of liquid in the inner lip, followed by a facilitated swallow: it is accomplished by placing a hand under the person's lower jaw, and raising it, thereby moving the tongue up and back in readiness for swallowing.

Re-learning swallowing Re-learning to swallow has been further helped by the development of a sensory stimulating loop which can be fitted to an upper denture if one is worn. If the patient has natural teeth, the loop is fitted to a dental plate. Nurses can also contribute more to the rehabilitation of people's post-stroke lip dysfunction by attending to 'food catches' on the lips during feeding, and the escape of food from the mouth. As each of these dysfunctions has social and psychological implications for the person, it is important for nurses to help with the re-learning of eating and drinking independently and with dignity.

A training programme which was originally developed by Heimlich was used to re-train swallowing in a 78-year-old man who in the previous 3 years had been fed by nasogastric tube (Axelsson et al, 1986).

Disabled people, whether it is a mental and/or physical disability, often have eating problems; these can be associated with hyposensitivity, hypersensitivity, sucking, biting, chewing, swallowing and drooling. When they have to be fed there is a potential problem of malnutrition (Sines, 1992). Anderson's book (1991), mentioned on p. 182 in the context of 'Problems associated with physical dependence', is equally applicable here in the context of 'Feeding and swallowing problems related to eating and drinking'.

Nausea This condition is easily recognized by the person experiencing it, but is difficult to describe. It occurs in waves, may be accompanied by excess salivation, pallor and sweating, and is often a precursor of vomiting. Almost always there is loss of appetite.

Causes Nausea may merely be a manifestation of over-indulgence in food and drink, but can also occur associated with anxiety states, post-anaesthesia, jaundice, dysfunction in the digestive tract, or the ingestion of drugs which irritate the lining of the digestive tract, or pain anywhere in the body. It may also be a symptom in the early months of pregnancy probably due to hormonal changes in the mother's body. It may also occur as an undesirable side-effect after administration of, for example, morphine or digoxin, in which case the drug may be stopped, or given in a reduced dose. Nausea can also be a reaction to cytotoxic drugs. Patients with cancer may be debilitated and the additional problem of nausea is very distressing.

Treatment To relieve nausea, acupressure is being used. One small project was carried out on 19 males undergoing elective urological surgery and the acupressure was applied to prevent postoperative nausea. The results were encouraging, but the project needs to be repeated (Rogers, 1990). A larger study of 80 females undergoing gynaecological operations gave similar encouraging results, but the report stated 'Further research should be undertaken to quantify the savings that could be effected if Sea-Bands were used routinely' (Phillips & Gill, 1993).

Nausea is distressing to the sufferer and the nurse should be comforting and supportive. Some people find it helpful to suck ice when feeling nauseated, others prefer a peppermint flavour, still others find it helpful to lie down in a quiet, well ventilated room. For some a modification of diet, avoiding the nausea-producing food or drink is all that is required. For others an anti-emetic drug may be medically prescribed to be given subcutaneously to relieve the discomfort until the cause is isolated and treated.

Some anti-emetic drugs are very expensive; they can be used prophylactically, for instance as a preoperative injection or as a patient-controlled administration adjuvant to cancer therapy. They can be combined with various 'complementary techniques' (Adams, 1993; Knapman, 1993; Pervan, 1993). It is pertinent that nurses and other members of the multidisciplinary team continue to research this subject, as with the increase of laser surgery enabling an increase in 'day surgery', preventing the potential problem of postoperative nausea from becoming an actual one is not only desirable but essential, and probably cost-effective.

Vomiting Nausea may be followed by expulsion of the stomach contents. In instances where vomiting is persistent it can lead to dehydration because of the excessive loss of body fluids. It is important for the nurse to make observations (Box 7.4).

Whatever the form, the nurse should procure, and help the person to hold the vomit bowl; and assist by wiping

---

Box 7.4 Observations which should be made when vomiting occurs

Time of occurrence
— early morning: related to pregnancy, renal disease
— soon after a meal and giving relief from pain: related to gastric ulceration

Character and appearance
— containing undigested food: related to indiscretion of food and drink
— containing red blood: related to rupture of a blood vessel in the upper digestive tract
— containing dark red digested blood ('coffee grounds'): related to gastric ulceration
— containing brown foul-smelling material ('faecal vomit'): related to intestinal obstruction

Manner of ejection
— effortless and in small quantities: related to intestinal obstruction
— with much pain and retching: related to gastritis and gastric ulceration
— projectile and without warning: related to head injuries, pyloric stenosis (obstruction due to narrowing of the pyloric orifice)

Any accompanying diarrhoea/constipation

---

the mouth with a tissue. The bed should be screened. Usually people find it comforting if a hand is placed on their forehead and such nurses' behaviour conveys assurance and sympathy without disgust at such episodes which are undoubtedly unpleasant for both patient and nurse. Most people find it easier if in a sitting position with the head over a basin but if it is necessary to lie flat, the head should be turned to one side and supported, and the person should be helped into a side-lying position.

It is important to remove vomitus and any soiled linen from the vicinity as quickly as possible. Should the vomit contain frank blood, or the linen be soiled with blood, then the nurse must carry out the procedure recommended by the health authority when removing the vomit bowl and soiled linen. These are now called 'universal precautions' because they are implemented whenever there is a possibility of contact with blood (or other body fluid) regardless of the known/unknown infectivity of that blood.

Facilities should be provided for sponging the face and having a refreshing mouthwash. A specimen of vomitus should be retained for inspection, as it may be helpful in diagnosis of the cause.

Observation of people who are in an impaired level of consciousness which includes recovering from an anaesthetic is of critical importance. Death can readily result because of respiratory obstruction caused by vomit being sucked/aspirated into the airway during such states. Patients are momentarily totally dependent on the nurse for immediate action. They should be turned on to one side in the semiprone position with all pillows removed until consciousness is regained and with it, the protective cough reflex.

Heartburn A burning sensation behind the sternum, often accompanied by regurgitation of an acid-like fluid into the mouth is called heartburn. Other terms used for the condition are pyrosis and waterbrash. Usually it occurs following meals and is frequently associated with a gastric ulcer or a hiatus hernia (herniation of abdominal contents into the thorax) but clears up when the ulcer heals or the hernia is repaired. It may be alleviated however by maintaining a sitting position following meals and sometimes, taking an oral alkaline mixture effectively prevents its occurrence. If these measures are unsuccessful a mouthwash helps to counteract the discomfort.

Flatulence Some patients complain of 'wind' or flatulence. Two types are recognized. Inevitably some air is swallowed when eating and sometimes when the stomach contracts, the air can be expelled up the oesophagus and produces what is termed belching. In some cultures it is a mark of appreciation following an enjoyable meal; in Western culture belching is usually considered to be an embarrassment. As a single feature, gastric flatulence is not generally considered to be pathological but can cause a great deal of discomfort or even pain and may be relieved by taking a peppermint sweet, or a drink of peppermint water which is usually more effective when given in hot water. Intestinal flatulence is discussed later.

Halitosis Halitosis literally means a foul-smelling breath and although the sufferer may not be aware of the condition, it is apparent to those in the vicinity. The condition is being discussed in this section of problems related to the AL of eating and drinking because it can be caused by infected gums or decayed teeth and dental attention may be indicated. It also occurs in very ill patients or those who are not taking sufficient fluid and food to keep the mouth clean and healthy. In such instances, the mouth and tongue become coated with a film consisting of bacteria, dead cells and decaying food and it is a nursing responsibility to provide frequent mouth care (p. 244) which will prevent or reduce halitosis and help the patient to feel more comfortable. Unless contraindicated, the patient should be helped to drink as much fluid as possible.

Exhaustion, emaciation, cachexia The word cachexia, in the last 2 decades has been associated with cancer. Gross loss of weight can be the person's problem which motivates a visit to the doctor. On the other hand, the loss of weight may occur after the first course of treatment whether it is radiotherapy alone or combined with cytotoxic chemotherapy. Cancer involves a proliferation of cells which requires increased metabolism. In the current state of knowledge there can be a place for aggressive use of parenteral nutrition (p. 191) in these people to allow better tolerance of chemotherapy and radiotherapy.

In HIV-positive people, once the seropositive stage progresses to active AIDS, loss of weight is one of many characteristics. It can be disconcerting to the person, partner, relatives, friends and professional staff. Oral and pharyngeal candidiasis can make swallowing difficult. Individualized nursing is certainly required. Some people may be able to swallow thickened fluids and it is essential to have advice about how these can be made as nutritious as possible.

Demented elderly people are another group who may experience gross loss of weight. This can be in spite of an adequate intake of nutrients (Watson, 1990). Should relatives challenge nurses, believing the weight loss to be synonymous with inadequate dietary intake, the nurses only defence is written evidence of the amount of food consumed at each meal.

Food allergy Many authors of scientific papers prefer to retain the term 'allergy' for reference to immunological mechanisms only, and suggest the use of 'idiosyncrasy' or 'food intolerance' to describe adverse reactions to food (Holmes 1993, 1994; Patchell, 1993). For the people who suffer, the terms will seem irrelevant. They may experience swelling in different parts of the body; heavy perspiration unrelated to exercise; fatigue not helped by rest; bouts of tachycardia; fluctuations in weight; and the symptoms come and go. Although some patients will have strong suspicions as to which foods provoke the symptoms, history alone should not be relied on and is no substitute for controlled clinical observation and dietary manipulation with suspected foods.

Pain Pain in the digestive tract may occur because of an inflammatory condition, an obstruction, a hiatus hernia, an unusual growth, and may be accompanied by vomiting.

Varying degrees of pain occur in most diseases of the upper gastrointestinal tract, often related to the intake of food and often at a specific time interval after meals. Foods which are difficult to digest — fried foods, rich carbohydrates and highly spiced foods — are particularly liable to cause pain and most frequently it is experienced in the epigastric region. The degree or duration of pain from gastric ulceration can often be reduced by taking an oral dose of an alkaline mixture, but in principle, pain should be dealt with by treating the cause.

Pain in a hollow muscular tube like the digestive tract can be experienced as *colic*, a severe sharp shooting pain. Colic is a discomfort not uncommonly experienced by babies and it may accompany many disorders of the digestive tract, of which, irritable bowel syndrome (IBS) is the most common, affecting 25 per cent of the population (Hogston, 1993). He discusses the nursing management of this condition.

Referred pain (p. 132) can be a feature of gallbladder disease, and the patient feels the pain in the region of his scapula (shoulder blade).

Toothache was mentioned on p. 185.

Anxiety about investigations   To assess deviations in the capacity to eat and drink, and any pain/discomfort in the digestive tract, various investigations are carried out, some of them very elaborate and requiring sophisticated equipment. The most commonly used in relation to this AL of eating and drinking are probably X-ray, which may or may not be combined with a barium swallow or barium meal; gastric secretion tests, and gastroscopy, with or without a biopsy. The actual technique of X-ray is not painful; the barium swallow and barium meal are distasteful; the gastric secretion test causes discomfort but the gastroscopy can be alarming and may even be painful. Nevertheless in all circumstances, people will have some anxiety about what they will be expected to do, how they will react and what the result will be.

The nurse must therefore take time to explain any preparation involved prior to the procedure and what to expect during and after. Any relevant instructions about the person's expected behaviour should be stated clearly and simply. Factual information about the preparation and technique will be found in the ward's procedure book but nurses must interpret it to patients.

Patients are dependent on the doctor or nurse in charge of the ward/clinic/health centre for an adequate account of what the tests have revealed. It is important to elicit that the person has understood what has been said.

These are a selection of the sort of actual and potential problems which people can experience in relation to their AL of eating and drinking because of a change in dependence/independence status.

CHANGE IN EATING AND DRINKING HABIT

Most people find even temporary change in dietary habits problematic, but sometimes people have to be helped to re-educate themselves about eating and drinking habits on a life-long basis.

Modification of habitual food intake

During illness appetite may range from extreme hunger as is found in uncontrolled diabetes mellitus to utter lack of interest in food when, for example, a person, has a high fever. When in hospital, the range of need is catered for by providing meals which vary in texture and quantity.

The variations can be described broadly as normal diet; light diet which contains no fatty, highly-seasoned foods; soft and fluid diets which are 'light' but are in semi-solid or liquid form and used for ill people or those who have ingestion, digestion and absorption problems.

Some people, however, whether at home or in hospital, are advised to accept modifications in diet as part of the treatment for a specific disease condition and some may rebel against this suggested restriction of food choice. When people are grossly overweight for example, it should be ascertained whether or not they are willing to accept a diet which is reduced in its daily kilojoule value, perhaps as low as 4000 kJ, and although this entails an overall reduction in dietary intake it usually involves a gross reduction in foodstuffs which have a high carbohydrate content. People often find great difficulty in altering life-long eating habits which involve shunning foods they enjoy, and also they feel hungry. They need much encouragement to resist unsuitable food and drink, and need help to learn about a balanced food intake even after a successful loss of weight. The amount of self-discipline required by people to maintain a *low carbohydrate/low kilojoule* diet should not be underestimated and their efforts require frequent reinforcement (Gatenby, 1991).

Diet diary   Before making a plan, it is helpful if overweight people keep a diary of everything eaten and the fluids taken; whether or not they were hungry at the time, as well as their mood. This usually highlights the snacks taken without noticing and when they felt vulnerable. Naturally height will be measured and a weight chart is a visible reminder of any change. Overweight people are then encouraged to make a diet plan; some cope better if they take a small meal at a 3- or 4- hourly interval. Foods containing fibre provide bulk and usually diminish the feeling of hunger. Some people manage best if they join a slimming club, all of which aim at permanent behavioural change related to eating and drinking habits. In recent years, proprietary preparations of Very Low Calorie Diets (VLCDs) have gained in popularity. They are particularly tempting to morbidly obese people who can buy these products without going to the doctor. Of course they do not help people to change their eating and drinking habits and this is essential for maintenance of the reduced weight.

Diabetic diet   Young people who are diagnosed as having diabetes mellitus, however, need to develop slightly modified eating and drinking habits on a lifetime basis. A diet with very restricted carbohydrate was recommended up to 1982. Since then, the British Diabetic Association's recommendations allow greater carbohydrate intake, while restricting fat, and continuing to restrict sucrose and other simple sugars. There is more emphasis on controlling total energy intake, which means controlling all food intake, instead of the previous restriction of only carbohydate foods. Indeed the modern diabetic diet is similar to the advocated healthy diet, which means that family cooking need not be so complicated.

Initially these people may be brought into hospital for tests but once diagnosed and on a regime where they understand the need to balance diet/insulin/exercise, the injections of insulin will deal with the defective carbohydrate metabolism provided the carbohydrate intake is controlled. These people can lead a normal life once they are educated to cope with the diabetic state — and it is a lifelong state. Those who develop diabetes when in the older age bracket are usually obese and the diabetic state can often be contained with a *low carbohydrate/low kilojoule* diet.

Low fat diet Obesity and diabetes mellitus are examples of conditions which necessitate modification in carbohydrate/kilojoule intake but sometimes the fat intake presents a problem. People, who have infective hepatitis (a form of jaundice) have this type of problem so a *low fat* diet is indicated until the liver recovers from the infection. The problem may be with a specific aspect of fat metabolism, however. People with coronary artery disease may be advised to omit a particular form of fat from the diet, namely saturated fat which is found in lard, butter and other animals fats. It has been found that when dietary intake of saturated fats is greatly reduced the level of blood cholesterol is reduced. High blood cholesterol seems to be associated with the deposition of fatty plaques in the arterial wall and this is conducive to coronary artery disease and myocardial infarction. Those who have had 'heart attacks' are therefore advised to take unsaturated rather than saturated fats in the diet and as with diabetics, this diet is usually advocated for the remainder of the person's life.

Pre-anaesthetic/investigation fasting

There are occasions when *food and fluid intake is prohibited*; before an anaesthetic and before certain investigations, the person may be asked to fast for several hours. Many investigations are carried out in Outpatient Departments, particularly in X-ray Departments. It is important to ascertain whether or not the written word has been understood by asking questions about the necessary dietary changes on the days prior to, and the morning of the clinic appointment. And of course the same applies to day surgery patients.

In hospital, an explanation with clear instructions about timing is usually all that is required for most adult patients though in *Nil by Mouth?*, Hamilton-Smith as long ago as 1972, deplored the great variations in practice many of which have no scientific basis. 20 years later, in 1992, Hung reported a similar study and found that no substantial changes had occurred. However Hunt (1987) reported an ongoing operational research project highlighting the complexity of a multidisciplinary approach that was necessary to overcome many of the 'planning' problems which require to be solved before nurses at clinical level can use research findings related to a research-based period of preoperative fasting.

An unnecessary length of preoperative fasting means that patients may arrive in the operating theatre in an (albeit temporary) malnourished state, but in the ensuing postoperative days, they may not be able to take adequate nourishment, thereby continuing the malnourishment which is not conducive to wound healing (Shireff, 1990; Benton & Avery, 1993). Hunt's project was based on the physiological necessity for fasting from food for 6 hours, and from fluid for 4 hours prior to an anaesthetic.

In 1990 it was established that the stomach contents of children aspirated at 2 hours and 6 hours after ingestion of clear fluid, revealed no difference in either volume or acidity (Bates, 1994). He describes the development and audit of an individual fasting plan for children attending a day surgery unit, with the objective of an optimum 2-hour fast from clear fluids, an excellent example of nurse-led practice development. He intends to repeat the audit annually to demonstrate further improvement or detect lapses into the old practice.

Prior to surgery, a patient is often given an injection of atropine which reduces secretion in the mouth and respiratory tract and therefore reduces the danger of inhalation of fluid during anaesthesia. Patients should be told to expect that they will feel thirsty and experience a feeling of dryness in the mouth.

Modification of habitual fluid intake

Problems with fluid intake are often more urgent than those associated with food intake. Fluid deprivation can only be tolerated for a few days and in a 24-hour period the adult human requires about 2500 ml of fluid. However Burns (1992) reviewed several physiology texts and concluded that a mean daily intake of 1500 ml was adequate.

Dehydration There are obvious reductions in fluid intake when it is impossible to procure drinking water — in dramatic shipwreck and desert rescues for example — but excessive fluid output from the body is the usual cause of *dehydration*. It may be found in any condition featuring high fever, vomiting or diarrhoea and these commonly occur in food poisoning, which in Great Britain increased from just less than 20 000 cases in 1981 to over 60 000 in 1992 (OPCS, 1992). Dehydration also occurs when there is severe haemorrhage, severe burns, untreated diabetes mellitus and untreated diabetes insipidus.

It may occur in milder form. Some elderly people with weak bladder control may deliberately reduce their intake in the hope that it will reduce the need to ask for a bedpan; or the person with a learning disability may be unable to make decisions about the adequacy of intake.

In the early stages of dehydration fluid is withdrawn from the skin and tissues in order to maintain the blood volume while simultaneously the kidneys excrete less urine in order to conserve body fluid. If the cause of dehydration is not treated effectively however, more serious effects ensue. Such people are thirsty and the tongue looks dry and leathery. There is lethargy, and the eyes (and fontanelle in a baby) appear sunken. The skin loses its natural elasticity and has a wrinkled appearance. Urinary output is not only reduced, but the urine is highly concentrated. In extreme cases, blood volume is reduced causing deficient circulation, and in turn the kidneys fail to excrete waste products. Renal failure and death may ensue.

Treatment Where there is mild dehydration, the nurse should encourage the person to drink and ensure that freshly procured drinks of a desired flavour, perhaps with ice, are available. Nutrients are added to the fluid and advice from a dietitian is essential. When there is gross dehydration, intravenous fluids will be required as well, usually in the form of a saline infusion as salt will have been lost along with body fluid.

It is important to understand that loss of body weight is due to lack of nutrients, hence the fluid balance chart should describe the fluid taken as well as the amount. The weight loss is indicative of usage of the body's store of fat, then protein from cellular structures. Records must be maintained of weight, fluid intake, all forms of output — urine, faeces, vomitus — and note made of excessive perspiration. Daffurn et al (1994) investigated the accuracy of fluid balance charts and the use made of the information. The usual treatment of dehydration is oral rehydration using sachets which contain salt and glucose to correct electrolyte imbalance; they are available without prescription.

The complex problem of parenteral rehydration of people who are terminally ill is mentioned in the context of the AL of dying (p. 413). Malone (1994) discusses hydration in the terminally ill patient, and Noble-Adams (1995) describes the method of subcutaneous fluid administration as treatment for dehydration.

Oedema In contradistinction to dehydration a person's body may retain an excess amount of fluid and the condition is called *oedema*. Oedema is most commonly seen when the heart, as a pump, is not functioning normally. The resulting swelling — it is recognizable by the way the skin in affected areas 'pits' on pressure — is most obvious in the dependent parts of the body such as the feet, ankles and legs. If the person is sitting in bed or on a chair, the swelling is in the sacral area. The person may be distressed by the ugly appearance of swollen ankles, the discomfort, the reduced mobility. If pressure sores are to be prevented, the stretched 'devitalized' skin in affected areas requires special care. When

there is gross imbalance fluid will also collect in the pleural and peritoneal cavities causing respiratory difficulty and the person will then be breathless and uncomfortable, so a procedure to aspirate the fluid may be medically prescribed to alleviate the distress: this will necessitate specific nursing interventions.

It is logical to expect that a person who has oedema should take a *low fluid/low salt* diet. Again, individual likes and dislikes regarding time and content of fluid intake should be discussed with the person and a suitable regime adopted. These people often appreciate a pleasant tasting mouthwash at hand even during the night. Regarding salt intake, condiments are removed from the table but salt substitutes may be used for flavouring.

Complexity of change

Only a few examples have been cited which involve changes in eating and drinking habits, but in all instances it must be remembered that merely imparting information to people does not guarantee advice will be followed. Explaining the reason for a special diet is essential and should take into account the person's socioeconomic, cultural, religious, moral and ethical values. Wherever possible advice should be related to the usual dietary habits of the individual and modifications rather than drastic change should be attempted.

If the person must continue a special diet for some time, advice may be required in relation to purchase of certain foods, perhaps unaccustomed foods, and home budgeting may need to be adjusted. When a dietitian is not available to provide such a service, the nurse must inform and assist the person thereby providing an excellent opportunity to offer health education related to nutrition and food handling should this be necessary. It is important to remember too that a long-term dietary alteration may affect not only the individual but the family, and the nurse should be able to make helpful suggestions about food preparation so that people do not feel ostracized at meal times or that they are creating extra work because of changes in their daily activity of eating and drinking.

The foregoing is a brief introduction to the sort of actual problems which can be experienced, and potential problems which can be prevented from becoming actual problems, related to a change in eating and drinking habit.

CHANGE IN MODE OF EATING AND DRINKING

Some people, either temporarily for a short or long period, or permanently, are confronted by problems, because they are deprived of their usual mode of eating and drinking. If, for any reason, food cannot be ingested, nutrients can be introduced into the digestive tract and the term 'enteral feeding' is used.

Enteral feeding

A fine 'nasogastric' tube is passed along the floor of one nostril, through the oropharynx and via the oesophagus into the stomach; sometimes it is passed into the duodenum and occasionally as far as the jejunum. To avoid people having to cope with a nasogastric tube in situ, a surgical opening, that is a stoma, can be made into the stomach, duodenum or jejunum creating a gastrostomy, duodenostomy or jejunostomy via which enteral feeds (Reilly, 1993) can be introduced. Feeding via these routes provides people with different sorts of problems and these will be discussed.

Nasogastric feeding When nasogastric feeding is required, the problem for conscious people is that they are deprived of the sensual pleasure of smell, taste, temperature and texture of food which normally stimulates the flow of saliva and starts the first stage of digestion as well as maintaining moistness of the mouth for comfort and for speaking. Mouth care is therefore very important (p. 244), and a little Vaseline applied to the nostril is usually comforting. Proprietary feeds are available for nasogastric feeding through a fine bore tube and feed contamination has to be avoided (Jamieson et al, 1992; Williams, 1992). Food and drink can be swallowed in the presence of a nasogastric tube and some nutritionists suggest this 'weaning' process before final removal of the tube. Frank, sensitive discussion with these people is necessary about how they are going to cope with the social and cultural dimensions of this AL. If the treatment has to be prolonged, discharge from hospital to home needs very careful planning and implementing (Arrowsmith, 1994; Bruce, 1994).

Gastrostomy feeding After the surgical formation of a fistula between, for example the stomach or jejunum and the skin, nutrients are introduced via a catheter which stays in the fistula (Jamieson et al, 1992). One distinct advantage of 'ostomy' over nasogastric feeding is that patients can usually learn to feed themselves and quickly become independent for feeding and mouth care, although they are dependent on the apparatus and the commercial feeds.

An increasing number of children are being fed by gastrostomy (Coldicutt, 1994). Even if the child learns to be independent for feeding, members of the family require psychological support.

Parenteral (intravenous) feeding

The foregoing methods, although not using the usual oral route for the ingestion of food and fluid, do involve direct entry of nourishment to some part of the digestive tract. In some instances when it is not possible to provide nutrition via the tract itself, food nutrients dissolved in fluid to prevent malnutrition and dehydration, may have to be administered straight into the bloodstream by means of an intravenous infusion — parenteral feeding. The term 'total parenteral feeding' is used when all nutrients are introduced intravenously — nil by mouth — so meticulous oral hygiene is essential. The choice to be made by the nutrition team is whether to infuse into a peripheral vein or a central vein (Jamieson et al, 1992). A disadvantage when using a peripheral vein is that the solutions used are often hypertonic and can damage the lining of the vein causing phlebitis and thrombosis. The past tense might be more appropriate now because in the last decade knowledge about the elements in food and fluids has increased and some isotonic solutions are available, but they are expensive. Peripheral venous feeding continues to be used; combinations of fat with either amino acids and/or glucose in solution are infused and these substances are less hypertonic than previously (Taylor, 1994).

Central venous feeding is now more common than previously and the subclavian vein is the most frequently used route. A small number of people have to rely on central venous feeding permanently and when they become independent in using this process are discharged into the community with close liaison between the hospital nutrition team and the community services (Friend, 1992). These programmes can be likened to those of home dialysis for people with chronic kidney failure. It has to be remembered that these people are deprived, not only of the sensual pleasure of eating and drinking, but also of the social and psychological pleasures associated with family meals, as well as dining out. Some of them benefit from chewing food and discreetly disposing of it into a tissue.

Oral and dental hygiene was mentioned in the context of nasogastric feeding; they are no less important in people who are being fed intravenously, either peripherally or centrally; temporarily or permanently. Care of the mouth is discussed on p. 244.

The solutions which can be infused are numerous, and decisions about which to use for each individual are made by a multidisciplinary nutrition team. Some fluids contain soluble fibre to prevent constipation.

CHANGE OF ENVIRONMENT AND ROUTINE

Probably the biggest change of environment and routine which can cause actual or potential problems with the AL of eating and drinking is that of changing residence, may be from home to hospital or frail people moving into a nursing home, and so on.

Nursing homes

Nursing homes are increasingly important in care of the elderly in the UK. They vary from large purpose built 'homes' where a dietitian can be consulted, and the food is prepared by a chef, to small domestic residences where the food is prepared by a cook who may have little knowledge of nutrition (Nazarko, 1993). Initial dietary assessment and continuous ongoing assessment is the means by which the potential problem of suboptimal nutrition will be prevented from becoming overt clinical malnutrition.

Hospitals

Obviously the age of people may have special influence. Toddlers who have just become independent for actually feeding themselves may not have achieved 'clean' feeding. Ideally a family member could provide continuity, but if unable to do so, then the nurse needs to collect relevant information so that mealtimes will be changed as little as possible. Ongoing assessment will provide information about the adequacy of intake. The child should be praised each time there is less mess.

For young children, the change in environment and routine in hospital will be bewildering, even if one parent can be resident in the hospital or stay nearby. For others the enforced separation from mother and family will probably be traumatic, leading to unhappiness and confusion. Parents may not be able to be present at mealtimes. Essential pre-anaesthetic/investigation fasting has to be managed on an individual basis.

However individualist a mother has been about her children's diet, once they go to school, they may acquire habits of eating convenience foods; a large quantity and variety of such foods is usually available in nearby stores. There is no research evidence as to whether or not this plays any part in the staggering number of people who are malnourished on admission to hospital (Lennard-Jones, 1992).

An increasing number of authors write about 'hospital-induced malnutrition' (Alderman, 1990; Carr & Mitchell, 1991; Day, 1994). They provide evidence that nurses are less involved in the delivery and supervision of meals. The Patient's Association (1993) has submitted the result of its survey to the UKCC, with the recommendation that in order to monitor patients' nutrition intake, nurses should collect trays after meals to see what food has been left on the crockery. All food offered to patients should contain the minimum requirements set out in the Department of Health, COMA report (1991).

Most people are well accustomed to changes of diet while on holiday or during business trips but in these instances, they are usually in control of their decisions about eating and drinking. In hospital however this is not usually so.

Timing of meals People newly admitted to hospital often have no idea of the mealtime programme: whether to expect a cooked or a continental breakfast; whether the main meal is served in the middle of the day or in the evening; whether they will be allowed to have snacks between meals. Some people may have heard of the need to fast prior to surgery and certain tests, and be concerned about the discomfort of feeling hungry or thirsty.

Nurses can allay some of the anxiety by offering information and also by providing opportunities for people to ask questions so that they can feel reassured about what they are expected to do in continuing this important AL. Most people, understand that in an establishment as complex as a hospital, it is usually necessary to have set mealtimes; indeed, some find that meals give a certain degree of order to the day, providing stable time-points in an otherwise bewildering situation.

However, in the interests of financial economy, meal preparation for several hospitals is increasingly being centralized, leaving nursing staff in the wards with little control over the timing of meals. Appetite is often fickle during illness, and a person may be ready to eat an hour after the routine meal has been served. Or a person may be away from the ward, perhaps in another department, at the mealtime and may be hungry on return. Some hospitals are solving these problems by installing a microwave oven in the ward kitchen, so that meals precooked in the central kitchen can be re-heated. When the cook-chill process was introduced into some hospitals in the early 1980s, there were high hopes that it would provide cheaper, hot, nutritional meals, at the times people required them. The food is cooked and then fast-chilled and stored for up to 5 days in controlled low temperatures, and reheated immediately before eating. The method gives flexibility to kitchen staff regarding time of cooking, types of food served, and individual ward mealtimes. However, there is debate about the possibility of this method transmitting pathogenic microorganisms such as *Salmonella*, *Listeria monocytogenes* and *Campylobacter*. The debate continues providing an example of the necessity for nurses to continually update their knowledge.

Serving of meals In hospital, people may find that the way of serving meals is a problem because it is so different from their usual routine. Even though most people are accustomed to 'tray' meals in self-service restaurants, few are used to having all meals served in this manner.

People do not usually choose to be in bed while taking a meal, so for the minority of patients who are bedfast, eating and drinking may become a formidable task especially if they must remain in a recumbent position, or attached to various pieces of equipment associated with their treatment.

If bedfast people can sit up at mealtimes, the nurse should help them into a comfortable position and ensure that they are adequately supported with pillows before placing the bedtable in an appropriate position ready for the mealtray. Many people like to drink with a meal and, unless it is contraindicated, most patients have a water-jug and glass on the bedside locker so the nurse should check that it is within easy reach.

Functionally-designed hospital furniture has improved over the last few decades. Chairfast people can have a bedtable lowered to receive the mealtray so that they are in the usual position for eating and drinking. They can then eat and drink in their usual style, which might be using modified cutlery and crockery, or even being fed by another person. Ambulant people will enjoy meals more if sitting at a table; in fact, in new and upgraded wards, a dining area is frequently included in the design of the ward unit.

Meals should be served in a calm, unhurried manner if people are to enjoy what is really a social event in their day. The nurse should appreciate the symbolism attached to food, indicative of hospitality and caring. Associated with this symbolism, the very acts of serving and accepting food provide an opportunity for establishing and maintaining the important relationship between nurse and patient.

Particularly in a psychiatric hospital, group dining may be a deliberate therapeutic measure to give patients an opportunity to solve some of their problems by practising the social behaviour associated with mealtimes.

Alteration in appetite Most people have personal idiosyncrasies about food choice and even when an appropriate, attractive meal is served, patients may not feel inclined to eat. If they are feeling unwell, or homesick, or unused to the type of food served, they may not eat adequately and the nurse must be interested in the 'used' tray. Over a century ago (1974, 1859) Florence Nightingale observed:

> 'A nurse will often have patients loathing all food and incapable of any will to get well who just tumble over the contents of the plate or dip the spoon into the cup to deceive the nurse and she will take it away without ever seeing that there is just the same quantity of food as when she brought it, and she will tell the doctor too that the patient has eaten all his diets as usual when all she ought to have meant is that she has taken away his diets as usual.'

The stress and anxiety associated with admission to hospital may result in lack of appetite, albeit temporarily. Early establishment of rapport with newly admitted people may help to minimize it. Unpleasant sights and odours may diminish appetite and nursing activities need to be planned so that the ward atmosphere is free from malodour at mealtimes. Pain, particularly of a chronic nature, can interfere with appetite and if it is possible, pain-control regimes could take mealtimes into consideration so that patients are relaxed, free from pain and can anticipate the meal with pleasure. Loss of appetite occurs when there is nausea and/or vomiting and these are discussed on p. 185 to 186.

Anorexia (loss of appetite) is a symptom of several diseases, and when the disease is treated, normal appetite is usually re-established. Reduction in appetite can affect the body's response to medication therapy. Conversely, both the side- and therapeutic effects of medications can interfere with food intake by either increasing or decreasing appetite.

Anorexia is a common and serious symptom in patients with cancer. They experience such unpleasant changes in taste sensation, that they can reject food which relatives have carefully prepared especially for them, and this can cause family tension. Warning relatives that this might happen, and assuring them that the rejection is not personal, usually helps them to cope with the problem. The study reported by Stubbs (1989) is still pertinent. Items causing the greatest taste changes (in descending order) were meat, bacon and ham, fried eggs, tea, coffee, alcohol, sweets and chocolates. A nursing contribution is to encourage patients to regard food as an essential medicine to be taken at regular intervals throughout the day until treatment is successful. A high-protein breakfast may help with the problem of meat aversion which has been found to increase as the day progresses. Helping people who are experiencing changed taste sensation demands individualized nursing.

Anorexia nervosa, over-eating, obesity, compulsive over-eating, binge-eating and bulimia nervosa are all related to alteration in appetite. As they have a psychological dimension, they are discussed in the section 'Psychological factors influencing eating and drinking' (p. 177); and they were mentioned in the context of experiencing a problem because of psychological dependence on p. 183. Here they are mentioned in the context of experiencing a change of environment and routine.

As nutrients are essential for the repair of body tissue, it is imperative that nurses know about the therapeutic value of food, and either report verbally on patients' appetites and food intake at the 'end of shift' handover, or record the information on the patients' nursing notes.

Hospital meals Some hospitals continue to serve food from a mobile heated trolley and those patients who are able, make their decision when they are told what is available. This avoids the problem of removal of heavy covers and cling film inherent in a mealtray service; it provides for size of helping to be adjusted to current appetite, and patients may well be reassured to see nursing staff serving food, and taking an interest in the meals.

In those hospitals in which a menu provides an assortment of food, it is customary for the desired items for meals on the following day to be ticked on a menu card in the evening. Some provide for the selection of a large, average or small portion. Helping patients to choose meals from the next day's menu can offer nurses an opportunity to talk about the important links between nutrition and health. However, this means having a sufficient number of nurses on the evening shift. Some hospitals cope with the anticipated lack of evening staff by helping the patients fill in the menu cards in the afternoon. If there are visitors present, they too could benefit from the discussion about choice of diet. But, there are instances of patients who, having forgotten what they ordered the day before, refuse to eat the food. A clinical nurse specialist in a nutrition team states her reservations about the designation of 'non-nursing duties' to mealtime activities, and says that in some cases the ward clerk or maid fills in the menu cards, and removes the uneaten food (Carlisle, 1988).

However, even when hospital meals are adequate, some people will complain about them. There may be cause for dissatisfaction but grumbling about food may be a manifestation of some more covert need, for example lack of information about the treatment programme, upset of usual routine, lack of attention; the discerning nurse will investigate the significance of dietary complaints.

Pre- and post-meal activities   The majority of people who are not bedfast will be able to continue their habitual pre- and post-meal routines such as handwashing, visiting the toilet and cleaning the teeth. Bedfast people may experience considerable concern because they are no longer independent for these activities but nurses can reduce anxiety by ensuring that these facilities are made available.

Patients will be reassured if they actually see members of the nursing staff wash their hands in preparation for serving meals and/or helping with feeding activities. This is important for general hygiene reasons, but it is also important in order that food will be free from contamination by pathogenic microorganisms. Prior to meal-serving, the nurse may have been dressing wounds, or helping a person who is vomiting or she may have been handling a bedpan. In an establishment such as a hospital, it is crucial that all food-handlers should be scrupulously careful about hand cleanliness because potentially they can infect the food of many people, and people who are more susceptible to infection because they are already suffering from some disorder which has precipitated entry to hospital.

As a pre-meal activity, it is important for nurses to plan their work so that unpleasant sights, sounds and smells will not ruin the patient's appetite for food and drink. As far as possible, treatment appointments in other departments of the hospital should be scheduled for other times of the day, and doctors' rounds should avoid mealtimes. A general introduction has been given in this section to the sorts of actual and potential problems which people can experience with their AL of eating and drinking using four broad categories.

PLANNING AND IMPLEMENTING NURSING ACTIVITIES AND EVALUATING OUTCOMES

The large number of problems which can be experienced in relation to the AL of eating and drinking is indicative of the complexity of the apparently simple activity. 'Planning', 'implementing' and 'evaluating' will be recognized as the last three phases of the process of nursing, the means by which in our model, individualizing nursing is accomplished. Already the three words have occurred many times in the context of the so-called first two phases — assessing and identifying people's actual and potential problems.

It is indicative of the fact the phases are not linear, sequential or discrete. Only for learning and descriptive purposes is it useful to think of four (or five) phases. In the real world of nursing the sequence is everchanging for various reasons. In any one encounter with a person, all phases may be interacting. When the principles of the process are grasped, the interaction of the phases becomes increasingly apparent.

The general context in which this AL is set has to be considered throughout the nursing of a particular person. Information about this was provided at the beginning of the chapter in the discussion about the relationship of the lifespan to the person's eating and drinking; and its relationship to the person's dependence/independence status. And the five factors influencing the AL of eating and drinking are pertinent to discover for each person as they will have contributed to the person's individuality in eating and drinking, essential activities for the continuance of life.

In keeping with our conceptualization of nursing, the objectives of the nursing plan is to help the person:

- to prevent any potential problem from becoming actual
- to solve or alleviate any actual problems
- to prevent recurrence of a treated condition
- to develop positive coping mechanisms for those problems which cannot be alleviated or solved.

Planning and implementing nursing activities

The cognitive dimension of the process has undoubtedly helped many nurses to a better understanding of the planning, implementing and evaluating aspects of their nursing. This is particularly so, when there are identifiable problems with this AL for which there are recognized nurse-initiated interventions. Of course there are nursing practices which are influenced by multidisciplinary decisions, for example the fluid to be administered in both enteral and parenteral feeding.

The majority of people who seek treatment in the health service, in this instance the nursing part of that service, whether at primary or secondary level do not report a problem with the AL of eating and drinking. Yet nurses at both these levels are being asked to discover (in the words of the process by assessing) the nutritional intake and alcohol consumption of all patients. Nurses were identified in The Health of the Nation (Department of Health, 1992) as being able to play a key role in helping to improve the health of the nation by the year 2000 by paying attention to these two 'assessments'.

When nurses find a deficiency in nutritional intake and/or over consumption of alcohol (which may be confined to the weekends), then a plan for health education/ promotion to achieve a change in lifestyle needs to be implemented and evaluated. This could be achieved by using some of the leaflets and booklets produced by the Health Education Authority for information giving, always preceded by discovering (assessing) that the person can see and read the written word. At follow up clinics there can be further estimation (ongoing assessment/evaluating) of what action has been taken (implemented). From the research evidence about malnourishment in patients admitted to hospital, it is evident that nurses wherever they are working outwith hospitals, have an identified role in planning and implementing such activities as information giving and educating in relation to the AL of eating and drinking.

Again from research evidence already mentioned it is important for nurses to recognize that all patients in hospital who do not have an actual problem with eating and drinking, have a potential one of becoming malnourished during a stay of longer than two weeks (Dickerson, 1995). Whatever type of meal service is provided, it is evident that pressure resulting from a survey carried out by the Patients' Association will result in nurses having to accept the responsibility of planning their work so that they are in the vicinity of patients during mealtimes, and implementing that plan, which includes evaluating how much patients have eaten, and how much has been left on the plates – which may be covered by a lid.

Nursing's body of knowledge acknowledges that people who have a wound of any kind (including pressure sores) require adequate dietary intake, and planning may well include fortified drinks to achieve this (Wells, 1994). Such people may also be incontinent and they may reduce their fluid intake in the misplaced hope that it will be minimized. The interactiveness of assessing, planning, implementing and evaluating should cope with this misplaced belief (Oliver, 1994).

There are many conditions for which teaching/learning sessions have to be planned and implemented, for example, people newly diagnosed as diabetic. Not only has knowledge about dietary control to be imparted/acquired, but also the practical skills of preparing and injecting insulin, measuring blood glucose and testing

urine. The latter measurements are in fact evaluations of the body's metabolism.

Although this short section is headed 'Planning and implementing nursing activities' the word 'evaluating' has occurred five times. This is further evidence of the inseparability of the phases of what since the 1970s in the UK has been known as the process of nursing and the interactivity of the phases cannot be stressed too strongly. However a few words need to be said about evaluating as it pertains to the AL of eating and drinking.

Evaluating outcomes

There was generalized discussion about individualizing nursing by using the process (pp. 51 to 60). In this chapter some specific aspects of the process have been focused to the AL of eating and drinking. It cannot be said too often that evaluating is entirely dependent on the prior statement of the outcome/s which are to be achieved. They may include educational objectives, acquisition of practical skills or change of beliefs and attitudes to bring about a change in behaviour, and in many instances all three might be involved. And most texts advise that the person should participate in the setting of outcomes. However there may well be people who do not want to be involved in such decisions.

Evaluating is straightforward when measuring tools such as height, weight, skin callipers, upper arm circumference and volume of intake and output were used in the assessing phase. For those elderly people whose eating and drinking is not a problem, the expected outcome is that their weight will be unchanged. Those who are overweight may wish to participate in reduction of dietary intake to lose weight.

Outcomes are set with a view to people being rehabilitated to their optimum independence for this AL. When evaluation reveals that, for instance people on enteral or parenteral feeding have achieved the educational and skill acquisition objectives, they can be discharged from hospital to manage their feeding, supported by delivery of feeds, equipment and so on to their home. But evaluation also reveals that it is too soon to discontinue the nurse/patient relationship and such people are able to contact the ward whenever any queries arise.

Evaluating outcomes is a growing area in nursing as the current ethos of the health service is providing an efficient, cost-effective service which satisfies the 'consumers'. Nursing's contribution is by collecting data in process format as illustrated in Figure 3.9, p. 60.

This chapter has been concerned with discussion of the concepts in our model for nursing focused to the particular AL of eating and drinking. The interactiveness of the phases of the process has been stressed. However it is equally important to understand the interactiveness of the 12 ALs. Familiarity with the conceptualization of nursing offered in our Activities of Living model increases awareness of such interactiveness. It is only for the purpose of description and learning that they can be separated.

REFERENCES

Adams L 1993 Managing chemotherapy-induced nausea and vomiting. Professional Nurse 9 (2) November: 91–94

Alderman C 1990 Best possible taste? Nursing Standard 4 (31) April 25: 22–23

Anderson A 1994 Eating for life. Pregnancy Diet. Nursing Times 90 (6) February 9: 44, 46, 48

Anderson C A 1991 Feeding — a guide to assessment and intervention with handicapped children. Jordanhill College of Education, Glasgow, Scotland

Arrowsmith H L 1994 Discharging patients receiving enteral nutrition. British Journal of Nursing 3 (11): 551–557

Arrowsmith H 1993 Nursing management of patients receiving a nasogastric feed. British Journal of Nursing 2 (21): 1053–1058

A worker from Al-Anon 1993 Living with a timebomb. Nursing Times 89 (22) June 2: 44–45

Axelsson K, Norberg A, Asplund K 1986 Relearning to eat late after a stroke by systematic nursing intervention: a case report. Journal of Advanced Nursing 11 (5) September: 553–559

Bates J 1994 Reducing fast times in paediatric day surgery. Nursing Times 90 (48) November 30: 38–39

Beadle L, Townsend S, Palmer D 1995 The management of dysphagia in stroke. Nursing Standard 9 (15) January 4: 37–39

Benton D, Avery G 1993 Quality, research and ritual in nursing. Preoperative fasting. Nursing Standard 7 (49) August 25: 29–30

Black P A 1993 A confident start to a new relationship. Breastfeeding. Professional Nurse 9 (3) December: 193–196

Brandt W 1980 North-South: a programme for survival. Pan Books, London

Briggs D 1992 Baby milks and the E C. Nursing Times 88 (32) August 5: 24, 26

Bruce J A W 1994 Clinical enteral nutrition. Nursing Standard 8 (32) May 4: RCN Nursing Update, 3–8

Burns D 1992 Working up a thirst. Nursing Times 88 (26) June 24: 44–45

Buxton V 1993 A healthy start in life. Nursing Standard 8 (10) November 24: 18–20

Cabell C 1990 Regaining a basic pleasure. Nursing Times 86 (47) November 21: 27–29

Campbell J 1995 Making sense of the effects of alcohol. Nursing Times 91 (5) February 1: 38–39

Carlisle D 1988 Food for thought (hospital food does not have a sparkling reputation). Nursing Standard 2 (15) January 16: 28

Carr E K, Mitchell J R A 1991 A comparison of mealtime care given to patients by nurses using two different delivery systems. Journal of International Nursing Studies 28 (1): 19–25

Charalambous L 1993 A healthy approach. Nursing Times 89 (20) May 19: 58–60 (Nutrition score)

Chilvers C E D 1993 Breast feeding and risk of breast cancer in young women. British Medical Journal 307: 17–20

Clarke L 1991 Breastfeeding initiatives. Nursing Standard 5 (49) August 28: 49–50

Coldicutt P 1994 Children's options. Gastrostomy. Nursing Times 90 (13) March 30: 54, 56

Cooper D 1994 Problem drinking. Alcohol survey results. Nursing Times 90 (14) April 6: 36–39

Curtis H 1992 HIV testing for pregnant women. Letter to the Editor. The Independent, December 21

Day M 1994 Deals on meals. Nursing Times 90 (20) May 18: 16–17

Department of Health 1991 Reference Values for Food Energy and Nutrients for the United Kingdom. COMA report, HMSO, London

Department of Health 1994 Weaning and the weaning diet. HMSO, London

Department of Health 1991 The Health of the Nation: A consultative document for health in England. HMSO, London CM 1523

DHSS 1988 Present day practice in infant feeding. Third report. Reports on health and social subjects No. 32, HMSO, London. Report of a working party of the panel on Child Nutrition, Committee on Medical Aspects of Food Policy (COMA) HMSO, London

Dickerson J 1995 The problem of hospital-induced malnutrition. Nursing Times 91 (4) January 25: 44–45

Fretwell A 1991 Causes of anorexia nervosa. Nursing 4 (35) May 23–June 12: 15–17

Friend B 1992b A sobering issue. SCAD. Nursing Times 88 (4) January 22: 14–15

Friend B 1992a Drink drive. Nursing Times 88 (38) September 16: 19

Friend B 1992 Self-service. Person on total parenteral nutrition living independently at home. Nursing Times 88 (44) October 28: 26–28

Gatenby S J 1991 A positive change for a healthier life. Professional Nurse 6 (9) June: 524–527.

George M 1993 Poverty, diet and health. Nursing Standard 7 (49) August 29: 21–23

Greenhorn T 1992 Fed up? (Dependent for feeding) Nursing Times 88 (30) July 22: 32–33

Hamilton–Smith S 1972 Nil by mouth? Royal College of Nursing, London

Harrison M 1991 Weighty concerns. Nursing Times 87 (42) October 16: 40–42

Hogston R 1993 Nursing management of irritable bowel syndrome. British Journal of Nursing 2 (4): 215–217

Holmes S 1993 A positive response to an adverse reaction. Professional Nurse 8 (7) April: 423, 424, 426–428

Holmes S 1994 Food intolerance defined. Nursing Times 90 (42) October 19: 33–35

Holmes S 1991 Planning for the best start in life. Professional Nurse 6 (4) January: 202, 204, 205

Holmes S 1991a Support can boost the body's defences. Professional Nurse 7 (2) November: 83, 84, 86, 88, 89

Hung P 1992 Pre-operative fasting. Nursing Times 88 (48) November 25: 57–60. Occasional Paper

Hunt M 1987 The process of translating research findings into nursing practice. Journal of Advanced Nursing 12: January: 101–110

Jamieson E M, McCall J M, Blythe R 1992 Guidelines for clinical nursing practices related to a model for nursing. Churchill Livingstone, Edinburgh

Jamieson L 1994 Getting it together. Teaching package for breastfeeding. Nursing Times 90 (17) April 27: 68–69

Jones A, Stone S 1992 Beating bulimia. Nursing Times 88 (46) November 11: 30–32

Kenny T 1991 Anorexia nervosa — a nursing challenge that can bring results. Professional Nurse 6 (11) August: 666–669

Knapman J 1993 Controlling emesis after chemotherapy. Nursing Standard 7 (15) January 6: 38–39

Laurent C 1993 Private function? National Opinion Poll (for the Royal College of Midwives) of 924 men re their attitudes to breastfeeding. Nursing Times 89 (47) November 24: 14–15

Lennard-Jones J E 1992 A positive approach to nutrition as treatment. King's Fund Centre, London

Le Page P et al 1987 Postnatal transmission of HIV from mother to child. Lancet ii: 400

Leslie H, Learmonth L 1994 Alcohol counselling in a general hospital. Nursing Standard 8 (27) March 30: 25–29

Lindsay W, Allen R 1992 The art of positive drinking. Nursing Times 88 (25) June 17: 46–48

Lyall J 1991 Starting young. Nursing Times 87 (32) August 7: 16–17

Mairis E 1992 An appetite for life. Assessing and meeting nutritional needs. Professional Nurse 7 (11) August: 732–734, 736–737

Malone N 1994 Hydration in the terminally ill patient. Nursing Standard 8 (43) July 20: 29–32

Mathieson A 1995 Infant weaning: the COMA report. Nursing Standard 9 (16) January 11: 25–29

Meades S 1993 Suggested community psychiatric nursing interventions with clients suffering from anorexia nervosa and bulimia nervosa. Journal of Advanced Nursing 18: 364–370

Mitchell E, Scragg R, Stewart A W et al 1991 Cot death supplement. Results from the first year of the New Zealand cot death study. New Zealand Medical Journal 104 (906): 71–76

McMillan I 1994 Consuming anxieties. Nursing Times 90 (23) June 8: 14–15

Morley D 1994 Midwives and HIV: the case for continuing education. Nursing Times 90 (36) September 7: 48–49

Nazarko L 1993 Nutritional problems in nursing homes. Nursing Standard 7 (27) March 2: 33–36

Nightingale F 1974 Notes on nursing. Blackie, London (original 1859)

Noble-Adams R 1995 Dehydration: subcutaneous fluid administration. British Journal of Nursing 4 (9) May 12–24: 488, 490, 492, 493, 494

Nursing Standard 1994 Alcohol information for primary school children. Nursing Standard 8 (23) March 2: 16

Nursing Times 1993 New laws on baby milk. Nursing Times 89 (49) December 8: 6

Oliver E 1994 Maintaining nutritional support in the community. Journal of tissue viability 4 (1): 28–32

OPCS 1994 Social Trends 24. Central Statistical Office. HMSO, London

Patients' Association 1993 Catering for patients in hospital: guidelines on hospital food. Patients' Association, London

Perry M 1992 Learning disabilities: community nutrition. Nursing Standard 7 (11) December 2: 38–40

Pervan V 1993 Understanding anti-emetics. Nursing Times 89 (10) March 10: 36–38

Phillips K, Gill L 1993 A point of pressure. Nursing Times 89 (45) November 10: 44–45

Plant M 1990 Advising on alcohol. Pregnancy. Nursing Times 86 (12) March 21: 64–65

Purtell M 1994 Teenage girls' attitude to breast feeding. Health Visitor 67 (5): 156–157

Reid L 1992 Teaching what comes naturally. Breastfeeding. Nursing Times 88 (30) July 22: 45

Reilly H 1993 Role of dietary supplements in nutritional support. British Journal of Nursing 2 (11): 558, 560–562, 564, 566

Richardson N 1993 Fit for the future (Learning disabilities). Nursing. Times 89 (44) November 3: 36–38

Rogers P 1990 Using acupressure bands for postoperative nausea. Nursing Times 86 (20) May 16: 52–53

Schwarz T 1990 Bottle or breast. The first BIG decision. Nursing Times 86 (35) August 29: 63–65

Shireff A 1990 Pre-operative nutritional assessment. Nursing Times 86 (8) February 21: 68, 70, 72

Sines D 1992 Meeting the nutritional needs of people with multiple handicaps. Journal of Clinical Nursing 1 (2) March: 57

Social Survey Division 1992 Infant feeding survey 1990 (OPCS). HMSO, London

Stubbs L 1989 Taste changes in cancer patients. Nursing Times 85 (3) January 18: 49–50

Taylor M 1994 Total parenteral nutrition (Part 1). Nursing Standard 8 (23) March 2: 25–28

Thomson R 1991 Breastfeeding shame? Nursing Standard 6 (5) October 23: 42

Todd S 1992 Weaning without sugar. Nursing Times 88 (32) August 5: 27–28

Wallace E 1993 The effects of malnutrition in hospital. British Journal of Nursing 2 (1): 66–69, 71

Waller G 1991 Sexual abuse as a factor in eating disorders. British Journal of Psychiatry 159: 664–671

Watson H 1992 Identification and minimal intervention for at-risk and early problem drinkers in general hospital wards — a role for nurses? University of Strathclyde, Glasgow

Watson R 1990 Feeding patients who are demented. Nursing Standard 4 (44) July 25: 28–30

Way S 1991 Food for Asian mothers-to-be. Nursing Times 87 (49) December 4: 50, 52

Wells L 1994 At the front line of care. Nutrition in wound management. Professional Nurse 9 (8) May: 525, 526, 528–530

While A 1990 Getting it right. Community Outlook October: 14, 18

Williams C 1995 Causes and management of nausea and vomiting. Nursing Times 90 (44) November 2: 38–41

Williams G 1992 Hard to swallow. Enteral feeding. Nursing Times 88 (17) April 22: 63–65, 67

Williams J 1990 Food presentation and the terminally ill. Nursing Standard 4 (51) September 12: 29–32

World Health Organization 1992 Global programme on AIDS. WHO, Geneva

ADDITIONAL READING

Daffurn K, Hillman K L, Bauman A, Lum M, Crispin C, Ince L 1994 Fluid balance charts: do they measure up? British Journal of Nursing 3 (16) September 8–21: 816–820

Fawcett H 1991 A new specialist for nutritional care. The role of the nutrition nurse specialist. Professional Nurse 6 (5) February: 246, 248, 250

Fawcett H 1993 Interpreting a moral right. Ethical dilemmas in nutritional support for terminally ill patients. Professional Nurse 8 (6) March: 380–383

Field J 1992 A specialist role in patient nutrition. Nursing Standard 6 (38) June 10: 38–39

Holmes S 1993 Building blocks. Foods. Metabolism. Nursing Times 89 (21) May 26: 28–31

McPherson G 1993 Lifelines. Babies. Parenteral feeding. Nursing Times 89 (17) April 28: 70–72

Negus E 1994 Stroke-induced dysphagia in hospital: the nutritional perspective. British Journal of Nursing 3 (6): 263–267, 269, 270

Roberts P H 1993 Simply a case of good practice. Avoiding catheter-related sepsis in total parenteral nutrition. Professional Nurse 8 (12) September: 775, 776, 778, 779

Skelton J 1994 Dysphagia in motor neurone disease. Nursing Standard 8 (37) June 8: 57–62

Springett J, Murray C 1994 Direct input. Central line feeding for total nutrition. Nursing Times 90 (17) April 27: 48–52

Tredger J 1994 Overview of the use of therapeutic and modified diets. Nursing Times 90 (34) August 24: 46–47

Thompson J 1992 Parenteral nutrition. Nursing Times 88 (2) January 8: 62, 64

8

Eliminating

The AL of eliminating

Eliminating is an activity of living which all individuals perform with unfailing regularity throughout life. Whatever people are doing, wherever they are, and regardless of the time of day, they respond to the need to eliminate and this response is an integral activity of everyday life. One of the most interesting characteristics of this AL is that, by custom, it is performed in private. In public buildings, and even in the family home, the provision of a place affording privacy to the individual for eliminating is considered to be essential. Even in societies which emphasize the communal nature of activities of living, eliminating is normally a private activity and the products of elimination are concealed from the public eye.

So essential is eliminating that even a unicellular organism must eliminate the waste products of the metabolic processes which are constantly going on within it. In many multicellular organisms however, separate systems deal with the elimination of urine and faeces. In human beings the urinary system produces and excretes urine; whereas the large bowel or colon produces and excretes faeces — the colon has customarily been described as part of the 'digestive system' but in this text is called the defaecatory system.

In our conceptualization of nursing, the AL of eliminating is contextually related to the person's lifespan; dependence/independence status; the biological, psychological, sociocultural, environmental and politicoeconomic factors influencing it; producing individuality in carrying out this AL, which is the basis for individualizing nursing by assessing, planning, implementing and evaluating (Fig. 8.1).

Lifespan: relationship to the AL of eliminating

The lifespan clearly has relevance to eliminating and as a component of the model will now be focused to this AL.

Eliminating is so necessary that the newborn baby excretes waste matter (meconium) from the bowel, and urine from the urinary bladder shortly after birth by reflex (involuntary) response to a stretch stimulus from fullness in the

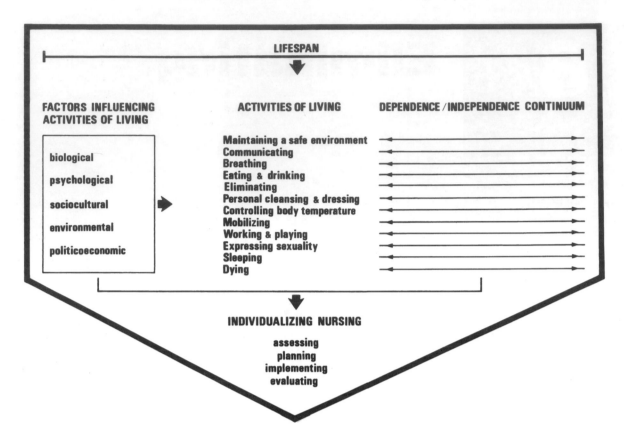

Fig. 8.1 The AL of eliminating within the model for nursing

bowel and bladder. Eventually voluntary control over reflex evacuation of the bladder and bowel is achieved.

Infancy and childhood

An important milestone in childhood is the acquisition of voluntary control over elimination. Although toilet training helps the child to learn to recognize the signals of the need to eliminate, it cannot really hasten the development of voluntary control because this is dependent on maturation of the required components of the nervous and musculoskeletal systems and learning ability.

The time to start toilet training a child depends partly on age, and partly on each individual child's 'readiness' to begin. One of the first indicators of 'readiness' for toilet training is awareness of having a full bladder. Soon the child begins to warn the mother that the potty is needed and at this stage can begin to do without nappies during the day. Control over defaecation is gained before control over urinary elimination.

By 3 years of age many children can go to the toilet on their own and are beginning to be able to do without toileting during the night. Children of 4 are usually competent in the social skills associated with elimination and, by school age, have developed independence and also a feeling of desire for privacy while eliminating.

Gradually when children have gained control of both

activities they can make decisions for themselves about where and when they will eliminate. Sometimes children may misuse these newly acquired skills to manipulate the parents, for example by 'wetting' to attract attention, or by referring to eliminating activities in company to cause embarrassment. Attitudes develop not only to the activities, but also to the products of the activities. Whereas society's attitude to ingestion of food is that it is pleasant, desirable and in the main carried out in the company of others; its attitude to elimination of the waste from food — faeces — is that it is unpleasant, sometimes offensive, intensely personal and carried out in privacy.

Adults and elderly people

The majority of adults can cope with the AL of eliminating even in diverse circumstances, for example while travelling when available toilet accommodation may not coincide with their normal pattern, or indeed may be different. Toward the end of the lifespan, eliminating habits established in childhood may undergo change. Often in the process of ageing the bladder loses its tone, and the kidneys become less efficient, so that older people sometimes need to eliminate smaller amounts of urine at a more frequent time interval than when younger. The process of ageing can also manifest in the bowel as sluggishness of muscular action and there can be decrease in the volume of faeces as many older people eat less; these conditions can predispose to chronic constipation.

Dependence/ independence in the AL of eliminating

The concept of lifespan is clearly relevant to the concept of dependence/independence for eliminating. For everyone there is a *natural dependence* in the early years and for some there is a return to a varying level of dependence in the later years. There are others who are not capable of achieving independence as they progress through the stages of the lifespan because of congenital conditions as diverse as abnormality of the bowel or bladder, of the nerves supplying them, or physical abnormality of the limbs, or learning disability.

Anywhere along the lifespan people's dependence/ independence status can change because of trauma to, or disease of, the bowel or urinary system, or indeed the cause may be in the nervous system. Because the AL of mobilizing is a necessary part of eliminating, trauma or disease affecting the musculoskeletal system can also change a person's status on the dependence/independence continuum for the AL of eliminating.

The concept of 'aided independence' is applicable to eliminating. People who experience physical decline in advancing years can be helped to retain their 'independence' by provision of a grab rail near the toilet to help them regain the standing position. Should there be stiffness of the hips which makes sitting difficult, a removable raised toilet seat can be used.

Factors influencing the AL of eliminating

So far two components of the model — the lifespan and the dependence/independence continuum — have been described in their relationship to the AL of eliminating. Here, the third component, 'Factors influencing the ALs', will be focused to eliminating; the factors are biological, psychological, socioeconomic, environmental and politicoeconomic and they will be described in that order.

BIOLOGICAL

The main purpose of eliminating urine is to dispose of unrequired fluid intake and dissolved chemicals which the body cells are not immediately requiring (and which cannot be stored) so that the body is correctly hydrated, in electrolyte balance and thereby in overall acid/base balance. The main purpose of excreting faeces is to rid the body of indigestible cellulose and unabsorbed food but faeces also contains shed endothelial cells, intestinal secretions, water and bacteria. The nature of the products of eliminating — urine and faeces — will now be discussed.

Urine

Urine is secreted throughout the 24 hours but production slows during sleep, and voiding is usually unnecessary during that period; so the first urine voided on waking is normally darker in colour due to its concentration. Otherwise the colour ranges from amber to straw-coloured.

Urine has a specific gravity of between 1.015 and 1.025 and is normally acidic with a pH (a hydrogen ion concentration) of about 6. It is composed of about 96% water, 2% salts (especially sodium and potassium) and 2% nitrogenous waste (urea). When recently voided it has only a slight smell but after exposure to air, it decomposes and begins to smell of ammonia.

A high fluid intake results in a high urine output and vice versa. However, the normal urine output is around 1 to 1½ litres in 24 hours; the usual frequency of micturition is from 5 to 10 times in that period.

Faeces

The first stool of the infant is a sticky, greenish-black substance called meconium which has accumulated in the bowel from about the fifth month of prenatal development. This consists of mucus, endothelial cells, amniotic fluid, bile pigments and fats. Meconium is passed several times in the first days of life. Then a brownish-green stool is passed and, a few days later, the baby's excreta become yellow in colour. A breast-fed baby has softer, brighter yellow stools than a bottle-fed baby whose stools are paler, more formed and with a slightly offensive smell. Once the infant is weaned and beginning to have a balanced diet of normal foodstuffs, the faeces begin to take on their familiar composition.

Faecal matter in the adult is normally brown in colour, soft in consistency and cylindrical in form. There is an odour from faeces due to the action of bacterial flora in the intestine and the smell varies according to the bacteria present and the type of food ingested. Faeces are normally composed of water (75%) and solid matter (25%) made up of quantities of dead bacteria, some fatty acids, inorganic matter, proteins and undigested dietary fibre. With regard to number and size of stools, the collection of epidemiological information shows that people in rural third world countries excrete two stools a day with a total weight of between 300 and 500 g, whereas the average for people in Western society is one stool daily weighing between 80 and 120 g (Burkitt, 1983).

In Burkitt's reference it is also stated that the time taken from ingestion of food to its output as faeces is termed 'intestinal transit time'. Again there is difference in this time between people in rural third world countries and Western societies — approximately 1–1½ days in the former; and about 3 days in young healthy adults in the latter, the time increasing in the elderly to 2 weeks. If carcinogens are formed in the bowel, their contact with the lining membrane will be minimized by rapid transit time.

An acid stool is produced by bacteria breaking down the unabsorbed dietary fibre, and faecal acidity is thought to be one of the factors which reduces the amount of potential carcinogens in the bowel.

It is likely that in the next few years more information will be available about the function of faeces in preventing not only bowel disease, but also disease in other parts of the body. This shows very clearly the importance of constant updating of knowledge.

The physical act of eliminating

To be able to eliminate in the normal way a person has to have fully functioning urinary and defaecatory systems. This not only means intactness of the organs comprising these systems but also of the sensory and motor nerves supplying them. Beginning students will acquire detailed knowledge of these body structures and functions in the biology component of the curriculum; it is important to integrate and synthesize the acquired knowledge into the 'nursing component'. Such knowledge of biology is necessary not only for understanding the pathological conditions which can occur in these systems, and the effect which they can have on the AL of eliminating; but also for understanding the nursing interventions ensuing from medical prescription for investigation and treatment of the pathology.

Gender influences this AL since usually men stand while passing urine and women sit; this is taken into consideration when providing facilities, particularly in public buildings.

However, the AL of eliminating involves much more than simply the physical acts of micturition and defaecation. The person must be able to reach the toilet (which often is situated upstairs in homes and public buildings), to adjust clothing, to sit on a toilet and rise from it. Post-elimination hygiene too, including the use of toilet paper and handwashing, has to be carried out. It is apparent that eliminating is closely related to the equally complex AL of mobilizing.

PSYCHOLOGICAL

A minimum level of intellectual ability is required to learn the many skills involved in eliminating. If the learning is started too early or is very strict some people think that it can contribute to a rigid personality.

If people are to achieve and maintain a healthy state of eliminating they require knowledge about the relationship of this AL to the amount of fluid taken into and lost from the body; the amount of fibre in the diet, and the type of exercise to keep the abdominal and pelvic floor muscles effective in the act of eliminating.

A person's attitudes and beliefs about this AL may well influence the way it is carried out. For example in a public toilet some people never sit on the 'communal' seat, as they believe that it can carry infection; others flush the cistern to drown the noise of their own eliminating.

The development of concepts of modesty and privacy are also important to enable a person to appreciate and conform to the prevailing social customs.

Certain emotions may affect the AL of eliminating. Most people have experienced the urgent need to empty the bladder when facing a stressful situation such as an examination. On the other hand depression often causes apathy and sluggishness and this can influence eliminating, usually resulting in constipation.

SOCIOCULTURAL

The fact that different words are used in different cultures for the process and products of eliminating is interesting. Alternatives such as nappy or diaper tend to be perpetuated from one generation to the next. Likewise the names used for the products of elimination are important, and those used by one cultural group might be considered vulgar by another. Indeed even within a culture, different words may be used by those in different social classes; and in many instances it is family convention which influences the words used. When children first start school they may well be exposed to those from a mix of social classes and as they discover some of these differences they may need help in continuing to use the words selected as family convention.

The child is eventually able to go to the particular place provided for eliminating and gradually there is socialization according to the concept of privacy and modesty for this AL. There can be differences in the name given to this place, and while the word 'toilet' has a wide acceptance, others such as lavatory and bathroom are used. In most cultures there are 'public toilets' or 'conveniences' for use by people who are away from home and they are usually labelled separately for males and females.

Some strict post-elimination activities are specified by several religions and are transmitted to each succeeding generation. Of course it is desirable that everyone is socialized into acquiring adequate and safe hygiene activities related to eliminating in the interest of preventing infection, particularly the diarrhoeal diseases.

ENVIRONMENTAL

It is all too easy for those who are used to flush toilets which are attached to a water carriage system of sewage disposal to think that these are the norm. But in some parts of the world people arc fortunate if they have chemical toilets, or indeed latrines (earth toilets) which will be discussed in the politicoeconomic section. All three types are designed so that the person can sit on them, but in some countries it is customary to provide a toilet which is a hole in the ground filled with water, on either side of which are foot plates, and elimination is achieved in the squatting position which is functionally efficient. In some parts of the world there is no amenity and people 'go into the bush' to defaecate where the surrounding earth may be too hard and dry to be scooped to cover the faeces; it is therefore an attraction for flies which can transmit infection to food causing one of the diarrhoeal diseases.

Whether or not an inside toilet is available in a home will obviously influence several aspects of this AL. Most homes have only one toilet and it may be within the bathroom or separate from it. If separate, unless the room has handwashing facilities within it, it may be less easy to uphold standards of hygiene. This applies equally if members of several households have to share a toilet which is not within the home. If to reach the toilet one has to go right outside, then in bad weather the feeling of the need to defaecate may go unheeded which could predispose to constipation.

POLITICOECONOMIC

It is difficult for us to realize that only a little more than 100 years ago cholera was rife in the UK and still is in some parts of the world. Mortality and morbidity from the diarrhoeal diseases of typhoid, paratyphoid, the dysenteries and enteritis was, and in some countries still is, high. The realization in the first half of the century that there is a faecal-oral route for spread of such infection led to the increasing introduction of water carriage systems of sewage disposal resulting in a gradual reduction in the incidence of diseases spread by this route. Of course such schemes cost money, and they are dependent on decisions made by a country's government.

In developing countries where the financial budget is not considered sufficient to warrant the implementation of an extensive water carriage system of sewage disposal (the water may not be available), local people in the villages are being encouraged to construct earth toilets. Some countries are using their economic aid from other countries to accelerate this programme in an attempt to

achieve the World Health Organization's goal 'Health for all by the year 2000'.

In many countries there is legislation about for example the sanitary requirements for campsites, public toilets, and toilets in public buildings. Minimally, cold water has to be provided for post-elimination handwashing in an attempt to prevent outbreaks of the diarrhoeal diseases. Providing water at a temperature higher than that which can comfortably be borne by the human hand can render the supplier vulnerable to prosecution should there be a scalding accident.

Individualizing nursing for the AL of eliminating

Individualizing nursing for this AL can only be accomplished by discovering a person's individual eliminating habits together with that person's attitudes and beliefs related to the AL of eliminating. This information can be collected in the assessing phase of the process of nursing which is an integral part of our conceptualization of nursing. Taking advantage of what has been discussed so far in this chapter, we have prepared an aide-memoire for the initial assessment (Box 8.1).

ASSESSING THE INDIVIDUAL IN THE AL

The majority of people enter the health service at primary level where they come into contact with nurses at various clinics. Consultation time is usually limited and conversation focused to the title of the clinic so that assessing the AL of eliminating may not have a high priority, even although some attenders may be experiencing a problem, for example constipation. Therefore realistically it is mainly nurses providing a service to people in their own homes, in hospital (particularly long-stay wards) or in nursing homes who are likely to fully assess this AL.

It is important that during an episode of illness the person's individual habits of eliminating are changed as little as possible, unless they are detrimental to health. It is therefore imperative that nurses know about these individual habits and use this knowledge to implement an individualized nursing plan. The information can be gleaned by nurses bearing in mind the topics noted in the preceding résumé while discussing the AL of eliminating with the person. It is useful, particularly during the initial assessment phase of the process of nursing if the nurse has in mind the following questions:

- how often and when does the individual eliminate urine/faeces?
- what factors influence the way the individual carries out the AL of eliminating?

Box 8.1 Assessing the individual in the AL of eliminating

Lifespan: effect on eliminating

- Involuntary voiding in infancy
- Childhood training for continence
- Loss of muscle tone in old age

Dependence/independence in eliminating

- Relevant to lifespan
- Congenital conditions
- Disease/trauma
- Dependence on aids/on people
- Total dependence

Factors influencing eliminating

- Biological
  - — fully functioning urinary and defaecatory systems
  - — ability to reach the toilet, manipulate clothing, carry out post-eliminating toilet, wash hands
- Psychological
  - — intellectual ability
  - — concept of modesty, privacy
  - — response to toilet training
  - — attitude to eliminating
- Sociocultural
  - — knowledge about diet/eliminating
  - — word for products of elimination
  - — cultural group/social class/family convention
  - — word for place of eliminating
  - — post-elimination hygiene/religion
- Environmental
  - — type of toilet
  - — handwashing facilities
- Politicoeconomic
  - — money available for prevention of diarrhoeal diseases

- what does the individual know about eliminating urine/faeces and post-eliminating hygiene?
- what is the individual's attitude to eliminating?
- has the individual any longstanding problems with eliminating urine and faeces, and if so, how have these been coped with?
- what problems if any does the individual have at present with eliminating urine/faeces and are any likely to develop?

The emphasis during assessment is on the discovery of the patient's usual routines, determining what can be done independently and noting exactly what cannot be done independently, and any coping mechanisms that have been used previously for problems or discomforts which might well be of a chronic or recurring nature. Relevant information from medical records will be noted to avoid duplication. In collaboration with the person whenever possible, any actual problems with the AL of eliminating will be identified.

The nurse may well recognize potential problems which may or may not be recognized by the person and these will of course be discussed with the person. Mutual realistic goals will be set, to prevent potential problems from becoming actual ones; to alleviate or solve the actual problems; or help the person cope with those which cannot be alleviated or solved.

The nursing interventions and when relevant any activities which the person agrees to do to achieve the set goals will be selected according to local circumstances and available resources. These will be written on the nursing plan together with the date on which evaluation will be carried out to discern whether or not they are achieving or have achieved the stated goals. As the interventions are implemented, it will be written in the patient's nursing notes. All these activities are necessary in order to carry out individualized nursing related to the AL of eliminating.

IDENTIFYING ACTUAL AND POTENTIAL PROBLEMS

However, before nurses can begin to think in terms of individualized nursing they need to have a generalized idea of the kind of problems which people can experience related to the AL of eliminating. These will be discussed together with relevant nursing activities which are encountered early in a nursing career. They are grouped together under four headings:

- change of dependence/independence status for eliminating
- change in eliminating habit
- change in mode of eliminating
- change of environment and routine.

CHANGE OF DEPENDENCE/INDEPENDENCE STATUS

The concept of a dependence/independence continuum is useful when focused to the AL of eliminating because movement can be in either direction. Many people are only temporarily dependent on the nurse for example for giving an enema and they quickly regain independence. On the other hand when a person succumbs to disease of the urinary or defaecatory system the dependence may be for information and advice about the condition; it may be about short-term changes, for example in diet and fluid intake and how abatement of the condition can be evaluated until the previous state of independence has been regained.

Availability of public toilets

In recent years another dimension of dependence has been recognized. People who develop urge incontinence of urine, become dependent on the availability of public toilets when they are, for instance, out shopping. There are three million people in the UK who have continence problems (Langford, 1994), but the Market and Operational Research Institute (MORI, 1991), after extensive polling estimated the number as 10.5 million. It can be assumed that another group that will be dependent on public toilets will be the homeless. Local authorities do not have a duty to provide public toilets, and Langford (1994) says that one third have been closed over the past decade. An organization has been formed to campaign for sufficient toilets and the subject has been discussed by the government (Pottle, 1994a).

Inadequacy of hospital toilets

There are inadequacies in hospital toilets 'which could result in loss of patients' independence' (Travers, Burns, Penn et al, 1992). In a survey of hospital toilets, none of them met the recommendations set by the British Standards Institute. They were too narrow, did not have rails or alarms; they were neither signposted nor labelled and did not have non-slip floors.

For other people, the change in dependence/independence status can be caused by limited mobility, confinement to bed, psychological disturbance, learning disability and unconsciousness. These will now be discussed.

Limited mobility

As mentioned earlier (p. 202) several physical skills are involved in the AL of eliminating. Any limitation on mobilizing obviously reduces a person's potential for independence. A person who is unable to walk easily, or for any distance, will have difficulty in getting to and from the toilet, especially one which is situated upstairs or outside. Someone with an arm in plaster or with hands badly affected by arthritis has a different problem. That person will be able to get to the toilet but may be unable to undress and dress or use toilet paper.

Those confined to a wheelchair may have problems when having to rely on public toilets unless there are facilities specially designed with an entrance ramp and the cubicle door wide enough to allow the wheelchair through. Also many people with severe disabilities are unable to leave their wheelchairs quickly enough, or often enough to use a toilet (Fader, 1994). Her article illustrates eight resources which can be used to enable hygienic micturition while remaining in the wheelchair, thus facilitating 'aided independence' for outings to the theatre and other public places.

Particular problems arise for the person in hospital whose mobility is completely restricted on account of confinement to bed.

Confinement to bed

When for any reason confinement to bed is prolonged, there may be loss of tone in the gastrointestinal and trunk muscles which may predispose to constipation. Urinary stasis can occur especially if the person is nursed in the supine position, since urinary flow from the kidneys to the bladder is assisted by the force of gravity. The attendant sluggish flow of urine is conducive to the formation of stones (calculi). In addition, when there is reduced muscular activity, there are fewer acid waste products in the urine so it tends to be alkaline — another condition which favours stone formation.

Nursing activities include supervising an adequate fluid and dietary fibre intake and encouraging the person to use all muscles as much as possible. Some people may require help from the physiotherapist in learning to exercise their abdominal and pelvic floor muscles.

People confined to bed or the bedside area may be totally dependent on the nurse or carer for help with the AL of eliminating. Unless a person is too ill or incapacitated to move, a commode at the bedside causes no more cardiovascular stress than using a bedpan. However in a community-based study, 140 commode-users and 105 carers were interviewed at home. The users' independence was assessed and on various criteria commode use was unacceptable (Naylor & Mulley, 1993).

Being perched on a bedpan is not very comfortable and it is almost impossible for a woman to use toilet paper to dry the perineum without her hand coming into contact with the urine in the pan. Handwashing facilities or moist finger wipes must be provided. Frequent removal of transient hand flora is the single most important method of infection control (p. 94).

However, there are people for whom there is no alternative to a bedpan, such as those on traction, or attached to monitors. They need to be helped on and off the bedpan (remembering the 'safe handling' advocated on p. 303) and the nurse needs to carry out post-elimination hygiene in such a way as to minimize their embarrassment because they probably have not been helped in this way since they were small children.

Whether using a bedpan or a commode at the bedside, people will probably experience embarrassment knowing that the bedcurtains do not mask either smell or noise when urine, faeces and flatus are being passed. Whenever possible it would seem to be desirable to transfer patients to the toilet in a wheelchair or a Sanichair.

Psychological disturbance

Various mental abilities are necessary for people to appreciate and conform to the various social customs associated with elimination. Knowledge is also needed to understand the importance of disposing of excreta hygienically, to recognize abnormalities of urine and faeces which may indicate the presence of disease, and to prevent the occurrence of problems such as constipation and urinary infection.

Psychological disturbance which results in confusion, depression or disorientation may mean that people do not remember, for example, when they last went to toilet, so they may keep returning absent-mindedly or else forget to go again when necessary. Other people become incontinent because they fail to recognize the signals of a full bladder or rectum, or recognizing them, fail to respond to them. Sometimes people who are disorientated, particularly at night, cannot find their way to the toilet and others may be so confused that they eliminate indiscriminately in their beds or on the floor.

Learning disability

People who have a learning disability are by definition slow learners. At one time their incontinence was accepted as inevitable. However, many of them are now helped to achieve both urinary and faecal continence by the use of behavioural modification techniques which are mentioned on p. 214.

Unconsciousness

Loss of consciousness results in loss of the ability to respond to a full bladder or bowel and the unconscious person becomes totally dependent on others for ensuring that urine and faeces are removed and disposed of. The nurse should carry this out in a manner that acknowledges the human dignity of the unconscious person. Some unconscious people become dependent on a closed urinary drainage system (p. 219), and the addition of a stool softener to the enteral feed (p. 191), or the parenteral feed (p. 191).

Pain related to eliminating

Pain inevitably causes some movement towards the dependent pole for the AL. The general discussion of pain is on p. 130; here it will be focused to the AL of eliminat-

ing, and considered as pain which can be experienced in any part of the urinary or defaecatory systems. The pain from an overfull bladder, and pain experienced when trying to expel hard, dry faeces have already been mentioned.

Dysuria Dysuria is the name given to painful micturition. The problem for the patient is a burning sensation as urine is passed and a constant feeling of an overfull bladder and a frequent urge to pass urine. There may be a constant dull ache in the groin. The person may be able to help with assessing/measuring the pain by keeping a diary of how it is being experienced and when. Some preventive and comforting activities for this condition are mentioned on p. 232 in the context of perineal toilet.

Ureteric colic Ureteric colic is usually caused by a stone moving in one of the ureters and the muscular contractions on, and the irritation caused by the stone produces the patient's problems which are excruciating pain, restlessness and sweating. The condition usually constitutes an emergency admission to hospital where muscle relaxant and pain killing medicines will be prescribed by the doctor unless surgery is imminent when the prescription will be for preoperative medications.

Tenesmus Tenesmus is the medical name for painful, ineffectual straining to empty the bowel. People with this problem should be advised to seek medical help because the cause can be as diverse as proctitis, prolapse of the rectum, rectal tumour or irritable bowel syndrome. Meantime, a warm bath may be comforting.

Flatulence Flatulence is gaseous intestinal distension. The intestinal flora produce some gas which is normally expelled per rectum. Some people experience excessive gas production which can be embarrassing as it produces borborygmi — rumbling noises caused by the movement of gas in the intestines; it can also cause abdominal distension which can be painful. It can sometimes be moved towards the rectum by contraction of the abdominal muscles. Carminatives taken orally may be effective, the most usual one being peppermint in the form of sweets or peppermint water; others are cinnamon, cloves, ginger and nutmeg. Sometimes a warm bath can result in the passing of flatus.

Alternatively a long hollow lubricated tube can be passed along the colon while the free end is immersed in water, through which the flatus can be seen to bubble (Jamieson et al, 1992). This is an intimate procedure and patients require not only an explanation of what to expect, but also an empathetic approach by nursing staff.

Haemorrhoidal pain Haemorrhoidal pain is increased on defaecation. Haemorrhoids ('piles') are dilations of the terminal parts of the veins which lie in the submucosa of the anal canal. The doctor can prescribe medication, which when applied locally reduces the inflammation and discomfort. People can buy rectal suppositories for this condition at a chemist's shop/drug store. A doctor's prescription is not required and they are

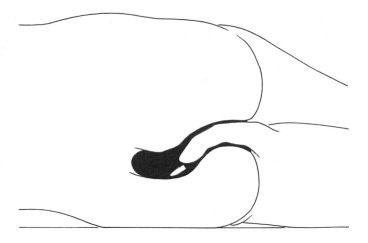

Fig. 8.2 Left lateral position for insertion of a suppository

classified as 'over the counter' medicaments. They are inserted via the anus (Fig. 8.2). They are cone-shaped and common sense would suggest insertion of the conical end first, but findings from a research project carried out in Egypt and summarized in the Nursing Times (1992c) suggest that base-foremost is more effective. Bleeding piles are recognized by the passage of fresh blood at the end of defaecation. Prolapsed piles constitute a surgical emergency; the application of a cold compress may provide some relief pending admission to hospital.

Constipation predisposes to haemorrhoids: should a nursing assessment reveal this problem it is pertinent to enquire what the person knows about constipation/piles/diet/exercise. A teaching/learning programme may need to be planned, implemented and evaluated. The desired outcome would be a biological change to evacuation of soft bulky faeces.

Postoperative pain Postoperative pain on defaecation is feared by many people after abdominal or urogenital operations and this may predispose to the problem of constipation. Discomfort will be alleviated to some extent by ensuring that faeces are soft and as easy as possible to pass without straining. The person can also be advised to lean forward while sitting on the toilet, folding the arms against the abdomen to give support to the wound and increase intra-abdominal pressure.

Anxiety about investigations/surgery

In the diagnosis of the cause of a problem related to eliminating, the doctor may require to carry out certain medical investigations many of which, being concerned with intimate parts of the body, are anxiety-producing and distressing for patients. The fact that patients do experience discomfort and anxiety related to investigations was highlighted several years ago by Wilson-Barnett (1980). She points out that the level of anxiety is not necessarily related to the seriousness or invasiveness of the particular

test and urges nurses to pay attention to the feelings of individual people. The research also attempted to assess whether information and explanations about scheduled investigations would reduce anxiety. Barium enema was one of the investigations studied and it was found that explanation of the preparation for, and procedure of, a barium enema did help to make the person feel less anxious.

Evacuant enemas An evacuant enema is still, in some hospitals, part of the routine preoperative preparation for surgery not involving the urinary and defaecatory systems. However, with the emphasis on holistic medicine it is gradually becoming a more selective procedure. There are a number of disposable evacuant enemas available; the microenema contains 5 ml of fluid and the hypertonic saline enemas contain 128 ml. Either, or both of these may be medically prescribed and thereafter, planning, implementing, evaluating and documenting the intervention is a nursing responsibility.

The administration of evacuant enema prior to labour has become a controversial subject and many women are becoming more voluble about their objections. However, studies reveal that some women are so anxious about soiling during labour that they prefer to have an enema. The state of the bowel must be assessed for each woman in labour and a mutual decision made as to whether or not an enema will be given.

Rectal lavage When investigation or surgery involves the defaecatory system it is obviously necessary to remove faeces from the bowel, and the enemas just mentioned may suffice or they may be combined with rectal lavage. This involves passing a wide bore catheter into the rectum through which a funnel full of water runs and is then returned into a bucket on the floor by lowering and inverting the funnel over it. This process is repeated until the returned fluid is clear and free from faecal flakes or stain and it can take up to 1 hour to achieve this.

Whole gut irrigation Another bowel preparation introduced in the 1970s is whole gut irrigation. From a flask containing either saline or mannitol, fluid drips through a nasogastric tube into the stomach while the patient sits on a commode for several hours. It is regarded as the most efficient remover of faeces from the gut but there are some adverse physiological changes and lack of patient acceptability.

Barium enema Some of these various methods are used prior to a barium enema and a low residue diet is often prescribed for the previous few days. Patients need to understand that another enema containing barium will be administered in the X-ray department and that after the X-rays are taken they can go immediately to the toilet to get rid of most of the heavy white chalk-like substance. Any residual barium will be passed in the next stool and the nurse needs to know and document when and how often there is a bowel movement. Many people remain as 'out patients' while bowel investigations are carried out. They receive a written preparatory programme. It is a nursing responsibility to evaluate that the instructions have been understood.

Sigmoidoscopy Sigmoidoscopy usually requires some bowel preparation and possibly dietary modification before passage of a tube-like instrument into the bowel via the anus, through which the rectum and sigmoid colon can be viewed. The actual procedure is uncomfortable rather than painful, but understandably some people find it difficult to relax the anus in the presence of others. Sigmoidoscopy is gradually being replaced by colonoscopy for which whole gut irrigation is usually necessary. The new fibreoptic colonoscopes can be manoeuvred through the colon to the caecum; light is transmitted by means of very fine glass fibres; photography and biopsy can be carried out if necessary. Whole gut irrigation, mentioned previously, is being done increasingly prior to any form of colorectal surgery.

Bowel preparation for urinary investigation Bowel preparation may be necessary when investigating urinary problems, because of the proximity of the colon. If the kidneys and ureters require to be X-rayed, an empty bowel as well as an intravenous injection of a radiopaque fluid gives a clearer X-ray. Many patients will not connect these procedures with investigation of their urinary problem, so they need an explanation. However, the radiopaque liquid may be injected directly into the renal pelvis by way of a fine catheter introduced through a cystoscope, an instrument which is introduced into the bladder via the urethra, and obviously patients require a different explanation in preparation for such an intimate procedure. It may be the bladder which has to be investigated after it has been filled with a radiopaque liquid introduced via a urethral catheter (see catheterization p. 219). Or the examination may involve a micturating cystogram in which, after injection of a radiopaque liquid, sequential X-rays are taken during micturition. This can be part of an investigation into urinary incontinence, when an already demoralized person requires extra psychological support. It may be provided by explanation of what to expect, and how the knowledge gained from breaking the social convention of privacy when passing urine, will enable realistic planning of interventions to relieve the distressing incontinence.

Change of dependence/independence status is a useful broad classification which helps nurses to identify people's actual and potential problems with the AL of eliminating. Change in eliminating habit is another classification and it will now be discussed.

CHANGE IN ELIMINATING HABIT

Even if conscious, deliberate attention were not paid, for example to how frequently the bladder was emptied, a person probably would experience a problem if there were a marked increase or decrease in the frequency of passing urine and faeces. Should there be a marked change in the colour, odour or consistency of either urine or faeces a person would be likely to notice it too.

As changes in eliminating habit are often indicators of some dysfunction of the urinary or defaecatory systems (or even other body systems) nurses have a responsibility to be able to recognize any change in a person's urine or its elimination, and faeces and their elimination. Recognition of changes is only possible if the nurse understands what constitutes 'normal' and has data from assessment on the individual person's norm.

Changes in urine and its elimination

Change in colour Several factors can cause a change in colour, sometimes transient and not necessarily pathological.

Pale urine may be due to temporary diuresis as a result of excessive fluid intake, or it can result from taking a diuretic drug, or it may be of a continuous nature as in the condition of diabetes mellitus.

Dark urine may mean that it is concentrated as a result of dehydration (p. 189) when less urine is excreted; the colour will lighten as the person increases fluid intake. Or it may be caused by the presence of bile pigments (urobilin or bilirubin) due to disease of the liver or gallbladder. The urine will become pigment-free as the disease responds to treatment.

Coloured urine can result from the intake of some foods. Carotene contained in carrots as well as other vegetables and fruits can make urine a bright yellow; beetroot and blackberries can make the urine red.

Medications can also change the colour of urine; an antibiotic called rifamycin makes it an orange-red colour. Naturally, people should be warned about this.

A smoky colour is indicative of 'occult' (hidden) blood from high in the urinary tract; it is so mixed with the urine that it has lost its identity as blood. On the other hand, urine which is red from frank blood usually means that the bleeding is lower in the urinary tract.

For students who require further information about colour changes in urine, Ford (1992) produced a four column table, the headings being — Colour, Drugs, Food, Disease/Condition.

Change in odour The characteristic odour of urine may change to sweet-smelling, a manifestation of diabetes mellitus. Part of the treatment of diabetic people is teaching them to test their urine to make sure that it does not contain excess glucose. Decomposing urine smells like ammonia. An infected urine has an offensive fishy smell, and there may be frank pus (pyuria) in the case of severe urinary infection. The person may need to increase perineal hygiene (p. 232), and be meticulous about changing underwear to prevent odour. In the case of dependent people this of course would be a nursing activity.

Change in frequency A change in the number of times a person passes urine may or may not be accompanied by an alteration in the total amount of urine voided in 24 hours and accurate data from intake and output charts are required to establish this.

Increased frequency can vary from that due to the anxiety associated with admission to hospital, and special procedures, tests and so on, to a totally demanding 'urgency' that dominates the person's life, even disturbing sleep. This type is a very disabling condition. It is often a manifestation of urinary infection (cystitis), a common problem of women and older people.

Many of the women are in the 20 to 50 age group who are sexually active. 'Honeymoon cystitis' is in the lay vocabulary. There are some self-help procedures which can be carried out to minimize cystitis after sexual intercourse (Gibbons, 1990).

The frequent voiding of small amounts of urine, although an inconvenience to the person, is actually helpful in combating the infection. The pathogenic microorganisms are not allowed to remain for long in the urinary tract and so excessive multiplication is prevented. When increased frequency of micturition in an older person is not due to urinary infection, it may be attributed to loss of muscle elasticity reducing sphincter control or deterioration in cerebral function.

Decreased frequency is closely associated with decreased output and it can result from obstruction, water retention (oedema), kidney disease and dehydration. It is particularly important for nurses to recognize decreased frequency in older people, since impairment of their thirst mechanism can put them at risk of dehydration. If suspected, the nurse can examine the lips and mouth for dryness, another clue to dehydration (p. 189).

Change in quantity Marked deviation from a person's norm is dangerous because it can result in fluid imbalance. As soon as ongoing assessment reveals a change, the nursing plan will request measuring of the fluid intake and output. This is a nursing initiative but depending on competence, the person may be able to help with the measuring and recording on a fluid balance chart.

A decreased output (oliguria) or total absence of urine (anuria) indicates that either urine is not being produced normally by the kidneys as in renal failure, or that its excretion from the bladder is being blocked. In the case of blockage which can be caused by prostatic enlargement, there is retention of urine in the bladder causing a midline abdominal swelling over which there is a dull sound on percussion. It is potentially dangerous and most uncomfortable; indeed, it can be very painful. Sometimes the pressure in the overfull bladder forces urine through the urethral sphincters when the condition is referred to

as 'retention with overflow'. Because of the mechanical nature of the blockage, the bladder has to be drained by a catheter (p. 219). The condition can also arise postoperatively when some patients experience difficulty in re-establishing micturition and it is standard practice for the nurse to document whether or not the patient has passed urine early in the postoperative period.

An increased output can be expected when people are taking diuretic pills, their purpose being to increase urinary output in people with oedema. Many of these people are treated at primary level so the nursing assessment should include toilet facilities available in the home to cope with increased frequency of micturition (Jay, 1989). Several of the hypotensive drugs are combined with a diuretic, and nurses need to be aware of this when planning individualized nursing for patients with high blood pressure. Over 2 litres in 24 hours constitutes a pathologically increased output of urine (polyuria). This condition is often associated with excessive thirst (polydipsia) and increased fluid intake, characteristic of the diabetic condition.

Collecting specimens of urine

This is a common nursing activity but the nurse should remember that it is probably a new experience for the patient. Careful instruction is therefore necessary and ascertainment of whether or not it has been understood. Explanation of the reason for the procedure will help the person to accept it, and of course privacy and dignity should be maintained throughout.

Mainstream specimens A specimen of urine can be collected in a clean container at any time — in the toilet at home, in a health clinic, outpatients' department or a hospital ward. Unless the urine has to be cultured for the presence of microorganisms it is not usually necessary for this to be mainstream urine (Nursing Times, 1992b). 'Mainstream' means that the first flow is passed into the toilet, the mainstream of approximately 30 ml is collected in the clean container, and the remainder passed into the toilet. It is necessary for the nurse to know whether or not a woman is menstruating, as if so, it may give a false-positive reading for blood in the urine.

Midstream specimen A midstream specimen of urine is collected when bacteriological examination in the laboratory is necessary to confirm or deny the presence of pathogenic microorganisms, and to identify their sensitivity to different antibiotics. Obviously the goal is to collect urine which is uncontaminated by microorganisms from the lower end of the urethra and the perineum. To accomplish this, the first flow is passed into the toilet (or other vessel), the midstream of approximately 30 ml is passed into a sterile jar and the remainder into the toilet. A research report states that vulval cleaning with swabs and soapy water prior to taking midstream urine specimens for laboratory culture, provided no more reliable results than specimens obtained without preparation (Baerheim et al, 1992). From their eight month study of 110 women who each provided eight consecutive early morning samples following different instructions, there was a highly significant result for no cleansing but holding the labia apart during micturition and catching the midstream flow.

Brown, Meikle and Webb (1991) analysed the content of medical and nursing articles published between 1956 and 1989 about collecting midstream specimens. From the analysis they were unable to define a standard method and stated '. . . the practice is still more affected by traditions, myths and assumptions than it is by research evidence'. Baerheim et al's results should help to remedy this.

However, health authorities vary as to instruction about this procedure. Should an antiseptic be advocated for pre-specimen swabbing, then the area must be thoroughly rinsed to prevent any of it contaminating the specimen, there to continue its bactericidal action resulting in a false report.

Procuring urine specimens from babies is notoriously difficult. A leakproof nappy is available, which on trial resulted in satisfactory specimens from babies in hospital and at home, in the first 6 weeks after birth (Goodinson, 1986). It can be used for a random specimen, or for a 24-hour specimen, explained below.

Early morning specimen of urine As the name implies it is the first urine excreted in the morning: it is more concentrated than daytime urine and is particularly useful for pregnancy tests and tuberculosis tests.

24-hour collection of urine Required when the test involves detection of a substance which is not secreted at an even rate throughout the 24 hours. The first urine passed at, for example 08.00 hours, is discarded. All urine is collected in a vessel, from which it is poured into a large container. At 08.00 hours the next day, the bladder is emptied and the urine added to the collection. For some tests, the contents of the container are stirred and a specimen poured into a glass jar for transfer to the laboratory. In other instances the container and its contents are sent to the laboratory.

Strict cleanliness is essential when collecting any of these specimens. When urine is being collected for bacteriological culture, there is a danger of the hands becoming contaminated with transient flora; and the environment and nurse's uniform can be contaminated from urine splash.

A catheter specimen of urine Collected by introducing a catheter into the bladder using an aseptic technique. The vessel into which the urine flows must also be sterile and capped immediately. As soon as the flow ceases, the catheter should be withdrawn to prevent microorganisms gaining access to the catheter lumen and travelling to the bladder.

Urine specimens from an indwelling catheter are collected from the apparatus attached to an indwelling catheter (p. 220). It may be a single specimen which is required or a 24-hour one.

Testing urine Several different types of reagent tests are available as 'dipsticks' or 'labsticks'. They can detect urinary tract infection much more quickly and cheaply than standard laboratory tests and their reliability has been tested (Thompson, 1991). She also discusses the significance of urine testing, as does the Continuing Education (CE) Article 343 (1995).

Changes in faeces and their elimination

Changes in appearance A disorder of the digestive system may be indicated by a change in the appearance of faeces. Absence of bile, as in biliary obstruction, produces putty-coloured stools. Some obstructive, infective, inflammatory or malignant diseases can cause the faeces to contain blood, which if not visible to the naked eye but detectable by chemical testing is called 'occult blood'. If blood is mixed with the faeces, causing it to look black and shiny, it is known as melaena and comes from a distal site such as the stomach or small intestine. Or it may be evident as frank red blood which, if on the surface of stools, comes from a local site, and most commonly from bleeding haemorrhoids. Steatorrhoeaic stools, those mixed with mucus and fats, occur in some metabolic disorders. Bulky stools containing undigested food materials indicate faulty absorption. Medications may affect the colour of faecal matter; iron products stain the stool black. Malformed stools, often pencil-like, are indicative of obstruction in the bowel.

Changes in frequency A healthy person normally has a fairly regular pattern of defaecation. The faeces should be of such a consistency that they are easily evacuated in response to a sensory stimulus caused by collection of faeces in the rectum. A deviation from this to a decreased frequency and difficulty in passing faeces is called constipation; change to an increased frequency of passing a more fluid stool is diarrhoea.

Constipation Lack of unabsorbable fibre in the large bowel results in constipation which is acknowledged as a common problem (Department of Health, 1990). However the British Nutrition Foundation (1990) says the view that constipation is simply a disease of fibre deficiency is no longer tenable; it should also be viewed as a disturbance of colonic motility. Nevertheless it goes on to say that constipation in many people, particularly those who are elderly, responds to the laxative effect of unabsorbable fibre (non-starch polysaccharides).

There is a dearth of recent data about constipation but Mallillin (1985) confirmed the high correlation between low fibre intake and constipation in hospital patients. Other studies report a reduction in the use of aperients and enemata after increasing the fibre content of hospital diets (Beveridge, 1986; Thomas, 1987). Dietary fibre is important because it adds bulk to the faeces, making defaecation easy and more frequent. Cereal fibre is more effective than fruit or green vegetable fibre and the easiest way to improve the diet is to take a bran cereal or add small amounts of millers' bran to fruit or cereal.

Whether constipation is an actual or a potential problem, the goal will be to re-establish the patient's usual frequency of defaecation (unless it was unsatisfactory), and promote ease of defaecation. The nursing intervention would be to ensure that the person understands the following preventive activities shown in Box 8.2.

Nurses can do a great deal to prevent constipation by educating people to follow this routine.

For the treatment of constipation most people think of taking medicine — aperients or laxatives — and unfortunately this is a widespread practice in the Western world. For some people it becomes a frequent, even a daily habit; this is dangerous because the bowel muscle loses its natural tone. But of course aperients are useful when constipation is a temporary problem, for example in response to a change of environment and routine. They should never be taken when there is accompanying abdominal pain, nausea or vomiting. Although aperients can be bought without a medical prescription, it is still the custom in most hospitals for them to be prescribed by the doctor but they are administered, evaluated and documented by the nurse. White (1995) discusses their use in terminal illness.

Passmore et al (1993) report a study in which 85 elderly patients with a history of chronic constipation participated. They received either a senna/fibre preparation with a lactulose placebo, or lactulose with a senna/fibre placebo for two weeks. After a rest period they received the other treatment for two weeks. On two criteria — stool consistency and ease of evacuation, the senna/fibre produced better results. The authors concluded that as well as being more effective, it was cheaper — an impor-

tant point when health professionals are being exhorted to provide a cost-effective service!

People who are severely disabled from cerebral palsy or learning difficulties are prone to chronic constipation, and for those who cannot be helped by the advice in Box 8.2, enemas, usually microenemas have to be used. Abdominal massage has been used successfully. It is described and illustrated by Emly (1993). A responding letter from Sheffrin (1993) urged nurses not to practice techniques for which they had not received instruction. In reply, Emly outlined the preparation provided by physiotherapists for nurses and assistants to achieve competency.

Constipation postoperatively is common, particularly after surgery affecting the gastrointestinal tract. This occurs because there is temporary loss of peristalsis, and for this reason it is important that bowel movements are recorded on the nursing documents. If this loss persists longer than the initial postoperative period, it develops into a serious condition called paralytic ileus.

However, a much more common complication of constipation is faecal impaction.

Faecal impaction This condition has already been mentioned; faeces harden and accumulate in the colon and rectum, making defaecation difficult or impossible. It is a distressing condition for patients because, although they may feel the need to defaecate, they are unable to, and abdominal distension and rectal pain cause severe discomfort. Sometimes small amounts of liquid faecal matter bypass the hardened faeces and leak from the anus and this may be wrongly diagnosed as faecal incontinence. When the problem is recognized, the nursing plan will indicate the individualized treatment. In some instances, if the chemical action of one or more evacuant microenemas does not break up the faecal mass, an olive oil microenema may be introduced into the rectum and retained for as long as possible in order to soften the faeces thereby facilitating manual removal using a gloved hand. Gentle hand movement is essential to avoid damaging the mucous membrane. It is an unpleasant procedure for both patient and nurse, and great sensitivity is necessary to preserve the patient's privacy and dignity.

Diarrhoea This is yet another change in eliminating habit; it is the condition in which faeces contain excess water and the frequency of defaecation is markedly increased. Diarrhoea is a common symptom and may be the result of something as benign and self-limiting as pre-examination nerves or something as serious as carcinoma of the colon.

Acute diarrhoea has a sudden onset and usually ends rapidly. It is often the result of an infection such as food poisoning, or it may occur from an infectious disease such as typhoid which affects the digestive tract. On the other hand there are some chronic conditions which cause frequent attacks of diarrhoea and abdominal pain.

Box 8.2 Preventive activities for constipation

- Eat a balanced diet which includes fibre-containing foodstuffs (e.g. wholemeal bread, bran cereals, green vegetables, salad and fruits)
- Maintain an adequate fluid intake
- Take as much exercise as possible
- Maintain usual habits of defaecation or establish satisfactory habits
- Respond to the sensation of a full bowel
- Avoid undue worry about bowel habit
- Promote ease of defaecation by using abdominal and pelvic floor muscles

They are classified as 'Inflammatory bowel disease'; ulcerative colitis and Crohn's disease are two examples. During an attack the bowel will be emptied 10 or 12 times per day. Such people are usually cared for in the community, but need time off from school or work to attend clinics. On occasions they may be admitted to hospital for a couple of weeks to stabilize their nutritional status. A minority have to undergo stoma surgery. As well as coping with their physical condition, some of these people suffer discrimination (Mayberry & Mayberry, 1993).

Over time, diarrhoea poses a danger to health because of the excessive loss of fluids and salts, incomplete absorption of nutrients from food, and incomplete synthesis of vitamins. If untreated, these people will suffer from a multitude of problems. They will become dehydrated and suffer from fluid and electrolyte imbalance, and will lose weight and strength. Medical management may include intravenous administration of fluids and dietary supplements.

Children require special mention — as diarrhoeal diseases are still a major cause of morbidity and mortality, more so in the developing countries, but still so in the Western world. The currently correct treatment for diarrhoea aims to prevent dehydration by adequate feeding combined with 'oral rehydration' (p. 190) when necessary. Antibiotics and antiparasitic drugs are only necessary in suspected cholera and dysentery. Antidiarrhoeal and antiemetic medications should not be used since they are without proven value (WHO, 1990).

There is currently a worrying trend in England and Wales. The number of people with dysentery was 2756 in 1990 and it had increased sixfold by 1992 to 17 019. The instances are fairly evenly spread across the social classes with only a slightly higher increase in the lowest income group (The Independent, 1993).

In the last two decades a condition known as 'antibiotic acquired' diarrhoea has been increasingly diagnosed. The bacterium *Clostridium difficile* is responsible and it is relatively resistant to chemical disinfectants. Antibiotic therapy can eliminate normal bowel flora allowing overgrowth of *C. difficile*. Diarrhoea occurs between five and 10 days after commencing a course of antibiotics. There can be an asymptomatic carrier state, yet another reason for considering all faeces as infected which means wearing a disposable plastic apron and non-sterile gloves, followed by meticulous handwashing (Griffiths-Jones, 1992; Robinson, 1993). The local multidisciplinary Control of Infection Committee will have a policy for students to adhere to.

Nursing activities, based on assessment of the individual, vary according to the severity and duration of the diarrhoea. Feeling the need to defaecate urgently can be distressing for older children and adults, so, to alleviate fear of soiling, availability of a toilet or commode is essential. The person should be encouraged to drink more than usual in order to replace fluid lost and to take a nourishing diet which is reduced in fibre-containing foods. Washing of the perianal area and the application of cream can help to alleviate skin soreness around the anus which is caused by the liquid faeces.

Because diarrhoea is often caused by infection, great care must be taken in the disposal of the patient's faeces. Regular handwashing (p. 94) is necessary by both patient and nurse to prevent spreading the infection. Of course, handwashing is necessary whenever faeces are dealt with, such as when collecting a specimen of this excrement.

Collecting a specimen of faeces

A specimen for bacteriological laboratory examination is obtained by asking the patient to defaecate (without also passing urine) into a clean bedpan and, using a spatula or disposable spoon, a small portion of faeces is put into a special sterile container. When faeces are to be cultured for microorganisms they should reach the laboratory and be examined within two hours. If this is not possible it should be kept below 40°C and transferred to the laboratory within 24 hours (Macleod, 1992).

Stool collections for several days may sometimes be required, for example in cases of steatorrhoea when estimations of amounts of fat in the faeces are made while fat intake in food is controlled. Whenever nurses are involved in the collection of specimens of faeces they must take care to avoid contamination of themselves and their clothes, and adopt a meticulous handwashing technique.

Incontinence of urine

By custom the word incontinence refers to the involuntary excretion of urine. Incontinence of faeces will be discussed later. When there is both urinary and faecal incontinence, the term 'double incontinence' is used.

When considering the subject of incontinence, few people give any thought to the very complicated phenomenon whereby throughout the day and night most children achieve continence by the age of 3. Norton (1988) gives an account of the complexities which all continent adults have mastered, yet about which the majority of both lay and professional people know very little. However there are some children who do not achieve continence and 1–2% of adults continue to be bed wetters.

Enuresis The definition of enuresis used by the Enuresis Resource and Information Centre (ERIC) is:

'an involuntary discharge of urine by day or night or by both, in a child aged five years or older, in the absence of congenital or acquired defects of the nervous system or urinary tract'

It is obvious from the literature that it is difficult to estimate the size of the problem for several reasons. Much of it is unreported because shame and embarrassment causes the subject to be kept secret within the family. There is lack of consistency in the data, often due to lack of definition, and method of collecting data, as well as style of reporting results. For example Norton (1994) in RCN Update (quoting information from ERIC) gives the size of the problem for nocturnal enuresis as 1 in 6 five year olds, 5% of 10 year olds and 1–2% adults over 15 years. Up to the age of nine there are about twice as many boys as girls. Daytime wetting is much less common, affecting more girls than boys (Dobson, 1990). Norton (1986) describes the complexity of acquiring night-time dryness and offers practical advice for helping families with the problem of nocturnal enuresis. She also provides an assessment guide, an essential requisite before planning treatment. Another assessment guide is provided by Ross (1994).

The most effective treatment for bedwetting is based on conditioning principles. A urine-sensitive pad is connected to a battery-operated alarm by the bedside; urine in the pad completes the electrical circuit, activates the alarm and wakes the child who then goes to the toilet. It can be used successfully for children who have a learning disability, and for those who are physically disabled as well as with 'normal' children. The use of an alarm is not an easy option; it needs patience and perseverance as it sometimes takes three months before the child is consistently continent at night, although many achieve success in a month. Some authorities issue alarms for one month only and in some areas there is a long waiting list for alarms (Sadler, 1990).

The incidence of incontinence   Incontinence is a condition which all nurses will have to deal with at some time in their career. Many incontinent people require help from the nursing service at primary level, for example in their own home, or their health centre or at a continence clinic. At secondary level the clinical label of the ward might be:

- gynaecology
- medical
- surgical
- long-stay (geriatric)
- urology
- paediatric
- psychogeriatric
- orthopaedic
- learning disability
- physical disability.

A comparison of the number of incontinent people in different age ranges and institutional or community settings is difficult to obtain. As long ago as 1988, Egan et al reported an extensive 4-year survey which revealed that of those in the 5–14 age range, 15.3% were in an institu-

tion while 84.7% were cared for at home; of those in the 15–64 age range, 44.4% were in institutions while 55.6% were at home; and in the 65+ range, 54.3% were in institutions and 45.7% were at home.

The total number of incontinent people is also difficult to estimate as so many of them are not in the care of the health or social services, but the experts working in this field give the figure of 3 million in the UK (Norton, 1995). Another part of the incontinence problem is in defining the different types arising from, for instance, a neurogenic bladder. However a poll carried out by Market and Opinion Research International (MORI) in 1991 indicated that 10.5 million people over 30 years of age were incontinent in the UK.

Neurogenic bladder   To begin to understand the complexities of incontinence one can examine the term 'neurogenic bladder'. It is used when there is interference with the nerve supply to the bladder, and it can result in various types of incontinence. In one type the desire to pass urine may be appreciated but there is no cerebral inhibition so the bladder contracts resulting in urge incontinence, and evacuation of the full bladder. In another type the full bladder empties reflexly with no sensation. Yet another variation is the atonic bladder which fills so full that the pressure stretches the sphincters and urine dribbles out continuously (overflow incontinence or retention with overflow). Such dribbling incontinence can also occur when the sphincters are incompetent and the bladder no longer acts as a reservoir. The medical diagnosis for people with these different types of incontinence can be as diverse as a stroke (cerebrovascular accident), spina bifida, paraplegia, peripheral neuropathy in diabetes mellitus, multiple sclerosis, a brain tumour, dementia or a head injury. This list shows clearly that incontinence is a symptom and not a disease; it presents the patient with a problem related to the AL of eliminating and the patient requires nursing help to cope with it since the damage to the nervous system cannot be cured. Woodward (1995) discusses assessment of these 'neuroscience' patients. Clean intermittent self-catheterization (p. 216) is probably the single most significant advance in the management of patients with a neurogenic bladder (Norton, 1994).

Dribbling incontinence   Dribbling incontinence can come from the non-neurogenic bladder if there is obstruction in or pressure on the urethra from such conditions as an enlarged prostate gland, a full rectum, or a cystocele. There is therefore a mechanical reason for the ensuing retention of urine and when there is sufficient pressure in the bladder it stretches the sphincters and produces dribbling incontinence. The treatment of the cause will theoretically cure the incontinence but in a few instances it is followed by a different type of incontinence.

Urge incontinence   Urge incontinence can also occur in the non-neurogenic bladder. Awareness of the desire to pass urine is immediately followed by passage of urine; this can be a small or large amount while the person is on the way to the toilet. Naturally people are very distressed about this problem and the more anxious they become the worse the condition gets. They perceive bladder fullness at a smaller and smaller volume of urine until they can be voiding every 10 or 15 minutes: the bladder musculature (detrusor) is unstable, and current thinking favours a plan for bladder training. It starts at the person's frequency, and aims to increase the time interval between passage of urine, after evaluation reveals that each short-term goal has been achieved, until eventually the long-term goal of voiding at a 3- or even 4-hourly interval is achieved. Obviously this demands committed patient participation and meticulous recording of constantly changing short-term goals, and their achievements. It may be that some people with urge incontinence could manage such a programme at home; others may need hospital admission for such a detailed and quickly changing plan.

Stress incontinence   Stress incontinence occurs because of insufficiency of the urethral sphincter mechanism; it is known to be the commonest form of incontinence in women of all ages (Norton, 1995). Should coughing or sneezing or running for a bus — indeed anything which increases intraabdominal pressure occur — the compromised sphincters permit escape of urine. Return of competence to the sphincters can be accomplished by perseverance with pelvic floor exercises (Turner, 1994). Midstream interruption of the flow of urine contributes to strengthening of pelvic floor muscles.

Stress incontinence can occur in the context of midwifery particularly in those who have had an epidural anaesthetic. Accurate documentation of urinary output in the postnatal stage should be perceived as diagnosing a potential problem of stress incontinence, and pelvic floor exercises can be planned, implemented and evaluated (Dolman, 1992). Assessment of women should include a full obstetric history, the circumstances in which urine escapes, urinalysis to exclude urinary tract infection, and a urodynamic assessment to measure bladder pressure and function.

Although the foregoing is a short account of different types of incontinence for the sole purpose of understanding the subject, in reality there can be mixed causes of a person's incontinence.

Incontinence and learning disability   There is a high incidence of incontinence among those who have learning difficulties because there is often damage to the nervous system and this may impair the individual's ability to exercise voluntary control over elimination. Even if there is no physical defect, those with learning disability usually have difficulty in coping independently with the AL of eliminating. However, if they are helped to learn the skills of independent toileting, incontinence often can be overcome. An effective method of toilet training is by the use of behaviour modification procedures.

This approach to teaching involves very careful and gradual shaping of new behaviour using reinforcement techniques. Detailed behavioural assessment is carried out first and, from evaluation, changes in behaviour are monitored. More than two decades ago, the effectiveness of behaviour modification toilet training with severely disabled children in a ward environment was evaluated as part of a research project carried out by Tierney (1973). She found that nurses once trained in the techniques involved had considerable success in toilet training children by this method.

Promoting urinary continence

There is a preventive dimension to promoting continence. For frail people, as well as those with limited mobility, poor balance, or painful joints, managing to reach the toilet, manipulate clothing and lower the body on to the seat can be problematic (White, 1994). She describes clearly several environmental aids which can help with such problems, thereby preventing them from contributing to incontinence.

'Fitness' of the pelvic floor muscles reduces the likelihood of stress incontinence. Because these muscles are stretched during childbirth, teaching pelvic floor exercises forms part of the midwives' acute and postnatal programmes. But when the mother arrives home with her new baby, the practice may not be continued. However, there is now a movement towards teaching these exercises as part of normal sex education in schools stressing the part these muscles play in sexual relationships rather than as a deterrent against incontinence in later life (Candy, 1994). Box 8.3 contains information about simplified exercises.

The pelvic floor muscles act as a sling across the pelvic floor which allows passage of the urethra, vagina and anus in the female (Fig. 8.3).

Box 8.3 Exercise instructions to strengthen pelvic floor muscles

- The exercises can be carried out when sitting, standing or lying
- Tighten muscles around anus/back passage as if preventing the bowel from opening
- Tighten muscles as if preventing the passage of urine
- Incorporate both these exercises into daily living, for example when washing hands, waiting for a bus or watching television
- When passing urine, stop and restart a couple of times

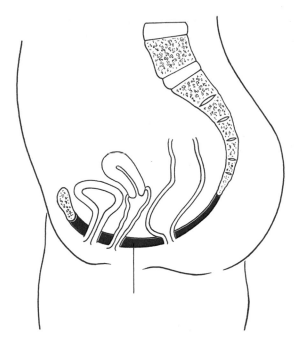

Fig. 8.3 Diagrammatic lateral view of the pelvic floor

Strengthening pelvic floor muscles can be further assisted by use of vaginal cones, perineometers with biofeedback, and electrical stimulation (Wells, 1990, 1991; Laycock, 1991).

As well as the size of the incontinence problem in people of all ages, both at home and in institutions, there is the financial cost of the nursing service and the equipment required, the major part of the money being spent on pads and pants to contain incontinence (Department of Health, 1993). Promoting continence also has a financial cost, but with its successful implementation, it may well be that it can be financed by the money saved on containing incontinence.

Added to this there is the personal psychological cost to incontinent people and their carers. In childhood, for example, the natural progression to continence is linked with 'being good', so the adult's denial is a defence against unacceptable feelings of weakness or 'badness'. Yet another explanation is that denial may help to protect self-image. These mechanisms can lead to hostility. Llewelyn (1992) discusses this subject and offers nurses advice about how to deal with it. Continence can only be promoted if the person acknowledges it as a problem.

There can also be a devastating effect on people's social life and it is therefore essential that nurses learn to use sensitivity and empathy when communicating with them.

There is now considerable literature about this subject and if the available knowledge were translated into practice using a positive attitude, many incontinent people would regain continence. Blannin (1992) wrote:

'Failure to promote continence is attributed to the disability

or frailty of the individual — rarely is it seen as being the result of poor nursing practice, ward routine or ignorance.'

An individualized approach is absolutely essential if success is to be achieved and the framework of the nursing process — assessing, planning, implementing and evaluating — can accomplish this.

Detailed information about the characteristics of the person's incontinence is essential before a plan can be devised for promoting continence. 'Toilet charting' defines the pattern of the problem and provides baseline data about, for example, time of passing urine into a receptacle and time of incontinence episodes. In the discussion about stress incontinence on p. 214, the quickly changing short-term goals were mentioned; toilet charts can be used for recording the achievement of each short-term goal; the setting of the next goal and so on.

Information about fluid intake is relevant because some incontinent people think that by restricting intake the problem will improve, whereas it may be exacerbated by the resultant concentrated urine which is a bladder irritant. Impaired mobilizing, manual dexterity, eyesight and hearing may all be contributing factors and should be borne in mind at the initial, and during ongoing, assessment (Chance, 1994). Incontinence cannot be assessed without considering the person and the context in which the incontinence occurs (Box 8.4). It is also important to know about the toilet facilities in the home environment in order to set realistic goals (Jay, 1989).

From what has already been written it is obvious that a strategy is needed to dispel the widely held belief that urinary incontinence is a taboo subject, and to get the people who 'suffer in silence' to come forward so that their condition can be assessed and an individualized programme planned and implemented with the objective of promoting urinary continence.

Continuous awareness As long ago as 1991 the Department of Health published 'An agenda for action on continence services' and in 1994 sponsored a 'Continence Awareness Week' (Pottle, 1994b; The Independent, 1994). The objective was involvement of all the media, national as well as local to inform the public about the taboo subject and to publicize the various forms of help available, such as telephone helplines, resource centres, drop-in clinics as well as continence clinics (Brown, 1994; Brown, Thomas, McCallum & White, 1991; Gibson, 1990; Nursing Standard, 1992). There are a few urodynamic clinics where special equipment is used to diagnose the cause of incontinence (Abbott, 1992).

Habit training Habit training to promote continence was mentioned in relation to urge incontinence and stress incontinence occurring from the non-neurogenic bladder (p. 214). And there is no doubt from the literature that many people have regained continence by using this method. However as far as a research base for using the

Box 8.4 Points to include in assessing a person who has urinary incontinence

- baseline data (p. 215)
- relevant medical history
- current medication
- current problems related to passing urine
  - number of times per day/night toilet used
  - number of times clothes/bedding wet
  - any change in volume of urine passed
  - any events precipitating incontinence
  - any discomfort/pain
  - date of onset
  - aids/appliances used
  - any change in odour of urine
  - any change in colour of urine
  - attitude to the problem
  - carer's attitude
- related circumstances
  - fluid intake
  - bowel habit
  - mobilizing ability
  - home toilet facilities
  - dexterity
  - hearing
  - sight
  - mental ability
- support services
- urinalysis (p. 210)

behavioural interventions, variously referred to as habit training, toilet training, bladder training and continence training, there are acknowledged difficulties. Cheater (1991) found that even Nurse Continence Advisers interpreted the terms differently. In her 'Conclusion' to the study she stated:

> 'Considerably more research however, is needed to evaluate the efficacy of these approaches. It is clear that if comparisons between studies are to be meaningful, the need to standardize terms used to describe the range of continence training approaches available must be addressed.'

Undoubtedly '. . . the UK is to be credited for its health service developments to meet the needs of people who suffer incontinence' (Roe, 1994). She describes her current three year research programme which will be completed in 1996 — a very good reason for students to acquire the habit of reading nursing journals!

There is now sufficient information from descriptive studies to enable health authorities to prepare 'Guidelines for an efficient service to incontinent people' so that members of the multidisciplinary group can translate them into action.

Intermittent self-catheterization Some people who are incontinent from, for example, a neurogenic bladder, may, after careful and detailed assessment be suitable for implementing an intermittent self-catheterization plan. Intermittent emptying of the bladder protects the kidneys from the effects of back pressure and infection as well as improving the quality of life (Professional Nurse, 1991). A 'clean' as opposed to a 'sterile' catheter is passed via the urethra into the bladder. Self-catheterizing enables people to control their bladders rather than their bladders controlling their lives, for example the bladder can be emptied before sexual intercourse (Winder, 1994). People learn to pass the catheter when sitting on a toilet or in a wheelchair, or in any comfortable position depending on physical ability. In the absence of/or reduced manual dexterity another person may carry out this procedure. Further research into good practice is needed (Winder, 1994). She advocates that after use the catheter is flushed with tap water, drained in the vertical position before replacement in a bag which is carried on the person so that it can be used at intervals throughout the day. But Deegan (1991) states the 'Children are instructed to rinse the catheter under a tap before and after use and place it in a bowl of hypochlorite solution overnight. A plastic envelope is provided as a daytime container and each catheter is used for one week'. The unit in which she works has used this method successfully since 1976.

For people who can manage it, self-catheterization is preferable to indwelling drainage systems and it is being used more and more as its successful use is reported in the nursing literature (Winder, 1994; Haynes, 1994).

Indwelling catheter drainage By common usage this term applies to drainage per urethra. The indwelling catheter is attached to a drainage system to promote continence, but only as a last resort (Britton & Wright, 1990). At the very beginning an experienced nurse has to make the decision regarding the type of catheter to be used. It is important that it caters for the person's comfort during initial insertion and subsequent changes which may be anything from a three-weekly to a three-monthly interval. It should minimize secondary complications such as tissue inflammation, colonization by microorganisms and encrustation by mineral deposits (Getliffe, 1993a; Kohler-Ockmore, 1993). Both authors make the pertinent point that it is the responsibility of nurses to match choice with the person.

In another article, Getliffe (1993b) describes her research which identified several criteria by which blockage of indwelling catheters occurred. Some people are not troubled by this phenomenon (non-blockers) and their nursing plan can safely request for example a three-monthly change of catheter. Other people's catheter encrusts more frequently (blockers) giving rise to a crisis. Collection of individualized data will identify a 'safe' time interval for change of catheter thus preventing the unpleasant and detrimental crisis.

Indwelling drainage can also be accomplished by surgical insertion of a catheter via the suprapubic route. This may be more comfortable and easier to manage for some people confined to a wheelchair and for those who are sexually active (Getliffe, 1993a).

Many people who have an indwelling catheter drainage system remain in their own home and either manage independently or with the help of a carer. A randomized controlled trial was undertaken to evaluate an educational programme on both these groups (Roe, 1990). It significantly improved handwashing after bag emptying, and before and after bag changing, although this effect did not persist over time. This clearly highlights a need for nursing surveillance of these two groups of people in their own homes.

From this albeit brief introduction to the subject of assessing, planning, implementing and evaluating the promotion of urinary continence, there cannot be any doubt about its diversity and complexity. However, for some people, urinary incontinence remains an intractable problem and they need help from a multidisciplinary team to cope with it.

Managing urinary incontinence

There are people whose incontinence cannot be cured but it can be contained in a sensitive manner. For both ambulant and bedfast patients bodyworn and bed drainage fabrics can be used, so that the skin is no longer in constant contact with urine. There are several different 'pad and pant' systems on the market, none of which is universally suitable for all incontinent people.

Disposable products   New products are increasingly available and researchers are conducting consumer studies using 'testers' for collection of data. Published articles confirm the fact that all people using pads (and pants) have needs as individual as their lifestyle. Consequently the initial and ongoing assessments not only take account of people's sensitivity, attitude, motivation, expectation and so on, but also their physical ability and lifestyle. Most of these people live in their own homes, some are in residential accommodation, some in nursing homes and others in hospices. Disposing of the disposables poses problems, and embarrassment is included in the list.

Currently re-usable garments have a high profile and a reputation for environmental friendliness but this is being questioned. Many of these and other complex issues are discussed by researchers Philp, Cottenden and Ledger (1992, 1993a,b,c,d). Philp and Cottenden (1993) discussing re-usables say that products should be visually attractive and as near in pattern to current underclothing for both men and women.

In an ideal world, all types would be available to nurses helping these people, so that the one best suited to, and most acceptable by the wearer would be an individualized decision after trying several of them. In the real world nurses need to discover which pads and pants are available locally to help achieve the patient's goal of containing incontinence. A trial to determine whether local people would find a re-usable garment to be as effective and acceptable as disposables is reported (Nursing Times, 1992a). The data revealed an unexpected difficulty in keeping mini pads in place. This was reported to the manufacturers and their design has since been modified.

However some intractable male incontinence can be coped with by penile sheath drainage (Watson, 1989). It is evident that careful assessment of the person is important, general factors being mental competence, manual dexterity and efficient personal hygiene, and local factors such as length of penis and whether or not it retracts when sitting and lying, and the presence of an inguinal hernia (Unsworth & Rowell, 1994).

In hospital a drawsheet over a plastic sheet is used less frequently, even for people who are incontinent of urine. In their favour they allowed easy replacement of one item of linen with minimum disturbance to the person in bed. However, drawsheets tend to allow urine to pool under the patient; they also slip and crease readily which is particularly undesirable if pressure sores are to be avoided. The use of incontinence pads is not an ideal solution either because they are seldom effective in containing the urine in one area and frequently cause irritation to the skin and therefore they too may contribute to pressure sore development. Sudocrem is better for treating incontinence-related dermatitis than conventionally used zinc cream; it also has bactericidal properties.

At home, however, protection of the bed is very necessary because most families are without a large resource of linen, and laundering wet and soiled linen becomes a major task for relatives, one which may be impossible if they are elderly or infirm. In the UK some areas have a laundry service through which bed linen is loaned and laundered and this is a tremendous help for a family when coping with an ill member at home.

Supporting the person   The importance of the nurse showing discretion, tact and kindness when helping people who have problems with the AL of eliminating cannot be overemphasized. It is especially important when nursing dependent, incontinent people. Some nurses do not find it a pleasant activity and it is sometimes difficult for them not to feel annoyed or disgusted at having to deal with another person's excreta. However, such a feeling must not be conveyed to the person who should never be scolded or made to feel like a child. Realizing that it is probably equally distasteful to dependent, incontinent people, communicating an understanding of their feelings by sympathetic and tactful nursing can turn what might otherwise be an unpleasant nursing activity into a satisfying and important aspect of nursing.

Because incontinence may make people feel ashamed and cause them to lose dignity it may cause loss of interest in personal appearance which can mean being less attractive to other people including those of the opposite sex. For those who are sexually active there is an even bigger problem. Nurses are becoming less reticent than previously to discuss with incontinent people how to continue expressing their sexuality, including being sexually active if they so desire.

Incontinence of faeces (encopresis)

Despite the increasing publicity now given to urinary incontinence, faecal incontinence still carries a high degree of social stigma. Supporting faecally incontinent people is equally important. When there is incontinence of faeces the person does need to be changed immediately. In many ways it is easier to manage an episode of faecal incontinence in a bedfast person. Coping with such an episode in an ambulant patient is a more problematic task: this was highlighted some time ago, in the research done by Reid (1976). Her observations of the nursing management of incontinence revealed how ill-equipped are many hospital wards for enabling nurses to adequately wash patients and change their day clothes. Either the patient needs to be taken to bed if this is to be managed properly, or the toilet facilities require to be adapted to provide the nurse with appropriate facilities. Some modern hospitals are equipped with bidets and these permit thorough washing of the perineum and indeed enable many patients to carry out this personal cleansing procedure themselves.

Unfortunate psychological associations can be made in the early period of life which can result in constipation. Lack of dietary fibre and fluid can further predispose to constipation in children. Faecal soiling in childen calls for careful and detailed assessment of the child in the context of other family members. Sometimes the condition is diagnosed as one of psychological origin and certain patterns or types of soiling might benefit from psychiatric attention. For many children their soiling is a readily understood consequence of colorectal loading which may be the result of long-standing constipation or an anal fissure, or discomfort associated with sexual abuse (Hill, 1991).

In adults the problem of faecal incontinence is probably under-reported because, not only is it a taboo subject, but the afflicted person can only interpret it as regression to a status associated with the early years of life, and feel bewildered and demoralized. Norton

(1986), estimates that about one adult in 200 living in the community suffers regular faecal incontinence.

Faecal incontinence may be the presenting feature, or a postoperative complication, of rectal or colonic disease which can occur at any age, but faecal impaction is the commonest cause of faecal incontinence in elderly people. 'Impaction' is misleading as elderly people can have massive faecal loading with soft or even liquid stools (Barrett, 1990). He says that treatment of the faecally incontinent demented person must be carefully planned. Knowledge of the causes and treatment are now sufficiently advanced, that faecal incontinence should be seen as a preventable and curable problem. It must not be accepted as inevitable (Barrett, 1990).

Continence advisers

In this section the term 'continence adviser' has been mentioned several times, and merits some amplification. The Association of Continence Advisers in the UK started in 1981 as a multidisciplinary group of professionals. Each member of the multidisciplinary group has a role in assisting the incontinent person. In alphabetical order the team consists of chiropodists, doctors, nurses, occupational therapists, physiotherapist, radiologists, supplies officers and technicians. In 1991 the name was changed to the Association of Continence Advice. The Association played an important part in the government sponsored 'Continence awareness' week mentioned on p. 215. The role of the nurse continence adviser is described by Rhodes and Parker (1994), but there is variation in interpretation of the role to suit local circumstances.

The Association also helped in getting television advertising time for products associated with continence/incontinence. Currently pressure is being applied at government level for local authority provision of public toilets to be statutory. At present it is voluntary and some have been closed because of the increasing cost of maintenance due to such social changes as increased vandalism. The Association produces a journal in association with the Nursing Times. It contains up-to-date information about the latest research-based knowledge related to promoting continence of urine and faeces.

From this albeit brief introduction to the subject of individualizing the promotion of urinary/faecal continence, there cannot be any doubt about its diversity and complexity. Nor can there be any doubt about the nurse being the focus of multidisciplinary activity in providing an efficient, effective and cost-effective service to each individual requiring it.

CHANGE IN MODE OF ELIMINATING

For various reasons it sometimes becomes necessary for

urine or faeces to be removed from the body by an alternative or artificial route. For the person, this causes problems arising from the imposed change in mode of eliminating.

Urinary catheterization

As already mentioned urine can be drained to the exterior through a tube — a catheter — inserted into the bladder via the urethra. This may be required once only as a preventive activity, for example to ensure an empty bladder preoperatively, or to relieve a distended bladder postoperatively. Catheterization may be required intermittently, perhaps to measure the amount of urine remaining in the bladder after normal emptying.

The procedure of catheterization An aseptic technique must be used in order to prevent the introduction of pathogenic microorganisms into the urinary bladder. Infection is a common and potentially dangerous complication of catheterization, urinary tract infection being the commonest hospital-acquired infection. It accounts for approximately 30% of all such infections and at least 500 deaths per year in the UK. Urinary tract infection is especially troublesome when an indwelling catheter is in situ, although when using a closed system of urinary drainage the likelihood of urinary infection is significantly lessened.

The range of catheters for short and long-term use are now much more sophisticated (Nursing Times, 1995). Bacterial colonization may be influenced by the properties of the catheter surface, thereby reducing the incidence of bacteriuria and encrustation ('biofilm') which can precipitate catheter blockage (Roe, 1993; Gould, 1994b). The word 'biofilm' has entered the medical vocabulary and it refers to the bacteria which can colonize all parts of urinary drainage systems, even the external surfaces. The bacteria secrete extracellular products which form an adherent film creating resistance to antibiotics.

Traditionally in the UK only men catheterized men, but with changing social mores, a movement is afoot to make it acceptable for a person who has no objection, to be catheterized by a nurse of the opposite sex (Pomfret, 1993, 1994).

Information about short-term indwelling urethral catheter drainage is contained in Box 8.5 and long-term drainage in Box 8.6.

Closed urinary drainage system The five points at which bacteria can enter what was previously and often still is, called a closed urinary drainage system are illustrated in Figure 8.4 and will now be mentioned briefly.

1. *The urethral orifice,* also called the meatal space and the pericatheter space. Microorganisms entering via the urethral orifice travel along the potential space between the outer catheter surface and the urethral mucosa. It

---

Box 8.5 Short-term indwelling urethral catheter drainage

Providing a service for people who have an indwelling urethral catheter is a common feature of clinical practice (Roe, 1993). Between 10 and 12% of patients admitted to hospital will have a short-term (median duration four days) insertion. Urinary tract infection has been the most researched aspect, and patients in gynaecological and urological wards are the most frequent subjects (Roe, 1993). The urethral/urinary catheter is attached to a closed urinary drainage system (Fig. 8.4) which was mentioned on p. 216 in relation to 'Promoting urinary continence'.

Box 8.6 Long-term indwelling urethral catheter drainage

A median duration for patients with long-term urethral catheter drainage is four years. Some have been known to use catheter drainage for up to 17 years (Roe, 1993). Several aspects of this practice were mentioned on p. 216. The prevalence of those nursed at home was established at four per cent, with as many as 16 to 28% being in chronic care facilities (Roe, 1993). She discusses in detail the interrelationship of urinary tract infection and other catheter-related problems. 'Biofilm' is a concept which is being used more frequently related to this subject. Mulhall (1991) defines it as a collection of microorganisms and their extracellular products bound to a solid surface. In the context of this brief discussion that means the catheter — its external surface as well as that of its lumen, and the same applies to the drainage tube; and it includes both the inside and outside of the drainage bag and its outlet tap. It is still pertinent to consider that there are five points at which bacteria can enter (Fig. 8.4).

---

has to be remembered that the urethra has a natural bacterial flora of commensals, that is, it is colonized; some commensals are potentially pathogenic, and any injury by catheter to the urethral mucosa will encourage the change of state from colonization to auto-infection. Cleansing of the meatal region would seem to be desirable on social grounds. However, there is no firm existing evidence to support the use of antiseptics for this procedure. It is obvious that further research is required to guide acceptable intervention on 'social grounds', or on validated grounds for 'prevention of urinary tract infection'. Application of knowledge from microbiology suggests that 4-hourly washing of the perineum would keep

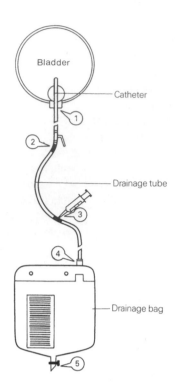

Fig. 8.4 Points at which bacteria can enter a urinary drainage system 1- the urethral orifice; 2- connection of catheter and drainage tube; 3- where sample of urine taken; 4- connection of drainage tube and collecting bag; 5- drainage bag outlet

the natural flora within the limits with which the body's defence system can cope.

2. *Connection of catheter and drainage tube.* The logical reasons for breaking this seal are when a substance has to be injected into the bladder, or when a bladder washout becomes necessary. Bladder washout/irrigation is now acknowledged to be of dubious benefit (Stickler, 1990). However a variety of substances are still frequently injected/instilled via this route but there is no sound rationale for their use (Roe, 1993). Both these interventions would be carried out using aseptic technique. Inadvertent breaking of this seal is not specifically reported in the literature.

3. *Where sample of urine taken.* A specimen of urine can be withdrawn by steadying the tube and piercing it with a sterile widebored needle attached to a large sterile syringe. The nurse's hands must have been washed to remove both resident and particularly transient flora, some of which may be pathogenic organisms, particularly in a hospital setting. A plastic apron will protect the nurse's uniform from any splash while transferring urine into a specimen jar. Afterwards meticulous hand washing

is obviously essential to prevent cross-infecting another patient. *The drainage tube* requires mention. Its purpose is to provide an uninterrupted downhill flow of urine, so it should never be above bladder level. The downhill flow is necessary to prevent stasis of urine in the bladder, especially important if the urine is known to be infected (bacteriuria).

4. *Connection of drainage tube and collecting bag.* It is necessary to break this seal when changing the collecting bag, whether it is of the single use type, or of the reusable type in which there is an outlet at the base for emptying urine. Before separating the drainage tube and collecting bag, placement of a clamp on each, helps to minimize urine splash. Biofilm will have collected on the inside and outside of both, and the 'film' renders the microorganisms more resistant to antiseptics. As soon as they are separated, the end of the drainage tube is in contact with the atmosphere which may contain pathogenic microorganisms, so time-wise minimal exposure is desirable. The nurse's hands require to have been effectively washed both before and after replacement of a collecting bag.

5. *Drainage bag outlet.* These are only present on the reusable bags and there are several types available. The results of one study indicated that nurses can contaminate their hands with microorganisms during bag emptying (Glenister, 1987). Assessment of visible hand contamination on emptying seven different types of drainage bag was achieved by the addition of methylene blue to the urine bag, and measuring the area of splash. After bag emptying, a drop of blue dye remained on the end of the outlet tap; Glenister suggests that the outlet needs to be wiped with an absorbent/disinfection cloth at the end of the procedure, but Mulhall et al (1988) state that 'There is very little evidence in existing literature concerning the value of disinfecting taps on drainage bags'. They consider that a sensible precaution would be to dry the tap thoroughly to prevent multiplication of bacteria.

Ascending infection along the surface of the urethra to the bladder has been mentioned; it can also occur via a contaminated drainage system (Blenkharn, 1988). In an attempt to avoid it, prevention of backflow during bag emptying is accomplished by the bag remaining below the level of the bladder. There are now several devices fitted to drainage bags to prevent backflow but scientific and clinical evidence of their effectiveness is inadequate (Mulhall et al, 1988). Although the various drainage systems are visually 'closed', and the term 'closed urinary drainage system' is still in common use, Lanara (1987) calls these 'open drainage systems' — they are open in a microbiological context because, on emptying they are open to the air. Closed systems have a second collection bag below the first and separated from it by a valve. The valve is opened to drain urine from the upper to the lower bag; it is then closed before the tap at the bottom of the lower bag is opened, thereby preventing access of air to the system. Evidence to support the microbiological 'openness' of the outlet tap in a single bag drainage system is provided by Blenkharn (1988).

The patient's problems with urethral drainage In this section so far, the emphasis has been on the equipment available and the technique of catheterization, rather than on the patient, but consideration of the patient is all-important whichever type of catheterization is used. Patients who are catheterized have a variety of problems to contend with. They are subjected to the embarrassment of the procedure and then have to put up with the inconvenience of having a tube and bag attached to the body. Patients have to get used to the difficulties this presents when carrying out such activities as bathing, walking or getting in and out of bed. They may also be embarrassed about explaining the appliance to visitors. Not least, such patients are at risk of developing a urinary infection. Helping patients to come to terms with such varied problems demands sympathetic and skilful nursing.

People with indwelling urethral drainage systems are being discharged home, and of course before they leave hospital they, and where relevant their carers need information about their catheter system and practice in managing it to prevent urinary tract infection. Roe (1990) carried out a study to discover patients' and carers' knowledge about catheter care (p. 216).

As long ago as 1989 another experienced nurse (Wright) developed a teaching programme for nurses to help them in their role as health educators. She also produced a written guide for catheterized patients who are being discharged with a catheter in situ: permission is given for it to be photocopied. It is evident from the literature that patients require to have opportunities for practising self-care before discharge from hospital.

While briefly surveying this complex subject of catheterization, which provides many actual and potential problems, several research-based references were provided, but Roe (1993) discusses the current level of research evidence for managing people with indwelling urethral drainage systems and considers that it is unsatisfactory. It obviously is a field for on-going research.

When people are experiencing other serious problems with the excretion of urine, other changes in the mode of eliminating become necessary, for example when conventional treatment for 'chronic renal failure' is not adequately removing waste products from the blood. The medical diagnosis changes to 'end-stage renal failure' and other means of removal become necessary for these people who have not enjoyed good health, probably for many years. The generic name for these treatments is 'renal replacement therapy' and it includes peritoneal

dialysis, haemodialysis (renal dialysis) and renal transplantation, and these will be discussed albeit briefly.

Peritoneal dialysis

In the UK at the end of 1990 over 1900 individuals with renal disease were alive on dialysis or had a functioning kidney transplant. This equates with 330 per million (European Dialysis and Transplant Association, 1991 quoted by Thomas, 1992). For many people peritoneal dialysis is the first line of treatment and is the most rapidly expanding area in renal replacement therapy (Martin, 1993). Many of them prefer it to haemodialysis because it allows greater freedom and independence (Bloe, 1990). A simple explanation of how it works is given in Box 8.7.

Continuous ambulatory peritoneal dialysis The person is admitted to hospital for insertion of a special catheter into the lower peritoneal space; it is anchored at skin level. As with any invasive technique, there is a risk of infection and people on peritoneal dialysis need to be able to recognize it, and what to do if it occurs (Fair, 1994). Renal units use individualized teaching plans (Jerrum, 1991; Wild, 1991). The goals can be stated as what the person will be able to do; Box 8.8 is an example. The title of this technique shows that it is compatible with people carrying out their daily routine, obviously modified to accommodate infusion and withdrawal of fluid. However such people need a lot of support and encouragement as their life literally depends on their commitment to complying with the exacting routine.

Continuous cycle peritoneal dialysis The principles are the same but the person is connected to a machine which performs 10 to 12 exchanges during the night, thus leaving the day free from dialysis (Martin, 1993; Gartland, 1993).

Box 8.7 How peritoneal dialysis works

The peritoneum is used as the dialysing membrane and the dialysing fluid is introduced via a catheter passed through the abdominal wall and anchored there. Fluid from a plastic bag passes through the catheter and remains in the abdomen for 4–5 hours, after which it is drained back into the bag. The process is repeated four or five times daily and the continuous clearance of waste products maintains a more stable blood chemistry and avoids the peaks and troughs which can occur with haemodialysis. This lessens the feeling of exhaustion experienced by people in end-stage renal failure, and gives greater dietary freedom and often a free fluid intake.

> **Box 8.8** Goals to be achieved by a person (or carer) learning home peritoneal dialysis
>
> - Care for the catheter exit site
> - Identify peritonitis
> - Identify infection at catheter site
> - Recognize other potential problems
> - Maintain fluid balance and recognise dehydration and fluid overload
> - Understand dietary requirements and restrictions
> - Manage the organization of fluid and supplies deliveries

Intermittent peritoneal dialysis This form is the least popular. The person is connected to a machine for 10 to 12 hours, three or four times weekly. Between treatments the abdomen is left empty of dialysate. It is useful for people who can no longer cope with their manual exchange programme (Martin, 1993).

Haemodialysis (renal dialysis)

Haemodialysis may be the treatment of choice for acute renal failure but as this is a reversible condition it is usually a short-term, life-saving treatment. It can also be used for short periods to rest the peritoneum when infection supervenes in that form of dialysis. Haemodialysis involves the continual removal of blood from an artery into a closed circuit containing a thin membrane which is bathed with dialysing fluid. This, just like the kidney nephrons, removes urea and other waste products from the blood before it returns to a vein and into the general circulation. The process is usually carried out overnight, several nights a week. All people requiring any form of dialysis are stabilized in a hospital dialysis unit where many learn to be independent. Some return to the unit to carry out their treatment independently; others return because they require supervision during treatment.

Approximately two-thirds become independent on home dialysis. Another person, usually a family member, learns to manage the technique and this can strain family relationships. Some people on haemodialysis experience almost immobilizing exhaustion at times, others tire easily. As well as coming to terms with the essential demanding routine, there is usually restriction of diet and this may affect not only appetite but also put certain constraints on socializing and family relationships. But since the stark alternative is death, this unrelenting routine has to be continued for life or until a kidney transplant is available. A few special holiday centres provide dialysis machines and people on renal dialysis can go to these centres, dialyse at night and enjoy a holiday during the day.

Unfortunately, few countries can afford to provide dialysis treatment and kidney machines for all those who require them. Without them many people die each year. When economic resources for health care are limited, many moral dilemmas face those responsible for allocating finance, as in this case, deciding who should have the available machines.

Renal transplantation

Renal transplantation offers a new hope for people with end stage renal failure, but it is not a first treatment for many, because there are insufficient donor kidneys available.

Opt-in/opt-out systems The system in some countries is distribution of donor cards (opt-in), so that people can carry with them notification of their willingness to have their kidneys used in the event of sudden death. But only 26% of adults in the UK have one, and only 18% admit to carrying one (Ward, 1993).

Some other countries have an 'opt-out' system whereby, unless a person carries an opt-out card, in the case of sudden death, the kidneys can be removed for donation.

Required request system Currently a system of 'required request' is being discussed in many countries. In the case of an unconscious dying patient, the doctor would be required to ask the family whether or not the patient had expressed any objection to his/her organs being used for transplant. If the patient's wishes are not known, the doctors would be required to ask the 'family' if they had any objection (Durman & Hudson, 1993; Christey, 1993). The public are being encouraged to think about these possibilities, so that, should a family tragedy occur, the 'required request' from the doctor will not be perceived as meddlesome or offensive, but as a duty which has to be carried out.

Donor families Organ transplant coordinators are, whenever possible, available to families before and after consent to donation. There are little data about how these bereaved families perceive the experience of losing a loved one, granting permission for donation, and the function of the coordinator. One small study is reported by Cunningham (1993).

Summarizing, there is no doubt that treatment for people with end-stage renal disease has improved over the last two decades, and some of them on dialysis live for years even without a kidney transplant. It is possible that ever increasing periods of dialysis will become necessary. At what point is death allowed to intervene? Janes (1990a) discusses this and other ethical issues.

It is pertinent to consider that during the years of dialysis, people do not become asexual and every encouragement should be given to help them enjoy expressing their sexuality by such things as attention to clothes, hair style, jewellery and bath additives. There may be actual problems related to sexual intercourse because of the chronic nature of the condition. These include loss of sexual drive (libido), capacity for orgasm, reduced fertility and inability to sustain an erection (Janes, 1990b). Referral to a sex counsellor or therapist may be appropriate.

Stomas/ostomies

For some people, excretion of either urine or faeces may require a permanent method of diversion (Allison, 1995; Crooks, 1994). Both excretions can be diverted to a stoma on the abdominal wall called a urostomy (urine), ileostomy (fluid faeces) or colostomy (formed faeces). They are being discussed under the generic term 'stomas' followed by a brief introduction to the particular types. The excretion flows involuntarily into a bag-like appliance which is fitted over the stoma and adheres to the surrounding skin. There are more than 100 000 people in England and Wales with a permanent stoma and 18 500 people will require stoma surgery each year (Hughes, 1991).

People at an early stage on the lifespan may need to have a stoma. They may be newborn babies, children and teenagers (Lyall, 1990). If the stoma is permanent, children incorporate it into their body image, but the older child or adolescent may go through the same sort of psychological grieving experiences as adults (p. 404). Health visitors, community nurses, school nurses and occupational health nurses all make an important contribution to the adjustment of this group to 'being different' yet still valued as an individual, and having an important contribution to make in developing their potential talents. Parents and school nurses should ensure that the teaching staff are aware of the implications of stoma surgery. Children express their sexuality in many different ways; however, after puberty, for most people who are confronted with needing a stoma, the AL of expressing sexuality assumes importance (p. 364). They experience fear and anxiety about matters such as: whether they will still look attractive; will the appliance show under their clothes; will they smell; will they be able to have sex; and will they be able to conceive? (Taylor, 1994; Anders, 1993).

Adults requiring this type of surgery may well have been ill for some time and may be depressed that the condition is not improving. Communication with them needs to be especially sensitive and empathic as they try to come to terms with a change in body image related to the AL of eliminating, which in itself has such private and personal overtones (Kelly, 1994).

Those belonging to an ethnic minority group may have rituals and beliefs about the AL of eliminating which need to be considered should a member require an individualized nursing plan for stoma surgery and after-care (Black, 1994). And another minority group who require consideration is that of homosexual men and their partners who engage in anal intercourse. They will probably need relevant information and counselling should one of them become an ostomist (Corless, 1992).

Potential and actual problems The person undergoing stoma surgery has many potential and actual problems with which to contend. Students of nursing require to explore their feelings about stomas. They should be forewarned that even a coloured picture may not prepare them for viewing a real stoma. If revolt is experienced as a result of the sight or smell, it should not be indicated in the patient's presence (Black, 1994). She goes on to say that postoperative nursing can allay patients' fears of rejection, mutilation and degradation, as well as promote confidence in preparing equipment and changing the appliance prior to discharge into the care of nurses at primary level.

Appliances Currently a vast selection of appliances is available to ostomists and most can be tailored to suit individual requirements (Jeffries, 1993; Thomas, 1991). Some are designed to accommodate leisure activities, and others for travelling — for example to minimize discomfort when wearing a seat belt. There are deodorant drops and powders, and air fresheners which can be used whenever the pouch is emptied or changed. In spite of improvements in materials and design, people's main problems continue to be skin soreness, leakage from the bag, the odour and sound of involuntary passage of flatus, as well as disposal of bags and their contents, and the skin appliances.

Stoma care nurses/clinical specialists Interest in and concern for people who have any kind of stoma has been demonstrated by nurses specializing in stoma care. The trend began in the USA in 1958 but the first stomatherapist was not a nurse but an 'ileostomist'; stoma care nursing was pioneered in the UK at St Bartholomew's Hospital in London in 1969, and it is estimated that there are now upwards of 380 stoma care nurses in the UK (Dulfer, 1992).

Given the previously mentioned number of people with a stoma, it is obvious that not all of them can have access to a specialist nurse. Surveys of patients and trained nurses about the teaching and counselling support for new stoma patients have confirmed that many wards do not have access to the services of a full-time specialist nurse. To help nurses in these wards, to help patients who are undergoing stoma surgery, the specialist stoma nurses share their up-to-date attitudes, knowledge and skills by publishing articles in appropriate journals.

Originally stoma nurses were employed by health authorities. Currently almost a third are funded by companies making stoma appliances and therefore it is pertinent to ask 'Are stomatists getting a fair deal?'. Commercial firms also employ stoma nurses to sell their products (under the name of service) to ostomists in places like nursing homes, their own homes and residential homes. They also visit nurses in hospital especially where a stoma nurse is not employed. North (1990), and Payne and Gardner (1992) discuss their perception of sponsorship and stoma nurses. In 1992 an association known as the Campaign for Impartial Stoma Care was formed. Members obviously feel that patients are not necessarily well served by sponsorship.

The foregoing text uses the generic heading of stomas, but a brief discussion of the particular stomas follows.

Urostomy Various surgical procedures can be used so that the ureters drain into a newly created 'bladder', sometimes called an ileal conduit, with its stoma opening on the abdominal wall. The urostomy bag has a tap at the base for emptying the urine, so what was said about teaching people to manage an indwelling catheter drainage system is pertinent here. The apparatus also has an anti-reflux valve to prevent back-flow of urine when the person lies down.

There is a Urostomy Association in the UK where people can gain and give support by sharing for instance, a practical detail about care of the appliance which has been found useful.

In the last decade surgery has developed a 'continent' urinary diversion. The stoma is much smaller, 0.5 to 1.0 cm in diameter. Through it the person passes a special tube at a 3 to 4 hourly interval and drains the urine into the toilet (Horn, 1990).

Ileostomy With regard to ileostomy, the effluent is fluid, so the external appliance may have an outlet tap at its base via which the contents of the bag can be emptied into the toilet, thus reducing the frequency of application of a clean bag to the skin. The fluid is strongly alkaline and may contain proteolytic enzymes, so prevention of leakage from the appliance, and extra protection of the peristomal skin are essential.

Patients requiring an ileostomy have usually endured an inflammatory bowel disease for many years and will probably be malnourished. Assessment will reveal the type of diet taken. Strong religious and cultural beliefs may have guided which foods were, and were not acceptable and it is wise to build on these. Prejudices, beliefs and anxieties may need to be aired, with the goal of providing a well-balanced diet (Farbrother, 1993). Ileostomists often lose five times more water and 10 times more salt daily than the rest of the population, as well as a small amount of potassium (Andrews, 1993), and acceptable ways of supplementing these losses are essential.

Colostomy Regarding a colostomy, its site will determine consistency of the effluent; from a transverse colostomy it will be a semisolid stool which collects involuntarily in a closed bag which is removed daily, followed by application of a clean bag. The faecal content of the used bag has to be flushed away in the toilet.

Some people with a colostomy eventually manage a daily evacuation at a particular time and are sufficiently confident to wear only a dressing over the stoma or a stoma cap. Others irrigate the bowel above the stoma each morning to minimize involuntary passing of faeces into the appliance during the day and between irrigations some only wear a stoma cap. These groups have less skin soreness, probably from minimization of leakage.

Disposal of stoma bags and appliances Bags are changed more frequently than the appliance which adheres to the skin. Urine or faeces adhering to the bag will quickly decompose increasing the unpleasantness of their odour. Ostomists are advised to wrap the bag (and when necessary the appliance) in newspaper, sealing, and placing in the household refuse system. The effluent from a sigmoid colostomy resembles a normal stool and cleansing of the bag before disposal requires cutting and eversion before flushing, wrapping, sealing and placing in the refuse bin. It is little wonder that many adults and elderly people find it aesthetically unacceptable. Harlow, as long ago as 1988, investigated the disposal of used stoma bags and stated:

> 'So we not only have physical and psychological problems with disposal of soiled stoma bags, but also social and ecological ones.
>
> Stoma care nurses spend much of their time reassuring patients that they can lead a virtually normal life postoperatively, and yet we are still in the Dark Ages when it comes to disposal. We could make a start by insisting that every public lavatory has a bin for disposal of soiled appliances. . . . It should be mandatory for all toilets in public buildings, hotels, guest houses and restaurants to have adequate facilities.'

It is hoped work will progress on the biodegradable bags and perhaps surgical techniques will also improve so that permanent stomas requiring bags will be things of the past.

However four years after Harlow's work a qualitative study (Kelly & Henry, 1992) found that the most frequently reported problem was disposal of used equipment! Some people had tried using airline sick bags, bin liners and nappy bags but found them unsatisfactory. These people considered that their need for advice about disposal had not been met. However a handout 'Living with a stoma' published by Professional Nurse (1993) advised that some local authorities operate a collection service of stoma appliances, and many appliance companies supply sealable plastic bags for disposal.

Meantime, however, we need to promote a sense of social responsibility for those people who do have a stoma so that they can experience an acceptable quality of living.

It can be seen that there are people who have many

and varied actual and potential problems with eliminating which can influence their dependence/independence status. The last broad classification which can change a person's dependence/independence is change of environment and routine a discussion of which follows.

CHANGE OF ENVIRONMENT AND ROUTINE

From time to time most people experience some disruption to their individualized eliminating habits as a result of a change in environment and routine. Going on holiday inevitably means adapting to a different timetable, doing different things, and making do with whatever toilet facilities are available, even if sometimes these are unfamiliar and unsavoury! If the holiday is a lazy one, it is possible that the less active routine will cause constipation; on the other hand, diarrhoea may be the result of sampling unfamiliar foods. The same sort of problems can be experienced by people who are admitted to hospital.

Admission to hospital

Disruption to established eliminating habits seems to be a common consequence of admission to hospital.

When people are admitted because of problems associated with urinary elimination or faecal elimination, doctors and nurses ask all sorts of questions about these activities; specimens of urine or faeces are collected and tested and sometimes special procedures such as catheterization are a necessary part of treatment. Certain communications between patients and staff centre round eliminating. These body functions are no longer private and personal; they seem to the patients to have become everybody's business and not unnaturally they may feel anxious and embarrassed.

Even those patients whose reason for admission is not specifically related to eliminating problems may at assessment be found to be experiencing a problem with this AL. Other patients may encounter difficulties with this AL because of the hospital environment. In particular many patients become bothered by the lack of privacy.

Lack of privacy

Previously in people's adult life nobody has asked whether or not they have had a bowel movement. This is still a routine in some hospitals and some patients who have not been admitted because of a bowel complaint may well consider this an invasion of their privacy.

Curtains round beds may provide visual privacy but they do not provide aural privacy for those patients experiencing urinary or defaecatory problems when giving related information to doctors and nurses. Nurses can help by modulating their voices; choosing to talk with the person when the beds on either side are empty; or inviting the person into a room in which they can talk without interruption.

For ambulant patients, in many hospital wards which were built in the days when the majority of patients were nursed in bed, toilet facilities are inadequate for the needs of today. Often there are too few toilets or those available are too far away to be readily reached; many are too small for wheelchairs or walking aids; and some are too cold for comfort, or so public that they deny any real privacy. A research project highlighting these and other inadequacies was mentioned on p. 205.

Nurses in a medium-term dependency ward for 20 males with a learning disability used the Dynamic Standard Setting System and identified lack of privacy particularly in the bathroom, bedroom and toilet areas (Marr & Pirie, 1990). An unexpected but valuable outcome was preparation of these residents for their move into the community.

Nurses may not be able to do much about the inadequacy of facilities in the ward, but they can make the most of what exists. For example, toilets should be kept clean and free from the clutter of sluice equipment, and air fresheners can be used to minimize malodour. (Aerosols are not recommended as some contribute to destruction of the ozone layer which is currently a cause of international concern.) Patients using the toilet should be afforded as much privacy as possible. How often do nurses thoughtlessly 'pop in' to ask if patients are ready to be helped back to bed when a call system could be provided which would avoid this situation?

Unfamiliar routine

If the imposed ward routine for the patients' AL of eliminating is not the same as their individual habit then they are more than likely to have a problem. For example, individuals who usually have a bowel movement immediately after breakfast may find this is not possible because they are expected to stay in bed awaiting the doctor's round. Some people, accustomed to getting up during the night to pass urine, may feel apprehensive about continuing this routine for fear of disturbing other patients.

When showing the newly admitted patient where the toilet facilities are, and discussing things such as when it may be necessary to use a bedpan or provide a specimen of urine, the nurse can take the opportunity to find out as much as possible about the patient's eliminating habits and later to record any relevant information. It is only when an assessment has been carried out that potential problems can be identified and the necessary nursing planned.

As far as possible, patients should be enabled to maintain any deeply ingrained individual habits of eliminating. Bedpan or urinal 'rounds' impose a routine on all patients and it is much better to accommodate each individual's accustomed routine whenever possible. This is more easily accomplished when 'primary nursing' is the system being used for provision of the nursing service, rather than task allocation.

Identifying people's actual and potential problems is a useful concept when applied to clinical nursing. It is a wide-ranging subject made more manageable by using our four broad categories referred to on p. 204. But identifying problems leads to planning and implementing nursing activities and evaluating outcomes which will now be discussed.

PLANNING AND IMPLEMENTING NURSING ACTIVITIES AND EVALUATING OUTCOMES

Throughout this chapter the words assessing, identifying people's problems, planning, implementing and evaluating have been used at appropriate places, confirming that these widely accepted 'phases' of the process of nursing do not have to be confined to discussion under their own heading, but can all be used in discussing a particular problem being experienced by a particular person. But the process of nursing is only a part of our model for conceptualizing nursing, the other concepts being the relationship of the lifespan to eliminating, dependence/independence in eliminating, factors influencing eliminating (biological, psychological, socioeconomic, environmental and politicoeconomic), and these have been mentioned where they were relevant. Their interaction results in individuality in eliminating which is of prime concern when writing an individual nursing plan about the nursing activities which have to be implemented to achieve the stated expected outcomes.

Educational dimension

There is no doubt from the preceding text that many nursing activities have an educational dimension for which nurses may have difficulty in stating expected outcomes. Many of the activities were mentioned in the context of identifying those problems for which they were required. Here they will be introduced, together with suggestions about possible stated expected outcomes, under three headings: information giving/receiving, acquisition of practical skills, and change of attitude.

Information giving/receiving

Some parts of the nurse's role involve providing information about preventing a particular condition, which might be preventing a potential problem from becoming an actual problem, or preventing the recurrence of a successfully treated condition. For imparting the information, a time has to be planned in the nursing programme when the nurse and patient can be together, preferably in an unhurried and private environment. It has to be ascertained that the person is 'hearing' adequately. 'Hard of hearing' is an invisible disability and many people are reluctant (perhaps not sufficiently assertive) to say that they have not adequately heard what was said. Education is a two-way process and the nursing responsibility is to observe non-verbal reaction and ask for feedback. So 'Understands the information' could be the stated expected outcome.

Providing verbal information may be accompanied by giving out leaflets, charts and so on. Again it cannot be taken for granted that the person has adequate vision, and can read and understand the written word. For non-English speaking people, identification of their language will permit selection of appropriate reading material, and on some occasions an interpreter will be required. It is no longer sufficient for the nurse to think that she has carried out her responsibility by speaking and providing the written word. 'Understands the verbal and written information' might be the stated expected outcome.

Acquisition of practical skills

Another educational dimension of the nursing role is enabling people to acquire practical skills such as those needed for intermittent self-catheterization, management of an indwelling catheter urinary drainage system and management of a stoma. Several of the references advocated self-catheterization as the preferred option to an indwelling drainage system but as yet no large scale patient satisfaction survey has been reported in the nursing press.

The survey of people who had a urinary drainage system and were living at home (referred to on p. 217) found lack of handwashing after emptying and changing the bag, presumably non-compliance with the teaching programme. A video package is available for people whose problem requires this method of managing intractable urinary incontinence. As yet there are no published evaluations of its effectiveness. It may be that there is no substitute for one-to-one teaching and learning of the knowledge required, and demonstration/practice evaluation of the required techniques to achieve effective management of such a complex system. Undesirable outcomes are infection of the bladder, ascending to the kidney where it can cause end-stage renal failure requiring dialysis.

Instruction for pelvic floor exercises is usually given in a hospital or at a clinic; thereafter the people continue to live in the community. They are probably aware of the expected outcome that doing them will prevent/improve the number of incidents of stress incontinence. Evaluation can be provided by the person keeping (and producing at the next clinic visit) a chart of incidents of stress incontinence with the time, estimate of the amount of urine passed involuntarily, and any immediately preceding activity such as coughing.

Provision of a pad and pant system to an incontinent person is not the end of the nurse's responsibility; there has to be evaluation of whether or not it is achieving the goal for that particular person — individuality is the basis of nursing. The expected outcomes from providing a pad and pant system to a person in the community could be:

- will be able to wear the pad and pant
- will receive adequate supplies regularly
- will feel sufficiently confident to continue/renew social life
- surrounding skin will remain unblemished
- safe disposal of used pads and pants.

The relevant references show that the last outcome is infrequently achieved.

Change of attitude

Even for people whose AL of eliminating is problem free, it has a private and personal dimension. Development of problems increases this, and if the problem results in a change of body image, the initial change of attitude will probably be a negative one. People with for instance a newly created stoma or the realization that they will need dialysis for the rest of their life need time to accept this change and to integrate, not only the practical details of the new condition, but how they feel about their changed 'self' and what this will mean in their social relationships. In the body structure the organs required for eliminating are near those of reproductive function so in stating expected outcomes it is pertinent that the person understands that sexual life can be resumed if so desired. The person should not have to ask; offering this information should be part of the nursing plan which is implemented and evaluated.

And 'implementing' is being interpreted in a wider context, an example being nurses joining the pressure group for provision for disposal of such things as incontinence pads, ostomy bags and appliances in public toilets. Another example is the pressure group that is opposed to sponsorship in relation to stoma nurses. When nurses find that the quality of their nursing is compromised because on evaluation, the ostomy bags and appliances provided by the employer are not adequate for some of the ostomy people in their care, they may be compromising the Code of Practice required by their Nurse-Registering Council.

'Implementing' has always been the part of nursing which nurses are most familiar with and, in the main

do well. However currently health and social services throughout the world are financially constrained and for nursing to receive its fair allocation of money, nurses need to be able to present data from assessing, identifying problems, planning (goals set may not be achievable — note the waiting list for equipment to treat people with enuresis on p. 213), implementing and evaluating.

This chapter has been concerned specifically with the AL of eliminating. But eliminating is just one of the 12 ALs which are part of our conceptualization of nursing. Its possible interaction with the AL of expressing sexuality has been mentioned in this section. And in previous sections of this chapter 'an assessment of nutritional status' was advocated implicating the AL of eating and drinking thus making it obvious that it is only for the purposes of discussion and learning that the ALs can be separated.

Our model for nursing provides a conceptual framework for nurses in the clinical areas to individualize their nursing by using the now widely accepted phases of the process (Fig. 3.9, p. 60).

REFERENCES

Abbott D 1992 Objective assessment ensures improved diagnosis. Principles and techniques of urodynamics. Professional Nurse 7 (11) August: 738, 740–742

Anders K 1993 Open communication can restore self-esteem. Sexuality and stoma. Professional Nurse July: 638, 640–643

Andrews C 1993 Mixed meals. Ileostomy diet. Nursing Times 89 (43) October 27: 56, 58

Allison M 1995 Comparing methods of stoma formation. Nursing Standard 9 (24) March 8: 25–28

Baerheim A, Digranes A, Hunskaar S 1992 Evaluation of urine sampling technique: bacterial contamination of samples from women students. British Journal of General Practice 42: 241–243

Barrett J 1990 Treating faecal incontinence. Nursing Times 86 (33) August 15: 66, 68, 70

Beveridge C 1986 Catering for health can save money. The Health Service Journal 8: 1118

Black P K 1994a Hidden problems of stoma care. British Journal of Nursing 3 (14) 28 July – 10 August: 707–711

Black P K 1994b Management of patients undergoing stoma surgery. British Journal of Nursing 3 (5): 211, 212, 214, 215, 216

Black P K 1995 Stoma care: finding the most appropriate appliance. British Journal of Nursing 4 (4) February 23–March 8: 188–192

Blannin J 1992 Breaking point. Poor provision of continence advice. Nursing Times 88 (5) January 29: 61, 62, 64

Blenkarn I 1988 Urinary drainage systems: a new look. Nursing Times 84 (9) March 2: 72, 74, 76 (The Journal of Infection Control Nursing)

Bliss J, Watson E 1992 Continence: a basis for change. Nursing Times 88 (13) March 25: 69–70

Bloe C G 1990 Peritoneal dialysis. Professional Nurse April: 345–349

British Nutrition Foundation 1990 Complex carbohydrates in foods. The report of the British Nutrition Foundation's Task Force. Chapman and Hall, London

Britton P M, Wright E S 1990 Catheters: making an informed choice. Professional Nurse 5 (4) January: 194, 196–198

Brown C 1994 Community centre (continence). Nursing Times 90 (4) January 26: 86, 89

Brown J, Thomas E, McCallum A, White H 1991 Campaigning for continence (a telephone helpline). Nursing Times 87 (14) April 3: 66, 68

Brown J, Thomas E, White H 1991 An incontinence helpline service. Nursing Standard 5 (38) June 12: 25

Brown J, Meikle J, Webb C 1991 Collecting midstream specimens of urine — the research base. Nursing Times 87 (13) March 27: 49–52

Burkitt D 1983 Don't forget fibre in your diet. Positive health guide. Martin Dunitz, London

Candy M 1994 Raising awareness of a hidden problem. Pelvic floor promotion. Professional Nurse 9 (4) January: 278, 280, 282, 284

CE Continuing Education 1995 Article 343 Urinalysis. Nursing Standard 9 (28) April 5: 32–35

Chance R 1994 A problem we need not take for granted. (Incontinence). Professional Nurse 9 (7) April: 498, 500, 502, 504

Cheater F 1991 Continence training programmes: need for standardisation. Nursing Standard 6 (8) November 13: 24–27

Christey K 1993 Overcoming staff fears. Organ retrieval. Nursing Times 89 (47) November 24: 36–37

Corless R 1992 Caring for a homosexual man undergoing a colostomy formation. British Journal of Nursing 1 (10): 501, 503–506

Crooks S 1994 Foresight that leads to improved outcome. (Siting stomas) Professional Nurse 10 (2) November: 89, 90, 92

Cunningham P 1993 A comforting approach. Donor families. Nursing Times 89 (33) August 18: 50–51

Deegan S 1991 Close to normality. Clean intermittent catheterisation. Nursing Times 87 (44) October 30: 65, 67

Department of Health 1993 Clinical audit. Meeting and improving standards in health care. HMSO, London

Department of Health 1990 The annual report of the Chief Medical Officer of the Department of Health for the year 1990. HMSO, London

Department of Health 1991 An agenda for action on continence services. HMSO, London

Dobson P 1990 Bedwetting — the last taboo. Nursing Standard 4 (44) July 25: 25–27

Dolman M 1992 Midwive's recording of urinary output. Nursing Standard 6 (27) March 25: 25–27

Dulfer S 1992 CIS sponsor debate flawed. Nursing 5 (1) January 9–22: 4

Durman R, Hudson S 1993 Protocol for loss. Organ retrieval. Nursing Times 89 (45) November 10: 50–52

Egan M, Thomas T M, Meade T W 1988 Incontinence: who cares? The Professional Nurse 3 (7) April: 238, 240–242

Emly M 1993 Abdominal massage. Nursing Times 89 (3) January 20: 34–36

Fader M 1994 From wheelchair to toilet. Nursing Times 90 (15) April 13: 76, 78, 80

Fair P A 1994 Hygiene for health. CAPD at home. Nursing Times 90 (5) February 2: 71–72

Farbrother M 1993 What can I eat? Ileostomy diet. Nursing Times 89 (14) April 7: 63

Ford H 1992 Some possible causes of colour change in urine. Nursing Times 88 (5) January 29: 66, 68

Gartland C 1993 Partners in care. Children on peritoneal dialysis. Nursing Times 89 (30) July 28: 34–36

Gaze H 1992 Stoma care? Sponsorship. Nursing Times 88 (15) January 29: 18

Getliffe K 1993a Informed choices for long-term benefits. The management of catheters in continence care. Professional Nurse 9 (2) November: 122, 124–126

Getliffe K 1993b Freeing the system. Catheter 'blockers' and 'non-blockers'. Nursing Standard 8 (7) November 3: 16–18

Gibbons P 1990 Cystitis in the sexually active female. Nursing Times 86 (2) January 10: 33–35

Gibson E 1990 An exhibition to eradicate ignorance. Setting up a continence resource centre. Professional Nurse 6 (1) October: 38, 40, 42

Glenister H 1987 The passage of infection. Nursing Times 83 (22) June 3: 68, 71, 73

Goodinson S M 1986 The nurse as innovator. Professional Nurse 2 (3) December: 87–90

Gould D 1994a Controlling infection spread from excreta. Nursing Standard 8 (33) May 11: 29–31

Gould D 1994b Keeping on tract. Nursing Times 90 (40) October 5: 58, 60, 62, 64

Griffiths-Jones A 1992 The safe disposal of excreta. Nursing Standard 6 (22) February 19: 28–29

Harlow 1988 Stoma care: waste disposal. Nursing Times 84 (8) February 24: 72, 75

Haynes S 1994 Intermittent self-catheterisation — the key facts. Professional Nurse 10 (2) November: 100, 102, 104

Hill P 1991 Assessing faecal soiling in children. Nursing Times 87 (14) April 3: 61, 62, 64

Horn S 1990 Nursing patients with a continent urinary diversion. Nursing Standard 4 (21) February 14: 24–26

Hughes A 1991 Life with a stoma. Nursing Times 87 (25) June 19: 67–68

Jamieson E M, McCall J M, Blythe R 1992 Guidelines for clinical nursing practices related to a model for nursing. Churchill Livingstone, Edinburgh

Janes G 1990a A better life than before. Renal patients. Professional Nurse 6 (1) October: 26–28

Janes G 1990b An open approach to minimise the effect. Sexuality and renal patients. Professional Nurse, November: 69–71

Jay P 1989 Community patients' toilet needs. Nursing 3 (35) March: 28–30

Jeffries E 1993 At home with stoma care. Appliances and services available. Nursing Times 89 (14) April 7: 59, 60, 62

Jerrum C 1991 CAPD: The state of the art. Nursing 4 (30) March 14–27: 28–30

Kelly M 1994 Mind and body (Stoma). Nursing Times 90 (42) October 19: 48–51

Kelly M P, Henry T 1992 A thirst for practical knowledge. Stoma patients' opinions of the services they receive. Professional Nurse 7 (6) March: 350–352, 355, 356

Kohler-Ockmore J 1993 Catheter concerns. Making long-term catheterisation safer and more comfortable. Nursing Times 89 (2) January 13: 34–36

Lanara V 1987 Catching infection from catheters. (Conference Report) Nursing Standard 1 (1) September 12: 6

Langford R 1994 A public inconvenience. Nursing Times 90 (27) July 6: 62

Laycock J 1991 Pelvic floor re-education. Nursing 4 (39) August 21: 15–17

Llewelyn S 1992 Attitude problems. Nursing Times 88 (31) July 29: 65–66

Lyall J 1990 A simple solution. Children with stomas and their parents. Nursing Times 86 (19) May 9: 16–17

Macaulay M, Henry G 1990 Drop in and do well. Community continence clinic. Nursing Times 86 (46) November 14: 65–66

Macleod J A 1992 Collecting specimen for laboratory tests. Nursing Standard 6 (20) February 5: 36–37

Mallillin E 1985 Facts about fibre. Nursing Times 81 (47) November 20: 32

Marr H, Pirie 1990 Protecting privacy. People with learning disability. Nursing Times 86 (13) March 28: 58–59

Martin J 1993 Peritoneal dialysis: prescription for the 90s. British Journal of Nursing 2 (3): 162, 164–166

Mayberry M K, Mayberry J F 1993 An information booklet for schools to help teachers deal with students with inflammatory bowel disease. Journal of Clinical Nursing 2: 19–22

MORI 1991 MORI-6040 Health Survey Questionnaire. BACC Books

Mulhall A 1991 Biofilms and urethral catheter infections. Nursing Standard 5 (18): 26–28

Mulhall A, Chapman R, Crow R 1988 Emptying urinary drainage bags. Nursing Times 84 (4) January 27: 64, 66

Naylor J R, Mulley G P 1993 Commodes: inconvenient conveniences. British Medical Journal 307, 6914, 1258–1260

Norton C 1994 Asking simple questions: promoting continence. RCN Nursing Update. Nursing Standard 8 (23) March 2: 4

Norton C 1988 Incontinence can be prevented at all ages. Professional Nurse 4 (1) October: 22, 24, 26

Norton C 1995 Nursing for continence. Beaconsfield Publishers, Beaconsfield

North K 1990 Sponsorship: the current dilemma. Nursing 4 (18) September 13–16: 15, 16, 18, 19

Nursing Standard 1992 Continence centre earns positive client feedback. Nursing Standard 6 (30) April 15: 16

Nursing Times 1995 (Special report.) Catheters. NT 91 (9) March 1: 45–46

Nursing Times 1992a Choosing garments to aid incontinence. Nursing Times 88 (27) July 1: 50, 51

Nursing Times 1992b Obtaining clean urine samples. Nursing Times 88 (39) September 23: 56

Nursing Times 1992c The best way to insert rectal suppositories. Nursing Times 88 (10) March 4: 50

Passmore A P, Wilson-Davies K, Stoker C et al 1993 Chronic constipation in long-stay elderly patients: a comparison of lactulose and a senna-fibre combination. British Medical Journal 307, 6907: 769–771

Payne C, Gardner J H 1992 Ensuring quality for ostomists. Commercial sponsorship. Nursing 5 (1) January 9–22: 19–20, 22

Pearson A 1993 Nursing, technology and the human condition (Guest editorial). Organ donation. Journal of Advanced Nursing 18: 165–167

Philp J, Cottenden A, Ledger D 1992 The re-user's guide. Nursing Times 88 (44) October 28: 66, 68, 70, 72

Philp J, Cottenden A, Ledger D 1993a A testing time. Choice of materials and designs available for re-usable garments and pads. Nursing Times 89 (4) January 27: 59, 61, 62

Philp J, Cottenden A, Ledger D 1993b Well disposed? Are re-usables as green as they seem? Nursing Times 89 (16) April 21: 65, 66, 68

Philp J, Cottenden A, Ledger D 1993c Mix and match. Continence aids. Patient assessment. Nursing Times 89 (16) April 21: 79, 72, 74

Philp J, Cottenden A, Ledger D 1993d Wash and wear. Nursing Times 89 (21) May 26: 63, 64, 66

Philp J, Cottenden A 1993 Picking and choosing. Four pages of reusable continence products. Nursing Times 89 (30) July 28: 70, 72, 74, 76, 78, 80

Pomfret I 1994 An unsuitable job for a woman? Male catheterisation. Nursing Times 90 (22) June 1: 46, 48

Pomfret I 1993 Men only. Nursing Times 89 (8) February 24: 55–57

Pottle B 1994a Stand up and be counted. Nursing Times 90 (27) July 6: 70

Pottle B 1994b Help is at hand. Continence awareness week. Nursing Times 90 (10) March 9: 71

Professional Nurse 1993 Living with a stoma. Professional Nurse 9 (2) November: 108, 110

Professional Nurse 1991 ISC (Intermittent Self Catheterization) can improve quality of life. Professional Nurse (2) July: 604

Reid E A 1976 The problem of incontinence. Nursing Mirror 142 (14) April 1: 49–52

Rhodes P, Parker G 1994 Profile of an adviser. Nursing Times 90 (4) January 26: 75, 76, 78

Robinson B 1993 Be alert to an avoidable problem. Professional Nurse 8 (8) May: 510, 512

Roe B 1994 Clinical developments in continence care. Nursing Standard 8 (24) March 9: 27–30

Roe B 1993 Catheter-associated urinary tract infection — a review. Journal of Clinical Nursing 2: 197–203

Roe B H 1990 Study of the effects of education on the management of urine drainage systems by patients and carers. Journal of Advanced Nursing 15 (5) May: 517–524

Ross J 1994 A plan of action. Continence assessment. Nursing Times 90 (27) July 6: 64, 66

Sadler C 1990 Getting dry. Community Outlook (Nursing Times) September: 33, 35

Sanderson P J, Weissler S 1992 Recovery of coliforms from the hands of nurses and patients: activities leading to contamination. Journal of Hospital Infection 21: 85–93

Sheffrin P 1993 Abdominal massage. Nursing Times 89 (7) February 17: 14

Stickler D J 1990 The role of antiseptics in the management of patients undergoing short term indwelling bladder catheterisation. Journal of Hospital Infection 16: 89–108

Taylor P 1994 Beating the taboo. Sexuality, stoma, patient education. Nursing Times 90 (13) March 30: 51–53

Tierney A J 1973 Toilet training. Nursing Times 69 (51/52) December 20/27: 1

The Independent 1994 Health chiefs target incontinence 'taboo'. The Independent

The Independent 1993 Dysentery cases show a sixfold increase. The Independent, April 2

Thomas M 1987 More fibre makes sense. Nursing Times 83 (3) January 21: 39

Thomas B 1991 Nurses' prescription of stoma appliances. Nursing Standard 5 (17) January 16: 25–27

Thomas N 1992 Measurement of quality of life for elderly people on dialysis. British Journal of Nursing 1 (6): 281, 282, 284, 285

Thompson J 1991 The significance of urine testing. Nursing Standard 5 (25) March 13: 39–40

Travers A F, Burns E, Penn N D et al 1992 A survey of hospital toilet facilities. British Medical Journal 304, 6831: 878–879

Turner T 1994 Muscle control: pelvic floor exercises. Nursing Times 90 (10) March 9: 64, 66, 69

Unsworth J, Rowell R 1994 Containing incontinence in men: an extra dimension. British Journal of Nursing 3 (18) October 13–26: 936, 938–940

Ward E 1993 Opting out. Organ donation. Nursing Times 89 (20) May 19: 44–45

Watson R 1989 In praise of sheaths. Geriatric Nursing and Home Care. 9 (3) March: 10–11

Wells M 1991 A tangible means of assessing progress. Biofeedback in the management of urinary incontinence. Professional Nurse April: 396, 397, 399

Wells M 1990 Stress incontinence and pelvic floor exercises. Professional Nurse 6 (3) December: 151, 154, 155

White H M 1994 Choosing continence aids. (Environmental) British Journal of Nursing 3 (22) December 8–January 11: 1158, 1160, 1162, 1163

White T 1995 Palliative care: dealing with constipation. Nursing Times 91 (4) April 5: 57, 58, 60

Wilson–Barnett J 1980 Prevention and alleviation of stress in patients. Nursing 10 February: 432–436

Wild J 1992 Dialysis without tears. 88 (18) April 29: 50–51

Winder A 1994 Achieving independence. Intermittent self-catheterisation. Nursing Times 90 (22) June 1: 50, 52

Woodward S 1995 Assessment of urinary incontinence in neuroscience patients. British Journal of Nursing 4 (5) March 9–22: 254–258

World Health Organization 1990 The rational use of drugs in the management of acute diarrhoea in children. World Health Organization, Geneva

Wright E 1989 Teaching patients to cope with catheters at home. The Professional Nurse 4 (4) January: 191, 192, 194

ADDITIONAL READING

Black P K 1994 History and evolution of stomas. British Journal of Nursing 3 (1): 6, 8–11

Bond L 1990 Altered image. 'Temporary' colostomy. Nursing Times 86 (18) May 2: 72, 75

Booth B 1992 Life savers. Organ donation. Nursing Times 88 (44) October 28: 16–17

Evans M 1993 Moral costs. Nursing Times 89 (37) September 15: 34–35

Evans M 1992 Ethical organs. Nursing 5 (2) January 23–February 12: 10–11

Hagland M 1994 Making sense of continuous renal replacement therapy. Nursing Times 90 (40) October 5: 37–39

Higgins C 1995 Microbiological examination of urine in urinary tract infection. Nursing Times 91 (11) March 15: 33–35

Kelly M P, Henry P 1993 Open discussion can lead to acceptance. The psychosocial effects of stoma surgery. Professional Nurse 9 (2) November: 101–102, 104, 106

Killingworth A 1993 Psychosocial impact of end-stage renal disease. British Journal of Nursing 2 (18): 905–908

Kuula V 1990 Eye of the beholder. 85 year old woman's change of body image after ureterostomy. Nursing Times 86 (48) November 28: 57, 59–60

Model G 1990 A new image to accept. Professional Nurse 5 (6) March: 310–312, 314, 316

Morrall S E 1990 The shock of the new. Altered body image: stoma. Professional Nurse 5 (10) July: 529, 532, 534, 537

Norton C 1995 Continence: a challenge for us all. British Journal of Nursing 4 (6): 307–308

Norton C, Brown J, Thomas E 1995 A phone call away. Nursing Standard 9 (25) March 15: 22–23

Nursing Standard 1993 Harvesting of organs: the nursing issues. Nursing Standard 7 (40) July: 25–26

Nursing Standard 1992 Testing renal patients for HIV: guidelines. Nursing Standard 6 (46) August 5: 32

Phillips S 1995 Gut reaction (Inflammatory bowel disease). Nursing Times 91 (1) January 4: 44–45

Richmond J 1994 The tyranny of interstitial cystitis. Nursing Times 90 (43) October 26: 72

Summerton H 1995 End-stage renal failure: the challenge to the nurse. Nursing Times 91 (6) February 6: 27–29

Wade B 1989 A stoma is for life. Scutari Press, London

Watson R 1990 The influence of component parts on the performance of urinary sheath systems. Journal of Advanced Nursing 15 (4) April: 417–422

White H M 1995 In control with incontinence aids. British Journal of Nursing 4 (6) March 23–April 12: 334–338

Wright A 1992 Routine assessment will identify problems. Professional Nurse 7 (4) January: 233, 234, 236

9

Personal cleansing and dressing

The AL of personal cleansing and dressing

Through the ages man has paid attention to his personal hygiene; there is archaeological evidence of the means whereby these activities were performed by members of previous civilizations. In each historical period there has been a gradual refinement of the articles used for cleansing the skin, hair, nails and teeth. Today, the ever increasing advertising of the cosmetic and hairdressing industries has increased most people's interest in personal grooming.

The clothing and fashion industries have developed equally expansively. Clothes today are very different from past times; clothing worn by members of previous generations on formal occasions is evident from paintings. Also depicted are the clothes worn for leisure time activities and for different sorts of work. Progress in manufacturing processes has resulted today in a wide variety of 'easy-care' clothes for every conceivable occasion so that people can now enjoy this part of everyday living with less effort and greater variety.

From the model of living (p. 21) and the model for nursing (p. 26) students will have gained a basic appreciation of this AL as part of our conceptualization of nursing. This chapter emphasizes the AL as a specific entity within the model illustrated in Figure 9.1.

The objective in most cultures is to socialize children into independent performance of personal cleansing and dressing activities, usually in privacy and in rooms set aside for these purposes. Even for those children who do not have their own bedroom, the bed and bedside area are symbols of privacy, and they usually dislike other members of the family 'interfering' with this area. For most people the attitude is inculcated from an early age that cleansing and clothing one's body is a personal concern, which if not carried out in privacy is accomplished in the presence of close family members only.

But the end result is observable by others, cleanliness and good grooming being commended in most cultures, while lack of these is deplored, particularly if accompanied by malodour and infestation. As there are several different activities concerned with personal cleansing, they will be discussed separately.

WASHING AND BATHING

Most people clean the skin by washing with soap and water, rinsing and drying.

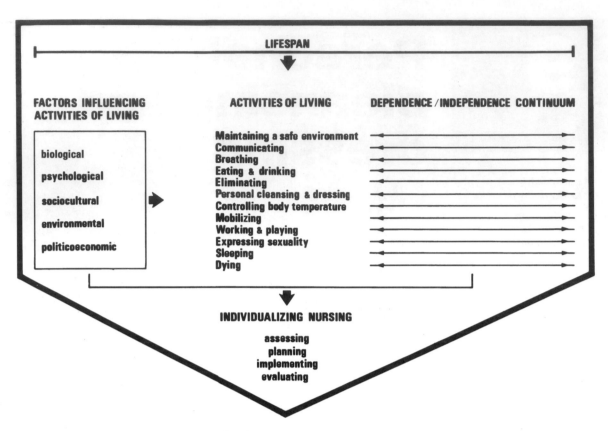

Fig. 9.1 The AL of personal cleansing and dressing within the model for nursing

It can be an 'all-over' wash using a basin of water, an immersion bath or a shower. The disadvantage of the immersion bath is that the bather is surrounded by the debris which is washed off the skin, and as the bath empties, some of this adheres and has to be removed. The shower, in contrast, is said to be more hygienic and has the advantage that it saves space and water. Children are socialized by membership in the family into a frequency norm for their 'all-over' cleansing, such as daily or weekly, however it is accomplished.

Even the apparently simple activity of washing is implicated as important in the prevention of the spread of HIV infection and AIDS. In the event of blood (or other body fluid) splashes to the skin, immediate washing with soap and water should be carried out (Royal College of Nursing, 1994).

HAND WASHING

Everyone is now encouraged to wash their hands before preparing or eating food and after going to the toilet. It is important that people are vigilant about the temperature of water issuing from hot water taps in public places. Increased hot water temperatures were recommended by safety executives to combat legionella that cause Legionnaire's disease which can be fatal. Thermostatic mixer valves are now being recommended (Nursing Times, 1991).

Hot air hand dryers can blow pathogenic microorganisms onto the newly washed hands. This information resulted from a comparative study of dryers, use of paper hand towels and pull down linen towels in public washrooms in hospitals, fast-food restaurants, shops and railway stations (Journal of Nursing Management, 1994). Hand washing assumes a particular importance in the context of hospital (Sneddon, 1990; Gould, 1994) and it is discussed on p. 94.

Frequent removal of the skin's natural oily secretion (sebum) may produce chafing, and broken skin is a route of entry for microorganisms which can lead to local infection. Dryness can be counteracted by using an emollient hand lotion after washing and adequate drying; when applied before sleeping it has maximum time to act (Thompson, 1994).

PERINEAL TOILET

The moist membranes in the female perineal area require special attention to maintain health and comfort and to avoid malodour. Females are encouraged to cleanse this area from front to back after elimination, especially of faeces. Microbiological data has confirmed that the majority of infections of the female bladder (cystitis) are caused by microorganisms that normally inhabit the bowel and are present in faeces and can therefore be in close proximity to the short urethra. Such organisms do no harm in their natural habitat but are pathogenic (disease-producing) in other organs.

CARE OF HAIR

A healthy condition is achieved by at least daily combing and/or brushing with a clean comb and brush; weekly hair washing is the norm for many people although daily washing is becoming more common in the younger age groups. Of all the personal cleansing activities, hair washing over the years has become the least 'private' (witness modern hairdressing salons). To cater for every kind of hair, there are numerous lotions and shampoos many of which help to keep the scalp free from dandruff. Spraying water over hair is thought to be the best way of completely removing shampoo, but many people still manage with a basin of clean water. Since hair grows daily, albeit slowly, most people have their hair cut at frequent intervals. Hair styles, which change with the fashion, are an important aspect of self-image and expressing sexuality.

CARE OF NAILS

Cleanliness can be achieved by removing any obvious dirt with a blunt instrument before using a nail brush while hand washing. After drying, while the cuticle is still soft it can be gently pushed backward with the towel to prevent it growing down on to the nail. A ragged cuticle can provide an entry point for microorganisms and a whitlow can result. Cuticle cream helps prevent raggedness. Finger nails are usually rounded to the shape of the finger end, although some people wear their nails long and pointed. A few occupations cannot be performed safely for the client by a person with long nails. For instance bakers, hairdressers and nurses are strongly encouraged to have short clean finger nails.

For toe nails it is thought that if they are cut in a straight line, any pressure on the middle of the nail from the shoes will slightly raise the two sides and avoid an ingrowing toe nail.

CARE OF TEETH AND MOUTH

Whereas many of the cells in the human body, if damaged, can be replaced the teeth cannot be. The best that can be done for decayed teeth is to remove the carious part by drilling and to fill the space with a suitable substance. To avoid dental caries, people must follow a rigorous routine of teeth and mouth care.

Fluoride protects the teeth (Jones, 1992); it is present naturally in some drinking water supplies throughout the world and is added artificially to others (in some countries). Where it is not present or has not been added, fluoride-containing toothpaste should be used by all age groups.

Brushing the teeth with a slightly abrasive alkaline paste or powder helps to remove plaque from the exposed tooth surfaces. Plaque is a sticky film of food and saliva deposits, cells shed from the mucous membrane and microorganisms; it adheres to the surface of the teeth and is not easily removed. The presence of plaque still adhering to the teeth after cleaning can be revealed by using a dye disclosing agent. Plaque builds up quickly in the absence of cleaning and starts attacking the teeth shortly after the ingestion of sugars or refined carbohydrates. Therefore it is important that the teeth are cleaned immediately after eating and drinking sweet things which acidifies the mouth and it takes two hours for saliva to neutralize it (Jones, 1992). A good 3-minute brush at least once a day is recommended to remove plaque, best carried out before sleeping.

Vigorous up and down movement when brushing teeth is now discouraged and stroking from the gum to the lower edge of the teeth is recommended, not forgetting the backs of the teeth. The gums are also damaged by plaque and gum disease accounts for the loss of more teeth than any other cause in adulthood (Barnett, 1991; Thurgood, 1994). Regular dental care, flossing between the teeth and adequate and proper brushing help to prevent gum disease. Recession of the gum, common in older age groups, encourages dental caries; desensitizing toothpaste enables brushing to be accomplished without discomfort if the gums are painful.

Ideally food debris should be removed from the teeth after each meal. When tooth brushing is not feasible at these times, the abrasive action from chewing something fibrous like an apple or orange is helpful. A drink of water removes food particles from the mouth but is not so effective in removing them from between the teeth; dental floss or a tooth-pick can accomplish this.

In spite of improved knowledge about the causes and prevention of dental caries, many countries are experiencing an increased incidence of dental caries and a lowering of the average age at which people become edentulous and require dentures. The social changes whereby fizzy drinks and ice cream are readily available to children who eat and drink these simple sugar-containing confections between meals contributes to the problem. Sticky sugar adheres to the teeth; it breaks down into acid more readily than starch; acid in contact with tooth enamel for a sufficient time erodes it, and dental caries ensues.

Halitosis is another disturbing problem for some people. It is usually described as malodour of the breath ('mouth air' in the research literature). The person may or may not be aware of the condition. A full dental and oral assessment by a specialist is necessary, and individual treatment will probably be prescribed. Nurses can help by assessing the person's knowledge of mouth care and correcting any inaccuracies or deficiencies, as well as encouraging the person to allocate sufficient time to mouth care. Measurement with a portable sulphide monitor provides objective assessment data (Scully, Porter & Greenman, 1994).

DRESSING

Changes in tradition and culture are reflected in clothes and each succeeding generation modifies dress to suit the changing environment and social conditions. Victorian crinolines would be difficult to manage as everyday clothes in today's fast-moving world and would certainly not fit in with the present-day attitude that clothes should be easy to launder and require minimal pressing and ironing.

Clothes are a medium of non-verbal communication. They can signify ethnic origin, level of income and social status, as well as personal preference of colour, style and fashion. They can convey mood: when well, people keep their clothes in good condition; when dejected, they frequently do not seem to notice stained clothes and down-at-heel shoes.

The manual skills required for independence in dressing are achieved by most people, but dressing includes much more than simply learning how to put clothes on. Children usually accept the type of clothing worn by members of the community in which they grow up. They learn that different clothes are worn for different occasions, such as for school and sport, and that a 'uniform' is worn by employees in many occupations.

Clothes which are next to the skin are in contact with sweat, sebum, epithelial scales; and also microorganisms which have optimal conditions for rapid multiplication, consequently clothes worn during waking hours should not be worn for sleeping and ideally should be changed daily. Microorganisms are attached to the scales of the skin and are shed into the atmosphere which can be a means of spreading infection.

Sensible selection of clothing can reduce strain on the heat-regulating centre in the brain by the protection afforded against rain, wind, cold, heat and sun. Clothing can also protect from injury, an example being crash helmets. Most people dress for personal adornment and get great satisfaction from doing so. The activity of dressing offers the opportunity for making decisions which help to develop a feeling of self-direction, an important part of self-fulfilment. And last but by no means least as already mentioned, clothes are a vehicle of communication.

Lifespan: relationship to the AL of personal cleansing and dressing

The AL of personal cleansing and dressing is performed throughout the lifespan but, in its various stages, there are some different concerns and preferences, and these are described in this section.

Infancy

During infancy, another person — usually a parent — attends daily to personal hygiene and dressing activities. For bathing the water is prepared at body temperature as an infant's skin is sensitive to heat. As well as a daily bath babies need to have any milk spillage removed immediately to prevent a sour odour. Because of their incontinent state the perineum and buttocks must be sponged and properly dried after elimination of urine and faeces, followed by application of a clean nappy or diaper which is non-irritant and absorbent. Excessive thickness between the legs should be avoided as the bones at this stage are still quite soft, being mainly organic matter. Loose-fitting and cross-over garments are chosen for the very young baby because even momentary confinement and darkening (as when clothes are drawn over the head) are frightening. Also the blinking reflex and tear glands do not work efficiently in early life.

At the crawling stage all-in-one suits are the most suitable daytime wear, for they will not impede the first attempts at standing unaided. As toddling is achieved, dungarees are useful as they afford some protection against the inevitable grazed knees. Gradually clothes characteristic of the culture are introduced. Night clothes should be made of non-inflammable material and pyjamas are safer than gowns which more easily catch fire.

The toddler can progress to the family bath where there is space to enjoy playing with toys so that bathing is associated with pleasure and relaxation. The cold water is run first to avoid overheating of the bath itself and scalding of the child. There are other dangers, too, for children at bathtime and so adult supervision is necessary throughout.

All clothes for children should fasten at the front and children should be able to dress themselves by the time they go to school. Children's clothes are now much more geared towards encouraging independence; for example, Velcro fasteners are provided instead of buttons and laces. Outdoor safety is also a concern of clothes' manufacturers these days. Road safety authorities are concerned about small children wearing coats with hoods, which can restrict hearing and vision as the wearer steps out on to the road. A fluorescent garment should be worn when children travel to and from school in inadequate daylight.

Care of the teeth is an extremely important aspect of this AL in the early years of the lifespan. There is considerable variation in the age at which a baby's first tooth appears but the usual teething period occurs when the baby is 6–9 months old, a time which can be somewhat trying for parents. While parents can help during this phase, they are vital in helping establish lifelong teeth care habits.

The habit of regular and proper brushing of teeth can be established as soon as a young child is able to hold a toothbrush and, indeed, at that early stage, it is fun rather than a chore. Dental education is increasingly being brought to young children through playgroups and nursery schools, and to their parents through the mass media and child health clinics. The main recommendations are proper brushing; regular dental inspection; and minimum intake of sugar-containing foods (and drinks) and refined carbohydrates. Sweets are better given following a meal and should be avoided altogether for snacks between meals; preferable alternatives are savoury foods and fruit. Started at an early age, it is more likely that habits which avoid harm to the teeth can be established.

Childhood

Increasing development of the neuromuscular system allows children gradually to master the technique of attending to their own personal hygiene and dressing with supervision. Increasing psychological development permits practice in decision making about these activities resulting in eventual independence and individuality. During these stages children gradually develop a concept of modesty in relation to the AL of personal cleansing and dressing.

Adolescence

As adolescence is reached there are several changes in the skin activity which may require specific attention. There is usually increasing under-arm perspiration and most people need to use a deodorant and antiperspirant. Dandruff on the scalp can occur. Many adolescents, particularly males, have to contend with acne, sometimes sufficiently severe to warrant medical treatment. Obesity creates a risk of maceration in the skin folds, for example under the breasts and in the groins which can affect care of the skin and choice of garments. Also excessive tissue on the upper inner aspects of each leg can cause unpleasant chafing from the friction produced when walking.

Adolescence can be the period for experimenting with way-out fashions and new hairstyles and provided that they do not cause any harm, tolerance and good humour reap better rewards all round than continual derisory remarks. It can be seen as part of the young person's bid for independence and a means of communication, both with peers and other groups.

Adulthood

As adult years are reached the reasons for and time of personal cleansing activities, such as bathing, may vary according to work and recreation. The choice might be an invigorating cold bath on waking or a soothing hot bath before sleeping. A whole lifestyle is reflected in a person's clothes: those for work, for formal social occasions, for informal social occasions, for relaxation, for leisure time activities and for sleeping. Most adults have acquired the ability to dress according to the socially acceptable norm for their culture, whatever the occasion, and to derive pleasure from so doing. Hair styling, grooming and use of cosmetics are ways of expressing personality and sexuality.

The elderly

In the declining years, elderly people may have increasing difficulty in managing some of the physical activities involved in cleansing and dressing, perhaps particularly getting into and out of the bath. Many gadgets are now available to enable older people to maintain their standards of personal cleanliness. Skin dryness may make moisturizing lotions necessary to prevent excessive flaking. Failing eyesight and shaking hands may make it increasingly difficult for older people to retain their independence with conventional clothing. Back fastenings of garments are difficult to reach and front fastenings are therefore preferable; zips and Velcro tapes are easier to manipulate than small buttons or hooks and eyes. Many older people more readily feel the cold and may need to wear extra clothing to keep warm. Two layers of thin material (because of the entrapped air which is a bad conductor of heat) are warmer than one thick layer. Adequately warm clothing is a simple, but important, means of preventing hypothermia (p. 277) which is a particular threat to old people in severe winter weather.

Problems with the mouth and teeth are also common in old age. Geissler & McCord (1986) mention statistics which indicate that 74% of those over 65 and 87% of those over 75 are toothless and, of those who do retain their own teeth, the majority have gum disease and caries. They recommend that the elderly should be encouraged to receive regular dental care and to ensure that oral health is maintained by proper cleansing of dentures and regular brushing of natural teeth.

Dependence/ independence in the AL of personal cleansing and dressing

The close relationship within the model of the dependence/independence continuum and the lifespan is reflected in almost all of the Activities of Living, and the AL of personal cleansing and dressing is no exception. In infancy there is almost total dependence on others for cleansing and dressing activities; childhood is characterized by ever-increasing independence; and independence is expected in adolescence and throughout adulthood, except for those unable on account of physical or learning disability, or during a period of illness. Declining physical and mental ability in the final stage of the lifespan may render the person dependent on help, for example with bathing or cutting nails. A variety of aids are available on the market which can help people to cope independently with cleansing and dressing activities which they would otherwise be unable to manage. Some of the available aids are described later in this chapter in the context of problems created by a change in dependence/independence status.

Factors influencing the AL of personal cleansing and dressing

The way the AL of personal cleansing and dressing is performed varies among individuals and many different factors are responsible for this. In keeping with the model, this section is subdivided into biological, psychological, sociocultural, environmental and politicoeconomic factors which influence the AL.

BIOLOGICAL

The largest physical body structure which relates directly to the AL of personal cleansing and dressing is the skin (the integumentary system). For centuries various medicaments have been applied to it for local effect. Today there are medicaments in the form of 'patches', which are absorbed into the blood for their general effect (Kelly, 1994). The skin's appendages (nails and hair), and the teeth are structures also related to

this AL. However, apart from these physical structures, the many activities associated with this AL require adequate functioning of the nervous, musculoskeletal and cardiopulmonary systems, among others.

Skin pigmentation

Skin colour is genetically determined and varies from being very pale in the case of albinos, through varying shades from 'fair' to black. In the UK an increasing number of Asian and black people are using potentially dangerous and disfiguring skin-lightening creams. Some contain hydroquinine and others contain mercury. Why should people in the UK want to use lightening creams? Are they receiving a message that only white skin is valued? Nurses, particularly those working in the primary sector are being urged to help in identifying lightening cream users (Godlee, 1992), and acquainting them with the dangers.

Hair

Hair colour is genetically determined and varies from white in albinos through varying shades from blond to black. Whatever the genetic inheritance hair becomes 'grey' with increasing age regardless of skin pigmentation. Hair also manifests ethnicity. Some people who were born and live in the west have tight curly hair and they spend a fortune having it straightened. Whereas white-skinned people born in the west with straight hair spend a similar fortune having it made wavy or curly. Apart from the occasional accident of skin injury from chemicals, straightening or curling hair is not a health hazard, and indeed may be health promoting by improving self-image.

Physical changes with ageing

Concerning the skin, nails, hair and teeth in particular, it is important to understand the physical changes which occur in the normal process of ageing. These changes have a direct as well as indirect influence on the ways in which personal cleansing and dressing activities are carried out. In adult years, care of the gums assumes as much importance as dental care because of the gradual shrinking of the gums with ageing. And, in later years, the loss of teeth and their replacement with dentures requires yet another form of attention.

　Similarly, changes occur in the course of the lifespan in the physical properties of the skin, hair and nails. Again, these changes mean that personal cleansing and dressing requirements are different at different stages of the lifespan. In adolescence, for example, there are the problems of acne and greasy hair; whereas, in old age, it is dryness of the skin and hair — and brittleness of the nails — which pose different problems, requiring different solutions.

Individual physical differences

The changes in the skin, hair, nails and teeth which occur in the normal process of physical ageing give rise to differences in physical appearance at various stages in the lifespan. In turn, people alter personal cleansing and dressing activities; for example, by modifying make-up to suit skin changes and altering hair styles as hair changes in condition and thickness.

Even among people of the same age, there are individual physical differences in terms of appearance which, to a large extent, is portrayed in the colouring and characteristics of the skin and hair. Individuality is portrayed by such things as the propensity for blushing and the presence of freckles, moles or birthmarks.

Physical hazards

Fair-skinned people are particularly at risk to one form of physical hazard, namely, the harmful elements of sunrays (p. 255). They have less pigment in their skin and, therefore, less protection. While suntanning had become fashionable with the advent of summer holidays abroad, more recently attention has turned to its dangers. Skin cancer, particularly in the serious form of malignant melanoma, is on the increase in many countries, including the UK (p. 255). The risk is higher in fair-skinned people and also in those with a large number of moles. Since malignant melanoma is potentially curable if treated early, a major effort has been put into public education in recent years, both to encourage early detection as well as prevention (Perkins, 1992); the most recent of these endeavours is about clothes.

Several governments are in the process of developing a labelling system to show which fabrics protect against harmful ultraviolet rays, to reduce the increasing incidence of skin cancer. Numbers will be given to 'clothing protection factors' — CPF numbers, comparable to those on suntan creams. Arms and legs should be covered with dark-coloured clothing of tightly woven fabric and loose fitting for comfort in hot weather. Head covering should be dark coloured and include neck protection. More than 40 000 people in the UK are diagnosed as having skin cancer every year. About 4 500 of these are malignant melanoma, the most dangerous form which kills 1 300 people in Britain a year. Incidence has increased by 50% in 10 years. Non-melanoma cancers, also associated with ultraviolet radiation rose from 19 000 cases in 1974 to 36 000 in 1988. These cancers rarely kill, but necessary surgery can be disfiguring (The Independent, 1994).

Another skin sensitivity to sun is being increasingly recognized. It is called polymorphic light eruption (PLE) and manifests as a recurrent itchy rash on light-exposed parts of the body, and recurs year after year. People with the condition can be reassured that it is benign and not associated with any internal medical problems, and does not cause scarring. Again nurses working in the primary sector need to be aware of the condition. Some patients will also be treated as outpatients at a dermatology clinic. Most sunscreens are against the B rays of the ultraviolet spectrum (UVB) and are not effective for PLE, indeed they usually worsen it. Recently a UVA/UVB screen arrived on the market and has proven to be effective in preventing PLE (Morton, 1993).

Sun is not the only form of physical hazard which can have an adverse, even dangerous, effect on the skin. Excessive heat, fire, cold, wind, pressure, friction and a whole range of chemical substances and diseases (e.g. infections and parasitic conditions) are other examples of physical hazards from which the skin requires to be protected.

Biological sex differences

The physical differences between females and males are relevant to discuss in relation to personal cleansing activities.

Female   Knowledge of the reason for effective perineal toilet (p. 232) will help to motivate girls to carry out this preventive technique. As the breasts develop, extra care is needed to avoid maceration in the lower skin fold; daily washing, powdering and support in a brassiere usually is sufficient preventive action. Girls require knowledge about the structure of their external genital organs so that they can remove excess secretion from the folds of skin and mucous membrane before it decomposes and causes an unpleasant odour. Psychological preparation for the onset of menstruation will help them to cope with its occurrence; during menstruation all glands are more active and a daily bath or all over wash is even more necessary. Girls acquire the behaviour of their cultural setting related to body hair; it can include removal of unwanted hair from the upper lip and legs, and from the female pubic area before the marriage ceremony.

Male   The bulbous end of the penis is the glans and the foreskin is the prepuce. Between the glans and foreskin at birth there are fine adhesions which prevent retraction of the foreskin and the necessity for cleansing under it. The adhesions dissolve in 6 months to 5 years when retraction of the foreskin is easily accomplished. If it is forcibly pulled back before this, the adhesions may be broken down and infection introduced. Boys are then taught to draw the foreskin daily over the glans and cleanse the circular skin fold. Like girls, boys must be taught that this cleansing is a necessary part of their personal hygiene to prevent unpleasant odour and infection. Before puberty boys need to be psychologically prepared for the possibility of 'wet dreams' (ejaculation of semen during sleep); they may wish to bath on waking to remove the characteristic odour of semen. At puberty they acquire the culturally determined behaviour of shaving or having a beard.

It is customary in some cultures for baby boys to have the foreskin removed (circumcision) shortly after birth. In other instances when parents wish to have a son circumcised they are usually advised to wait until he is toilet trained as this reduces the risk of infection. There is some evidence that there is less cervical cancer in women whose husbands have been circumcised.

Physical disability

Obviously, an individual's level of physical ability will determine the extent to which the various activities involved in personal cleansing and dressing can be carried out adequately; and people who are physically disabled may have difficulty in some aspects of this AL. Some are so severely disabled that they cannot participate in any of the activities comprising personal cleansing and dressing.

PSYCHOLOGICAL

Although modern society in general pays less attention to such things as dressing baby boys in blue and girls in pink, and adolescents nowadays tend to favour 'unisex' fashions, there are still basic differences in psychological outlook between the sexes with regard to the AL of personal cleansing and dressing.

Girls do tend to be more concerned with cleanliness and appearance, and boys may require greater encouragement to carry out personal cleansing activities with sufficient rigour. Adolescents of either sex may deliberately lower their standards of cleanliness as a form of protest against the authority of parents and teachers. On the other hand, their desire to be sexually attractive may result in a somewhat obsessional interest in appearance, make-up, hairstyle and clothes.

In adult years, too, standards of cleanliness and dress often reflect personality and emotion; an extrovert is more likely to wear bright colours and the latest fashion than a shy person; and a person who is depressed is likely to lose interest in appearance, sometimes even to the point of neglecting essential basic hygiene.

Attending properly to the AL of personal cleansing and dressing does require knowledge, for example about the importance of handwashing and the measures involved in preventive dental care. Therefore, lack of knowledge is likely to result in inadequate attention to cleansing and dressing activities which, in turn, may

result in problems such as infection, infestation, skin disease and dental caries. People who have a learning disability are by definition slow to learn, and require patient and repeated teaching in order to gain confidence and individual optimal independence in personal cleansing and dressing activities.

SOCIOCULTURAL

Not all cultures place the same value on cleanliness, and the personal cleansing pattern into which a person is socialized becomes deeply ingrained. Those used to a daily bath, shower or sauna may experience discomfort when facilities do not permit them to follow this pattern; conversely, people not accustomed to such patterns may find it strange to be in a country where this seems to be expected of everyone. Similarly, while some cultures place great value on cleanliness, others believe that the 'natural' smell of the body is normal and is part of sexual attractiveness.

There are ranges of norms for shampooing the hair (dryness or greasiness often being the deciding factor) and for cleaning the teeth, although many dentists would prefer that everyone accepted as their norm cleaning after meals and before going to bed at night. From a health point of view there is an essential norm for handwashing which is before touching food, and after elimination to prevent food poisoning and diseases spread by ingesting microorganisms from faeces.

There are still instances where culture dictates the type of clothing worn. In the West it has become acceptable for women as well as men to wear trousers; in some cultures it is customary for the men to wear robes and for the women to wear trousers. Religion still influences dress, for instance the clothing worn by monks and nuns. In most countries, not only culture and religion but also the law determine those parts of the body which must be clothed when in public. All of these sociocultural variations are more widely appreciated nowadays through the influence of the mass media and as a result of international travel.

ENVIRONMENTAL

It is easy for those whose homes have a piped supply of hot water and a fixed bath or shower to presume that these facilities are available to all people. Again it is presumed that water will be available from a tap until the threat or reality of a water shortage reminds people that even such a basic amenity cannot be taken for granted. The AL of personal cleansing and dressing does require the availability of certain amenities in the home environment if the activities involved are to be adequately carried out.

This is true also of the work environment. Some industries expose the skin to risk from such things as coal dust, tar, soot, asbestos and other cancer-producing agents. Showers are considered to be more efficient than baths and the workers are encouraged to shower before going home. In some countries protective clothing may be obligatory if there is a known health risk to the workers (p. 318).

The climate of the surrounding environment is another factor which influences the AL of personal cleansing and dressing. For example, in tropical climates there may be the need for more frequent bathing or showering to remove excessive perspiration. Many people in hot climates find that they are more comfortable in clothes made of cotton because it absorbs perspiration, and less comfortable in man-made fibres which are less absorbent. Garments made from man-made fibres and wool are useful for providing warmth in colder climates. White and light colours are chosen by people in sunny regions, since theoretically they reflect the sun's rays but this is challenged by the cancer coding for clothing (p. 237). In contrast dark colours, because they absorb the rays and are therefore warmer, are traditionally the choice of people in cold climates.

POLITICOECONOMIC

With the world shortage and consequent high cost of fuel, many people who have the facilities for a hot water supply are experiencing difficulty in affording it. This can apply especially to a nation's disadvantaged groups such as those on a fixed income, be it a pension or unemployment benefit. Some governments consider the amenity of a fixed bath sufficiently important to warrant a financial grant towards its installation in old property.

The importance of preventive dental care and treatment is recognized by those governments which provide a free (or subsidized) service for people unable to afford to pay for it themselves and/or who most need it: such as children, pregnant women, the elderly and the unemployed. The possible addition of fluoride to the water supply is something of a political issue.

There is certainly an economic dimension to the AL of personal cleansing and dressing at the individual level. Personal income determines the amount of money which can be spent on articles used for personal cleansing, such basic things as soap, shampoo, comb, hairbrush, toothbrush, toothpaste and manicure tools. In several countries pressure groups have succeeded in preventing tax increases on women's sanitary protection articles. When income is limited, emphasis is less on appearance and more on basic health issues — the prevention of infection, skin irritation or disease, dental caries and infestation with lice.

Economics also enters into the number of clothes a person can buy: minimally a person needs to possess enough clothes to wash or dry clean them sufficiently often to prevent odour from dried perspiration or irritation to the skin from dirty fabric. For those who are impoverished, clothes become simply a matter of basic necessity and the person is denied the pleasure of attractive clothes and variety in dressing.

Each of these factors contribute to the pattern and style of each person's individuality in attending to the AL of personal cleansing and dressing to which a variable proportion of time is allocated each day.

Individualizing nursing for the AL of personal cleansing and dressing

Taking into account all the issues described in the foregoing discussion of the various components of the model, it should be easy to appreciate that people develop marked individuality in relation to the various components of this AL. The components are predicated by the fact that in our model, the biological factors which are juxtaposed with the AL of personal cleansing and dressing are the skin, hair, nails, teeth and mouth.

Detailed knowledge about a person's individual habits related to personal cleansing and dressing activities is necessary if this important aspect of everyday living is to be given due emphasis in individualized nursing. Some people bath in the morning, others at night; some never have a bath, always a shower (and vice versa); and while some people bath only once or twice a week, others like to do so twice a day. Whatever the habits, they often become so ingrained that the person may strive to ensure that they can be kept up, for example while staying in a hotel or in lodgings or in hospitals.

ASSESSING THE INDIVIDUAL IN THE AL

If individuality and independence in the AL of personal cleansing and dressing are to be encouraged within the context of individualized nursing, nurses need to have information about the patient's usual routines; what can and cannot be done independently; what previous coping mechanisms have been employed; and what problems exist or may develop. Such information can be obtained through nursing assessment of a patient. Nurses can discuss the AL of personal cleansing and dressing with the person, using the résumé in Box 9.1 as a guide to relevant topics, and bearing in mind the following questions:

- what are the individual's usual personal cleansing and dressing habits?

Box 9.1 Assessing the individual in the AL of personal cleansing and dressing

Lifespan: effect on personal cleansing and dressing
- Infancy
  — skin care (incontinent state)
  — suitable clothing for mobility/safety
  — growth of teeth
- Childhood
  — developing independence and individuality
  — developing concept of modesty
  — importance of care of teeth
- Adolescence
  — increased underarm perspiration
  — problems of acne, greasy hair, dandruff
  — expression of feelings/individuality/ sexuality through clothes, make-up, hairstyle
  — puberty (menstruation/ejaculation)
- Adulthood
  — routines related to working and playing
  — reflection of personality in appearance and clothes
- Old age
  — skin dryness
  — difficulties with bathing, care of nails and feet
  — difficulties with dressing
  — physical disability

Dependence/independence in personal cleansing and dressing
- Dependence in infancy/old age/illness
  — on people
  — on aids and equipment

Factors influencing personal cleansing and dressing
- Biological
  — stage of physical development
  — physical changes with ageing
  — individual physical differences
  — skin state colour bruising/scars/ blemishes dry/moist turgid/wrinkled areas of discontinuity cleanliness
  — state of hands and nails cleanliness handwashing habits
  — state of mouth and teeth moist/dry mouth odour of breath

  teeth (number/condition, dentures)
  teeth-cleaning routine
  — condition/style of hair type (dry/ greasy) dandruff/lice hair washing routine
  — dress style/appropriateness standard of cleanliness/odour quality/suitability of footwear special clothing for work/play
  — physical hazards
  — physical sex differences
    female: perineal toilet breast care menstruation body hair
    male: cleansing foreskin shaving
- Psychological
  — sex differences/sexuality
  — standards related to personality/ emotional state
  — knowledge (e.g. handwashing, dental care)
  — intelligence
- Sociocultural
  — values concerning cleanliness/ appearance
  — social norms for cleansing/dressing routines
  — cultural influences/rules on dress
  — religious influences/rules on cleansing/dressing
- Environmental
  — bath/shower in the home
  — piped hot/cold water in the home
  — exposure at work to substances damaging to the skin
  — availability of bathing/handwashing facilities at work
  — climate
- Politicoeconomic
  — adequacy of necessary facilities for low income groups
  — personal income for articles for personal cleansing
  — personal income for essential clothing and footwear

- when and how often are the various activities performed?
- what factors influence the individual's personal cleansing and dressing habits?
- what does the individual know about the relationship of personal cleansing and dressing to health?
- what are the individual's attitudes to personal cleansing and dressing?
- does the individual have any longstanding difficulties regarding personal cleansing and dressing activities and, if so, how have these been coped with?

- what problems does the individual have now (or is likely to develop) with the AL of personal cleansing and dressing?

Of course, the nurse may not have to actually *ask* these questions. More often than not the answers are obtained in the course of discussion, or in what the person chooses to say in response to a general, open-ended question from the nurse. And, of course, all the questions should not come only from the nurse — valuable information can be gleaned from questions the person asks, and this is something to be encouraged. An assessment, perhaps especially on admission to hospital, has the purpose of *obtaining* information from patients but, equally, it is an opportunity to *give* information to them as well. And, of course, assessment involves much more than use of interview technique. Use of all the senses, especially observation, is vital and it may be that some people's problems are self-evident, requiring discussion only for corroboration.

Various tools have been devised for assessing the need for mouth care (p. 245), the risk of developing pressure sores (p. 248) and the risk of wound infection (p. 252) and they will be discussed in the context of change in dependence/independence status.

IDENTIFYING ACTUAL AND POTENTIAL PROBLEMS

There are dramatic circumstances when extensive burns and scalds wherever they occur on the body constitute a surgical emergency and immediate transfer to hospital is essential. The priorities will be to save life and prevent infection. Only from reflection of what nursing interventions were required, and from ongoing assessment will the person's problems per se begin to be recognized. A pain management programme will be an early requisite. As will enabling the person to come to terms with any change in self-image.

In less dramatic circumstances many of the people who are experiencing problems related to the skin, hair, nails, teeth and mouth will be encountered by nurses working at primary level. The problems might well be caused by skin disease or infestation, warts, moles, ingrowing toenails, minor burns including sunburn, and leg ulcers. Also people are being discharged home as soon as possible after surgery and nurses at primary level are involved in continuing the nursing plan for these people as well as those who have had 'day surgery'. They all need to understand that hands can transmit microorganisms to discontinuous skin thereby providing a potential problem of infection, so the nurse's educational role regarding prevention is foremost. The problems which a person may experience in relation to personal cleansing and dressing are many and varied; recognizing and solving them calls for sensitivity, empathy and ingenuity on the part of the nurse.

But not all actual problems can be solved, some can only be alleviated, and when this is the case, then the nursing role is to enable the person to develop positive coping strategies. And of course potential problems have to be prevented from becoming actual problems.

The problems which students are likely to encounter early in their careers are discussed in three categories:

- change of dependence/independence status
- change in mode of personal cleansing and dressing
- change of environment and routine.

The change of dependence/independence status is longer than the other two because it includes:

- causes of dependence
- aids to independence
- dependence for mouth care
- dependence for prevention of pressure sores
- dependence for management of pressure sores
- dependence for management of wounds
- psychological problems.

CHANGE OF DEPENDENCE/INDEPENDENCE STATUS

Acquisition of the skills for independent performance of the many activities related to personal cleansing and dressing requires an adequately functioning nervous system, not only to control movement in the lower limbs and to facilitate precision movements in the upper limbs, but also to enable learning about the rationale of the skills. Integrity of the musculoskeletal system is simultaneously necessary for carrying out the many manual skills involved. Inadequacies in these systems at birth may prevent the child from achieving independence for this AL; any dysfunction in the systems can prevent people maintaining independence even to the point of rendering them dependent for one or more of the activities which are part of personal cleansing and dressing.

The nature of the problems in achieving and maintaining independence for this AL varies according to whether the impediment is congenital, immediate, or of gradual onset. Gradual onset permits the person time to become psychologically adjusted to the changes and to develop physical manoeuvres for coping. Similarly there is a difference in the nature of the problems according to whether the impediment is short- or long-term. Personal hygiene problems experienced by people vary according to whether one or more limbs are involved, whether they are upper or lower ones or an upper and lower limb on the same side.

Causes of dependence

There is no easy method of classifying the numerous impediments to independence in carrying out the many skills involved in personal cleansing and dressing. Partly because there are so many skills and partly because such a variety of factors can affect the nervous, musculoskeletal and integumentary systems, there cannot be an exhaustive classification of causes of dependence. To help beginning students to develop this concept, the ensuing discussion uses the following headings:

- limited mobility
- absence of limbs
- involuntary movements

- sensory deficits
- unconsciousness
- psychological disturbance
- illness.

Limited mobility   The sites at which people experience limitation of movement determine the particular problems which they experience in performing some or all of the skills necessary for personal cleansing and dressing. A person with a frozen shoulder should be encouraged to put garments over the arm on the affected side first. Crippled hands cannot hold conventional articles for cleaning teeth, manicuring nails, combing hair; nor can they manage to fasten small buttons or zips. A stiff spine on the other hand interferes with getting into and out of the bath and applying garments to the lower limbs. Immobility of the jaw renders the patient dependent for mouth care but usually all the other skills of personal cleansing and dressing can be carried out independently.

Absence of limbs   Congenitally deficient children may not feel the absence of limbs to be a problem because a limb-deficient body has become 'normal'. Should admission to hospital be required there will already be an established regime of managing personal hygiene. It is important to record this regime and in particular exactly what nursing help is needed so that staff on successive shifts offer the same sort of help. On the other hand a person who loses one or more limbs, is faced with learning alternative techniques according to which limbs are absent. In the early stages there is increased risk of accident should the person even momentarily forget the limb deficiency; it is not unusual for the phenomenon of 'phantom' limb to be experienced (p. 132).

Involuntary movements   It is difficult for those who have achieved coordination of movement brought about by the smooth, sequential contraction and relaxation of various muscle groups to realise the many difficulties that can be experienced by not being able to control movement. To give an example: exaggerated uncontrollable hand movements (such as caused by Parkinson's disease) make such apparently simple tasks as dressing, shaving, putting paste on a tooth-brush, and even combing the hair, arduous.

Being patient, allowing such people time to carry out their activities, and praising the effort (even if the result is not as 'tidy' as the nurse would wish) are a means of providing psychological support, as well as enabling them to retain their optimal independence.

Sensory deficits   When for any reason the brain is not receiving warning stimuli from the skin about the temperature of the water being used for bathing, there is increased risk of scalding. Lack of pressure stimuli can mean that tissues are subjected to increased pressure which may result in pressure sores (p. 246). Many blind people achieve the necessary skills to attend to all aspects of their personal cleansing and dressing; others require some help with some of the activities related to this AL. Particularly, at the initial assessment, nurses need to be very sensitive when collecting data from a person with a sensory deficit.

Unconsciousness   Unconscious patients are totally dependent on the nurse for preserving their dignity and for ensuring the safety and integrity of the body during all aspects of personal cleansing and dressing. The limbs will probably be stiff and spastic and will need to be supported by one nurse without stretching the muscles and tendons, while the other nurse washes and dries the skin. Pressure sores (p. 246) are a potential problem.

Psychological disturbance   Even after healthy habits of personal cleansing and dressing have been established, these can be disrupted during psychological disturbance, whether this is caused by cognitive impairment or psychiatric illness of one kind or another. There may be a general deterioriation in the standard of personal cleansing skills and an apparent disregard for dirty malodorous clothing. Development of a nursing plan for such patients usually requires goal setting in small gradations to achieve the final goal of regaining healthy personal hygiene habits.

Illness   Illness can interfere with independence in several ways. Sometimes it is sheer exhaustion which prevents people attending to themselves; sometimes it is breathlessness, when the slightest movement causes further respiratory embarrassment. When the illness dictates that people are attached to various machines or gadgets, this can be yet another reason for dependence in some or all of the activities related to personal cleansing and dressing.

These are but a few examples of circumstances which can impede the many skills necessary for personal cleansing and dressing. There can be no hard and fast rules for nursing activities in this AL and a high degree of professional judgement is required to enable the development of an individual nursing plan and expertise in implementing and evaluating it.

Dependence for washing/bathing

It is obvious that on admission an accurate assessment of each person's manner of performance of this AL is imperative. Many disabled people have become experts at coping with their condition. Nurses should acknowledge this, listen to them and encourage them to continue to cope where this is permissible. In instances of psychological disturbance, and illness, the nurse may well have to take the lead in development of a nursing plan, and for an unconscious person it might be advisable to discuss previous hygiene habits with the relatives before devising a nursing plan. Unconscious patients, people with dementia and some people with learning disability are dependent on the nurses for preserving their right to privacy during personal cleansing and dressing activities.

The nursing plan indicates where the person's personal cleansing will take place: in bed or in the bathroom; what activities can be carried out independently and what sort of help is required with the other activities. There are many variables to consider when these decisions are made, and the following are some principles which nurses can bear in mind when helping dependent people to bath or be bathed in bed:

- each person is entitled to privacy during the activities of personal cleansing and dressing
- there is a possibility of lack of congruence between the nurses' and patient's concept of privacy and modesty
- activities related to patient's safety, integrity of their body systems, dignity and modesty are a nursing responsibility for which nurses are accountable
- most patients are entitled to make some decisions about aspects of their personal cleansing and dressing, and thus make an important contribution to preventing deterioration of self-image, and institutionalization.

Here it is appropriate to alert beginning students to the fact that there is a dearth of research on which washing and bathing dependent people can be based. As long ago as 1956, Boycott cultured potential pathogens including coliforms and *Staphylococcus aureus* from the water in which a person had bathed and from the deposits left in the bath. Maurer (1985) recommended 'vigorous cleaning with scouring powder' after each use of the bath. Currently many cleaning agents contain a hypochlorite which increases cost, but there is no research to support increased effectiveness in rendering the bath free from bacteria.

Greaves (1985) found that the hazards associated with bathing people in bed were even greater. She took samples of the water in the washbowl at various stages of the procedure (the bacteriological count was even higher than in Boycott's study). The face cloths and towels were also infected. She recommended that:

- patients should have their own bowl for the duration of their stay in hospital
- the water should be changed at least once during the procedure
- 'clean' areas should be washed before for example the perineum which harbours large numbers of bacteria
- disposable facecloths should be used.

It is customary in most hospitals in the UK for patients to provide their own facecloth. It should not be put back in the toilet bag but should be hung to dry — microorgan-

isms require moisture to multiply; deprived of it they die. If females bring only one cloth, it can provide a health education role for the nurse — a separate washcloth should be used for the perineum which should be washed from front to back to minimize the opportunity for bowel microorganisms to enter the short urethra. When a person is being nursed at home, a bowl should be reserved for washing and bathing. It is usually easier to arrange for drying of the face and washcloth between each use.

An alternative to bed bathing is the 'towel bath'. Wright (1990) illustrates and describes the procedure. In a small 'patient satisfaction' study, of the 25 patients, 23 preferred the towel bath, one preferred the bed bath and one did not enjoy either. Bacteriological data were not collected. A rudimentary costing was done for 500 towel and 500 bed baths. It was based on 1986 prices and salaries and showed that there was a saving of £345.49 when towel baths were used.

When patients are experiencing problems in relation to any or all of the activities necessary for personal cleansing and dressing, provision of relevant aids to independence can help both patients and nurses.

Aids to independence

Many types of equipment have been developed as aids to independence for personal cleansing and dressing activities.

For bathing and showering With an ageing population and a government policy of maintaining elderly people in their own homes for as long as possible, it is relevant for nurses to have some knowledge about equipment which can facilitate this. Many modern baths have a metal handle in each of the long sides; they are especially useful when the person is rising from the water. A grab rail can be fixed either on the wall, or across the taps, and this is also helpful when rising from the water.

Technologists have helped other people to maintain their independence for bathing by producing several types of compression/decompression devices whereby people can sit on the seat which is level with the top of the bath; swing their legs over the bath edge and press a handle which lowers them into the water. After bathing, exit from the bath is accomplished in reverse. There are people who can continue to bath themselves if they can be transported to the bath and lowered into the water. Various hoists can accomplish this, some of which are portable so that people can maintain their independence in their own homes. Various devices are illustrated in Nursing Times (1995).

For care of hair Extra large combs and brushes with modified handles may be helpful for people who have difficulty in gripping or with above-shoulder movement. Such a simple measure as positioning a mirror at sitting height may enable some people to brush and comb hair without help, for example those in a wheelchair or who have difficulty in standing or balancing. The use of dry shampoo is a substitute for wet hairwashing, enabling independence on occasions for patients who require to have their hair washed. People with 'Afro' type of thick, curly hair need to use particular combs, hairbrushes and techniques (Davis, 1977). People with cerebral palsy who have athetosis can be helped to acquire their optimal independence for drying hair by providing a towelling hood (Bush, 1984).

For care of nails With a total impediment of one hand there is usually no way in which a person can manicure unaided the nails of the other hand, though the person may be able to manicure the toe nails. Some people dislike filing their nails or having them filed; if unable to use nail scissors they may find that they can use nail clippers.

For care of teeth and mouth Electric tooth brushes may be more effective for disabled people's use. For people with shoulder deformities or arthritis who are unable to reach their mouths, it may be necessary to lengthen the toothbrush handle; this can be done simply with polyethylene tubing. Toothpaste can be dispensed from an inverted tube secured in a wall-attached device which helps some people to retain their independence. Dependence for mouth care is discussed on p. 244.

For dressing Velcro and long zip fastenings often help frail elderly and disabled people to continue dressing themselves or doing so with minimal help from another person. Where there is impediment of one arm or leg, the limb is put into the garment first so that maximum use can be made of the flexibility of the normal limb. When both upper limbs are disabled it may be that one sleeve can be drawn over one limb, the garment arranged over the front and back of the trunk and Velcro or a zip used along the second side. For those with disabled lower limbs it is usually preferable to put on trousers while lying on the bed. There are several gadgets which help them to be independent at this manoeuvre. Similar gadgets help with putting on pants and stockings.

The Disabled Living Foundation (1995) provides an illustrated step-by-step guide to dressing techniques. The local occupational therapists help people who have particular problems of dependence. Walker and Lincoln (1991) developed the Nottingham stroke dressing assessment and investigated the relationship between dressing abilities, and cognitive and physical problems.

Aids to independence for dressing are especially relevant when nursing elderly people, but it presumes that they have their own personal clothing. Authors writing about their disappointing experience when attempting to achieve this chose to remain Anonymous (1994).

Dependence for mouth care

The information under this heading proceeds from what was written about care of the mouth and teeth at the beginning of the chapter (p. 233), during the early stages of which there is a natural dependence. During the ensuing years, attitudes, values and beliefs, as well as knowledge about oral pH and the physical skills of oral brushing are acquired as part of the socializing process. Nurses in contact with young children have a preventive role, especially when these children have a physical disability such as uncontrollable arm movement which precludes acquisition of the physical skills. Children with a learning disability may not be able to acquire the cognitive dimension and will remain dependent on supervision to achieve oral health.

Having achieved independence, at any stage along the lifespan a person can become dependent for mouth care for a short or long period. Planning mouth care must be based on an understanding of oral pH (p. 233). There is a dearth of 'research' about mouth care for dependent people, but when those who have vigilantly carried out adequate mouth care become dependent even for a relatively short period they will not expect to have one or more carious teeth as a result.

Mouth care procedures in the UK were investigated for the first time by Howarth (1977). More recently there has been increased interest in care of the mouth, and several articles in nursing journals refer to Howarth's original work (Barnett, 1991; Clarke, 1993; Heals, 1993; Peate, 1993). People frequently develop oral problems as a result of chemotherapy, radiotherapy, immunosuppression and immunodeficiency. All people in these categories need regular oral assessment.

Since there can be a long period between people becoming seropositive for the human immunodeficiency virus (HIV) and manifestation of the infection, seropositive people need to be able to recognize white patches (thrush) on the oral mucosa which can be caused by *Candida*. When removed a reddened or bleeding surface is revealed (Pettifer, 1992).

Elderly people who have cognitive impairment or dementia may well be cared for in long-stay psychogeriatric wards or in nursing homes. They are often dependent on prompting to clean their mouth and teeth — either natural or dentures. Some are completely dependent for mouth care. In one study (Boyle, 1992) found that many members of the nursing staff rated cleaning mouths as the task they found most distasteful.

Assessing the need for mouth care A sore mouth can be symptomatic of disease within the mouth, or of pathology in another part of the body, pernicious anaemia being an example. Box 9.2 is not an exhaustive list of points to be considered in assessing mouth care, but it includes the main ones.

> **Box 9.2   Assessing the need for mouth care**
>
> • Current oral status
> • Physical and/or mental ability to achieve successful mouth brushing
> • Fluid and food intake
> • Nutritional status
> • Mouth breathing
> • Sore mouth
> • Oral pain
> • Dysphagia
> • Medications
> • Medical diagnosis

The number of published articles about this nursing practice has increased in the 1990s. Peate (1993), Clarke (1993) and Moore (1995) each provide an overview of relevant literature, as well as their experience in the wards. Buglass (1995) discusses the debate about use of a toothbrush versus foamsticks, among other aspects of mouth care. Barnett (1991) explores assessment of the mouth and methods of providing oral care, together with a discussion of the solutions (including toothpaste) used. Thurgood (1994) uses the phases of the process in his article and gives details about the agents used for mouth care.

Many of the people who develop a sore mouth from cytotoxic drug therapy attend Outpatients Clinics. Middleton (1994) developed a one-page ongoing assessment document which the patient keeps, fills in, and brings to the clinic where the current condition of the mouth is evaluated by a nurse and recorded. There is also a similar one for care of a sore mouth from *Candida* infection. See also Heals (1993).

The objectives of mouth care procedures are comfort, cleanliness, moistness, prevention of infection and encouragement of appetite. On the basis of available research evidence mouth care procedures, in the majority of instances, can be based on the following recommendations:

• use of a small headed, multi-tufted, childsize toothbrush
• use of fluoride toothpaste or, where the patient has particular problems, a chlorhexidine gel
• use of sodium bicarbonate for dry, encrusted mouths
• use of Vaseline for patients with dry mouth and lips
• use of chlorhexidine mouth washes for prophylactic purposes
• whole mouth brushing — which includes gums, palate and tongue as well as teeth (This requires to be stressed for patients who wear dentures and

who normally receive assistance only with denture cleaning).

It is suggested that a regime based on these recommendations will meet the objectives of mouth care procedures and will also be cheaper than use of prepacked mouth care trays, presently used by nurses in many hospital wards. These are important points in today's climate of providing an efficient, cost-effective nursing service.

Before leaving this section which deals with dependence for mouth care, it is necessary to mention those dental, medical and pharmaceutical professionals who have been lobbying for the removal of sugar from paediatric medications with the objective of helping to prevent dental caries. A particular group requiring paediatric medications are those who have learning disability (Manley, Sheiham & Eadsworth, 1994).

Dependence for preventing pressure sores

Before discussing the subject of dependence for preventing pressure sores, it is pertinent for students to know where they are likely to occur and what they are, even though there is some dubiety about what should be included in the term 'pressure sore'.

Pressure areas or sites   Body weight when sitting or lying is borne by the skin and supporting tissues overlying the bony prominences illustrated in Figure 9.2, and these are referred to as pressure areas or sites. Forty years ago the term 'bedsores' was used and it was indicative of the fact that the majority of patients in hospital and in the community were nursed in bed for the major portion of their indisposition. In the 1960s early ambulation was introduced with the objective of preventing 'pressure

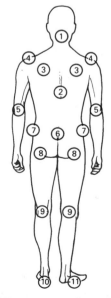

1. Occiput
2. Spinous processes
3. Scapula
4. Shoulder
5. Elbow
6. Sacrum
7. Iliac crest
8. Ischial tuberosity
9. Knee
10. Heel
11. Side of foot

Fig. 9.2 Pressure areas/sites

sores' (as well as several other possible complications of bedrest). But in one study there were more sores on the chairfast than on the bedfast patients, the site of the sore in the chairfast being over the sacrum not the ischial tuberosities (Clark et al, 1978). Further research is needed to investigate this phenomenon.

Defining pressure sores Some of the difficulty in defining pressure sores is definition of the word 'sore'. When pertaining to the skin it is usually interpreted as a break in its continuity. However the first sign that skin is reacting to pressure is redness, sometimes apparent on healthy people between the knees after sleeping and it quickly disappears. In some pressure sore grading systems this redness is classified as Grade 1, and if it does not blanch on finger pressure, as Grade 2. Logically if a preventive programme were planned and implemented at this stage there would not be any further skin deterioration. But there are so many factors contributing to pressure sores (which will be discussed) that this is not always the case. The ensuing Grades vary in different systems but here they will be discussed first as 'superficial sores' and 'deep sores'.

Superficial sores In these sores there is destruction of the epidermis with exposure of the dermis which can be caused by such things as creases in the bedclothes and/or personal clothes, crumbs, harsh linen, abrasion from bedpan or commode and persistent scratching. Superficial sores can be precipitated by excessive moisture from fever or incontinence which increases the friction between skin and the surface supporting it. Friction can produce blisters, which may be the first sign of damage. Once the epidermis is removed, the skin's protective function is lost and microorganisms can penetrate the exposed tissue which is moist with lymph. A semipermeable dressing can be applied using aseptic technique and secured in position to prevent entry of microorganisms (p. 69). Relief of pressure is essential until healing has occurred. There can be further destruction including the dermis and the sore is then classified as a deep one.

Deep sores In these sores there is destruction of the epidermis and dermis exposing deeper tissues which can include muscle and even bone. Unlike the superficial sore the damage can be established in the deep tissues before tracking out to the surface. Deep sores can become infected, discharging an exudate which results in protein and fluid loss so that there has to be reciprocal modification of the AL of eating and drinking. Deep sores can take many weeks, indeed months to heal and can require surgical closure to prevent further debility. The site, whether or not it is surgically dressed (and many new types of dressings and products have become available in recent years), must not be exposed to pressure and meticulous regular relief over the other pressure areas is essential.

Although classification has been discussed here simply in terms of distinguishing between 'superficial' and 'deep' sores, there is an emerging view that a more detailed and standardised classification system would be valuable, not only to guide practice but also as a basis for evaluative research. However the grades/classifications used by Milward (1993) and Wardman (1991) reveal the difficulties and are evidence of the need for a national grading system.

Factors contributing to pressure sores In order to understand the rationale of nursing activities which aim to prevent the development of pressure sores, it is essential to know about the various factors, both direct and indirect, which contribute to their development. Pressure sores result from an interruption of the tissue's blood supply, causing a local ischaemia and, if this continues, necrosis of the affected area. There are many predisposing factors but the main factors in pressure sore formation are continuous direct pressure and shearing force.

The various factors contributing to pressure sores are listed in Box 9.3 and hereafter are discussed in turn.

Compression of tissues Compression of tissues between two hard surfaces is the major cause of pressure sores. Compression of the skin and deeper tissues between the hard, bony skeleton and the unyielding surface of a bed is the most common example, but the same effect can result from the chair seat, stretcher, trolley, operating theatre table or X-ray table. The effect of compression is to reduce the blood supply to the cells so that they receive fewer nutrients and less oxygen, and there is less efficient removal of their waste products. Tissue death results from anoxia, not from mechanical damage to cells. It is understood that pressure evenly distributed over a larger area is less injurious than local 'point pressure', but prolonged low pressure is more hazardous than a short period of high pressure.

Shearing force When any part of the supported body is on a gradient, the deeper tissues (mainly muscle) near

---

Box 9.3 Factors contributing to pressure sores

- Compression of tissues
- Shearing force
- Heat
- Moisture
- Friction
- Poor skin hygiene
- Poor general nutrition
- Lack of oxygen
- Lack of spontaneous body movements
- Age
- Medical diagnosis

the bone 'slide' towards the lower gradient while the skin remains at its point of contact with the supporting surface because of friction which is increased in the presence of moisture. The blood vessels in the deeper sheared area are stretched and angulated, thus the deeper tissues become ischaemic with consequent necrosis. Shearing force can be created by badly executed moving of patients.

Heat Friction and pressure combine to produce a localized increase of temperature. The metabolic rate is raised which increases the demand for oxygen yet its supply is lessened by compression of blood vessels. Two hourly relief of pressure increases the blood supply and reduces the local temperature simultaneously.

Moisture Excessively moist skin from perspiration, urine or faeces encourages pressure sores which start as maceration of devitalised epithelium. It is therefore important to keep patients' skin as clean and as dry as possible. To this end, retraining for continence is planned and implemented for patients who are incontinent of urine.

Friction The adherence property of friction has already been mentioned. It can also cause injury resulting in the loss of epidermal cells (abrasion). Sometimes the first evidence of a frictional sore is a blister. It can occur on the heels, ankles and knees, especially in restless patients. Maintaining patients in a non-friction position is an important nursing activity.

Poor skin hygiene As noted previously skin has a natural flora of microorganisms which are constantly multiplying, so their number is higher if skin is unwashed. Consequently abrasion or maceration of unwashed skin is more likely to become infected.

Poor general nutrition Poor nutrition results in loss of subcutaneous tissue and muscle bulk, both of which normally act as mechanical padding. Lack of specific nutrients in the blood such as protein and vitamin C render a person more liable to pressure sores. Particular attention to the dietary intake of people at risk of developing sores is an important nursing activity (Wells, 1994).

Lack of oxygen Localized lack of oxygen due to lessened blood supply caused by compression and shearing has been mentioned. Anaemia is one cause for a generalized reduction in oxygen in the blood (hypoxaemia) and interference with oxygen absorption in the pulmonary membranes is another. People with hypoxaemia from any cause are at risk of developing pressure sores. Adequate intake of iron-containing foods such as red meat, egg yolk, green vegetables and salads is useful to maximize the blood's oxygen carrying function.

Lack of spontaneous body movements People when sitting, lying and sleeping make many small movements in response to sensory stimuli received by the brain. This is a protective physiological phenomenon to avoid excessive pressure on a particular part of the body. In any condition which prevents this protective mechanism, such as frailty, illness, anaesthesia, unconsciousness, loss of

sensation (as in paralysis or being under the influence of alcohol), drugs, or sleeping pills, predisposes to pressure sores.

Age In the Glasgow survey of 10 751 people in hospital and at home (Clark et al, 1978), 8.8% had at least one pressure sore and of these, the over 70s contributed the largest number. In another large survey of 885 patients (David et al, 1983), the prevalence was 6.7% and 85% of these were over 65 years of age. A consistent finding in smaller, more recent studies, some of which are referenced later, is that increasing age increases the prevalence rate. In a number of countries, there are many more people in their 80s who, should they become ill will be in the vulnerable group for developing pressure sores.

Medical diagnosis Although medical diagnosis was implicit in some of the foregoing 'factors contributing to pressure sores', it is useful to introduce the wide range explicitly. Poor general nutrition can result from any one of the chronic inflammatory bowel conditions such as Crohn's disease; or any of the malabsorption syndromes where the pathology can be in the small intestine or in the production of digestive enzymes. Cancer in different parts of the body can be characterized by gross loss of weight. And a compromised cardiovascular system can interfere with blood supply, especially to the feet putting the heels at special risk. The inexplicable loss of weight which can occur in people with dementia even when they are eating well was mentioned on p. 187. The Glasgow study (Clark et al, 1978) in its cross analysis of medical diagnosis and presence of at least one pressure sore, found that people of any age with multiple sclerosis, cerebral palsy, spina bifida or paraplegia were top of the list.

Identifying people 'at risk' Knowledge of the factors which contribute to the development of pressure sores leads to an appreciation of those groups of patients who are particularly at risk. The elderly, as already mentioned, constitute the single largest section of the patient population at risk of developing pressure sores. However, people who are bedfast or chairfast or otherwise immobilized should be considered as vulnerable. Crow (1988) comments that, while

'patient characteristics provide general indicators of vulnerability, there are more specific factors leading to irreversible damage in the tissue itself which need to be considered; aspects currently regarded as important concern damaging external loads which close the microcirculation and lymphatic system and intrinsic factors which weaken the tissue or its supporting network.'

Some of these various factors have been discussed in the earlier section on 'factors contributing to pressure sores'.

These factors provide the basis for tools which have been developed to identify patients 'at risk'. The Norton scoring system for identifying elderly people at risk of

Name	Date	Physical condition		Mental condition		Activity		Mobility		Incontinent		Total score
		Good	4	Alert	4	Ambulant	4	Full	4	Not	4	
		Fair	3	Apathetic	3	Walk/help	3	Sl. limited	3	Occasionally	3	
		Poor	2	Confused	2	Chairbound	2	V. limited	2	Usually/ur.	2	
		V. bad	1	Stuporous	1	Bedfast	1	Immobile	1	Doubly	1	

Instructions for use

- identify the most appropriate description of the patient (4, 3, 2, or 1) under each of the five headings and total the result
- record the 'score' with its date in patient's nursing notes or on a chart
- assess weekly and whenever any change in patient's condition and/or circumstances of care.

A 'score' of 14 or below denotes need for intensive care, that is, 1–2 hourly changes of posture and the use of pressure-relieving aids. Norton, in 1987, advised an increase of score from 14 to 15 or below.
Note: when oedema of sacral region has been present, a rise of score above 14 does not indicate less risk of a lesion.

Fig. 9.3 The Norton scoring system

developing pressure sores is illustrated in Figure 9.3. Although it is now many years since the initial publication of the score (Norton et al, 1962), widespread knowledge of it and its increasing use in nursing is a relatively recent development. The system is dependent on the subjective judgement of the assessor and, therefore, has limitations as a foolproof tool. The advantage of the Norton score is that it provides at least some means, which is not time-consuming, of assessing patients' risk of developing pressure sores and providing timely warning of the need to implement appropriate preventive nursing activities. Assessments should be repeated regularly (and frequently if the patient's medical condition deteriorates), preferably by the same nurse, and a downward trend in the score is particularly significant. The US Department of Health and Human Sciences recommended two risk assessment tools — Norton's and Braden's (Nursing Standard, 1992).

Since Norton's early work, numerous risk calculators have been devised and it now has several competitors, the best known is probably the one developed by Waterlow (1991).

Wardman (1991) compared the use of these two scoring systems on a small group of nursing home patients and recommended continuing use of the Norton scale. Bridel (1993a) provides an overview of a 'good' assessment tool and discusses the Norton, Waterlow and Braden scales. Birchall (1993) and Davies (1994) provide an overview of available tools. Some students may need more detailed analytical information and this is provided by Hamilton (1992) and Edwards (1994).

Since the general acknowledgement that a minimum two hourly relief of pressure is necessary, such areas as operating theatres, accident and emergency, and X-ray departments have become suspect. Bridel (1993b) explored use of the Braden assessment score for patients in operating theatres and Mullineaux (1993) explored use of the Norton score for elderly patients with fractured neck of femur in accident and emergency and X-ray departments.

Responding to the current and expected further increase in nursing patients in their own homes, the Kalsall Pressure Sore Calculator is available (Milward, 1993a,b,c). An educational leaflet is available to raise the level of awareness about the preventable nature of pressure sores among young wheelchair users living in the community. The most common reason for re-admission to a spinal unit is pressure sores (Stockton, 1994).

All of the assessment scoring systems are dependent on the subjective judgement of the assessor. Milward (1993a) states that many authors have highlighted discrepancies in scoring between individual nurses. Being aware of this should alert nurses to the reality that any selected scoring system should not be used as a substitute for good clinical judgement.

Preventing pressure sores Available knowledge about the cause of pressure sores has increased considerably over the last three decades. Indeed the literature is now so extensive that beginning students need help to reduce it to a manageable size for study. Knowledgeable people now realize that causation is so complex, no longer can 'poor nursing' be used as the scapegoat. This does not detract from the importance of the nursing contribution.

Pressure sore policies Increasing use of quality circles related to prevention of pressure sores in the 1980s and reports of their effectiveness in the professional press gave the subject higher visibility. Possibly there was an added impetus when the Department of Health recommended a reduction of 5 to 10% in the annual incidence of pressure sores.

General management became involved and in the process of developing a 'policy statement' there was gradual realization that 'pressure sores' was a complex issue requiring a multidisciplinary approach.

Multidisciplinary approach A preventive programme developed from local nursing research and led to a multidisciplinary decision to concentrate investment on proactive prevention as a more efficient use of available resources than confining spending to reactive treatment (St Clair, 1993; Callaghan, 1994; Milward, 1993b). A similar local nursing research project revealed that 70% of mattresses were unfit for continued use. It became evident that nurses needed guidance about matching the patient's level of risk to available equipment for relief of pressure (Benbow, 1993). 'Mattress fatigue' needs to be integrated into the concept of pressure sore prevention. Other professionals who can contribute to a multidisciplinary approach to the prevention and treatment of pressure sores are listed in Box 9.4.

Nursing contribution to relieving pressure On the basis of the knowledge that prolonged low pressure is hazardous to the compressed tissue, it is self-evident that relief of pressure is the single most important nursing activity in the prevention of pressure sores. Frequent, minor changes of position — which may be accomplished by the patient, if properly instructed — should be incorporated into the nursing plan as well as the more familiar intervention of 'regular turning'. For example, when a patient is bedfast but has some ability to move, a monkey pole or overhead trapeze is a simple means of achieving frequent relief of pressure by lifting the buttocks off the bed. When they are necessary, turning regimes are usually based on a 2-hourly schedule which to the best of our knowledge is the necessary frequency if those patients particularly at risk are to be adequately protected from developing pressure sores. Lowthian (1979) designed a turning clock to assist nurses in carrying out this preventive measure. The scheme is adaptable to suit each individual's routine and requirements; a list of scheduled times and a signature space accompanies the clock so that there is documentation of the actual implementation of the planned nursing intervention.

Torrance (1983) points out, however, that there are disadvantages in regular turning. First, there is the inconvenience to the patient of regular disturbance, disrupting sleep and perhaps causing pain. Second, it is a time-consuming activity for the nursing staff. In circumstances when regular turning is either undesirable or

---

Box 9.4 Other professionals who can contribute to a multidisciplinary approach to the prevention and treatment of pressure sores

Profession	Contribution
physicians	prescription for medicaments, dressings
surgeons	surgery for intractable sores
occupational therapists	teach transfer skills home assessment for bathing, washing cooking equipment
physiotherapists	mobilizing to relieve pressure deep breathing to increase O_2
dietitians	adequate nutritional intake for both prevention and healing
pharmacologists	oral and intravenous dietary supplements lotions and dressings
biotechnologists	research and development of: supporting surfaces for bedfast people and those who spend most of the day in a chair/wheelchair; pressure measuring devices
supplies officers laundry managers microbiologists directors of finance	contribute to the buying, hiring, servicing and disinfection of pressure relieving equipment

All members need to be aware that we are living in an increasingly litigation-conscious society (Richardson, 1991).

---

impossible to accomplish, or indeed as an adjunct to it, pressure-relieving devices can be employed.

Careful positioning and intelligent use of pillows can help to minimize tissue compression. Bed cradles strategically placed relieve the weight of the upper bedclothes from particular parts of the body. Sheepskins and synthetic fleeces used to be favoured as aids to reduce compression but are less frequently advocated for that purpose. Devices are also available which alternate the area of body under pressure, the most common example being the alternative pressure mattress or ripple bed. The basic system consists of a cellular air mattress connected to an electrical air pump and the air cells are alternately inflated and deflated. Most pump units can be adjusted to an appropriate weight setting, though in practice the heaviest setting is usually best for most patients. In addition to ripple mattresses, a variety of more recently-developed pressure-relieving beds and mattresses are now available; these include low air loss beds, air-fluidized beds, and the 'Vaperm' mattress.

Although there are many aids of various kinds available, the importance of regular change of position and manual turning where necessary cannot be overemphasized in relation to the prevention of tissue compression, the major cause of pressure sores.

Nursing activities to prevent shearing These include skilled moving of patients and positioning which will ensure prevention of sliding in any direction for patients in beds and chairs. Sliding down the bed can be prevented by adjusting the mattress or inserting pillows so that the knees are slightly bent and the thighs supported. A padded foot-board is also helpful. It is, of course, important that such measures do not discourage movement and patients should be asked to rotate each foot several times every hour or so.

The possibility of shearing in sacral, ischial and heel tissues should not be forgotten when patients spend some part of the day in chairs. The patient is less likely to slump in the chair if the back does not slant too much and if the feet are well supported.

The chair needs to match the patient's physique and be covered with a material which prevents downward sliding. Torrance (1983) identifies a number of factors which contribute to risk of pressure sores in the chairfast patient: slumped posture, badly fitting wheelchairs, or geriatric chairs, and poorly adjusted footrests or footstools. He advocates that patients should be taught to lift free of the chairseat (by hand push-ups) if no pressure-relieving cushions are employed. On the subject of cushions, he emphasizes that selection must be individual in relation to size and fit. Air, rubber and foam rings are not recommended.

As a summary of the foregoing discussion, which has been based on evidence from research as far as possible, there follows a statement of the principles of prevention of pressure sores:

- assessment of risk (based on knowledge of predisposing factors/use of tools, e.g. Norton score)
- relief of pressure to avoid damage by tissue compression — especially point pressure and prolonged low pressure (maximal exposure being 2 hours for those at highest risk)
- avoidance of shearing force (by skilled handling/ positioning in bed or chair to prevent sliding)
- avoidance of excessive heat, moisture and friction
- maintenance of adequate skin hygiene
- maintenance of adequate nutrition
- correction of oxygen lack/anaemia

- avoidance/correction of conditions which decrease spontaneous body movements.

As already mentioned the scenario is changing and nurses are increasingly taking the initiative and defining the size of the problem in their area, and gaining the support of members of other disciplines so that 'Pressure sore policies' can be devised and implemented throughout the area for which a Local Health Authority provides a service.

An increasing number of frail elderly people are being cared for in private nursing homes. Local Health Authorities have written standards with which they have to comply before they can be licensed, and thereafter they are inspected at regular intervals.

Proper management of the wound is, of course vital, and this will be discussed in the next section. But perhaps a reminder should be given that management of pressure sores is concerned with people and not just the sores! Individualized nursing is a vital aspect of the management of the complex issue of pressure sores.

Computer databases will increasingly contribute to quality monitoring of the prevention of pressure sores. Articles are beginning to appear in the nursing journals about nurses' experience of using a computer in this context (Kearsley, Little & Wiseman, 1994).

Dependence for management of pressure sores

If preventive measures are rigorously implemented, many pressure sores can be avoided and those which do occur, if noticed early enough as a result of regular assessment, can usually be treated successfully. Even though Torrance's book was published in 1983 it is still relevant and when pressure sores do occur he suggests that their management can be considered as comprising three aspects:

- removal of pressure (i.e. to keep the ulcerated area free of further pressure)
- treatment of predisposing factors (as described for prevention)
- care of the wound.

It is the third aspect — wound care — which remains one of nursing's controversial issues. Traditionally pressure sores were considered separately outside the concept of 'wounds'. However with the research that has been done, pressure sores which have resulted in destruction of deep tissues are now classified as cavity wounds, which can also occur from many causes other than pressure. Hollinworth's (1994) definition of a wound is applicable to deep pressure sores:

'A wound is a loss of continuity of the skin; soft tissue, muscle and bone may be involved.'

Members of several other disciplines as well as nurses are contributing to research about various types of wounds (including pressure sores). The title selected for this multidisciplinary group's 'organization' was 'The Tissue Viability Society' which is indicative of the many factors required to regain tissue viability as well as the inclusion of all types of wounds.

In the meantime in the nursing scenario, recognition of the complexities surrounding 'wound care' resulted in the appointment of wound care nurse specialists to disseminate research-based information to guide nursing practice. With increasing knowledge about the complex physiology of wound healing (Cutting, 1994; Cahill, 1994), it was realized that pressure sores were not an exception. So in the last few years an increasing number of tissue viability nurse specialists have been appointed. Hollinworth's definition of a wound (quoted above) does not take account of pressure-produced redness of skin over pressure areas which disappears on relief of pressure, and similar redness which does not blanch with finger pressure as warning signs before loss of continuity of the skin. 'Pressure sore' wounds, are now classified as chronic ulcerative wounds, sub-classified as pressure ulcers (Collier, 1993; Collier, 1994).

Dependence for management of wounds

Surgical operations mainly take place in hospitals where the policy is to admit people for elective surgery only one day prior to the surgery to minimize the possibility of colonization of the skin with 'hospital microorganisms' (Box 9.5), and to discharge them from hospital as soon as possible. So people have returned home and nurses may therefore attend to wounds in the person's own home, or in the health centre or at a clinic in the outpatients' department of a hospital.

Assessing wounds It is obvious that any person who has a wound (whatever the classification) is dependent on nurses for assessing it accurately, planning appropriate treatment, and evaluating at specified intervals until the summative evaluation of a healed wound. The points to be assessed regarding the person include such items as those illustrated in Figure 9.4; it also includes information about the wound. Various plastic measures are available which can be held above a wound to estimate its size and shape and is therefore useful as an assessment and evaluation tool (Fig. 9.5). The Wound Care Society (Flanagan, 1994) published assessment charts, and Morison (1994) devised two charts, one for surgically closed wounds and one for open wounds. In keeping with the concept of lifespan in our model readers are referred to a wound risk assessment chart for children (Bedi, 1993).

Risk assessment for *wound infection* is becoming part of nursing and in many areas it is incorporated into a

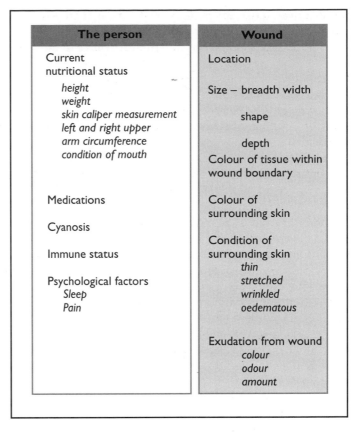

The person	Wound

Current nutritional status *height weight skin caliper measurement left and right upper arm circumference condition of mouth*	Location
	
	Size – breadth width
	
	   shape
	
	   depth
	Colour of tissue within wound boundary

Medications	Colour of surrounding skin
Cyanosis	Condition of surrounding skin *thin stretched wrinkled oedematous*
Immune status	
Psychological factors *Sleep Pain*	
	Exudation from wound *colour odour amount*

Fig. 9.4 Assessment factors related to the person and the wound

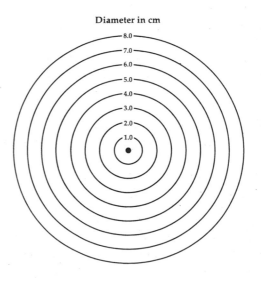

Diameter in cm

Fig. 9.5 Wound measurer

'written standard' or 'policy' or 'protocol'. One example of a 'risk assessment standard for preventing surgical wound infection' is set out in structure, process, outcome format (Kingsley, 1992).

It is difficult to cost the extra nursing hours required, as well as lotions and dressings needed because of wound infection, but the personal and emotional cost of pain, discomfort and inconvenience to the person is inestimable.

Staphylococcus aureus is often the organism responsible for surgical sepsis; most strains respond to antibiotics but increasingly the multiresistant strains are causing concern (Kalideen, 1990). Hence the need for several preoperative preparations.

Preoperative skin cleansing Traditionally patients had a 'preoperative bath' but critical thinking reveals that even if the immersion bath is previously disinfected, after the washing process, the water contains debris from the skin. The aim of preoperative skin cleansing is to remove the potentially pathogenic transient microorganisms and reduce the resident skin flora to the lowest possible level (Kalideen, 1990). But the removed microorganisms will be part of the debris just mentioned. There is a dearth of recent research on which to base nursing policy, but a study by van Dieman (1985) and quoted by Spencer and Bale (1990) showed that preoperative bathing with Hibiscrub (a detergent solution containing chlorhexidine gluconate) was effective in reducing hospital acquired wound infections.

Showering would seem to be preferable since any removed debris would go straight to the outlet. Kaiser et al (1988) quoted by Kalideen (1990) showed that showering with chlorhexidine reduced staphylococcal colony counts consistently, repeated application being more effective than one.

However Morison (1988) mentions the potential hazard of showering or bathing, namely that it may lead to the transfer of bacteria from areas such as the perineum and nose to other areas which are not colonized. She cites evidence of the value of whole body disinfection with an antiseptic solution in theatre as an adjunct to preoperative skin cleansing in the ward.

Morison also states that Hibiscrub is popular as a preoperative skin cleansing agent and that there is evidence of this being effective. On this basis she considers that 'two whole body preoperative washes with Hibiscrub, usually the night before and on the day of the operation would therefore seem cost effective and beneficial for patients'.

Hair removal Removal of hair from the skin around the site of incision is another nursing practice carried out in the preoperative period by many generations of nurses, and it still continues in some clinical areas. But according to Pettersson (1986) all of the research evidence points to one fact — that shaving ought to be avoided. The author, a Danish nurse, explains that nurses and doctors in Denmark have changed their attitude towards preoperative hair removal, considering it to be unnecessary unless hair around the operation site is copious, coarse or very long. If removal is necessary shaving is being replaced by depilation or clipping using hair clippers. Morison (1988) refers to evidence that clippers can nip the skin creases and, for this reason, and because of the hazard of cutting the skin when using a safety razor — she favours the use of depilatory creams. However, people may be sensitive to these and a patch test is recommended which can take several hours. Currently there are some hypoallergenic creams which only take one hour to patch test (Viney & Cheater, 1992).

If shaving is requested by the surgeon, Morison recommends that this is done as near as possible to the time of operation so that there is minimal opportunity for microscopic skin injury to become colonized with possibly pathogenic microorganisms.

To prevent infection, disposable razors are the first choice. Millward (1992) reports a project which investigated the cleaning/sterilizing of electric razors which were used communally and found practices to be very haphazard.

As will be apparent from the foregoing discussion, the issue of preoperative skin preparation is a complex and controversial one and nurses are responsible for keeping their knowledge up to date should any further research be done about this subject.

Other preoperative nursing practices In addition to preparation of the skin, further protection is afforded by the provision of special clothing for the patient's transfer to theatre. There is usually a complete change of bed linen while the person is bathing and putting on a theatre gown. A theatre cap is worn on the rationale that it decreases the possibility of microorganisms being shed from the hair. These modifications in the AL of personal cleansing and dressing can add to the normally raised anxiety level of the patient who requires surgery but adequate explanation of the rationale should help to allay fears.

Aseptic technique Whenever wounds are exposed, precautions are necessary to ensure the air contains minimal microorganisms. Sometimes a treatment room with special ventilation is available. If not the wound is dressed in the ward at least one hour after dust-producing activities have ceased during which time the dust will have settled out of the atmosphere.

Every hospital has its particular regime of 'aseptic technique' to prevent microorganisms gaining access to wounds, equipment and lotions. It is devised and kept up to date by the multidisciplinary Control of Infection Committee. Industry provides the market with an ever-increasing number of lotions and paper towels for hand hygiene; lotions and dressings to achieve a moist environment for wound healing (Koh, 1993; Moody, 1993;

Moody, 1992; Hollinworth, 1994). And as deep cavity wounds begin to heal, so the type of dressing needs to be changed. As already said, nurses need to understand the physiology of wound healing so that they can assess changes in the wound which signify that the current dressing is no longer appropriate. The Control of Infection Committee usually simplifies the list of products available in its area.

The National Control of Infection Nurses' Association and the Wound Care Society each publish a quarterly supplement in the Nursing Times and the Tissue Viability Society publishes similarly in the Nursing Standard. Reading these will help students to acquire up-to-date information.

Complex and controversial as the nursing practices related to preoperative skin preparation and wound care are, it is increasingly being recognized that other factors have to be taken into account in the context of reducing wound infection (Box 9.5) in the interest of patient comfort and cost-effectiveness.

Before ending this discussion of prevention of wound infection, some comment has to be made about transmission of virus infections (hepatitis B and HIV) in blood and body fluids (Royal College of Nursing, 1994). Since HIV seropositivity and AIDS has spread into the general population, each health authority will have itemized 'universal precautions' to which members of staff should adhere at all times. Because conversion to seropositivity can take weeks and even months, 'universal precautions' take account of the fact that transmission can be two way — from staff to patients and vice versa. In the context of doing surgical dressings, the possible route of virus transmission is blood to blood. Consequently any abrasion of a member of staff's skin of the arms and hands must be adequately covered with a waterproof adherent tape — otherwise adherence to the regime of aseptic technique is adequate precaution.

Psychological problems

The total surface area covered with skin is extensive and it is therefore not surprising that anything which causes 'difference' can produce problems for the person. The minimum areas of the skin which are exposed in most cultures and climates during the day are the face, neck and hands and they are customarily mutually observed when a person is in the company of others.

Naevi Some people have extensive birthmarks (naevi) and if they are on a part of the body normally covered by clothing during the day, they do not cause undue distress. Yet if they are on the face and neck they can be a source of psychological trauma. Nurses can help by having a positive not a discriminating attitude toward people with visible birthmarks or other disfigurement of the skin. Any visible stigma can produce psychological reaction in the

Box 9.5 Factors influencing risk of wound infection

Factor	Rationale
lifespan	the very young and very old can be at increased risk
nutritional status	malnourished tissue • less resistant to infection • receiving less nutrients for healing
required medications	their prescription denotes compromise in one or more biological systems
blood supply at: • operative site • chronic wound	a lessened blood supply decreases the oxygen and nutrients reaching the tissues increasing the risk of infection
psychological and emotional status	tension and anxiety: decreased maximizes biological functioning, increased minimizes biological functioning
time of admission	no sooner than necessary to avoid 'hospital' microorganisms colonizing patient's skin
preoperative skin cleansing	• to remove potentially pathogenic transient microorganisms • to reduce resident skin flora to lowest possible level
hair removal	if requested by the surgeon, the desired outcome is absence of skin abrasion
aseptic technique	to prevent microorganisms gaining access to: • wounds • equipment • lotions
immunocompromised from: • disease (including AIDS) • side-effects of therapeutic treatment	minimal resistance to pathogens

person bearing the stigma and in the observer. Either of them can react by being self-conscious, embarrassed, anxious, fearful, shocked and even repulsed if the sight is of extensive skin trauma.

Dentures People react differently to wearing dentures; most suffer initial self-consciousness and embarrassment and thereafter go to great lengths so that they are never seen without their dentures, perhaps not even by their spouse. Naturally for such people, admission to hospital presents them with a very special personal problem. Nurses need to be sensitive when caring for people who have such idiosyncrasies.

Hair loss Iatrogenic loss of hair can sometimes be accepted by cancer patients because they hope that the cytotoxic drugs will improve their condition (p. 258). Shock and anxiety can be precipitating factors in causing patchy baldness which a person finds disconcerting. If the condition can be accepted as a temporary one it will be remedied, but continuing anxiety can result in increasing baldness. Encouraging the person to talk about the anxiety and helping to identify its cause is an important part of treatment. Wearing a wig might be a helpful solution if baldness is severe.

Skin disease People with skin disease can become very depressed; indeed some skin diseases are a somatic expression of a psychological disturbance. Attending to the afflicted areas can be time-consuming and healing can be slow. Also in periods of excessive stress the condition can exacerbate which is disappointing to all concerned. If people with visible skin disease experience avoiding actions by others, they naturally feel uncomfortable and discriminated against. The external applications can stain and soil clothes demanding extra washing and drying. Can home facilities accommodate this? Can the financial budget cope with it?

Skin disorders in a child can be very distressing for both child and parents (Elliot, 1990). Currently there is interest in complementary therapy, particularly a Chinese herbal tea (Frost, 1994). A placebo-controlled, double blind trial showed promising results (Sadler, 1992). A larger study collected data when children were seven, 11 and 16 years old. It revealed that the point prevalence of observed eczema increased with rising social class at all three ages. The researchers suggested that this might be due to:

- positive health-related behaviour
- higher maternal age
- wall to wall carpets and central heating.

It would appear that sociocultural and environmental factors are not static but can change over a relatively short period.

Scars The formation of scars, an inevitable sequel to wound healing has both physical and psychological implications for the person. Disfiguring facial scars have particularly profound effects as do those which affect sexuality in a direct way; for example, scars on the breasts or genital area. It is especially important for patients to be realistically prepared in advance of surgery for what the scar will look like since research has indicated a relationship between expectations and adaptation.

The cosmetic appearance can be improved by daily application of an oil or cream. An increasing number of services teach cosmetic camouflage skills. The British Red Cross provides such a service using trained volunteers. Considering the importance of self-image to mental health it is a commendable contribution.

Burns Burn injuries can have an equally profound physical and psychological effect on the victim and Lowry and Gill (1992) consider that it is vital for nurses to fully understand the effect a scald or burn injury has on the skin and on the person who can be of any age. The area of body surface burned is assessed on a percentage basis and, initially, it is the extent of the burn which determines the severity of the injury and the threat to life; the depth of injury is also important in terms of the treatment plan. Prevention of infection and pain control are vital aspects of treatment, along with wound care and nutrition, all of which have been discussed.

In the long-term, many burns victims suffer psychological problems such as depression and anxiety. Not all professionals acknowledge that 'psychologically based methods of "healing".....' can include support in a mental/spiritual capacity, not only to help the person adjust to the permanency of extensive visible scarring (with possible limited movement such as inability to close the eyes) as well as promoting healing of the lesion (Shakespeare, 1993). Professional counselling services should be available to help such people integrate their changed body image in such a way that life is meaningful in pursuance of their optimum independence.

Excessive sweating (hyperhidrosis) There are changes in a patient's internal environment in response to such states as anxiety and fear. At whatever point they contact the health care system, whether at a doctor's surgery, clinic, health centre or hospital, and on going to such places as the X-ray department and the operating theatre, they will experience some degree of anxiety. One of the body's reactions is increased secretion of sweat. There may be added embarrassment at wet patches on clothing in the axillary region and damp footwear. A constant readiness on the nurse's part to give adequate preparatory explanation; to listen to the patient; and to observe non-verbal behaviour for clues as to the cause of anxiety is necessary. Arranging for a daily change of clothing will help to prevent odour which could cause further embarrassment. The person may benefit from knowledge about more effective anti-perspirants and deodorants.

Generalized hyperhidrosis can be a symptom of many conditions (including thyrotoxicosis, chronic infection, diabetes, acromegaly and gout) and so careful investigation is necessary if excessive sweating appears to be more than a temporary concomitant of fear, anxiety or increased metabolic rate!

Itching (pruritus)   Itching is not a disease per se but can be symptomatic of many diseases (Box 9.6). The problems experienced by the person (of any age) are crossness, irritability and inability to sleep because of the discomfort. A natural reaction is to scratch an itching part of the body; scratching can induce more itching and more scratching can break the skin so that there is a portal of entry for microorganisms increasing the possibility of permanent skin disfigurement. The sight of the broken skin may make the person feel guilty and this can add to the misery.

The nurse can help in a general way by offering suggestions that short clean nails will lessen trauma and risk of infection. Cotton gloves may help, especially if scratching during sleep is a problem. Use of bland non-perfumed talcum powder and soap may be helpful; soap, if used, should be well rinsed off before drying the skin. Soap substitutes in powder form can be made into a running liquid, applied to the skin and removed by water, preferably in a spray. Other people find application of aqueous cream helpful for cleansing itching skin. Polymorphic light eruption and its recurrent itchy rash was mentioned on p. 237. Over-spiced food and hot baths are best avoided. Overheating from any cause is undesirable. Loose clothing made of non-irritant material is advisable especially for night clothes. If the person's mental activity can be diverted to other interests, so much the better.

When itching may indicate the presence of a disorder which should be medically treated, the appropriate action should be taken; an example is the case of a mole which becomes itchy since this may be indicative of malignant melanoma.

Melanoma   Many countries in the west are having to cope with an increasing number of white residents who develop malignant melanoma. Morrison's (1992) article reports a small part of a larger study and deals with the participants' lifestyle regarding sun exposure and knowledge about, and use of skin protection. In a matched sample of 80 subjects with suspected sun related skin lesion and 80 with non sun related skin problems, 43% of the matched control group and 27% of the 'suspected' group wanted to acquire a tan while on holiday (Fig. 9.6). The popularity of sunbeds must also be remembered in this context.

Sun protection factor   The sun protection factor (SPF) is a guide to prevention of burning, the higher the number the longer the protection. The factors range from 2 to 20+ which is the highest sunscreen, blocking out approximately 90% of ultraviolet B radiation (UVB). But the skin also needs protection from ultraviolet A (UVA) radiation. There

---

Box 9.6 Categories of causes of itching

Allergic reaction to:
  topical application
  ingestion of specific medication or food

Infectious disease
  German measles
  chickenpox

Skin disease
  impetigo
  eczema/dermatitis
  psoriasis
  skin cancer/melanoma

Other disease
  jaundice
  diabetes

Infestation
  head lice
  body lice
  scabies
  threadworms

Discharge
  vaginal
  penile

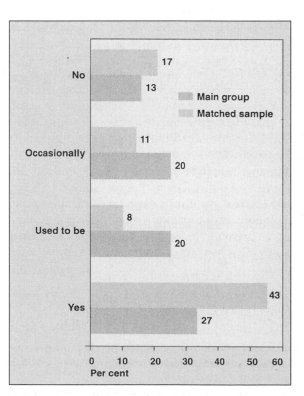

Fig. 9.6 Percentages of sample groups who desire to tan while on holiday (Reproduced with kind permission from Nursing Standard. First appeared on June 24 1992.)

are only a few creams available which protect from both, and they are relatively more expensive. Only 29% of the sunscreen users in the study applied a factor higher than nine when abroad, and only eight per cent when at home.

Health education Morrison (1992) encourages nurses to advise people to use a sunscreen which protects against UVB and UVA. The higher protection factor is better value because the protection lasts longer. Application at regular intervals particularly after swimming is essential, unless a waterproof product is used. Hats for men, women and children should shade the neck and face. Clothing should be to the wrists and ankles and the possibility of a cancer risk coding for fabrics as mentioned on p. 237 is under consideration.

EVERYONE should regularly inspect skin for any change in existing moles and the appearance of any new moles. Malignant melanoma is a potentially curable disease. Nurses are in a privileged position of being able to educate members of the public to take preventive action. Perkins (1992) advises a skin protection factor of 15 or more, together with using a parasol, and she says that swimming in T shirts is currently fashionable and should be encouraged.

Submammary intertrigo Intertrigo is 'superficial inflammation occurring in moist skin folds' (Roper, 1989). A point prevalence study of sores in female submammary skin folds in one district health authority on April 6, 1989 is reported by McMahon (1991). It was the first collection of data about this subject and revealed its size-five point three per cent. Elderly people and those with mental illness featured highly, suggesting that functional loss or self-neglect could be a predisposing factor. McMahon (1991) goes on to state that the prevalence makes intertrigo as common as pressure sores, and brings into question absence of discussion about this problem in nursing texts. A further research project revealed an unsatisfactory treatment situation and as nurses are the main 'prescribers' of treatment for such a condition, it makes further research essential (McMahon & Buckledee, 1992).

Skin reaction to radiotherapy With improved apparatus most skin reactions are less devastating than previously. A simple to a severe erythema frequently progresses to a dry or even a moist desquamation, with a few advancing to tissue necrosis, each of these stages requiring different treatment and the radiographers are researching this area (Crane, 1993; Barkham, 1993).

Most people requiring radiotherapy are already debilitated and a considerable number experience an increased degree of anxiety and depression. Nurse's observation of skin reaction needs to be described succinctly and accurately, so that nurses on succeeding shifts can evaluate any healing or worsening of the condition, as well as how the person is reacting to it.

This section discussing problems which can be experienced by people because of change in their dependence/independence status has been longer than the others due to the number of conditions which can produce change. Any change in mode of personal cleansing and dressing can also result in problems and an introduction to these follows.

CHANGE IN MODE OF PERSONAL CLEANSING AND DRESSING

Habits of personal cleansing and dressing are integral to a person's lifestyle and are important manifestations of self-image and self-esteem. Enforced change in the mode of carrying out any of the activities involved means that people have to cope with the change, and nursing activities aim at helping them to do so with minimum discomfort or distress.

Imposed non-bathing

Empathizing with people who are not permitted to bath is easier when one remembers the unpleasant 'grubby' feeling experienced at the end of a long journey. How much worse the feeling must be when for any reason a bath cannot be taken for a long time: for post-radiotherapy patients it can be weeks; for patients with extensive skin destruction it can be many months. Most people's objective when bathing is to feel refreshed and relaxed and prevent malodour.

The nurse can therefore make suggestions as to how these objectives might be achieved during a period of imposed non-bathing. Unless contraindicated, exposed skin areas (e.g. face, neck, hands and feet) and areas where sweat glands are concentrated (e.g. axillae and anogenital area) should be washed frequently. Anti-perspirants/deodorants and perfume/after-shave lotion, unless contraindicated on medical grounds, can help to promote a feeling of freshness and prevent malodour. Frequent changing of clothes and bedlinen would also increase the person's feeling of cleanliness and comfort.

Change in mode of bathing

Some people, for example those in a plaster cast, though unable to completely immerse themselves in water, might be able to bathe or shower at least some parts of the body if given appropriate help. Other people, particularly if confined to bed, can be bedbathed by the nurse. Provided this procedure is carried out in privacy and adequately (p. 243), it can be soothing for the patient.

Notwithstanding the hazards of the bedbath, Spiller (1992) was concerned with patients' views on bathing and, in particular, whether these were in accordance with nurses' views. Interestingly, the results of the study indicate that patients and nurses seem to hold different views on some issues, for example, patients seem to be less embarrassed at being bathed by a nurse than nurses think they will be.

Frequency was another point of difference between nurses and patients. If individualized nursing is based on the persons's individuality, daily bathing may not be appropriate. It is important that nurses do not impose daily bathing on patients provided the risk of cross infection will not be compromised.

Infestation

A change in mode of personal cleansing and dressing is required for treatment of infestation. Lice and scabies are the most common forms of infestation and are more common among people who, for any reason, have to be crowded together. Schools are notorious for the spread of head lice and, although previously thought to be more common among children from overcrowded, poorer homes, this is no longer the case. Health education should not only play a major part in preventing and controlling infestation but also in reducing the undeserved social stigma (Ward, 1992).

Knowledge of infestation and its treatment can be used by nurses in a wide variety of contexts, hence the following information.

Head lice The female lays tiny white eggs called 'nits' and cements them to the hairs near the scalp especially behind the ears. These hatch out in 1 week and are fully grown in 3. During a lifetime of 5 weeks they live on human blood. They cause intense irritation with consequent scratching; if this is performed with dirty finger nails infection can result and the resultant dried discharge and matted hair make detection and disinfestation difficult. There is loss of sleep with lowering of vitality; the sores may even give rise to enlarged lymph glands with possible abscess formation.

Head lice are impervious to washing and hair cutting, but a fine comb is effective. Malathion and Carbaryl are two effective insecticides for the treatment of head lice (Ward, 1992; Oliver, 1994). Lotions are preferred to shampoos because they are more effective and help to delay the emergence of resistance. The lotion should be applied to the scalp and hair exactly as instructed.

The hair is then tidied — not combed vigorously which would disturb the lice from the scalp. The nits will be killed but not loosened from the hair. There is protection from re-infestation for some weeks after application because malathion bonds to the hair.

It is recommended that the two insecticides should be rotated every three years to prevent the lice developing resistance to either of them. Some district health authorities have adopted this policy (Ward, 1992).

Body lice The female lays her eggs in the seams of clothing; but when day clothes are not changed for night clothes, the eggs can be attached to the body hair. They hatch out in one week, become mature in 2 and live for 4–5 weeks. They too live on human blood and their crawling and biting cause intense irritation with consequent scratching and danger of introducing infection.

No specific treatment is required other than a bath and normal laundering of personal clothes. During removal of an infested person's clothes, an apron and gloves should be worn and it should be done in a bright light as body lice only transfer in the dark (Ward, 1992).

Scabies The incidence of scabies in Britain is increasing (Nursing Standard, 1993). It is an allergic response to the excreta and saliva of the parasitic itch mite (*Sarcoptes scabiei*) which burrows in the skin. It favours those areas where the skin is thin: between the finger knuckles, around the axillae, round the waist, between the thighs, around and especially on the medial aspects of the ankles. The scratching and trauma to the skin can lead to infection. Healthy people can develop this 'itchy' reaction. There can also be a non-itchy manifestation which can occur in the elderly. Scaly lichenous plaques resembling eczema or psoriasis appear on the skin (de Selincourt, 1990).

After removal of clothes they are washed immediately. Two medicaments are available, lindane and malathion. Lindane is contraindicated during pregnancy, breastfeeding, in young children as well as people of low body weight or those with a history of epilepsy (Ward, 1992).

Application should be to the entire skin surface when it is clean, cool and dry. Twenty four hours later the person should have a bath, and if possible, a change of clothing. Disinfection of bedding and clothing will be required when people have crusted scabies, and treatment of all who have been in contact is essential to prevent a large outbreak in such places as long-stay wards and nursing homes for the elderly (Ward, 1992).

Whatever type of infestation is concerned, it is important that the nurse relates to the patient in a tactful and sympathetic manner. The person's cooperation is essential if treatment is to be effective, and receptiveness to education with a view to prevention of recurrence, is more likely if the nurse establishes a good rapport.

Modification of clothing

Even with a forearm or ankle in plaster, such things as fitted sleeves or narrow trousers are impossible to put on and clothing has to be modified accordingly. Stretch fabrics, and wide sleeves/trousers — whether or not they are in fashion — are easiest to manage. For a short period this is likely to be accepted by the patient and unlikely to cause undue distress.

However, as was mentioned in an earlier part of the chapter (p. 244), there may be reasons why some elderly people cannot manage to cope with conventional clothing: for example, necessitating wearing front rather than back-opening clothes. Similarly, disabled people may require to modify clothing in order to achieve maximum independence in the activity of dressing. Providing suitable clothing for elderly and disabled people is a basic but often neglected need, which Norton pointed out as long ago as 1983. She recalls how she became aware of this when, as a student nurse some 40 years earlier, she had inflicted pain on a crippled elderly person when trying to dress her in a hospital issue nightgown. Later, in the course of her research into geriatric nursing problems in hospital (Norton et al, 1962), items of night attire were subjected to systematic study for the first time. Since then there has been an increasing awareness of clothing problems and the production of all kinds of garments for all manner of disabilities. Undoubtedly there are problems inherent in the supply of clothing, storage and laundering in hospitals (Goodwin, 1994): how to overcome these problems and to introduce successfully a personalized clothing service is the subject of a Disabled Living Foundation publication and the DLF has a clothing adviser who can offer advice on all aspects of clothing.

Nurses, by virtue of their first-hand awareness of the problems, can help in this matter by specifying the clothing needs of individual people. In addition, empathy is necessary so that any person who has to wear modified clothing can be helped by the nurse and the occupational therapist to regain confidence and continue to use dressing as a source of self-esteem and a means of communication.

Wearing a prosthesis

There are various types of prostheses which can be worn, almost all of them resulting in some change in mode of personal cleansing and/or dressing.

Dentures The prediction that fluoridization of an increased number of water supplies and use of fluoride-containing toothpastes would decrease the number of elderly people requiring dentures in the future has been overtaken by the worrying increase in dental caries caused by young people's frequent ingestion of sugar-containing snacks and fluids which is likely to result in even more edentulous adults (Jones, 1992).

Some people are very sensitive about being seen without dentures, even for the short time of removal for cleaning. In older people with shrinking gums, dentures can become so loose that they may cause embarrassment in such activities as eating and speaking. Most dentists now advise that dentures are not removed before sleeping, although many older people still remove them. In contrast, those who have a plate with just one or two teeth attached are strongly advised to remove it before sleeping. In addition to denture cleaning, whole mouth brushing (teeth,

gums, palate and tongue) is necessary for oral and dental hygiene to be achieved. Some patients will require assistance to achieve this; McCord & Stalker (1988) provide guidance (which is still relevant) on oral hygiene for elderly disabled people.

Artificial limbs The term 'artificial limb' includes everything from what can reasonably be called a 'wooden leg' to a highly sophisticated powered prosthesis with electrodes placed on opposing muscles that transmit a signal to an electronic device which operates the prosthesis. With the latter device a member of the family is usually taught to help the person with personal cleansing and dressing activities. If the person has to be admitted to hospital, anxiety can be reduced if the family member is offered the opportunity to continue the helping role. If this is not possible, the patient can teach the nurse the method of coping with bathing and so on.

Artificial eyes People who wear an *artificial eye* become adept at caring for the prosthesis with the necessary apparatus and lotions in a hygienic manner. If for any reason a patient cannot continue to do this, a tissue is placed by the nurse at the outer corner of the eye, the artificial eye is removed on to it using a scoop with a slight curve and the eye is placed in its container and covered with a suitable lotion such as Optrex. The socket is then wiped with swabs wrung out of water or saline solution. Patients are naturally anxious about the safety of such a precious article, and it is reassuring if the nurse explains exactly what she has done with it and transmits to the patient a mutual desire for its safety.

Breast prostheses Various types of *breast prostheses* are available. Women who have had a mastectomy are helped to come to terms with the 'visible' assault on their femininity by discussing and handling these prostheses before operation. Indeed in some hospitals a person who has recovered from mastectomy and learned to cope with a prosthesis talks with a newly admitted person who is scheduled for mastectomy. It is increasingly recognized that an important nursing activity is the facilitation of such discussions. Another one is helping the person to realize that hygiene of the prosthesis is important because it is in contact with the skin, at least during waking hours. Clothes do not usually have to be modified.

Wigs Although wearing *a wig* may be indulged in as a 'fun activity', one's perspective may change if a wig has to be worn for medical reasons. Furthermore one of the most common reasons for having to wear a wig is loss of hair (alopecia) due to taking cytotoxic medications, an increasingly common treatment for cancer. In the case of some forms of cytotoxic therapy, hair loss can be a devastating experience. Early hopes of prevention by a procedure known as scalp cooling have not been sustained (Tierney, 1991). Chemotherapy-induced alopecia remains a problem for many people. Such people may already be debilitated in body and spirit, and loss of hair constitutes an extra problem, often perceived as a major one. Nurses can help by taking an interest in the choice of wig and commending the person's appearance when it is worn.

From the foregoing wide-ranging discussion, students will appreciate that there are many opportunities for practising the skills of assessing and identifying the person's problems, recognizing what nursing help is required to overcome or cope with the problems; writing a plan so that all nurses will provide equivalent nursing and evaluate whether or not the stated expected outcomes have been achieved.

However it has to be realized that it is unrealistic to expect that nurses can document an individualized plan for each person when they are working in such places as schools, occupational health departments, and 'drop-in' clinics for homeless people. Nevertheless the proposed conceptualization of assessing and identifying actual and potential problems which can arise because of a change in dependence/independence status for, or in mode of, personal cleansing and dressing can guide nurses as they contribute their nursing function in these areas.

In most countries the current emphasis is on providing people's health needs in the community setting, usually entitled 'at primary level'. But there will always be people whose episode of illness necessitates admission to a general or a special hospital for a short or a longer period, indeed some beds are allocated to 'long-term' care. For these people, problems can arise because of the change of environment and routine, and an introduction to possible problems because of these changes follows.

CHANGE OF ENVIRONMENT AND ROUTINE

Relatively few people are admitted to hospital because they are experiencing a problem with their AL of personal cleansing and dressing. But all people who are admitted require the many activities which comprise this AL to continue throughout their stay. There was discussion of admission to hospital in the context of the AL of communicating on p. 121 to p. 130. Here it will be focused to the AL of personal cleansing and dressing.

Unfamiliar ward routine

The newly admitted person cannot know the ward routine concerning personal cleansing and dressing activities unless information is given. It is common for people who are to be admitted from a waiting list to receive general information usually in leaflet form; generally this includes advice about toilet articles and night attire which they should bring with them, whether or not they can retain their daytime clothes, and if not, what alternative arrangements they should make. If this is not so, then relevant information requires to be provided on admission

and a function of the admitting nurse is to give this information and to create an atmosphere in which questions can be asked.

'Admission bath' Those people who are admitted from the waiting list and who have had a bath before setting off for the hospital will, to say the least, be surprised to be asked to have a bath as part of the admission procedure. Should the person be admitted for surgery, the explanation that frequent baths in the preoperative period reduce the number of microorganisms on the skin will be useful. Otherwise this part of the admission procedure should be used selectively, that is for those who have not bathed within the preceding 24 hours.

If all people must have baths on admission then the objective clearly must be for observation of their skin condition including bruising which is important for several reasons (Mairis, 1992). The person may subsequently have an accident and claim that it resulted in a bruise, which in fact was present on admission; or the person may have been subjected to ill-treatment, referred to as 'battering' or 'non-accidental injury'. Any evidence of pressure sores must also be carefully noted, together with the person's ability to perform the ALs of personal cleansing and dressing. Unless nurses explain that the condition of each person's skin has to be recorded, a patient is likely to feel disquiet at having to have an admission bath and to infer that the nurses think personal hygiene habits are deficient.

Personal clothing For most people clothes are important symbols of their independence and people can experience distress when their clothes are sent home or to the hospital store cupboard, in which case the nurse makes a detailed list of each item and asks the person to check the list and sign it. The person will feel less distressed if it is understood that the staff would prefer possessions to be kept in the ward and that the only reason for their removal is inadequate ward facilities for safe keeping. It is important that nurses understand the patient's problem: being without their own clothes creates a sense of 'depersonalization' and also means being deprived of the freedom to decide to leave the hospital, should there be any reason to do so.

Change from usual routine

For most people the ritual of personal hygiene is an essential part of caring for themselves. These hygiene habits are built into a routine which gives a pattern to the day, an important contribution to a feeling of security and stability. But most people realize that in hospital the routine will differ from their own. The ward routine must accommodate the needs of a group; it must be both expeditious and safe and must not put the patients at any risk.

When the nursing workload is heavy, time can be saved by alternative arrangements for personal cleansing and dressing activities; for example, finger wipes before meals if handbasins are difficult to provide; toothpicks and a drink of water after meals as a substitute for teeth cleaning; and a dry shampoo instead of a proper hairwash.

Most people, even those who are housebound, wear daytime clothes and change into night attire. It is now less common to see patients in night attire during the day. Ambulant people are being encouraged to wear daytime clothes; this not only improves their self-image but also gives temporal demarcation to being in bed and being 'up', and it also helps to create a sense of normality. In clinical areas where this has not been encouraged, nurses might consider whether wearing daytime clothes could be introduced, even on a trial basis to begin with.

Some of the difficulties inherent in the use of personal clothing in long-stay hospitals are now easier to overcome than in the past as a result of general improvements in clothing materials and styles. In particular, simple-to-fasten garments, the variety of stockings and tights and easy care underwear are all improvements which could be exploited, as well as velcro fastenings on footwear. It does not take much imagination to appreciate that an elderly woman with long-standing pride in her appearance is likely to lose her sense of dignity if deprived of personal underwear (albeit unseen clothing) and supplied with stockings which wrinkle or, even worse, are rolled down or fall down. Likewise, an elderly man may well wish to wear a collar and tie daily, and what reason is there why he should not? Apart from aiming to preserve self-esteem and dignity, personal clothing also provides the opportunity for people in long-term care to preserve their autonomy and exercise decision-making skills which also helps to prevent boredom, lack of motivation and 'institutionalization' (Nursing Standard, 1990).

Lessened decision-making

As already noted, most people have been used to making decisions about the simple activities of personal cleansing and dressing and this is something which should be encouraged as far as possible. There are not many decisions, however, which a bedfast person can make about personal hygiene. It is therefore important that nurses allow the patients to make the few decisions available to them, for instance whether or not they want soap on their face, or deodorant applied, what they would like to wear, and so on. It is equally important to recognize when patients are too exhausted or too ill to make decisions, or perhaps unable to make them because of confusion or intellectual impairment.

When all decision-making is removed from people, particularly those in long-term care, they cease to make

the effort to consider alternatives thereby losing initiative and accepting imposed routine; they become institutionalized (p. 243). When routine is rigid, members of staff cease to question and to consider alternatives; decision-making becomes unnecessary; they too lose their initiative, become bored and institutionalized thus compounding the patient's problem of lack of stimulation.

Lack of privacy

Most people prefer privacy when carrying out personal cleansing and dressing activities, as has been noted. Curtained washing cubicles or curtains round the bed do not provide the same security as the locked bathroom door, and some people feel threatened when using such facilities. Shrunken or incompletely drawn curtains can preclude privacy and some patients, particularly women, fail to attend to perineal toilet because of this. Should a nurse become aware of a patient's difficulties in this area she can arrange for use of a private facility or replacement of shrunken curtains; and at all times nurses should be vigilant in making sure that curtains are completely drawn.

In conclusion, there is no doubt that people who are admitted to hospital can experience problems related to their AL of personal cleansing and dressing.

Alerted to possible problems, students will be guided as to the sort of information to collect at the initial assessment and how to use it when writing and implementing a nursing plan.

For many short term patients who do not experience problems related to change of environment and routine, and who will remain independent during their stay, this AL need not necessarily appear on the plan, but the information gained while assessing (Appendix 1) will facilitate individualized conversation between nurse and patient.

Planning and implementing nursing activities and evaluating outcomes

Earlier in this chapter the components of our model — lifespan, dependence/independence continuum, factors influencing each AL — biological, psychological, sociocultural, environmental and politicoeconomic were focused to the AL of personal cleansing and dressing. It is important for students to realize that the abbreviations AL and ALs include all these components. This generalized background knowledge was then applied to this AL in the context of the process of nursing, starting with the assessing phase, the outcome of which is identifying people's actual and potential problems with this AL.

When such problems have been identified for a particular person, then the goals/outcomes have to be set, together with the necessary nurse-initiated interventions which have to be implemented to achieve them. Statement of the goals/outcomes is an essential prerequisite for evaluating whether or not they have, or are being achieved.

From the foregoing paragraph it might be assumed that the phases of the process are sequential and this is not the case. It is only for the purpose of description and learning that each has to be considered separately as they were in Chapter three. Already in this chapter each of the four phases has been mentioned many times highlighting their interactive nature. They are constantly interacting and indeed all four phases can be utilized by experienced nurses in one nursing intervention.

Experienced nurses do not consciously 'go through' the phases, but on reflection the phases were used. For example when doing a surgical dressing, ongoing assessment/evaluation might reveal that a stage of healing had been reached which required application of another type of dressing (changed plan implemented) to achieve further healing (no change in stated expected outcome). It is this cognitive complexity which accompanies so many psychomotor nursing tasks, not to mention the affective milieu that is difficult for nurses to explicate.

Health education

In relation to this AL, nurses have many opportunities to implement their health education (p. 257) role. For example practice nurses might be 'aware' of an increase in the number of people attending with sunburn and mole change. A scan of computer records would reveal actual numbers (assessment data); after teaching sessions on this subject (planning, implementing), ensuing numbers would provide data to be compared with those from assessment (evaluation). There are other areas of health education where the phases of the process can be applied to an individual, for instance, head infestation. Yet health education on this subject is an ongoing activity for school nurses, but it is difficult if not impossible to apply the phases of the process to each member of a school community.

The main objective when teaching about handwashing is prevention of those diseases which are spread by the faecal-oral route. Again practice nurses could utilize 'process thinking' and count the number of people attending the clinic because of diarrhoea/vomiting before and after a teaching programme. Nurses working with people who have learning disabilities in long stay

premises have to remember that outbreaks of dysentery can be a problem; they too could develop a programme based on the phases of the process.

Now that dental caries and other oral conditions are mainly preventable, nurses wherever they are working can think of their health education role in this area in the phases of the process.

Oral hygiene

For those who do not have an actual oral problem, it has to be remembered that when they have to move to such places as a hospital (including a special one for children), a nursing home or respite care, they continue to have potential problems, for instance dental caries and various periodontal conditions. It is therefore important that the nursing plan takes account of providing/implementing adequate preventive activities. Evaluation in the case of both short and long term stays would be evident if there had not been any oral discomfort or pain.

The factors to be borne in mind when carrying out an oral assessment were mentioned on p. 245. These assessment tools are helping nurses to explicate the complexity of applying the phases of the process to the task of mouth care. At the beginning of each session of oral hygiene there can be ongoing assessment of the current condition; after implementation of the planned nursing activity there can be ongoing evaluation of whether or not the mouth looks cleaner and more moist. This is subjective evaluation, the nurse using her previous experience and clinical judgement and the person can be asked how the mouth feels. 'Consumer satisfaction' is now part of the health service vocabulary.

Pressure sores

One of the various tools for identifying people who are at risk of developing pressure sores can be used at the initial assessment. If the risk score denotes a potential problem then the preventive nurse-initiated interventions will be written in the nursing plan. The stated expected outcome is likely to be 'skin over pressure areas unblemished'. It is important that nurses record the time of inspection, state of the skin and sign for each implementation. According to our current knowledge base, a minority of people develop a pressure sore despite the accepted standard of preventive nursing activities. Should there be a claim against the health service for such an occurrence, adequate records are nursing's only defence.

The same tool needs to be used at intervals and this provides ongoing assessment data about the risk which can increase, decrease or remain the same. Any decrease of risk is likely to cancel preventive activities in the nursing plan. Any increase of risk is likely to result in further planned nursing interventions which have to be implemented and evaluated. Accurate nursing records are essential because the local incidence of pressure sores has to be calculated before there can be evaluation of whether or not the national target for reduction (from 8 to 5%) set by the Department of Health (1991) is being or has been achieved. Implementing nursing activities and evaluating outcomes for actual pressure sores is now allocated to that of any other wound which will be discussed later.

Wounds

A stated expected outcome for people who have a clean stitched surgical wound is healing by first intention with minimal scarring. But healed wounds can improve in appearance for as long as 12 months, especially if moisturising lotion or cream is applied daily. Long term follow up about consumer satisfaction with wound appearance has not been carried out.

Progress has been made in identifying people who are at risk of developing wound infection. Several such tools were mentioned on p. 251. The preventive nursing activity to be implemented is commonly referred to as aseptic technique. An inflamed wound is not necessarily infected, it can be a manifestation of the tissues' reaction to assault; when infection occurs there is evidence of pus and there may be evidence of other symptoms such as fever, pain and restlessness. There will be planned nursing activities which have to be implemented and evaluated relating directly to the infected wound, but there may also be planned nursing activities which have to be implemented and evaluated to deal with the other symptoms. Fever can be factually assessed and evaluated by use of a thermometer; pain can be assessed and evaluated by the person experiencing it using a Likert type painometer; the degree of restlessness is observable by the nurse and of necessity it is a subjective evaluation, but the degree will probably be decreased by diminishing fever and pain experience.

When the wound involves destruction of skin then factual assessment of length, breadth, shape and depth is valuable, but fraught with difficulties. Whatever the planned nursing activity which has to be implemented, the evaluation will take account of the factual assessment for which Figure 9.5 provides some assistance.

Cavity wounds usually result from trauma and pressure sores are now included in this category. They become colonized by the skin's natural flora and in the warm, moist environment the multiplying microorganisms can become pathogenic and cause an infected deep cavity wound. All that has been said about other types of wounds which become infected applies to these wounds and to the person experiencing the wound.

From what has been written in this chapter there cannot be any doubt about the large number of the nurse-initiated activites which can be planned, implemented and evaluated for dealing with the problems which people can experience in relation to their AL of personal cleansing and dressing. But this AL is only one of 12, and problems with it can have repercussions in other ALs.

Congruent with our model for nursing the broad expected outcomes from selecting appropriate nursing interventions are:

- preventing potential problems from becoming actual problems
- solving or alleviating actual problems
- preventing recurrence of treated problems
- helping with development of positive coping mechanisms for those problems which cannot be solved.

And these outcomes are achieved by the method known as the process of nursing which is illustrated in Figure 3.9, p. 60.

REFERENCES

Anonymous 1994 The problems of providing a personal clothing service. Nursing Times 90 (30) July 27: 33

Barkham A M 1993 Radiotherapy skin reactions. Professional Nurse 8 (11) August: 732, 734, 736

Barnett J 1991 A reassessment of oral health care. Professional Nurse 6 (12) September: 703, 704, 706–708

Bedi A 1993 A tool to fill the gap. Professional Nurse 9 (2) November: 112, 114, 116, 118, 120

Benbow M 1993 Better than cure. Nursing Times 89 (34) August 25: 55–57

Birchall L 1993 Making sense of pressure sore prediction calculators. Nursing Times 89 (18) May 5: 34–37

Booth B 1994 Sore point. Nursing Times 90 (5) February 2: 20–21

Boycott J A 1956 A note on the disinfection of baths and basins. The Lancet 2: 678–679

Boyle S 1992 Assessing 1 Mouth care. Nursing Times 88 (15) April 8: 44–46

Bridel J 1993a Assessing the risk of pressure sores. Nursing Standard 7 (25) March 10: 32–35

Bridel J 1993b Pressure sore risk in operating theatres. Nursing Standard 7 (32) April 28: 4, 6, 7, 10

Buglass E A 1995 Oral hygiene. British Journal of Nursing 4 (9) May 12–24: 516–519

Bush T 1984 The sense of well-being. Nursing Times 80 (1) January 4: 31–32

Cahill J 1994 Is this the best intervention? Professional Nurse 9 (6) March: 394, 396–398

Callaghan C 1994 Audit changes. Nursing Times 90 (35) August 31: 69, 70, 74

Clark M O, Barbanel J C, Jordon M M, Nicol S M 1978 Pressure sores. Nursing Times 74 (9) March 2: 363–366

Clarke G 1993 Mouth care and the hospitalized patient. British Journal of Nursing 2 (4): 225–227

Clarke G 1993 Mouth care and the hospitalised patient. Professional Nurse 8 (6) March: 225–227

Collier M 1994 Assessing a wound. Nursing Standard 8 (49) August 31: RCN Nursing Update: 3–8

Collier M 1993 Assessing a wound. Nursing Standard 7 (20) February 3: RCN Nursing Update: 3–8

Crow R 1988 The challenge of pressure sores. Nursing Times 84 (38) September 21: 68–73

Cutting K 1994 Factors influencing wound healing. Nursing Standard 8 (50) September 7: 33–36

Davies K 1994 Pressure sores: aetiology, risk factors and assessment scales. British Journal of Nursing 3 (6): 256, 259, 260, 262

Dealey C 1991 The size of the pressure sore problem in a teaching hospital. Journal of Advanced Nursing 16 (6) June: 663–670

Department of Health 1991 The health of the nation. HMSO, London

de Selincourt K 1990 A disease of sympathy. Nursing Times 86 (34) August 22: 20–21

Disabled Living Foundation 1995 All dressed up. Disabled Living Foundation, London

Edwards M 1994 The rationale for the use of risk calculators in pressure sore prevention, and the evidence of the reliability and validity of published scales. Nursing Times 86 (20) May 16: 72

Elliot B 1990 Itching agony. Nursing Times 86 (20) May 16: 72

Flanagan M 1994 Assessment criteria. Nursing Times 90 (35) August 31: 76, 78, 80, 82, 84, 86, 88

Frost J 1994 Complementary treatments for eczema in children. Professional Nurse 9 (5) February: 330–332

Godlee F 1992 Skin lighteners cause permanent damage. British Medical Journal 305 (6849): 333

Goodwin S 1994 Personal laundry: an essential part of patient care. Nursing Times 90 (30) July 27: 31–32

Gould D 1994 Making sense of hand hygiene. Nursing Times 90 (30) July 27: 63–64

Greaves A 1985 We'll just freshen you up dear. Nursing Times 81 (36) March 6: 3–4, 7–8

Hamilton F 1992 An analysis of the literature pertaining to pressure sore risk-assessment scales. Journal of Clinical Nursing 1: 185–193

Heals D 1993 A key to wellbeing. Oral hygiene in patients with advanced cancer. Professional Nurse 8 (6) March: 391, 392, 394, 396, 398

Hollinworth H 1994 The healing process. Nursing Times 90 (7) February 16: 84, 86

Howarth H 1977 Mouth care procedures for the very ill. Nursing Times 73 (10) March 10: 354–355

Jones S 1992 Fluoride: spanning the health divide. Nursing Standard 7 (10) November 25: 36–39

Journal of Nursing Management 1994 Hand dryers emit bacteria claims University report. Journal of Nursing Management 2 (3) May: 149

Kalideen D 1990 Preparing skin for surgery. Nursing 4 (15) July 26–August 8: 28–29

Kelly J 1994 Understanding transdermal medication. Professional Nurse 10 (2) November: 121–125

Kingsley A 1992 Assessment allows action on risk factors. Professional Nurse 7 (10) July: 644–646, 648

Kearsley N, Little T, Wiseman C 1994 Realised potential. Nursing Times 90 (24) June 15: 44–45

Koh S 1993 Dressing practices. Nursing Times 89 (42) October 20: 82, 84, 86

Lowry M, Gill A 1992 Taking the heat out of burns. Professional Nurse October: 28–30

Lowthian P 1979 Turning clocks system to prevent pressure sores. Nursing Mirror 148 (21) May 24: 30–31

Mairis E 1992 Four senses for a full skin assessment. Professional Nurse 7 (6) March: 376–378, 380

Manley G, Sheiham A, Eadsforth W 1994 Sugar-coated care? Nursing Times 90 (7) February 16: 34–35

Maurer I 1985 Hospital hygiene. London, Edward Arnold

Middleton J M 1994 Putting care on the record. Professional Nurse 9 (4) January: 240–243

Millward S 1992 The hazards of communal razors. Nursing Times 88 (6) February 5: 58, 60, 62

Milward P 1993a Scoring pressure sore risk in the community. Nursing Standard 8 (7) November 3: 50, 51, 52, 54, 55

Milward P 1993b How to manage pressure sores in the community. British Journal of Nursing 2 (9): 488, 490, 492

Milward P 1993c How to manage sores in the community. British Journal of Nursing 2 (9): 488, 490, 492

Moody M 1993 Wound dressings: principles of choice. Nursing Standard 7 (35) May 19: RCN Nursing Update: 3–8

Moody M 1992 Problem wounds: a nursing challenge. Nursing Standard 7 (6) October 28: RCN Nursing Update: 3–8

Moore J 1995 Assessment of nurse-administered oral hygiene. Nursing Times 91 (9) March 1: 40–41

Morison M 1994 Wound care: a problem solving approach. Nursing Standard 8 (19) February 2: 3–8. RCN Nursing Update

Morison M 1988 How can the incidence of surgical wound infection be reduced? Professional Nurse December: 122, 124, 125

Morrison G 1992 Malignant melanoma and sun exposure. Nursing Standard 6 (40) June 24: 30–33

Morton O 1993 Here comes the sun. Nursing Times 89 (29) July 21: 52–54

Mullineaux J 1993 Cutting the delay reduces the risk. Professional Nurse 9 (1) October: 24, 26, 28, 30

McCord F, Stalker A 1988 Brushing up on oral care. Nursing Times 84 (13) March 30: 40–41

McMahon R 1991 The prevalence of skin problems beneath the breasts of in-patients. Nursing Times 87 (39) September 25: 48–51

McMahon R, Buckledee J 1992 Skin problems beneath the breasts of inpatients. Journal of Advanced Nursing 17 (10) October: 1243–1250

Norton D, McLaren R, Exton-Smith A 1962 An investigation of geriatric nursing problems in hospital. Churchill Livingstone, Edinburgh (Re-issued in 1975)

Nursing Standard 1993 Incidence of scabies doubles inside a year. Nursing Standard 7 (28) March 31: 16

Nursing Standard 1992 In Brief: The Norton scale. Nursing Standard 6 (47) August 12: 14

Nursing Standard 1990 Making clothing an issue. Nursing Standard 4 (27) March 28: 6

Nursing Times 1995 Bathing aids: handling and lifting in the home. Nursing Times 91 (8) February 22: 53–54

Nursing Times 1991 HVA warns of hot water risk. Nursing Times 87 (21) May 22: 5

Oliver P 1994 Making sense of . . . headlice. Nursing Times 90 (22) June 1: 34–35

Peate I 1993 Nurse-administered oral hygiene in the hospitalised patient. British Journal of Nursing 2 (9): 459–462

Perkins P 1992 Malignant melanoma: mole watching and the adolescent. Professional Nurse 7 (10) July: 678–680

Pettersson E 1986 Preoperative hair removal and infection control. In: Tierney A J (ed) Recent advances in clinical nursing practice. Churchill Livingstone, Edinburgh: 169–175

Pettifer A 1992 Oral candidiasis and HIV infection. Nursing Standard 6 (42) July 8: 34–35

Roper N 1989 Churchill Livingstone Nurses' Dictionary. Churchill Livingstone, Edinburgh

Royal College of Nursing 1994 2E AIDS nursing guidelines. Royal College of Nursing, London

Sadler C 1992 Time for tea? Nursing Times 88 (35) August 26: 34–36

Scully C, Porter S, Greenman J 1994 What to do about halitosis. British Medical Journal 308 (6923) January 22: 217–218

Shakespeare P 1993 Burn wound healing. Journal of Tissue Viability 3(1): 16–21

Sneddon J 1990 A preventable course of infection. Professional Nurse 6 (2) November: 98, 100, 102, 104

Spencer K E, Bale S 1990 A logical approach. Management of surgical wounds. Professional Nurse 5 (6) March: 303, 304, 306

Spiller J 1992 For whose sake — patient or nurse? Ritual practices in patient washing. Professional Nurse 7 (7) April: 431, 432, 434

St Clair M 1993 Keeping the pressure high on prevention. Nursing Standard 7 (21) February 10: 4, 6, 7, 10

Stockton L 1994 Preventing pressure sores in wheelchair users. Nursing Standard 8 (20) February 9: 54–56

The Independent 1994 Clothes to be given cancer-risk coding. The Independent, April 19

Thompson J 1994 Moisturising solution. Nursing Times 90 (8) February 23: 52, 54

Thompson J 1990 Foot and leg care. Community Outlook, February: 14, 16, 17

Thurgood G 1994 Nurse maintenance of oral hygiene. British Journal of Nursing 3 (7): 332–334, 351–353

Tierney A 1991 Chemotherapy-induced hair loss. Nursing Standard 5 (38) June 12: 29–31

Torrance C 1983 Pressure sores: aetiology, treatment and prevention. Croom Helm, London

Viney C, Cheater F 1992 Pre-operative shaving in gynaecology. Nursing Standard 7 (8) November 11: 25–27

Walker M F, Lincoln N B 1991 Factors influencing dressing performance after stroke. Journal of Neurology, Neurosurgery and Psychiatry 54 (8): 699–701

Ward K 1992 The management of skin infestations. Nursing Standard 6 (23) February 26: 28–30

Wardman C 1991 Norton v Waterlow. Nursing Times 87 (13) March 27: 74, 76, 78

Waterlow J 1991 A policy that protects. Professional Nurse 6 (5) February: 258, 260, 262, 264

Wells L 1994 At the front line of care. The importance of nutrition in wound management. Professional Nurse 9 (8) May: 525, 526, 528–530

Wright L 1991 Bathing by towel. Nursing Times 86 (4) January 24: 36, 37, 39

ADDITIONAL READING

Banfield K R, Shuttleworth E 1993 A systematic approach with lasting benefits. Professional Nurse 8 (4) January: 234, 236, 238

Crane J 1993 Extending the role of a new hydrogel. Journal of Tissue Viability 3 (3): 98–99

Davies K 1994 Pressure sores: aetiology, risk factors and assessment scales. British Journal of Nursing 3 (6): 256, 259, 260, 262

Gould D 1994 A study of glove use. Nursing Times 90 (30) July 27: 57, 58, 60, 62

Hamilton F 1992 An analysis of the literature pertaining to pressure sore risk-assessment scales. Journal of Clinical Nursing 1: 185–193

Hatton-Smith C K 1994 A last bastion of ritualised practice? Professional Nurse 9 (5) February: 304, 306–308

Holmes S, Mountain E 1993 Assessment of oral status: evaluation of three oral assessment guides. Journal of Clinical Nursing 2: 35–40

Jenkins D A 1989 Oral care in the ICU: an important nursing role. Nursing Standard 4 (7): 24–28

Livesley B 1987 Pressure sores: an expensive epidemic. Nursing Times 83 (6): 79

Lowthian P T 1993 Acute patient care: pressure areas. British Journal of Nursing 2 (9): 449–450, 452, 454–456

Moore J 1995 Assessment of nurse-administered oral hygiene. Nursing Times 91 (9) March 1: 40–41

McFarlane A 1990 Why do we forget to remember handwashing? Professional Nurse 5 (5) February: 250, 252

O'Dea K 1993 Prevalence of pressure damage in hospital patients in the UK. Journal of Wound Care 2 (4): 221–225

Osborne S 1987 A quality circle investigation. Nursing Times 83 (6) February 18: 73–76

Richardson B 1991 Pressure sores: the manager's role. Nursing Standard 5 (36) May 29: 7–9

Royal College of Nursing 1994 Guidelines on Infection Control. Royal College of Nursing, London

Tedder R 1980 Hepatitis B in hospitals. British Journal of Hospital Medicine March: 274–279

Thompson J 1990 Foot and leg care. Community Outlook February: 14, 16, 17

Waterlow J 1988 Prevention is cheaper than cure. Nursing Times 84 (25): 69–70

10

Controlling body temperature

The AL of controlling body temperature

Unlike the cold-blooded animals whose temperature fluctuates according to the changing temperature of their external environment, man is able to maintain body temperature at a constant level, independent of the degree of heat or cold in the surrounding environment.

For most of the time people are unaware of their body temperature and this is because it remains constantly at a comfortable level. This control of temperature is accomplished because a special regulating centre in the hypothalamus of the brain carefully balances the amount of heat produced and lost by the body. There are also behavioural aspects of controlling body temperature.

BEHAVIOURAL CONTROL

When the body temperature rises or falls outside the range of normal, a person is aware of feeling too hot or too cold. In either circumstance, the individual must perform certain activities to assist the physiological process of body temperature control. If people feel too hot when indoors, they can cease being active if that is the cause; or they can turn down heating appliances, open windows, draw curtains to keep out the sun, remove some clothing, take a cool shower or bath, or have a cold drink. If they are outside doing manual work they can remove some layers of clothing or can rest for a while until they cool down; if they are in direct sunshine they can move into the shade and, perhaps, use any suitable article as a fan to move the surrounding air thereby cooling themselves further.

When people feel too cold indoors or outdoors, they can perform various activities which are the converse of those indulged in by people when they are too hot. Physical activity quickly generates body heat and additional items of clothing provide extra warmth and protection from the chill of a wind. Materials made of fibres which trap air are warmer since air, being a poor conductor, preserves body heat. Use can also be made of the fact that dark colours absorb heat from the sun and so help to keep the body warm whereas light colours reflect heat.

Regulating the temperature of the atmosphere in homes and buildings is another activity which must be performed if body temperature is to be controlled satisfactorily. Any householder knows how expensive it is to equip a home so that it is capable of being cool in hot weather and warm in cold weather. Coal, electricity, gas and oil are all expensive commodities and, in addition, many countries are experiencing a shortage of energy resources. Some governments, in an attempt to minimize wastage of these important and scarce resources, provide financial aid to householders for double-glazing windows and insulating walls and roofs. Special publicity campaigns are also common, especially in work places, to remind the public to save these particular resources. When the temperature outside is low it is essential for health and comfort that homes are kept especially warm; this is particularly important for the very young and the elderly, but for many who are less well off, it can be a source of anxiety because of the high and increasing costs of heating a home (Reid, 1994).

PHYSIOLOGICAL CONTROL

Most of the numerous biochemical processes occurring within the body can only take place if the temperature of the body remains at a fairly constant level and within a relatively narrow range. The functioning of the nervous system is easily disturbed by temperatures outwith that narrow range of normal and, at the same time, many other systems of the body are adversely affected. Eventually, if the body temperature rises or falls excessively, there is permanent damage to body cells and the possibility of death. So essential is thermoregulation to health and survival that the body's own physiological control mechanisms are finely tuned.

The fact that body temperature remains constant within a relatively narrow range of normal, irrespective of the temperature of the external environment, enables man to adapt not only to very different climates but also to daily and seasonal variations in the environmental temperature. If this adaptation were not possible, the scope of human activity would be severely limited and the individual would suffer such discomfort from extremes of heat and cold that everyday living would be disrupted and miserable, and health would be threatened constantly.

In terms of physiological control of body temperature, the key factors are the temperature-regulating centre, heat production and heat loss; these are outlined briefly below.

Temperature-regulating centre

An area of nerve tissue in the anterior part of the hypothalamus of the brain acts as a centre which regulates body temperature. Nerve cells in this area respond to changes in the temperature of circulating blood. It is thought that the centre also responds to impulses from the temperature-sensitive receptors in the skin, muscles,

blood vessels, the abdominal cavity and various areas of the central nervous system.

The centre's function is to balance the amount of heat produced by the body and the amount of heat lost by the body. It works just like a thermostat; there is a constant 'set' temperature which is maintained as the centre responds by balancing heat production and heat loss. To achieve this the centre has two control mechanisms: its *heat-promoting centre* activates processes which increase heat production and reduce heat loss; conversely its *heat-losing centre* stimulates actions which reduce heat production and increase heat loss. These two centres work reciprocally; when one is activated, the other is depressed.

Heat production

All the metabolic processes continuously proceeding in the human body produce heat. At rest and during sleep the body is kept warm enough by the amount of energy produced at the basal metabolic rate. Additional heat production results mainly from skeletal muscle movement and, if this is not sufficient, the body initiates reflex muscular activity — shivering — which increases the rate of heat production up to fourfold. At the same time, stimulation of the sympathetic nervous system speeds up the process of cellular metabolism and raises the hairs on the skin, a vestigial mechanism in humans, which in hairier mammals traps the warm air next to the body, thereby insulating it.

The prevention of unnecessary heat loss is an important way of conserving body heat. Most heat loss occurs through the skin by evaporation, conduction, convection and radiation. Vasoconstriction, the constriction of blood vessels, minimizes this heat loss because less warm blood circulates in the subcutaneous tissue. At the same time sweating is greatly diminished, reducing heat loss by evaporation.

Heat loss

A variety of means are used by the human body to lose heat. Heat is lost from skin which is in direct contact with cooler air by the process called conduction; this is assisted by convection currents of air circulating around the body. Heat is also lost by evaporation of moisture from the skin surface, naturally increased by sweating. There is some loss of heat by radiation from the body into the cooler atmosphere. Vasodilation enhances loss of heat through the skin by bringing more blood to the surface of the body. Panting, more common in animals though it does occur in man, aids heat loss by increasing evaporative heat loss from the moist respiratory tract. At the same time the heat-losing centre depresses the mechanisms which result in heat production, metabolism is slowed down and muscular activity is decreased.

Heat loss/gain balance It is the balance between heat production and heat loss which must constantly be regulated to keep the body temperature within the limits of the range of normal. This fundamental concept of temperature control by balance is illustrated in Figure 10.1.

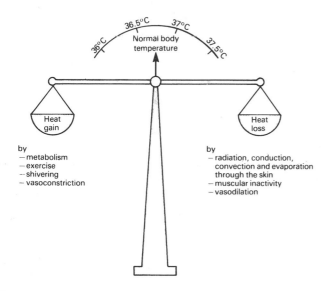

Fig. 10.1 Heat loss/gain balance

Lifespan: relationship to the AL of controlling body temperature

The lifespan component of the model (see Fig. 10.2) is especially relevant to the AL of controlling body temperature.

INFANCY

As long ago as 1900 a French neonatologist observed that the survival rate in the postnatal period was only 10% for infants whose body temperatures were 32.5 to 34°C and that survival rose to 77% when the infants were kept at 36 to 37°C (Drummond, 1979). Survival rates have improved among preterm and low birth weight babies and this is partly attributable to better artificial support of body temperature control in vulnerable newborn babies (Stewart, 1990).

Any newborn baby requires to have the skin dried immediately to prevent loss of heat by evaporation, and to be wrapped in warm clothing to prevent further loss of heat through conduction, convection and radiation. An infant's body weight comprises 2–6% brown fat (Drummond, 1979). This is richly supplied with blood

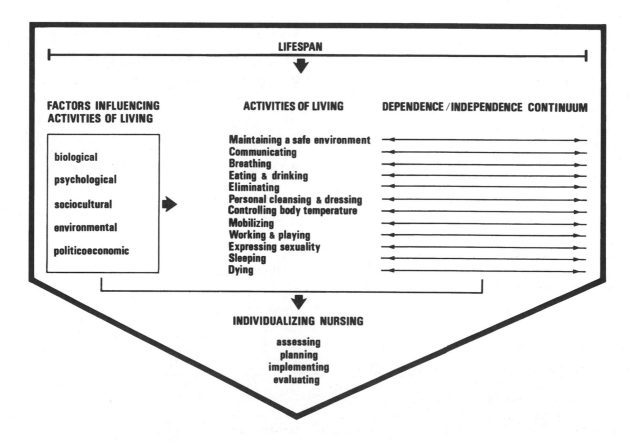

Fig. 10.2 The AL of controlling body temperature within the model for nursing

and has many nerve endings: these provide the stimulus for increased metabolism when the baby is exposed to cold, but prolonged exposure depletes the store of brown fat and this is undesirable. The heat receptors in the face are particularly sensitive and it is especially important that a baby is kept free from draughts and that the head is kept covered since significant heat loss can occur through exposure of that body surface area.

CHILDHOOD

In the first few months and indeed years of life, the heat regulating system continues to be highly sensitive to stimuli which cause heat production: for example, even the exertion of prolonged crying can raise the body temperature above the range of normal. Until the young child learns to associate, for instance, the discomfort of being hot and sweaty with the relief obtained by taking off a garment and sitting still for a while, parents need to be vigilant on the child's behalf to avoid unpleasant and potentially harmful excessive rises in body temperature. The same principle applies to falls in body temperature.

ADULTHOOD

Throughout a woman's fertile life there is a slight rise in temperature just after ovulation and until 2 days before menstruation but many women are not aware of it. A slight rise in temperature occurs during the early stages of pregnancy and is maintained until parturition. In later life, some women experience hot flushes as part of the menopause caused by the hormonal imbalance which occurs at this time.

OLDER AGE

Towards the end of the lifespan too, thermoregulation is less efficient due to impaired temperature discrimination, a reduction in the ability to constrict peripheral blood vessels, and a possible reduction in the shivering threshold (Collins et al, 1977; Macmillan et al, 1967). Older people can quickly suffer from the ill-effects of extreme heat or extreme cold. At the same time they may be less active and less well nourished so that it becomes important they have extra environmental warmth, to prevent hypothermia.

Dependence/ independence in the AL of controlling body temperature

The concept of a dependent/independent continuum as a

component of the model has relevance to the stages of the lifespan when considering the AL of controlling body temperature. As well as children's physiological control being highly sensitive to stimuli, the many behavioural aspects of this AL have to be learned, as well as the perception of when they are necessary. In the later years of life, some degree of dependence on others may return in terms of carrying out the various activities required for controlling body temperature.

However at any stage of the lifespan a person can have an infection when the body's response is to increase its temperature and make the person dependent on medication such as aspirin (an antipyretic) or antibiotics to reduce it, or on people to carry out cooling activities until normal temperature is regained. Conversely the body can respond to inadequate food, clothing and heating by lowering its temperature to dangerously low levels, rendering such a person dependent on others for gradually warming the body to restore it to normal temperature. If, at the other extreme, overheating renders a person exhausted there is a similar dependence on others for assistance to return body temperature to its normal level.

In a later section of the chapter more will be said about dependence/independence in circumstances of a person's loss of temperature control.

Factors influencing the AL of controlling body temperature

The factors influencing controlling body temperature will now be considered. The objective of this component of the model is to encourage consideration of how the five factors — biological, psychological, sociocultural, environmental and politicoeconomic — influence the way a person develops individuality in carrying out the AL of controlling body temperature and, therefore, should influence related nursing activity.

BIOLOGICAL

The mechanisms of thermoregulation have already been outlined. A number of factors influence the process of thermoregulation and also the individual's ability to assist with controlling body temperature. There are several factors in this category and they will be discussed under the headings of exercise, hormones, social drugs, food intake and time of day.

Exercise

Body heat is produced by skeletal movement and so the

body temperature is related to a person's activity level. The body temperature is highest during periods of great activity and lowest during periods of sleep.

Exercise, if overdone, can cause overheating and 'exertion-induced heat illness is now a recognized disorder which occurs in basically healthy individuals during or following prolonged strenuous exercise' (Walker, 1986). Heat cramps, heat exhaustion and heat stroke are now not uncommon occurrences at events such as fun-runs, marathons and athletic meetings and, given the potential danger of severe overheating, caution should be observed and proper precautions taken.

Hormones

The temperature variations which occur during the female fertility cycle (see earlier under 'Lifespan') are due to the influences of the female sex hormones.

An excess production of the hormone thyroxine results from over-activity of the thyroid gland and this increases the body's metabolic rate, thus raising the body temperature. Conversely with an underactive thyroid gland less thyroxin is produced and body temperature is lower than normal.

Social drugs

Caffeine increases the metabolic rate, although how it does so is not fully understood. Smoking cigarettes has a similar effect since nicotine stimulates the sympathetic nervous system. Alcohol can increase cooling since it causes vasodilatation of the blood vessels in the skin, resulting in a greater loss of heat from the body surface.

Food intake

Body heat is generated by the metabolism of food and the body's metabolic rate is increased directly as a result of ingestion of food. This is particularly so when the food eaten is high in protein and the stimulatory effect may last as long as 6 hours. Mothers who encourage their children to take a nourishing protein breakfast in order to keep warm in cold weather are therefore, albeit unknowingly, encouraging a practice which is based on sound knowledge of factors which influence body temperature.

Time of day

Variations in body temperature which are related to time of day are obviously influenced by the day and night pattern of activity and sleep. Body temperature is highest in the evening (1700 to 2000 hours GMT) and lowest in the early morning (0200 to 0800 hours GMT). The converse is true for people who regularly work at night and sleep during the day.

PSYCHOLOGICAL

Extremes of emotion sometimes affect the body's metabolic rate causing slight increase in body temperature. Excitement, excessive anxiety or anger may cause an elevation of temperature and, indeed, this fact is reflected in such phrases as 'flushed with excitement' and 'hot with rage'. On the other hand, apathy or depression may cause the body temperature to fall.

Knowledge acquired in the formative years about the sort of precautions to be taken when the outdoor temperature is very high or low will influence how a person carries out this dimension of the AL of controlling body temperature. Similarly the importance which a person attaches to making the home capable of being cool in hot weather and warm in cold weather will be reflected in efforts to achieve this, assuming the resources to do so.

A person's temperament and personality traits will have an effect on whether or not a person takes sensible precautions, or risks exposure to the potential problems of heatstroke or frostbite. Current mood will influence how a person carries out this AL; for example, when advised to wear a coat, a child may express resentment of adult interference by going outdoors inadequately clad.

SOCIOCULTURAL

The sociocultural factors which can have an effect on the AL of controlling body temperature are fairly limited but customs concerning clothes are certainly pertinent. Some religions, for example, dictate the wearing of a head cover at all times, regardless of the environmental temperature. Similarly, ceremonial occasions which are part of a certain culture may demand elaborate dress which is uncomfortably hot in summer weather; or, conversely, not warm enough on a cold day, as any British winter bride choosing conventional dress will testify! Everyone, too, no matter where in the world, is socialized into acceptance of norms regarding the extent to which clothing can be shed in the hottest weather; this varies between countries, and sometimes between the sexes, and is socioculturally determined rather than by the need for comfort and body temperature control.

ENVIRONMENTAL

As previously mentioned, changes or extremes of environmental temperature can cause the body temperature to vary and the person to feel warm or cold. In any extreme climate there can be dramatic temperature variations: for example, in parts of North Africa it can be bitterly cold during the night but as hot as 40°C in the mid-afternoon of the same day. Even in the so-called temperate climate of the UK there are considerable seasonal variations; the temperature can fall to −10°C or lower in winter and reach 40°C in summer. But heat waves in countries such as the UK, much as they are welcomed, catch the public unaware of the risks as Feinmann (1986) warned, mentioning hyperthermia in children and the elderly as one of the undesirable consequences. It is only by the process called acclimatization that the human body is capable of adaptation to very hot, very cold or very extreme climates. There is no chance for acclimatization to occur in sudden, short-term change of climate as happens in a heat wave or a brief summer holiday abroad. It is the popularity of such holidays which has increased the population's exposure to the problems of hyperthermia particularly; and, of course, also to the risk of skin cancer from excessive exposure to the sun's rays although that is not directly related to body temperature as such.

The body's ability to tolerate extremely high temperatures is closely related to the humidity of the atmosphere. A hot day which is dry and breezy, as opposed to one which is humid and still, is less uncomfortable because body heat is readily lost by convection and evaporation of sweat. Similarly, cold, dry weather is less chilling than cold, damp weather.

The availability of hot/cold baths and showers will determine whether or not a person can take advantage of these facilities in controlling body temperature. Likewise, whether or not a house has central heating, air conditioning and double glazing will influence the other activities which the occupants need to carry out to help control their body temperature on a day-to-day and season-to-season basis.

POLITICOECONOMIC

Many of the activities which individuals carry out in relation to the AL of controlling body temperature need money — to buy clothes, bedding and food; to heat a house and prevent loss of heat from it by excluding draughts, installing double glazing and insulating lofts. Inadequate provisions of this kind may mean that a person is vulnerable to the adverse effects of cold; the two most vulnerable groups in terms of the resultant condition of hypothermia are the young and the elderly. Although public and professional awareness of the problem of hypothermia is now widespread, it has taken a long time for the problem to be given the attention it merits.

A national survey of hospital admissions carried out by the Royal College of Physicians as early as 1965 showed that 0.68% of all patients admitted had temperatures below 35°C. Of these the highest incidence was in children aged 0–1 years which worked out at 82.2 cases per 1000 admissions. It has to be pointed out that hypothermia was not the reason for admission nor did the patients have clinical signs and symptoms of hypothermia; nevertheless they had an unacceptably low body temperature (Millard, 1977). In 1972 the UK Government recommended a temperature of 70°F for a living room when the temperature outside is 30°F. Yet in the early 1980s the Electricity Consumer Council's annual report stated that some elderly people were attempting to heat their homes on less than £1 per week, the inference being that such homes were inadequately heated. And now, in the 1990s, there is renewed concern in the UK that the government's imposition of VAT (valve added tax) on fuel bills may hamper hypothermia prevention (Reid, 1994).

Age Concern, a British voluntary organization, was in the forefront of early efforts towards seeking a better deal for the elderly to prevent deaths from hypothermia and to reduce other such cold-related deaths as coronary heart disease, stroke and chest infections (Taylor, 1982). Although less than 1000 deaths a year in the UK are certified as hypothermia, many more patients are seen in casualty departments with this diagnosis (Hillman, 1987). There are about 70 000 more deaths in Britain in winter than in summer and there is growing support for the theory that hypothermia is a significant contributory factor (Toulson, 1993). In other countries with equally cold or colder winters, such as Canada and Sweden, the numbers of deaths are spread more evenly across the year and, some argue, this is a reflection of their generally better standards of housing and more aggressive approach to the prevention of hypothermia. There is no doubt that prevention of hypothermia is essentially a politicoeconomic issue, at least in the UK situation.

Individualizing nursing for the AL of controlling body temperature

From the foregoing discussion it is evident that there are many dimensions of each component of the model which help us to describe how a particular person develops individuality in the AL of controlling body temperature. A résumé of these dimensions is provided in Box 10.1.

Knowledge about the person's individual habits in carrying out the AL of controlling body temperature is absolutely crucial for planning individualized nursing. The discussion so far will have given an idea of what nurses should keep in mind when engaged in the process of assessment.

ASSESSING THE INDIVIDUAL IN THE AL

The following questions will help the nurse to focus on

<table>
<tr><td>

Box 10.1 Assessing the individual in the AL of controlling body temperature

Lifespan: effect on controlling body temperature
- Infants: need to be kept dry, warm and out of draughts
- Young children: parental vigilance to avoid excessive rise/fall in temperature
- Adults: avoidance of adverse effects of excessive heat or cold
- Elderly people: requirement for adequate heating, clothing, exercise and nutrition to avoid hypothermia

Dependence/independence in controlling body temperature
- Infants/children dependent on adults for maintenance of temperature
- Elderly may be dependent on others for maintenance of temperature/prevention of hypothermia

Factors influencing controlling body temperature
- Biological
  - exercise
  - hormones
  - social drugs
  - food intake
  - time of day
- Psychological
  - knowledge about precautions in high or low outdoor temperature
  - value attached to making home appropriately warm/cool
  - temperament
  - personality traits
- Sociocultural — choice of clothing
- Environmental
  - extremes of environmental temperature
  - high/low humidity
  - air velocity
- Politicoeconomic
  - vulnerability of young, elderly
  - availability of money for heating, insulation, clothing, bedding, food
  - public education to prevent hypothermia

</td></tr>
</table>

- does the individual perceive body temperature to be comfortable, too high or too low?
- what factors influence the way the individual carries out the AL of controlling body temperature?
- what does the individual know about the behavioural and physiological aspects of controlling body temperature?
- are sensible precautions taken to avoid excessive rise or fall in body temperature, or does the individual take risks relating to, for example, the potential problems of hyperthermia, hypothermia and frostbite?
- what value does the individual put on adequate nutrition, clothing, bedding, heating and insulation in order to assist in controlling body temperature?
- is there any financial hardship which prevents the individual from attending to the AL of controlling body temperature?
- has the individual any longstanding problems with the AL of controlling body temperature and, if so, how have these been coped with?
- what problems, if any, does the individual have at present with controlling body temperature and/or are any likely to develop?

MEASURING BODY TEMPERATURE

In assessing the individual in relation to the AL of controlling body temperature it is self-evident that the ability to measure body temperature objectively is extremely helpful in the identification of an abnormal body temperature and, later, in the evaluation of the outcomes of related nursing intervention. While it may not be possible to measure body temperature with complete accuracy in the clinical situation, for reasons which will be discussed, careful measurements will provide the nurse with a useful assessment and evaluative tool. The subject of measuring body temperature is discussed in some detail because, although often considered to be a simple task, it is a time-consuming activity when undertaken routinely in hospital wards, and, further, there remains considerable controversy over the 'best' way to 'take temps' in spite of the innumerable research studies which have been undertaken over the years.

The aim of measuring body temperature

The aim is to identify deviations from the range of normal (and, in particular, from the individual's usual body temperature) or to monitor changes over time and to evaluate the outcome of specific interventions designed to return a raised or lowered temperature to normal. It is usual to take a patient's temperature on admission to hospital because, although many factors influence temperature control, this single measurement may not be meaningful.

the sort of information which might be sought in the course of assessing a person in the home or on admission to hospital with the objective of identifying problems (actual and/or potential) with the AL of controlling body temperature:

However, if a deviation from normal is found, or is anticipated, the procedure is repeated at regular intervals of 2, 4 or 12 hours. It has become less common for all hospital patients to have their temperature taken regularly as a matter of routine. This means that it is important for nurses to be alert to signs of pyrexia or hypothermia and to take a patient's temperature if she has reason to suspect any problem with body temperature control.

Most nurses still consider taking temperatures to be a simple basic procedure requiring little skill or knowledge, but the findings of research suggest that traditional practice is far from accurate and inappropriate practices are being continued in ignorance of the facts. Reviews of the relevant literature have been provided by Sims-Williams (1976), Erickson (1980), Brown (1990) and Fulbrook (1993a), among others. On the basis of research evidence, guidance can be given on the procedure which should be followed. It must be recognized, however, that there remain points of controversy and practice protocols require to be reviewed as new evidence is published. The main points which should be drawn out of the following discussion are shown in Box 10.2.

The clinical glass thermometer

This is the instrument still most commonly used in the home and in many health care settings for measuring body temperature. It is a simple, inexpensive instrument containing mercury which expands with heat. The amount of expansion, as indicated by calibrations marked on the glass, gives the measure of body temperature. On the Celsius scale (1°Celsius = 1°Centigrade) the standard thermometer registers temperatures between 35°C and 43.5°C. The low-reading thermometer, for use with patients at risk of or suffering from hypothermia, registers down to 21°C. All clinical thermometers have a constriction above the bulb so that when the mercury has risen it remains at the level reached until forcibly shaken down. The special thermometer for use in the rectal site only has a short, blunt bulb to prevent injury to the anal mucous membrane; it is coloured to distinguish it from those used in the oral or axillary sites.

Accurate measurement of body temperature is essential if the exercise is to be useful. To achieve this the nurse must use a reliable instrument, select an appropriate site, leave the instrument in situ for the necessary length of time and, finally, read the thermometer accurately. While all thermometers with the British Standard Kitemark are virtually guaranteed to be accurate, the site of the body used should be carefully considered since environmental influences can produce inaccurate readings.

Sites for temperature-taking

The oral site is most commonly selected because it is

Box 10.2 Temperature-taking

Main points

Routine temperature-taking is best done in the evening (7–8 pm)

Regular temperature-taking (e.g. 4 hourly) is only necessary when there is evidence or suspicion of an abnormally high or low temperature

Accurate measurement is essential and requires

- use of a reliable thermometer
- selection of an appropriate site
- adequate placement time
- accurate reading

Used correctly, the conventional glass thermometer is convenient and reliable

The oral (sub-lingual) site is convenient and familiar for adult patients who are conscious and alert but accuracy when using a glass thermometer depends crucially on an adequate placement time (i.e. absolute minimum of 3 minutes)

The axillary site, although long thought to be less accurate than other sites, is now considered as reliable as rectal recording for infants and as reliable as oral temperature-taking for adults, but requiring a 12 minute placement time in the case of the latter

The rectal site best approximates core temperature and is least affected by external influences but has the disadvantages of causing discomfort and embarrassment to the patient and cross-infection is a hazard

Electronic thermometers are accurate, time-saving and with low risk of cross-infection if disposable cover slips are used

There is still controversy over aspects of the procedure of temperature-taking and practice should be reviewed as new research evidence is published

Note: See text for supporting references and discussion

---

convenient and is considered to be the most sensitive to changes in the temperature of the blood in the arteries. It is certainly the most convenient site in the case of the fully conscious adult.

The exact placement of the bulb of the thermometer is

important. This should not go just anywhere in the sublingual cavity (under the tongue); the exact place where the maximum mouth temperature is ascertained is at the junction of the base of the tongue and the floor of the mouth either to the left or to the right of the frenulum. Areas of the mouth other than these two 'heat pockets' (Fig. 10.3) are lower in temperature and, therefore, are not an accurate reflection of the actual body temperature.

Still further precautions must be taken to ensure an accurate measurement. If the patient has taken a hot drink, it has been suggested that a time lapse of 6 minutes is needed prior to inserting the thermometer and 15 minutes if the drink is an iced one. A hot bath may raise body temperature and the effect can last up to 45 minutes; strenuous exercise has a similar effect. People who wear lower dentures require relatively longer to return to a stable oral temperature after such activities. Smoking does not appear to affect recordings.

Research recommendations have specified that, to ensure statistically reliable recordings, the optimum placement time is 8 minutes for men, and 9 minutes for women in room temperatures of 18–24°C (65–75°F). However, later research by Pugh Davies et al (1986) showed that no clinical advantage was gained when using a measurement time longer than 3 minutes. A 3-minute reading should therefore be regarded as the minimum.

The axillary site provides a measure of skin temperature and, therefore, less accurately reflects deep body temperature due to variations in both the temperature of the air and the blood flow to the skin. Values obtained therefore tend to be lower than those from the sublingual cavity or the rectum. It has been suggested (Closs, 1992) that this site should be used only when no other site is suitable and only a rough estimate of body temperature is required. The axillary site is, however, useful for babies, children or patients who are confused, breathless or unconscious. The thermometer must be maintained, according to research recommendations, in a secure underarm position for about 9 minutes in adults and 4–8 minutes in babies and children.

According to Fulbrook (1993b), however, the thermometer should be left in situ for a minimum of 12 minutes. His research shows that, recorded thus, the axillary site appears to be just as satisfactory as oral temperature-taking. He contends that invasive procedures (i.e. via mouth or rectum) are, therefore, unnecessary.

The rectal site is traditionally reserved for babies and those adults, particularly the elderly, whose temperature is highly variable, or suspected of being abnormally low. It is considered to be the site best able to provide a recording which is an accurate reflection of the temperature of the core of the body (although it is slower to respond to changes) because of the proximity of a good blood supply and the natural insulation from external influencing factors. The thermometer should be inserted to a depth of at least 4 cm past the anal sphincter in adults and 2–3 cm in babies. The thermometer should be left in place for 3 minutes to obtain an optimal rectal temperature. However, the procedure does subject the patient to considerable embarrassment and so should not be used unless essential. There is, in addition, the hazard of cross-infection when a thermometer is coming in contact with faeces. Brooks (1992) demonstrated from research that the risk of cross-infection was substantially reduced when electronic thermometers were replaced by single-use disposable thermometers for rectal temperature taking; and, compared with glass thermometers, even electronic ones are arguably safer because disposable protective sheaths are supplied.

The argument for using this site with babies is that environmental temperatures alter axillary temperatures more than anal temperatures. However, as Eoff et al (1974) pointed out, the environmental temperature of the nursery is usually kept stable and, in fact, subsequent research by Barrus (1983) confirmed that the axillary site is as reliable as the rectal site, given the environmental temperature is stable. Given this, use of the axillary site avoids two risks associated with the rectal site; firstly, reflex defaecation and secondly, there is no chance of accidental injury to the mucous membrane of the anus.

The otic site (i.e. ear), although rarely used, is said to be an ideal site for temperature-taking because the tympanic membrane provides a reliable indicator of core temperature. A special thermometer must be used. Davis (1993) recommends that the otic route be restricted to children over 3 years of age on the basis of US research which showed axillary temperature-taking to be more reliable with younger children.

The timing of temperature-taking

More often than not, ward routine has dictated the timing

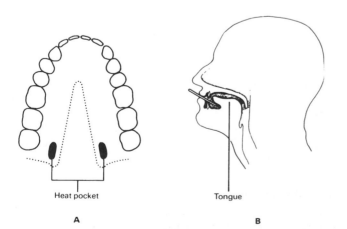

Fig. 10.3 The oral site (A) position of heat pockets on mouth floor (B) thermometer in position in a heat pocket

of temperature-taking rounds in hospital wards with mid-morning, for example, being chosen as a time when nurses could attend to this. However, in view of the fact that body temperature is higher in the evening than in the morning, Brown (1990) recommends strongly that any daily 'temp rounds' should be done as near as possible to 8 o'clock in the evening. Toms (1993) reiterates this advice, noting that research findings have shown that, for most patients, a daily temperature recording taken in the evening is adequate to screen for pyrexia and, therefore, more regular recording (i.e. 3 or 4 times per 24 hours) is necessary only for those patients who are found to be pyrexial on screening.

Newer temperature-recording equipment

Although the clinical glass thermometer continues to be used, especially in the home, alternative temperature-recording instruments have become increasingly popular in hospitals. This is not surprising as entrepreneurs in business are aware that many queries still remain about the satisfactory use of glass thermometers. A great range of equipment is now available, including infra-red thermometers, liquid crystal thermometers, tympanic membrane thermisters, pulmonary artery catheter thermisters and, of course, electronic thermometers.

Electronic thermometers work by the same principle as an ordinary glass thermometer, the probe being covered with a disposable cover slip before insertion and the audible signal given when the maximum temperature is recorded ensures that the thermometer is not removed prematurely. A digital display allows accurate reading of the recorded temperature. The electronic thermometer is favoured because it is said to be accurate, quicker to register and easier to read. Stronge & Newton (1980) carried out one of the early clinical trials to compare an electronic thermometer (the IVAC 821) with the standard system of glass thermometers in performance and cost. They concluded that the time saved using an electronic thermometer on the surgical ward equalled one extra nurse a week. Research conducted in the 1990s (Jensen et al, 1994) has suggested that *rectal* electronic thermometry is more accurate than *oral*, and should be used for daily routine measurements.

Infra-red thermometers are a more recent development (Shinozaki et al, 1988). These are accurate and give a reading within 2 seconds. Depending on cost, these may become available in clinical areas in the future. However, both electronic and British Standard glass and mercury thermometers are acceptably accurate for clinical use (Closs, 1987). The mercury thermometer is a safe, simple and inexpensive instrument but it is easily broken. This fact alone makes investing in expensive electronic thermometers a viable proposition. However, the debate continues over which type of thermometer is most

reliable and cost-effective for routine use in hospital wards.

Concluding comment

From the foregoing discussion, readers will realize the importance of basing nursing activities on the best available knowledge; and that this can change in the light of information as it becomes available from new research. Closs (1987) reviewed 27 nursing texts and found considerable variation in the temperature-taking procedures being recommended. More recently, Fulbrook (1993) has again drawn attention to the continuing inconsistencies between knowledge and practice in relation to temperature-taking; and, as he points out, there remain many points which still require clarification before the procedure of temperature-taking is conclusively defined.

IDENTIFYING ACTUAL AND POTENTIAL PROBLEMS

The information obtained from measuring body temperature and talking with the patient will be examined to identify, in collaboration with the patient whenever possible, any actual or potential problems with the AL of controlling body temperature. Many patients in hospital and in the community do not have a changed body temperature but if there is evidence of an increased or decreased body temperature, or a risk of either, then these actual or potential problems must be identified. The kinds of problems which patients can experience in carrying out this AL can all be discussed under two main headings:

- change of dependence/independence status for controlling body temperature
- change of environment and routine.

CHANGE OF DEPENDENCE/INDEPENDENCE STATUS

In the model of living the dependence/independence continuum for the AL of controlling body temperature is closely related to the lifespan, a greater level of dependence being a characteristic of those people at either end. This is also the case in a nursing context; many of the patients who have problems which change their dependence/independence status are children or are elderly. However, people can have a change in status when they are at any stage on the lifespan as a result of an increase or decrease of body temperature. When the stated goal of return to that particular patient's normal body temperature has been achieved, the patient is dependent on the nurse for encouraging return to the previous status of independence with (when appropriate) adequate knowledge to prevent recurrence of the condition which caused a

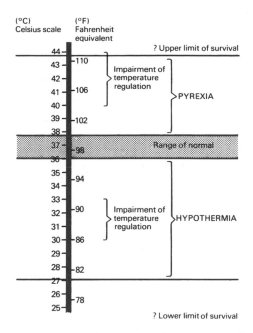

Fig. 10.4 Range of normal/abnormal body temperature showing pyrexia and hypothermia

Box 10.3 Causes of imbalance in body heat

Malfunction of the heat-regulating centre in the hypothalamus as a result of raised intracranial pressure from trauma or neoplasia.

Impairment of the heat dissipating mechanism. Heat is gained faster than homeostatic mechanism can remove it. This happens most often in conjunction with severe dehydration, when perspiration cannot take place.

Response to a pyrogen (agent causing fever). Pyrogens include foreign antigens — the products of tissue damage produced through inflammation or toxins released by microorganisms. There are two types: exotoxins and endotoxins.

(Gould, 1994)

change in status, particularly important in the case of hypothermia.

This important problem is discussed here along with other problematical changes in body temperature which render the patient dependent on the nurse, albeit sometimes only for a short period.

An abnormally high body temperature is referred to as *pyrexia*; an abnormally low temperature is the definition of *hypothermia*. The upper and lower limits of survival are not known exactly but are thought to be at temperatures of above 43°C and below 25°C (Edholm, 1978) respectively. Figure 10.4 illustrates these temperature ranges.

Pyrexia

The condition of pyrexia exists when the body temperature rises above the upper limit of the range of normal, that is above 37.5°C. It is one of the cardinal signs of physical illness, often the first indication that there is some disturbance of body function. Most commonly, pyrexia is a manifestation of infections, neoplasms, trauma (accidental and surgical), diseases of the nervous system, and metabolic disorders. There is reason to believe that pyrexia actually helps the body to combat infection because bacteria survive less readily, and production of immune bodies increases, when body temperature is raised above normal. The main reasons for imbalance in body heat are given in Box 10.3 after Gould (1994).

Pyrexia itself is a very debilitating condition and a dangerous one for young children, even if the associated disease condition is not particularly serious. The abnormally high body temperature is a source of discomfort

and anxiety for the patient and it places considerable strain on the body. These consequences are particularly undesirable in some instances, for example post-operatively when the excessive demands on body systems may impede recovery and wound healing. While a slight postoperative pyrexia is the normal response to surgical trauma, it may also be a warning sign of such diverse complications as infection of the wound, respiratory tract or urinary tract; or of formation of a blood clot in a vein (deep venous thrombosis). Postoperative pyrexia is debilitating: the increased metabolic activity resulting from the rise in temperature increases the body's need for oxygen which, in turn, increases the demands placed on the respiratory and circulatory systems, and it has been estimated that a 1°C temperature rise increases oxygen needs by 10% (Bruce & Grove, 1992).

Onset of pyrexia Although the onset of pyrexia is sometimes sudden, more often it is gradual and manifests as a feeling of unwellness. The person may complain of a headache, loss of appetite, lethargy and tiredness and, usually fairly quickly, begins to feel cold and shivery. This is what is referred to as *chill* and it can last for a few minutes or even an hour, depending on the speed of onset of the pyrexia.

Chill can be explained — the infection or causative factor raises the 'set' point of the body temperature and, to cope with this, heat production increases due to shivering and the metabolic rate increases; there is vasoconstriction and reduced sweating. The patient feels cold and often lies curled up, a position which reduces excess heat loss by conduction, convection and radiation. Once the body temperature is raised, the balancing mechanism keeps it at the new 'set' level.

Features of pyrexia Once the temperature stabilizes

at the higher than normal level, the patient's problem is now one of feeling uncomfortably hot. In an attempt to lower the temperature again, heat loss mechanisms are activated; vasodilation makes the skin warm and flushed and sweating increases which creates another problem. At this stage the hot patient tries to get cool by removing clothing and keeping as still as possible. Usually the patient will feel thirsty due to excess fluid loss through the skin, and dehydration can result quite quickly. Loss of appetite turns into loss of weight, contributing to the person's overall feeling of lethargy and weakness which are further problems.

There are also mental changes associated with pyrexia. The person becomes irritable and restless and this is very obvious in children, who cry, refuse to be comforted and toss and turn in bed. Sometimes severe headache, photophobia (sensitivity to light) and drowsiness may add to the patient's problems: sometimes disorientation ensues and it is known, for example that 'speeded time' perception can be caused by a high body temperature. The problem for the patient is that time seems to drag because the 'internal clock' runs more quickly than the watch. Sometimes mental processes are upset to such an extent that hallucinations may occur and delirium may result. Not infrequently convulsions occur in young children.

During the course of a fever, body temperature may fluctuate quite dramatically as there is continual adjustment to reduce the raised temperature. Alternating episodes of fever and chill are characteristic of pyrexia until the reduction of the 'set' level is permanently achieved. Usually the return of the body temperature to normal occurs gradually. A typical temperature chart of a pyrexial patient is shown in Figure 10.5.

Nursing a pyrexial patient If a raised body temperature is not lowered, it tends to get higher and higher; eventually the regulating mechanisms become impaired, damage to cells occurs and death ensues. The aims of nursing intervention are to:

• prevent any further increase of body temperature
• reduce body temperature to the patient's normal level
• prevent the onset of dehydration
• alleviate the discomforts associated with pyrexia

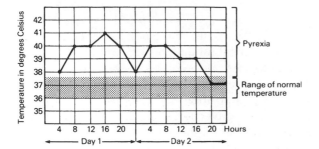

Fig. 10.5 Example of a typical temperature chart of a pyrexial patient

• assist with activities for which there is loss of independence.

The nursing activities that are carried out are based on the principles involved in the body's heat production and heat loss mechanisms. Which activities are appropriate depend on the stage and severity of the pyrexia and are decided on the basis of ongoing nursing assessment. Regular assessment of the patient is necessary as the condition changes and as the outcome of nursing intervention is ascertained by evaluation. Measurement of body temperature is, as discussed, an important tool for evaluation and it is essential that accuracy is ensured so that the progress of the fever is recorded and effectiveness of treatment ascertained.

Promotion of heat loss by radiation is encouraged by removing excess clothing, and heat loss by convection by using fans to circulate air. Body heat can be dispersed utilizing the principles of conduction and evaporation as when tepid sponging or applying cold wet sheets or ice packs. Cold water or ice should be applied with caution since they are likely to cause localized vasoconstriction; this would then reduce heat loss, the opposite of the desired effect. Although it seems radical, and in contradiction to a mother's instinct, a tepid immersion bath may be the most effective way of quickly reducing severe pyrexia in a child. Using cool or cold water to reduce pyrexia does not, however, appear to lower the raised setting of the hypothalamus (Bruce & Grove, 1992) and may induce shivering which, of course, will only serve to increase the body temperature (Castledine, 1994a) and, therefore, caution should be exercised.

Additional heat gain can be prevented by limiting the patient's activity and encouraging as much relaxation, rest and sleep as possible. For this reason, patients with pyrexia are usually nursed in bed; body temperature is lowest during periods of inactivity and sleep.

Alleviating discomforts associated with pyrexia involves a variety of nursing activities. Special help may be required with personal cleansing and dressing because, with excessive sweating, the patient will need to wash more frequently than usual. It is important to pay special attention to the skin folds and the genitalia, and to change the nightclothes and bedclothes when they are damp with perspiration.

To prevent dehydration, and the discomfort of a dry mouth, frequent drinks should be encouraged and opportunities made for cleaning the teeth and rinsing the mouth. Although unlikely to have a good appetite, the patient should continue to eat because while the temperature remains high, the metabolic rate is also high. An appetising well-balanced diet, containing protein and carbohydrate foods, should be provided. Being confined to bed, the patient will be unable to use the toilet facilities and a bedpan or commode will be required.

As pyrexial patients are often restless and irritable the nurse should be attentive to their needs, helping to minimize discomfort and anxiety. Understanding that disorientation to time can be caused by pyrexia should direct the nurse's interaction with the patient. Since any period of waiting, when there is speeded time perception, is likely to seem longer than it actually is, the nurse must try to be punctual in time-related activities, such as meals. The need to continually assist the pyrexial patient in time estimation was pointed out by Alderson (1974).

Hyperpyrexia

An extremely high fever, hyperpyrexia, is a feature of the condition of *heatstroke* which results from prolonged exposure to a very high environmental temperature.

Heatstroke   Heatstroke is a life-threatening condition and usually there is partial or total loss of consciousness. The heat-regulating centre loses control and as a result of the physical effect of heat on brain tissue and that of other large organs, various injurious processes are triggered off. The most important of these is clotting of blood in the capillaries which, in turn, reduces oxygenation of vital organs, such as the heart and liver. Without immediate treatment to cool the body and maintain functioning of the large organs the person affected by heatstroke will die. Walton (1994) underlines the seriousness of heatstroke, stating: 'Heatstroke must be recognized quickly as untreated heatstroke is fatal'.

Illness or death from heatstroke are not unusual in parts of the world where the temperature is very high during the hot season. But even in temperate climates a heatwave may cause some people (particularly the very young and the elderly) to succumb to heat exhaustion. The affected person becomes pale, complains of nausea and headache and shows signs of shock. Usually moving the person to a cool place and providing a cold drink are sufficient to relieve the discomfort.

When heat exhaustion turns to heatstroke there are signs of very high temperature: the skin is flushed, hot and dry, and there is impaired consciousness. Sometimes if the person has been exposed to excessive direct sunlight, there is accompanying sunburn which is extremely painful as well as hazardous. As a result of excessive loss of body fluid in perspiration, causing salt depletion, heat cramps may occur. These are severe muscle cramps and they are often accompanied by extreme thirst, nausea and dizziness. A long salt-containing drink usually gives relief.

Heat stress   Lack of acclimatization plays a major role in people's intolerance of heat, and illness due to heat is most likely to occur when there is excessive physical activity while working or playing in exceptionally hot or humid conditions. The nurse concerned with industrial health services, or with health education for the young

---

Box 10.4   Hyperthermia — Main points

Pyrexia and hyperpyrexia — or hyperthermia — is present when the body temperature rises above 37°C (98.4°F), sometimes reaching 43°C (110°F)

Hyperthermia is caused by two factors:
— the inability of the body to lose heat by the normal means (i.e. failure of the temperature-regulating mechanisms)
— situations which alter the set point of the hypothalamus, causing body temperature to rise

Hyperthermia can be induced by adverse *external* conditions (i.e. high ambient temperature, high humidity, radiant heat) or changes in the *internal* environment due to an infectious, inflammatory or immunological condition

The aims when treating a pyrexial patient are to:
— prevent further rise in body temperature
— reduce the temperature to the individual's normal level
— treat/prevent dehydration
— attend to discomforts and dependence

Heat stroke, the result of over-exposure to heat (e.g. during a heat wave), is life-threatening (especially for the young and old) and requires immediate treatment aimed at reducing the pyrexia

Key reference: Castledine (1994a)

---

and the elderly, can contribute to the prevention of illness due to heat by advising those at risk to limit activity, keep as cool as possible and maintain hydration when exposed to heat for any length of time. Barrett (1991) draws attention to the role of the occupational health nurse in actively screening workers for risk of illness due to heat, using the term 'heat stress disorder' to describe this condition and defining it as occurring when the heat of the environment added to the body's own metabolic heat exceeds the capacity for normal body functions to be maintained without strain. (See Box 10.4.)

Hypothermia

The problem of hypothermia has already been mentioned in relation to the lifespan (the susceptibility of the young and the elderly) and in terms of related politicoeconomic factors. Interestingly, hypothermia has only been a recognised clinical condition internationally since the 1970s (Hillman, 1987).

Literally, 'hypothermia' means lower than normal body temperature. In 1966 the Royal College of Physicians (UK) defined hypothermia as a 'deep body' or 'core' temperature of 35°C or under (Taylor, 1982).

Accidental hypothermia The most common cause of accidental hypothermia is prolonged exposure to a cold and damp environment. It is well-known that exposure in cold water or winter blizzard conditions can cause hypothermia to develop rapidly. Fishermen, sailors, farmers, skiers, climbers, yachtsmen and motorists are a few of the many people who, in the course of working or playing, are exposed to cold, wet and windy conditions. Without wearing special clothing and taking safety precautions they have little chance of staying alive when the weather conditions are severe. With increasing numbers of homeless people in the UK and other countries, hypothermia is an obvious risk for those who sleep out of doors with minimal protection from the cold and wet.

However, within the walls of a house, people can succumb to the dangerous effects of cold and dampness and recently, as already pointed out, it has been recognized that the elderly constitute a group particularly at risk of hypothermia. On low income, they are often forced to live without adequate heating or warm clothing; in addition, they are less active physically and tend to be less well nourished so that body heat production is lowered. Sometimes an elderly person, who lives alone, falls or suffers a stroke and, having lain in the cold all night, when discovered, is found to be hypothermic. Accidental hypothermia, however, can occur even if an elderly person is sitting in a chair, fully dressed and covered with a blanket because, over time, their body heat can be absorbed gradually by the surrounding cold air (Wright, 1991). In a survey conducted in the UK (reported in Reid, 1994), 81% of older people were living in homes where the temperature was below the World Health Organization's recommended level of 20°C, and one-third had living room temperatures at or below 16°C.

The risk is also great for those at the opposite end of the lifespan. Without stability of body temperature or the ability to increase heat production voluntarily very young babies are susceptible to hypothermia unless at all times they are kept warm, dry and out of draughts. Premature babies, or others considered to be at risk, may be nursed in an incubator so that a constant warm environment can be provided, thus preventing hypothermia.

Perioperative hypothermia Hypothermia as pointed out by Goldberg & Roe (1966) may also occur as a consequence of routine surgery, particularly when large body cavities are exposed and when the patient receives substantial volumes of blood and other intravenous fluids. In addition, hypothermia is deliberately induced during specific types of operation such as cardiac surgery, when the body's oxygen requirements are reduced by lowering its temperature.

Although inadvertant hypothermia caused by a cold environment in the operating department was recog-

nized as far back as the 1880s, Surkitt-Parr (1992) contends that there is still inadequate attention given to thermoregulation in the perioperative period. He outlines the cardiovascular, neurological, haematological, immunological and metabolic problems, as well as disturbances in fluid-electrolyte balance, which can result from hypothermia in surgical patients. Major contributing factors are identified as the witholding of oral intake preoperatively, diminished central nervous system activity due to premedicant drugs and inactivity and unconsciousness from the administration of a general anaesthetic. The type of surgery and the length of operation also contribute (see also Closs et al, 1986). The ambient operating room temperature, however, has been shown to have the greatest effect on the incidence of inadvertent hypothermia. Studies have confirmed that the ideal temperature (21°C) is not always achieved.

While a theatre manager in a British hospital, Surkitt-Parr (1992) undertook a study to ascertain staff's awareness and understanding of hypothermia in surgical patients. His survey and observations revealed that, although staff's theoretical knowledge was quite good, procedures to protect patients from hypothermia were not always followed. This suggests a need for at least occasional audit of practice in all operating departments.

Features of hypothermia The most significant feature of hypothermia is that even parts of the body well covered with clothing feel extremely cold to the touch. (If, in addition to exposure to a cold atmosphere, parts of the person's body actually come directly into contact with extreme cold, hypothermia is likely to be accompanied by frostbite.) As the body temperature falls, the whole of the body becomes cold to the touch, looks waxy and the face appears swollen. As the metabolic rate lowers, breathing becomes slower and more shallow and there is a progressive fall in heart rate, cardiac output and blood pressure.

The onset is often insidious; this is why people affected often have failed to recognize the serious cause of their feeling of lethargy and extreme tiredness. Whether a climber caught in a blizzard or an elderly person in their own home, all they want to do is to lie down and go to sleep which, of course, is the worst possible course of action. Quickly their drowsiness increases and eventually coma results. Then the body temperature falls even more rapidly and, if the condition remains untreated, death will occur.

In summary, Hillman (1987) lists the stages of hypothermia as:

1. Feeling of cold and shivering
2. Fall of body temperature to 35°C or below
3. Confusion
4. Dyspnoea

5. Irregular heart beat
6. Respiratory arrest
7. Cardiac arrest
8. Death.

Similar accounts of the signs, symptoms and clinical progression of hypothermia are provided in more recent articles by Toulson (1993) and Castledine (1994b).

Nursing a hypothermic patient

A nurse (or anyone else) who comes across a person who appears to be suffering from hypothermia should summon the assistance of a doctor or the emergency services. Immediate first-aid treatment of mild hypothermia should be in the form of passive rewarming. In the worst conditions resuscitation may be necessary and, in such circumstances, the priorities are (in order):

- respiration
- circulation
- warming
  (Hillman, 1987).

Rapid rewarming, however tempting, is dangerous because it may cause circulatory collapse. The aim should be slow rewarming of the body to return it to normal/usual temperature. Direct heat is inadvisable too, as this causes peripheral vasodilation which draws heat away from the vital organs in the core of the body. Slow rewarming, a rise of 0.5°C/hour, can best be achieved by putting the patient to bed, covered with lightweight blankets or a metal impregnated space blanket and warming the environmental temperature to 26–29°C (79–84°F), if possible. Regarding use of a space blanket, it is now recommended that this be placed over a warmed, ordinary blanket since this is more effective in optimizing rewarming and preventing loss of heat than using it on its own (Toulson, 1993).

Regular measurement of body temperature using a special low-reading thermometer is the method of evaluating the effectiveness of interventions aimed at re-warming the patient.

As the body temperature gradually rises (Fig. 10.6) and consciousness is regained, the patient can be encouraged to increase mobilizing and, by taking warm drinks and nourishing food, increase heat production further until the temperature reaches normal levels. Older people who survive accidental hypothermia apparently have a residual impairment of their thermoregulatory mechanisms which persists for up to 3 years, thus increasing their risk of a subsequent episode of hypothermia (Castledine, 1994b). This group, therefore, should be a particular target for education aimed at preventing hypothermia.

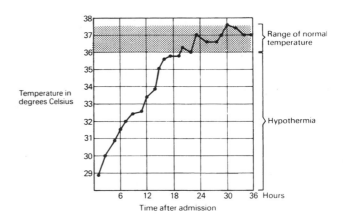

Fig. 10.6 Example of a typical temperature chart of patient with hypothermia

Preventing hypothermia

'Prevention is the key in the battle against hypothermia. It is not a disease, but a preventable condition often brought about by the state of mind and health of an individual, coupled with the effects of social and physical factors such as poverty, loneliness and a lack of knowledge of the risks' (Vyvyan, 1992).

There is scope for all nurses, in their role as health educators — whether in community or hospital settings — to attempt to educate people about how to prevent hypothermia and to detect those at risk. Key target groups are those who care for the young and the old, and independent elderly people themselves.

The elderly in the community must be helped to understand and implement the principles involved in prevention. A room temperature of at least 20°C (70°F) is recommended; it may be most economical if one room of a house is kept warm and used throughout the day and night. It must be remembered that the coldest time is just before daybreak. The amount and type of clothing worn are also important. Several layers of light but warm material provide more warmth and protection from cold than one heavy garment; heat is conducted away from the body when clothing is damp and so dryness of material is essential as well as warmth. For this reason, old people should be advised to dry themselves thoroughly after a bath. Warming the bed with a covered hot water bottle or electric blanket can help, as can wearing bedsocks and even a head cover of some sort.

In summary, key points to put across in health education for hypothermia prevention in the elderly are:

- Have at least one hot meal a day, and plenty of hot drinks (especially one before bed)
- Keep at least your main room well heated (to at least 20°C) and well insulated

- Seek help over problems with fuel bills
- Keep as active as possible
- Keep warm in bed at night, remembering the temperature is at its lowest just before daybreak
- Several layers of light clothing give more warmth and protection than one or two thick layers
- Wrap up when going outdoors on a cold day; wear a hat/cap, scarf and gloves
- Hypothermia is a serious, potentially fatal, condition.

Finally, by way of review of the main points made in the section on hypothermia as a whole, study Box 10.5.

CHANGE OF ENVIRONMENT AND ROUTINE

Although the problems which patients can experience with the AL of controlling body temperature have been outlined under the heading of 'change of dependence/independence status', they also can be considered as problems which arise from change of environment and routine.

At home

When people are confined to bed at home, whether it is for a short or long time, the problem may well be that

---

Box 10.5 Hypothermia — Main points

Hypothermia is present when the body temperature falls to 35°C (95°F) or below

Those most at risk of accidental hypothermia are elderly people (especially those who are frail, inactive, housebound, poorly nourished or mentally impaired), outdoor sportsmen/women, outdoor workers and the homeless

The main cause of accidental hypothermia is unprotected exposure to cold and damp, indoors as well as outdoors

Although most common in winter, hypothermia can occur at any time of year (e.g. on the mountains in summer)

Slow rewarming is the proper first-aid treatment for mild hypothermia

Severe hypothermia (i.e. temperature below 30°C/86°F) is a life-threatening condition and requires expert and immediate treatment

Nurses can play a part in educating 'at risk' groups, especially the elderly; hypothermia prevention is an important health and social issue

Toulson (1993), Castledine (1994b)

---

they exchange the atmosphere of the living room for the cooler atmosphere of most bedrooms, unless of course the central heating extends there or another form of heating is affordable. In addition, confinement to bed or any limitation on routine activity will decrease usual heat production levels and, as a result, the body temperature may fall below its usual norm.

In hospital

Those patients who are admitted to hospital almost invariably find the atmosphere of the ward environment warmer than that at home and this, equally, can be a problem. When people are ill, they become less tolerant of minor discomforts and are more quickly prone to feel miserable if the environment is too cold or too hot, draughty or stuffy, or changeable. Some people like to wear a lot of clothing and have the room well ventilated; others prefer to have the room well heated and wear less. In an open hospital ward, it is impossible to cater for each patient's particular preference.

However, it is essential for the nurse to find out from assessment each patient's usual habits. If any patient is feeling very uncomfortable, the nurse can help by adjusting the heating and ventilation for the majority, and advising extra or less clothing for individuals according to their needs and wishes. Older and immobile patients feel the cold more readily and may appreciate the extra warmth of a blanket around the shoulders or over the knees. Electric blankets and heating pads can also be offered; hot water bottles now tend to be discouraged due to their dangers but, if used, must be covered.

Body temperature falls during the night and patients should be encouraged to express their preference as to the amount of bedclothes they require in order to keep warm during sleep.

In helping to maintain a comfortable environmental temperature, nurses should always give first consideration to the patients' needs and remember that, being active in their work, they are less likely to appreciate that it may be cold for the patients when it seems warm to them.

PLANNING AND IMPLEMENTING NURSING ACTIVITIES AND EVALUATING OUTCOMES

In keeping with the components of the Roper, Logan and Tierney model for nursing, this chapter has discussed the relationship of the lifespan to the AL of controlling body temperature; the effect of the individual's dependence/independence status; the influence of biological, psychological, sociocultural, environmental and politicoeconomic factors on the AL; and the principles underpinning the process of individualizing nursing (i.e. individual assessment and identification of actual and potential problems relating to the AL of controlling body temperature) — by way of reminder, refer back to Figure 3.9 (p. 60). In the case of this AL, patients' problems have been discussed mainly in terms of a change of dependence/independence status arising from undesirable changes in body temperature — hyperthermia on the one hand, and hypothermia on the other. In relation to each, nursing activities have been identified and, in the case of both, some of these relate to the management of actual problems and others to the prevention of potential problems.

Implementing nursing activities which relate to the AL of controlling body temperature involve much the same practices, whether the patient is in a hospital ward or at home. Indeed, the community setting is of prime importance when considering the role of the nurse in relation to this AL, especially in terms of prevention (i.e. of heat-induced illness and hypothermia) by means of health education.

Evaluating the outcomes of nursing intervention requires that explicit goals, mutually agreed with the patient when this is possible, be set, whether to prevent potential problems from becoming actual ones; to alleviate or solve the actual problems; or to help the person cope with those which can not be alleviated or solved. On evaluation, if goals were not reached, they would then be revised or rescheduled, or even discontinued. In the case of the AL of controlling body temperature, there is one key objective measure for evaluating outcomes of nursing activities which are implemented when actual problems require management — i.e. the measurement of body temperature. It has been emphasized, however, that this is only a valid and reliable measurement when the procedure is undertaken with accuracy. There are, of course, other goals of nursing in relation to this AL which require other types of outcome evaluation: for example, goals which relate to the patient's comfort or to knowledge gains from health education.

It is worth repeating here that, although discussed in four phases — assessing, planning, implementing and evaluating — individualizing nursing is not a linear progression; it assumes a built-in responsiveness to feedback at any of the phases, with ample allowance for change within the overall framework.

This chapter has been concerned with the AL of controlling body temperature. However, as stated previously, it is only for the purpose of discussion that any AL can be considered on its own; in reality the various activities are so closely related and do not have distinct boundaries. Figure 10.2 (p. 267) is a reminder that the AL of controlling body temperature is related to the other ALs and also to the various components of the model for nursing. However, it must be repeated that it may not be relevant to consider this particular AL for every patient in every circumstance. Professional judgement is required to assess the relevance of each AL for each patient at any particular point in time.

REFERENCES

Alderson M J 1974 The effect of increased body temperature on the perception of time. Nursing Research 23(1) January/February: 42–49

Angerami E 1980 Epidemiological study of body temperature in patients in a teaching hospital. International Journal of Nursing Studies 17(2): 91–99

Barrett M V 1991 Heat stress disorders. American Journal of Occupational Health Nurses 39(8): 369–380 (as reported in Professional Nurse 1992 7(6): 390)

Barrus D H 1983 A comparison of rectal and axillary temperatures by electronic thermometer measurement in preschool children. Pediatric Nursing 9(6) November/December: 424–425

Brooks S 1992 Benefits of disposable thermometers. Nursing Times 88(33): 54

Brown S 1990 Temperature taking — getting it right. Nursing Standard 5(12): 4–5

Castledine G 1994a Nurse-aid management of hyperthermia. British Journal of Nursing 3(5): 239–242

Castledine G 1994b Nurse-aid management of hypothermia. British Journal of Nursing 3(4): 185–187

Closs S J, Macdonald I A, Hawthorn P J 1986 Factors affecting perioperative body temperature. Journal of Advanced Nursing 11: 739–744

Closs S J 1987 Oral temperature measurement. Nursing Times 83(1) January 7: 36–39

Closs S J 1992 Monitoring the body temperature of surgical patients. Surgical Nurse 5(1): 12–16

Collins K J, Dore C, Exton-Smith A N 1977 Accidental hypothermia and impaired temperature homeostasis in the elderly. British Medical Journal 1: 353–356

Davis K 1993 The accuracy of tympanic temperature measurement in children. Pediatric Nursing 19(3): 267–272

Drummond G 1979 Hypothermia: its causes, effects and treatment in the very young and the very old. Nursing Times 75(49) December 6: 2115–2116

Edholm O G 1978 Man — hot and cold. Edward Arnold, London

Eoff M J, Meier R S, Miller C 1974 Temperature measurement in infants. Nursing Research 23(6) November/December: 457–460

Erickson R 1980 A sourcebook for temperature taking. IVAC Corporation

Feinmann 1986 Some don't like it hot. Nursing Times 82(29) 16 July: 21–24

Fulbrook P 1993a Core temperature measurement in adults: a literature review. Journal of Advanced Nursing 18: 1451–1460

Fulbrook P 1993b Core temperature measurement: a comparison of rectal, axillary and pulmonary blood temperature. Intensive and Critical Care Nursing 9(4): 217–225

Goldberg M J, Roe C F 1966 Temperature changes during anaesthesia and operations. Archives of Surgery 93: 365–369

Gould D 1994 Controlling patients' body temperature. Nursing Standard 8(35): 29–31

Hillman H 1987 Hypothermia: the cold that kills. Nursing Times 83(4) 28 January: 19–20

Jensen B N, Jeppesen L J, Mortensen B B, Kjaergaard B, Andreasen H, Glavind K 1994 The superiority of rectal thermometry to oral thermometry with regard to accuracy. Journal of Advanced Nursing 20, 660–665

Macmillan A L, Corbett J L, Johnson R H, Crampton-Smith A, Spalding J M K, Wollner L 1967 Temperature regulation in survivors of accidental hypothermia of the elderly. Lancet 22 July: 165–169

Millard P H 1977 Hypothermia in the elderly. Nursing Mirror 145(18) November 3: 23–25

Moorat D S 1976 The cost of taking temperatures. Nursing Times 72: 767–770

Nichols G, Kucha D 1972 Oral measurements. American Journal of Nursing 72(6): 1091–1093

Pugh Davies S, Kassab J Y, Thrush A J, Smith P H S 1986 A comparison of mercury and digital clinical thermometers. Journal of Advanced Nursing 11(5): 535–543

Reid T 1994 Fuelling ill health. Nursing Times 90(13): 16

Shinozaki T, Deane R, Perkins F M 1988 Infrared tympanic thermometer: evaluation of a new clinical thermometer. Critical Care Medicine 16(2): 148–150

Sims R 1965 Temperature-taking in a teaching hospital. Lancet 2: 535–536

Sims-Williams A J 1976 Temperature taking with glass thermometers; a review. Journal of Advanced Nursing 1 November: 481–493

Stewart A J 1990 Special care baby units — maintaining the ideal temperature. Professional Nurse 5(10): 544–546

Stronge J L, Newton G 1980 Electronic thermometers. A costly rise in efficiency? Nursing Mirror 151(8) August 21: 29

Surkitt-Parr M 1992 Hypothermia in surgical patients. British Journal of Nursing 1(11): 539–545

Taylor G 1982 Cold comfort. Nursing Times 78(5) February 3: 181

Toms E 1993 Vital observations. Nursing Times 89(51): 32–34

Toulson S 1993 Treatment and prevention of hypothermia. British Journal of Nursing 2(13): 662–666

Vyvyan M Y T 1992 Making sense of hypothermia. Nursing Times 88(49): 38–40

Walker M 1986 When the going gets hot. Nursing Times 83(32) 6 August: 44–47

Wright J 1991 Accidental hypothermia. Professional Nurse 6(4): 197–199

Mobilizing

The AL of mobilizing

The capacity for movement is a characteristic of all living things and the ability to move the body freely is a necessary and much valued human activity. Everyday communication, for example, which is so vital to social life, is virtually impossible without movement, involving as it does the acts of speaking and listening; and the associated eye movements, facial expression, and head and body language.

Likewise, behaviour associated with the activities of breathing, eating, drinking, eliminating, working, playing and so on all involve movement, and when asleep, the body systems continue their ceaseless activity. Everyday living involves a multitude of complicated body movements in innumerable combinations, many of them internal and unseen, and many of them not at conscious level.

In the ensuing chapter, the AL of mobilizing will be discussed in the context of the concepts used in the Model for Nursing, namely: lifespan; the dependence/independence continuum; factors influencing mobilizing; and individualizing nursing (Fig. 11.1).

Lifespan: relationship to the AL of mobilizing

Infancy and childhood

Physical activity is a basic human drive and is important throughout life. Mobilizing as an intrinsic part of living is evidenced by the first movements of the baby's hands and feet, indeed even before birth, the pregnant woman is aware of fetal movement at around 16 weeks' gestation, and ultrasonic examination can identify movement at a much earlier stage. The kicking and arm-waving continue as older babies lie awake for periods and are increased during changing and bathing. Crawling is the next experiment then standing, walking, jumping and running are achieved sequentially. From the second year onwards, the mobilizing dimension of eliminating is mastered and for most children the many skills (involving dexterity as well as mobilizing) required for carrying out

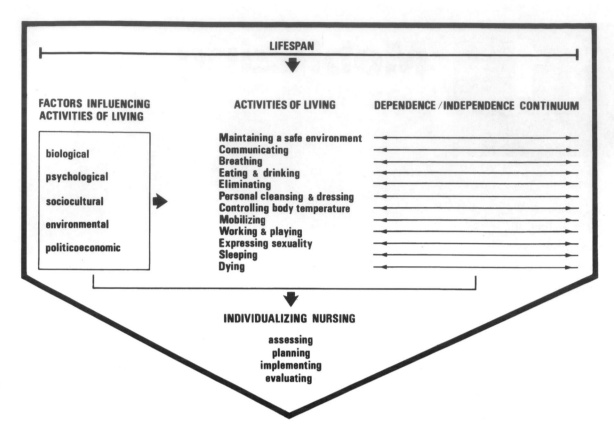

Fig. 11.1 The AL of mobilizing within the model for nursing

personal cleansing and dressing are acquired by 4–5 years of age, in anticipation of attending school.

The acquisition of these basic mobilizing skills, however, is a very complicated and lengthy process. At birth, the nervous system is not sufficiently developed to permit coordinated musculoskeletal movement, and even when the nervous system is in a state of readiness for learning to take place, human infants, if compared to young animals and birds, are relatively slow to adopt independent, coordinated movement. Observation of a baby trying to walk will indicate how many failures there are before there is management of standing and walking unsupported and even then, the sense of balance is unpredictable.

As the body systems develop with age, the healthy growing child is constantly adding to mobilizing skills, and good walking, standing and sitting positions should be cultivated (Fig. 11.2). As well as being aesthetically pleasing to the onlooker, they conserve energy when used in a variety of everyday activities at home, at school and at play, indeed many recreational activities such as gymnastics, dancing and ice-skating encourage good posture.

Adolescence and adulthood

For healthy adolescents, the teenage years are usually crowded with activity, often initiated as part of the school curriculum although as work interests take over, there may be a reduction in the range and intensity of sporting activities. By adulthood, decisions about mobilizing related to working and playing have often stabilized and phrases such as 'sedentary' and 'physically demanding' may apply to leisure activities as well as to income-generating work. However, these are the 'risk-taking' years and are associated with road traffic accidents and sporting casualties (p. 80) which may involve temporary or permanent mobilizing problems.

As far as women are concerned, pregnancy can affect mobilizing. At whatever stage of the lifespan's reproductive years it occurs, it is not difficult to recognize the gait of a pregnant woman in fact, the change in her centre of gravity, as the fetus enlarges, sometimes causes low back pain and in the later months, her capacity for mobilizing is usually reduced. In the postmenopausal phase, too, mobilizing may be potentially affected. Women are more prone than men to develop osteoporosis (loss of bone mineral density) which, in later years, can result in fracture following a fall involving application of a force which would not break normal bone (RCN Nursing Update, 1993). The discovery of a mutation in a gene may determine the cause of osteoporosis (O'Neill et al, 1994) and eventually possibilities for prevention and cure but meantime, recent studies have shown that its onset can be delayed (Box 11.1). Regarding the positive effects of

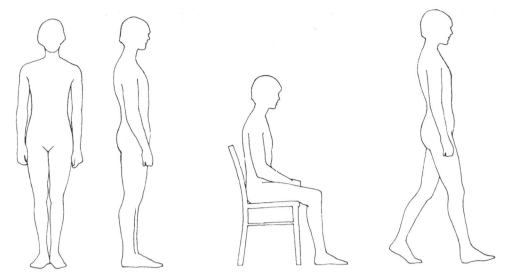

Fig. 11.2 Effective sitting, standing and walking positions

exercise Wolman (1994) provides an interesting account related to Sports Medicine, and Young and Dinan (1994) underscore the wide-ranging positive effects of regular exercise throughout life in preventing not only osteo-

porosis but a number of physical, psychological and social discomforts to which older people may be prone.

It is essential that nurses — so well placed to teach prevention — should be conversant with methods of delaying the onset of osteoporosis. The National Osteoporosis Society (NOS, 1993) has excellent literature about this disabling condition which reputedly affects two million people in the UK.

The elderly

Not only in the industrialized world, but also in developing countries, the number of people over 65 years of age is increasing — 145 million in the West, and 182 million in developing countries (WHO, 1993). For their general pleasure and well-being, the elderly should be encouraged to maintain their mobilizing routines and this has further mention in the following section about factors influencing mobilization. In addition, it is evident, even from an economic viewpoint, that more attention will have to be given to promoting good health in this group of people; there is a marked age-dependent demand on already financially-strained health services and encouraging them to remain healthier could reduce both the bed-occupancy and the budget allocation.

However, for most ageing people, there comes a time when they gradually lose body weight, have less energy and shrink in height. Not only does this directly affect the AL of mobilizing, but also the mobilizing dimensions of personal cleansing, eliminating, eating and drinking, working and playing. Each morning it takes longer to prepare for even everyday activities, and similarly in the evening, preparation for sleeping can be exhausting. Staged within the elderly person's energy level, thoughtfulness and imagination on the part of any helper can assist an older person to maintain some pleasure and dignity in the mobilizing dimension of so many ALs.

Dependence/ independence in the AL of mobilizing

Relationship to the lifespan

It is obvious that with regard to the AL of mobilizing, the dependence/independence component of the model is closely related to the lifespan component. For the majority of people, after a period of dependence in infancy, there is increasing independence in childhood. At the other end of the lifespan, the majority of old people experience a gradual decrease in the level of independence until many of them become dependent on some type of aid, often a walking stick, to broaden the base and take some of the body weight when walking.

Physical dependence

However there are some people who at birth do not have adequate body structure and function to achieve independence in mobilizing, as they progress through the stages of the lifespan. There are others, who having achieved independence, are deprived of it at a further stage on the lifespan, perhaps due to accident or disease. For them, aided independence may be a possibility by learning to use external aids such as walking frames, crutches, leg calipers, and artificial limbs which may be body worn aids although there may be dependence on another person for help with applying the aid. For those who cannot stand, the ability to mobilize may be achieved by dependence on a wheelchair and possibly another person to push it although some are able to use a self-propelled or a battery operated wheelchair. Some can also manage to drive a modified car and indeed become independent as they use a hoist to transfer from wheelchair to car. In recent years, disabled people have become more 'visible' in the community and nurses should be alert to opportunities for helping them to integrate as contributing members of society.

Intellectual and emotional dependence

Although a physical impediment is perhaps the most obvious circumstance which interferes with independence in mobilizing, people who have learning difficulties may experience varying degrees of dependence while mobilizing or while undertaking a variety of other ALs which involve mobilizing, for example eating and drinking, eliminating, dressing, working. Certain psychiatric

disorders too, can alter the individual's independence for movement often without any detectable, biological defect in the musculoskeletal and nervous systems (p. 289 and p. 299).

Factors influencing the AL of mobilizing

Important concepts in our models are the five factors — biological, psychological, sociocultural, environmental and politicoeconomic — which influence the way individuality in mobilizing develops and they will now be discussed in turn, although inevitably they are interrelated.

BIOLOGICAL

The intact musculoskeletal system

As well as many others, a fully functioning musculoskeletal system is essential for acquisition of the skills related to mobilizing. It is not the purpose of this book to provide biological detail of the human body systems; physiology and anatomy are studied in another part of the curriculum. Suffice it to say at this point that to achieve some understanding about the nature of mobilizing, there are several physical principles which are helpful and three examples have been selected — contraction and relaxation of muscle; leverage; and gravity.

Contraction and relaxation (extension) In health, all muscles fibres are in a state of what is called muscle tone, ready for instant, smooth movement. Muscles contract to produce action and are often arranged in pairs associated with two or more bones and a joint, such that the pair have opposing functions; as one muscle (the flexor) contracts and flexes, the other (the extensor) relaxes and extends to allow movement in the desired direction. When, for example, the flexor muscles on the anterior aspect of the upper arm contract to bring the forearm up towards the shoulder, the extensors on the posterior aspect relax to allow movement in the desired direction (Fig. 11.3). This diagram is a simplification of the highly sophisticated muscle activity in the human body, indeed muscles usually work not only in pairs, but in groups and Figure 11.3 merely demonstrates one of the principles of muscle action.

Leverage The principle of leverage, too, is useful in understanding the nature of mobilizing. A lever is a rigid bar which revolves around a fixed axis or fulcrum and a simple example of a lever is a see-saw. Two children of equal weight and equidistant from the middle will balance the see-saw but if one child moves further back, that end of the see-saw will move towards the ground assisted

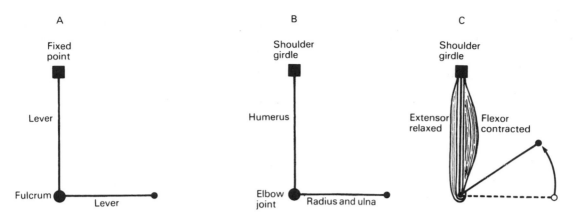

Fig. 11.3 Principles of muscle movement at the elbow joint

by the pull of gravity, and to elevate his end the child must push upwards against the force of gravity. By using the board as a lever it is possible for one child to lift the other quite some height off the ground, which would probably be impossible using only the arms. Utilizing the principle of leverage increases an individual's lifting, moving and handling power.

Law of gravity Knowledge about the law of gravity is also important in understanding the nature of mobilizing. Every object has a centre of gravity (in the human it is around the level of the second sacral vertebra) and it is possible to draw an imaginary line through the centre of gravity to the object's base of support. One merely needs to visualize a tall slender object and a low squat one to appreciate that the broader the base of support and the lower the centre of gravity, the more stable is the object (Fig. 11.4).

Similarly the baby who is starting to crawl has a low centre of gravity and wide base, and when he first stands, somewhat unsteadily, he places his feet wide apart. Likewise, patients out of bed after an illness hold on to furniture or lean on someone's arm or use a walking stick in an attempt to increase their base of support (Fig. 11.5).

It is now recognized, however, that effective mobilizing especially as related to moving and handling loads (including people) involves more than a knowledge of body mechanics.

Ergonomics and the musculoskeletal system

As already mentioned, a knowledge of body mechanics and its application can help people to acquire effective techniques of mobilizing, and of moving and handling loads without compromising the musculoskeletal system. However, this biologically weighted interpretation of mobilizing and handling, based on knowledge from the physical sciences, is restricted to muscular bulk and contracting power. There are other components to consider. The science of creating a match between people and their activities; the environment in which they find them-

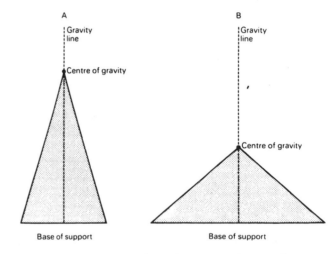

Fig. 11.4 Stability in objects: base of support and centre of gravity

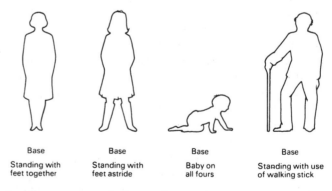

Fig. 11.5 Stability in the human frame

selves; and the equipment which they operate is called ergonomics. It is a mix of knowledge from human and physical sciences and is applicable to all human activity, but is of particular relevance to the working world. It looks at how things, jobs and environments are matched to people's sizes, strengths, abilities and other human attributes (Corlett et al, 1993), and is an example of the inter-relatedness of the five factors in our model. The use of ergonomics in nursing theory and practice is discussed in more detail on p. 303 and its use in the working world in general on p. 318.

Threats to musculoskeletal integrity

The healthy individual's ability for unaided physical mobility is often taken for granted until circumstances intervene which interfere with part of the musculoskeletal system and its associated pathways. Right at the point of birth, the midwife, as well as the obstetrician, plays an important role in assessing the newborn baby for the presence, normal appearance and function of all four limbs. Congenital dislocation of the hip (CDH) for example, may be detected. Although there is an abnormality of the skeletal system involving muscles surrounding the hip, an infant with CDH is not ill. Such children will usually be referred to an orthopaedic specialist, and the application of external splints over a period of time almost always prevents disability in mobilizing during childhood. But while acquiring individual mobilizing habits, this child has to learn to cope, in addition, with external aids.

Fractured or diseased bones are also threats to musculoskeletal integrity and can interfere with mobilizing in many different ways. Joints too may become diseased and so painful that movement is impeded. Should the hips, knees or ankles be affected, walking becomes difficult; when the small joints of the hands are involved there can be interference with many aspects of mobilizing for example those used in domestic activities, personal cleansing and dressing, and working and playing. A muscle sprain may cause swelling and thereby reduce movement. Any form of paralysis such as hemiplegia caused by a cerebrovascular accident (CVA), or paraplegia caused by an accident, severely restricts mobilizing. Of course, even someone with perfectly adequate musculoskeletal and nervous systems may have mobilizing difficulties because of, for example, breathlessness or vision defects, such is the relatedness of the ALs.

For those who have a permanent physical impairment which reduces mobility, the aim is to help them to enjoy everyday living to the optimum level. If physically impaired from birth, the goal will be the achievement of a lifestyle where they will have the maximum possible mobility. For those who succumb to an immobilizing disease or injury, it may mean adapting to a lifestyle which is less physically active but just as personally fulfilling, and the adaptation may be merely temporary or it may require to be a lifelong adjustment.

It is important that, whatever the age group, nurses can help those who use mobilizing aids — and their families and the general public — to understand that they are important as individuals and have equal rights with other members of society. The majority of these people are in the community and if the disability is likely to be permanent, they will seek optimal independent living within the context of their individual ability, not their disability.

PSYCHOLOGICAL

Developing self-image

It is the capacity for movement which first allows infants to explore themselves and their environment. If the child's movement is restricted or if they are deprived of opportunities to respond to stimuli in their surroundings, not only physical but also psychological growth may be impeded. This capacity to explore the environment is critical and lack of, or loss of mobility, or reduced mobility can have a devastating effect on the youngster's image of self, perhaps even affecting the capacity to take their place effectively in society as adults.

Balancing emotions

Some people use physical activity as an outlet for emotions, for reasons as diverse as boredom and aggression. Many 'normal' teenagers and young adults who engage in strenuous activities say that they do so to 'let off steam' and many admit that by so doing, they experience relaxation and recreation. In similar vein, physical activities are deliberately encouraged in social clubs for young offenders, so that energies may be expended in a way which is pleasurable to the individual rather than in uncontrolled and sometimes violent types of behaviour such as fighting, joy-riding and ram-riding. Balanced, goal-directed movement enables one to control one's environment thus enhancing feelings of independence and autonomy. Even when nursing potentially aggressive people who have mental health problems, recreation and vigorous games can channel aggression (Kinsella et al, 1993).

Reacting to emotional trauma

Emotionally disturbing experiences during the early formative years can affect adult behaviour and in some instances affect the AL of mobilizing. In a stable, loving home environment, children will outgrow isolated traumatic events. However if the child's early experiences involve prolonged insecurity or lack of love or if an overburdened parent imparts exaggerated anxieties to the child, there may be excessive timidity and an undermining of the child's self-confidence. This may not be immediately apparent but in later life, painful events such as unhappy love affairs, career disappointments or bereavement may cause a vulnerable person to succumb to feelings of anxiety which interfere with everyday living activities.

The state of anxiety, among other features, may affect mobilizing in the form of a continuous state of restlessness, tense musculature, tremors of the fingers, hyperactivity (especially of the hands shown as movements such as screwing up a handkerchief), dizziness and unsteadiness. On examination, there is no organic reason for the physical disability which interferes with the person's control of movement. In order to resolve such mobilizing problems, it is essential to help these individuals to confront and master the painful situation causing the anxiety and to recognize personally that the physical symptoms are related to particular aspects of their own private lives (p. 299).

Level of intelligence

As far as mobilizing is concerned, a minimum level of intelligence is required to learn the skills necessary for purposeful and safe mobilizing. Helping the child to learn, for example, about safe mobilizing begins in the home, progressing to school, usually including more formal health teaching (p. 77) and then on to adulthood where safety in the workplace assumes importance (p. 317). However for children with learning difficulties, the pace of acquiring the safe and dextrous mobilizing associated with many of the ALs may be much slower and in some instances, may not be achieved even in adulthood.

Attitudes to mobilizing

Attitudes can play an important role in behaviour. Attitudes to safety when mobilizing may, for example, determine compliance with speed regulations, or laws about limited alcohol consumption while driving a vehicle; or taking the time to use safety equipment at work. Perhaps a more subtle manifestation of attitudes is seen in behaviour towards people who have physical or mental disabilities, especially when they are dependent for the mobilizing activities which are associated with many of the ALs.

Attitudes to dependence in mobilizing

For many people, their concept of 'dependence' in a health context is of physical and/or mental disability. In the not too distant past, many such dependent people were segregated from the general public and were cared for in large, old fashioned institutions. Ordinary people therefore did not have an opportunity to develop a positive attitude to dependent people. More than a decade ago attempts to encourage a more positive approach were given international publicity when the World Health Organization designated 1981 as 'The Year of the Disabled Person'. People were made more aware of the many hobbies and sports in which disabled people can take part; these include shooting, bowling, archery, fencing, field and track events, snooker and weight lifting.

The Year of the Disabled Person also drew people's attention to the types of work which can be accomplished by disabled people and some of the opportunities open to them are mentioned in the chapter on working and playing under the headings 'Physical disability' (p. 322), 'Learning disability' (p. 324), 'Mental illness' (p. 326) and 'Sensory loss/impairment' (p. 328).

People who are dependent for mobilizing can be distressed by the public's attitude to their dependence. Some members of the public show their discomfort by using 'distancing' techniques which make disabled people feel uncomfortable; some may be embarrassingly over-solicitous; others manage a mature interaction, conveying that the disabled person is valued as a 'person', yet acknowledging, probably by non-verbal communications, the reality of the dependence (Box 11.2). For children who have a disability such as a leg amputation, the child's problem is also the problem of the parents, and the youngster may have to endure harsh teasing from their peer group.

It is desirable that able bodied people should become more aware of the ways in which such people can be helped to achieve a satisfactory life-style in work, leisure, recreation and family situations. Adequate provision for their needs will overcome their disadvantages to some extent and help them to make the positive contribution they are so competent to make in the community where they live.

The idea still persists that mentally and physically

Box 11.2 A 'large abnormality label'

A veterinary surgeon (Raw, 1993) who has multiple sclerosis and is confined to a wheelchair lives a very full life, but considers the wheelchair to be a 'large abnormality label'. When asked by medical students what annoyed her most about attitudes to the disabled, she replied 'Two things — being patronized and paternalism; the latter especially from the caring professions . . . . . the disabled must take responsibility for their own affairs'.

When asked about the biggest disadvantages of being disabled, she said 'Day-to-day living takes much longer than normal, but I do have equipment to help me. For example a machine enabling me to do things like open the front door, telephone, switch on lights and television; and a hoist to get me in and out of bed. Even so, much time is wasted because nothing can be done quickly — there is no rushing out of bed in the morning if you oversleep!'

disabled people should be protected from the rigours of everyday living. It is becoming more accepted, however, that instead of a passive role, it is preferable to assist them to face the stresses and risks of active participation in the life of the community. To help them to do this, a wide range of facilities must be available from health and social services, from housing agencies, from education and employment departments and from voluntary organizations. Different organizations offer help of various kinds and it is obvious that coordination of these services is needed if the person is to have maximum benefit. In an ideal world no one would be dependent, but in the real world there will always be a group of people who have some form of problem related to mobilizing which makes them dependent to a greater or lesser degree.

SOCIOCULTURAL

Mobilizing and mechanization

There are social and cultural variations in the degree of physical mobility involved in occupations and these affect lifestyle. Despite increasing mechanization, especially in the industrialized world, many people who work on building sites and in road-making, in mining operations or in farming, are involved in more strenuous mobilizing than those who work in more sedentary jobs, and this may prompt them to balance their physical output by choosing less energetic pastimes — and vice versa. For both livelihood and leisure, social class and economic status may determine the form of certain mobilizing activities dictating, for example, whether a person travels on foot or on public transport, by car or on private plane.

Unfortunately, increased mechanization in relation to both work and play, has introduced new problems; there is concern about the lack of exercise in everyday living. Currently, the importance of regular physical exercise is extolled in the media and advocated in the document The Health of the Nation (DoH, 1992) not only as a benefit to the musculoskeletal system, but to promote general physiological and psychological well-being; and Young and Dinan (1994) list what they call the 'preventive effects of exercise' (Box 11.3).

The sedentary lifestyle of many people in most industrialized countries is deplored; a lifestyle which is considered to be a major contributing factor to conditions such as hypertension, coronary heart disease and obesity. All of these have increased in incidence in the last few decades, indeed coronary heart disease is a major cause of death in most countries in the Western World (WHO, 1993). Recent research has shown appreciable protection from CVA in later years if the lifestyle adopted in early adulthood features vigorous exercise, especially if continued into the upper age groups (Shinton & Shagar, 1993).

Box 11.3 Preventive effects of exercise

Discussing the health of older people, Young and Dinan (1994) commend the value of exercise in preventing various diseases and discomforts, for example:

Disease, such as:
- Osteoporosis
- Non-insulin dependent diabetes
- Hypertension
- Ischaemic heart disease
- Stroke.

Disability caused by:
- Intermittent claudication
- Angina pectoris
- Heart failure
- Asthma
- Chronic bronchitis.

Immobility, which can cause:
- Faecal impaction
- Incontinence
- Deep vein thrombosis
- Pulmonary embolism
- Gravitational oedema
- Skin ulceration.

Isolation, which can cause:
- Loneliness
- Depression.

Mobilizing dependence and social role

Understandably, especially for adults, any circumstance which reduces the ability to mobilize, particularly when it diminishes independence, may influence the person's role in relation to family, work and leisure, although many such people compensate and/or adjust, and live lives which are just as fulfilling as their mobile, independent peers.

For people who have a pathological anxiety about venturing out-of-doors (agoraphobia — a fear of open spaces), there may be considerable social isolation; their inability to move out of the house inevitably interferes with work plans unless they can work from home, and it makes activities such as shopping an intolerable ordeal during extreme phases of the illness. The anxiety may fluctuate in intensity; sometimes a mild awareness of tension, but at other times a state of panic in which the person may be overwhelmed by a feeling of terror, but is unable to say just what it is that causes the fear. Understandably, such a distressing mobilizing problem has an effect on others who share the same house, even on neighbours who find it difficult to comprehend, and certainly on friends who strive to understand apparently illogical behaviour.

Mobilizing and rhythm

It is fascinating to consider some of the more recreative mobilizing activities which are influenced by sociocultural factors. Most countries of the world have national dances which are a much valued expression of national pride and patriotic fervour, many of them providing symbolic continuity as they are handed down from generation to generation. Often, they are performed to the accompaniment of music and it is interesting that even young children seem able, intuitively and uninhibitedly, to keep in time to rhythm and enjoy body movement as a response to music.

Many adults, too, seem to enjoy rhythmic body movement as reflected in social recreations such as dancing, ice-skating, gymnastics; and some religious groups show a strong link between music, singing, hand-clapping and body movement. Even at work, long before the advent of piped music, artisans were known to sing while busy at the weaving frame, or harvesting, or hauling in the fishing nets, indeed songs from the cultural heritage of many countries reflect this rhythmic association.

ENVIRONMENTAL

Home environment

The type of family residence is an important determinant of optimal achievement in mobilizing. For example, high rise flats are not conducive to a child's optimal development of the AL of mobilizing; even if an outdoor play area is available in the complex, it may be unsuitable for younger children who really require some direct supervision. At the other end of the lifespan, even a third floor flat which is not serviced by a lift may deter a frail elderly person from taking a daily walk. Available space within the home is another influencing factor and the type of furniture for toddlers and frail people to use as a support while walking is important. Ergonomists pay special attention to the design of furniture, particularly chairs so that for example a desirable sitting posture can be maintained.

Neighbourhood environment

There are many other environmental factors which influence the AL of mobilizing particularly for those with impaired vision, hearing or agility. These include having to cross busy streets, having to climb a gradient when setting out from or returning to the house, or lack of parks and open spaces in which to take exercise in an unhurried manner.

Climatic environment

One should not forget that local climate and terrain can affect mobilizing. The majority of people do not exercise strenuously in a hot and humid atmosphere, and where facilities are available are much more likely to go swimming for example. Obviously people who have a tendency to breathlessness fare badly in a windy climate and even although willing to be active may not get sufficient outdoor exercise.

Man-made energy and the environment

It is interesting to consider the impact of man's ability to control mobility in the environment with reference to the transport and transfer of people and goods. In industrialized countries, the capacity for personal physical movement from place to place is greatly enhanced by machines.

In the initial stages of man's existence on this planet he had to rely on his own body's energy to move himself and his goods from place to place, but as he learned to domesticate animals, he came to conserve his own energy by riding a horse or a bullock or an elephant. With the advent of the wheel, he was able to construct a carrier of sorts which could be drawn by animals. Making an immense chronological leap down to the industrial and technological revolutions, he was able to harness other forms of energy in devising fuel-powered vehicles such as cars, trains, ships and planes for rapid transit of people and vast quantities of goods — and in so doing, helped to create some disturbing problems of environmental pollution (p. 76).

Significantly man is now showing concern about the dwindling natural energy sources in the world and there is a drive to conserve existing supplies. There is also considerable activity in the development of nuclear power, and exploration of the possibilities for utilizing solar, wind and wave energy to man's advantage so that he can continue to augment his own capacity for physical mobility. Hopefully man will find the appropriate balance between exploiting the mobilizing power of machines, and maintaining a personal exercise level which is conducive to health and the enjoyment of everyday living.

POLITICOECONOMIC

Local government

Economic factors undoubtedly influence the facility for mobilizing. Every large city has its slums and areas of substandard housing indeed these are often owned by the local council or administrative body. The environs of such areas are frequently in bad repair and may be poorly lit so there are restrictions on young children in terms of possibilities for physically active pursuits. Also councils vary greatly in the provision of parks and open spaces, children's playgrounds, playing fields, swimming pools, sports arenas and leisure centres, and all these can directly influence the mobilizing habits of the population.

The local council is of course responsible for the state schools in which physical education is available. The range of sports can vary from one city to another, but if for instance the school does not have facilities for swimming, tuition arrangements can usually be made with the municipal swimming pool so that pupils are not deprived of this sport which is such a healthy form of mobilizing.

The council is also responsible for the state of city pavements so that pedestrians can walk safely. There is usually a kerb of several inches between pavement and street and these can be hazardous for both adult and child when a pushchair is being used. Such kerbs also present problems to those of all ages whose form of transport is a wheelchair whether it is manually wheeled by another person, or is self-propelled or battery driven. In some countries it is now mandatory to provide suitably placed ramps when new pavements are being constructed in order to cater for the special needs of these groups of people.

Pedestrian crossings are usually sited at traffic lights but where these are absent, for example on a long, straight road, it is not unknown for public-spirited citizens to succeed in persuading the council to instal a pedestrian-controlled crossing so that particularly those with an impediment in walking can take time to cross safely.

Central government and voluntary agencies

The government makes financial provision for people who have a disability to assist them — and thereby their carers — to cope with everyday living. The current allowance is not means-tested, not based on National Insurance contributions or taxed, and usually is paid on top of other benefits: up-to-date information and leaflets are procurable at social service departments.

The central government in the UK also encourages local councils to provide wheelchair access to public buildings, theatres, cinemas, banks and shopping precincts so that users of this form of mobilizing are not deprived of entry, and some councils have detailed written information about access to these places. For those not wheelchair-bound but with mobilizing problems there are Shopmobility Schemes in certain areas of larger cities where, on arrival at a shopping area, a wheelchair is available, free of charge, to enable the person to visit different stores. There are also Motability and Dial-a-Ride Schemes providing car transport usually with volunteer drivers; and a number of national volun-

tary bodies make provision for transport. For rail and air transport, special assistance is available, on request, and even some commercially-owned taxis now have a hydraulic lift or ramp for a wheelchair. Such is the growing awareness about provision for people who are disabled.

Of course some disabled people can drive their own car and if the vehicle displays the necessary sticker, they can park in areas which are normally forbidden to private vehicles, or restricted in some way.

However, the attitude still persists that disabled people are here to be looked after rather than taking control of their own lives. Fewster (1990) considers it is an historical attitude, derived from charity and from people being segregated into institutions; he labels it 'wheelchair apartheid'. Every effort must be made to dispel this myth. This is recognized by people who have a disability. A revolution in the way all able-bodied people and policy-makers think about disability was the call from 500 delegates attending Eur'able, the first European Conference of People with a Disability. The delegates agreed that disability must be treated as a human rights issue rather than an individual tragedy, sickness, or medical condition. They insisted that disability is a consequence of social prejudice and consider that disabled people are the experts on what kind of social and economic changes are necessary to meet their needs and end discrimination (Martell, 1993).

Individualizing nursing for the AL of mobilizing

Most people, when they waken each day, have the prospect of complete control over their mobilizing routines, but there are exceptions. For example, people with learning difficulties may require varying degrees of assistance or supervision in ALs which involve mobilizing. And in certain psychiatric disorders such as depression, the individual may need support and encouragement to initiate and/or complete several everyday activities requiring movement which they would normally perform unaided. For those who are physically disabled, especially for walking, it may be necessary to use a walking stick or frame, or a wheelchair or an adapted car; and by using these aids, retain considerable choice about when and where they will carry out the AL of mobilizing.

For the few people who do not have the freedom to decide about their everyday mobilizing activities, whether transiently or permanently, the curtailment in the person's capacity for movement almost always creates some problems. However, the manifestation of upset will depend on the degree and duration of the reduced activity; and with the ability to use 'coping mechanisms' and/or aids to deal with resulting deviations in the normal activities of everyday living which involve mobilizing.

The Roper, Logan & Tierney mode of conceptualizing the AL of mobilizing enables identification of individuality in mobilizing — the cornerstone of individualizing nursing for that AL — and individualizing nursing can be achieved by means of:

- assessing
- identifying clients' problems, actual and potential
- planning
- implementing
- evaluating.

ASSESSING THE INDIVIDUAL IN THE AL

Nurses are involved in assessing the individual's ability for mobilizing throughout the lifespan. For example, as already mentioned in Biological Factors, the midwife assesses mobilizing in the newborn baby in relation to general appearance and functional ability. Thereafter, the health visitor assesses the acquisition of normal childhood developmental milestones and advises, among other things, about promoting good posture. Then school nurses will continue surveillance and may be involved in coordinating attendance at specialist clinics for children who have congenital abnormalities related to mobilizing. Occupational health nurses assess ergonomic aspects related to the workplace and are vigilant about identifying circumstances which could lead to accidents, thus preventing potential hazards to an employee's ability to mobilize. Community nurses may make home visits to either children or adults who have mobilizing problems in order to assess progress towards independence; or their continuing ability to cope in the community; or their need for further rehabilitation or hospitalization.

When people come into contact with the health service, therefore, one of the nurse's initial responsibilities involves assessing. Whether or not the student is using the actual format of the Guideline document suggested by the authors (Appendix 1), information which could be categorized as 'Biographical and health data' is usually noted at first contact with the person and probably remains substantially unchanged. The main information, collected as soon as possible but perhaps over a series of contacts, is the 'Nursing Plan' related to the 12 ALs insofar as they are affected by lifespan, dependence/independence status and the five factors. Examples of this individuality in mobilizing have been cited in the preceding part of this chapter and are summarized in Box 11.4.

Assessing is achieved by various means such as observing the person and by acquiring information about usual habits, partly by asking appropriate questions;

Box 11.4 Assessing the individual in the AL of mobilizing

Lifespan: relationship to the AL of mobilizing
- Infancy and childhood — increasing skills
- Adolescence and young adulthood — peak performance
- Later years — decreasing agility and stamina

Dependence/independence in mobilizing
- Increasing independence in childhood, to adulthood
- Dependence on another person
- Body-worn aids / External aids } for aided independence
- Transport mode — to school, work, shops; for leisure

Factors influencing mobilizing
- Biological
  - adequacy of musculoskeletal and nervous systems
  - body posture/gait
  - muscle strength/mass/tone
  - congenital/hereditary interference with function
  - effects of trauma, disease
- Psychological
  - intelligence level; temperament; values; beliefs; motivation
  - knowledge about benefits of exercise and prevention of injury
  - general attitudes
  - attitudes to dependence and disability
- Sociocultural
  - social class: tradition: religion
  - work activities/transport
  - leisure activities/transport
  - effects of mechanical advances on lifestyle
  - dependence affecting role in relation to family, work, leisure
- Environmental
  - housing conditions and environs
  - local climate and terrain: influence on work/hobbies
  - effect of man-made energy on transport of people and goods
- Politicoeconomic
  - community amenities
  - safety of streets/crossings and prevention of injury
  - legal requirements for access to, and mobility in buildings
  - availability of exercise facilities for leisure

partly by listening to the patient and/or relatives/ friends; and partly by using relevant information from available sources. It can be useful to bear in mind the following questions:

- how much exercise does the individual take daily/ weekly?
- when does the individual exercise?
- what factors influence the way the individual mobilizes?
- what does the individual know about mobilizing particularly with regard to health?
- what is the individual's attitude to mobilizing?
- has the individual any long-standing problems with mobilizing, and if so, how have these been coped with?
- what problems, if any, does the individual have at present with mobilizing and are any likely to develop?

Of course answers to these questions may be evident from observation of the person or from medical/other records. Some may be revealed when the home environment is mentioned or when there is discussion about occupation. The nurse could ask, for example, about the distance of the workplace from home, and the type of transport used, indeed the AL of working and playing is so closely related to mobilizing that it may be appropriate to collect information about them simultaneously. It must be emphasized that eliciting information about usual routines is an important part of assessing especially in relation to coping mechanisms; the accent must be on promoting independence and making full use of 'aided independence' where appropriate.

Collated information can then be examined, in collaboration with the client when possible, to discover what the person can/cannot do independently and to identify any actual problems with the AL of mobilizing as well as relevant potential problems.

IDENTIFYING ACTUAL AND POTENTIAL PROBLEMS

The body structures associated with mobilizing are extensive and the psychological factors which directly affect the individual's physical capacity to actually move the body are numerous so it is understandable that people can experience a wide variety of problems related to this AL which involve many of the other ALs. The examples which will be mentioned in this section, however, will refer mainly to the manifestation of problems as reflected in musculoskeletal activity and will be coupled with examples of related solutions. They will be discussed under the following headings:

- change of dependence/independence status

- change in mobilizing habit
- change of environment and routine
- pain associated with mobilizing.

CHANGE OF DEPENDENCE/INDEPENDENCE STATUS

Upper limb problems

It is important to remember that change of dependence/ independence status for mobilizing can be in either direction along the continuum. For example after a Colles' fracture, the forearm, wrist and upper hand may be stabilized in a rigid cast, so the person at first is unable to carry out some activities. The early dependence is greater when the preferred hand is involved, but with ingenuity, some tasks can be carried out using the unpreferred hand, so the person becomes more independent for particular tasks. In instances where an amputation of an upper limb is required, similar changes in the dependence/ independence continuum occur because even with the availability of technologically improved prostheses, help may still be required with placement and removal of the prosthesis.

Of course, may actions carried out by the two hands can be performed by one hand. Often the second hand is merely used to hold an object steady. In principle therefore, if some other means can be used for 'steadying', for example securing vegetables on a spiked board, the good hand can be used to carry out the activity of peeling the vegetable. Similarly bread can be steadied ready for buttering; a grater can be fixed to the wall in a suitable position; clothes can be washed using one hand then wrung out by twisting them round the tap. When eating, a rubber pad under the plate will hold it securely, a guard on the plate will prevent food sliding on to the table and a fork with a cutting edge allows manipulation of food by one hand.

Less dramatic but more permanent problems with hand movements can be caused by, for example, rheumatoid arthritis; simple household tasks can become a painful ordeal. However quite apart from hand surgery which can offer dramatic relief (McHenry, 1991) there are now numerous gadgets to assist with most domestic jobs and the skill of the occupational therapist can individualize equipment to suit personal requirements (Waterlow, 1992).

It is possible to surmount the problem of decreased upper limb mobility at work too, and also for leisure activities. A paper-weight can secure writing paper and allow handwritten correspondence; a typewriter or personal computer can be manipulated with one hand; various aids have been devised to facilitate manual skills at the place of employment, and for hobbies such as knitting, sewing and gardening.

Lower limb problems

Nowadays, for fracture of the lower limb, various biotechnical plates, screws and nails may be used to approximate the ends of broken bone, and immobilize the affected part until healing occurs. These techniques shorten the period of immobility. Nichol (1993) discusses the importance of preventing infection when skeletal pins are used, a potential problem not only in hospital, but in the community because nowadays, patients are discharged home much more quickly.

The lower limb's activity is also temporarily compromised during hip and knee replacement surgery to relieve the pain of arthritic joints (Waterlow, 1992; Boon & Graham, 1992). The nurse and the physiotherapist play an important part in the post-surgery period to help the patient achieve maximum mobility. This is now such a successful procedure that patients can usually walk, unaided, within a few weeks; in contrast to their preoperative painful gait, often requiring the use of a stick.

When there is a mobilizing problem associated with one of the lower limbs, a walking stick with a rubber tip or a quadruped (light metal stick with four small feet) can increase the base of support and help to maintain balance. It is crucial that the stick is of the correct length for that person and it is useful to have a loop of elastic attached to the handle so that the person is free to grasp door knobs and open doors without dropping the stick.

On stairs there may be rails on both sides to assist ascending and descending but it is often better to use only one rail and walk sideways to maintain better balance. Until patients gain confidence, helpers should always stand below the patient when going up, and in front of them when they are coming down. When ascending, the patient should use the good leg first and when coming down, the affected leg first; and it should be remembered that manipulation of stairways may be particularly difficult for an elderly person who is more easily fatigued.

At home in the kitchen, a re-arrangement of storage space and adjustment of working heights can help to increase the person's independence, and articles such as long-handled dustpans can make floor cleaning relatively simple. A trolley can be used for transporting articles from one place to another.

Some people have a lower limb incapacity which necessitates use of a wheelchair. In the UK a wheelchair can be provided free, under the national health service arrangements, indeed more than one may be supplied if medically recommended: a transit chair to take in a car and another for use in the house. It is almost impossible to get all the desired features in one model and it is important to assess individual needs: width (important in relation to size of doorways, corridors, lifts, public toilets), depth, seat height, position of foot support, angle of back, wheel diameter, type of tyre, weight, fixed or detachable arm rests and so on.

When choosing a wheelchair for long-term use it is imperative to see the home surroundings. It will almost certainly be necessary to rearrange furniture and carpets, and it may be necessary to widen doorways or provide ramps, modifications which may qualify for a local authority grant in the UK. Devlin (1989) provides practical information for wheelchair-bound mothers (as well as for blind and deaf mothers) to help them cope with the day-to-day care of a new baby. Corlett et al (1993) provide considerable detail about wheelchair choice and use.

Hemiplegia, paraplegia and tetraplegia

Independence can be even more compromised following, for example, a CVA when one side of the trunk is affected along with the related arm and leg, and opposite side of face; and to an even greater degree if someone has, for example, severe muscular dystrophy or a cervical cord injury (Fig. 4.2, p. 88), when the capacity for mobilizing may be minimal. However, using biomedical engineering knowledge, apparatus involving computers has been devised which can be operated by means of the blink of an eyelid or an expiratory puff allowing the user to turn lights on and off, use radio, TV, a computer and so on, thus allowing considerable 'aided independence'.

Currently there is no mechanism for repairing nerve cells, but there is a ray of hope. At the International Conference of the Spinal Research Trust in June, 1993, it was announced that work by doctors and scientists is progressing towards stimulating the regrowth of nerve cells with the prospect of possible repair of spinal cords. In the UK, each year, about 600 people succumb to spinal cord injury and it is estimated that there are already 40 000 existing victims of traumatic paralysis. The initial impact of such an injury is described by Partridge (1994) who examines the nurse's role in providing psychological support, and Spooner (1995) emphasizes the importance of emotional care when a 'horse-riding accident catapulted her into a wheelchair'.

Musculoskeletal problems

For whatever reason, and in any part of the body, when muscles are inactive, atrophy (wasting) commences and this muscle degeneration in turn depletes the capacity for movement leading to further impairment and so the cycle continues. Exercises may be performed by the patient (active) or by the nurse helping the patient (passive or assisted). The muscle contraction involved not only increases muscle strength, it improves circulation and the movement preserves muscle tone and helps to prevent contracture (Fig. 11.6). In the bones too, lack of muscle action contributes to degenerative changes involving release of calcium from the bones (osteoporosis); and even if halted, it may take months for the bone to

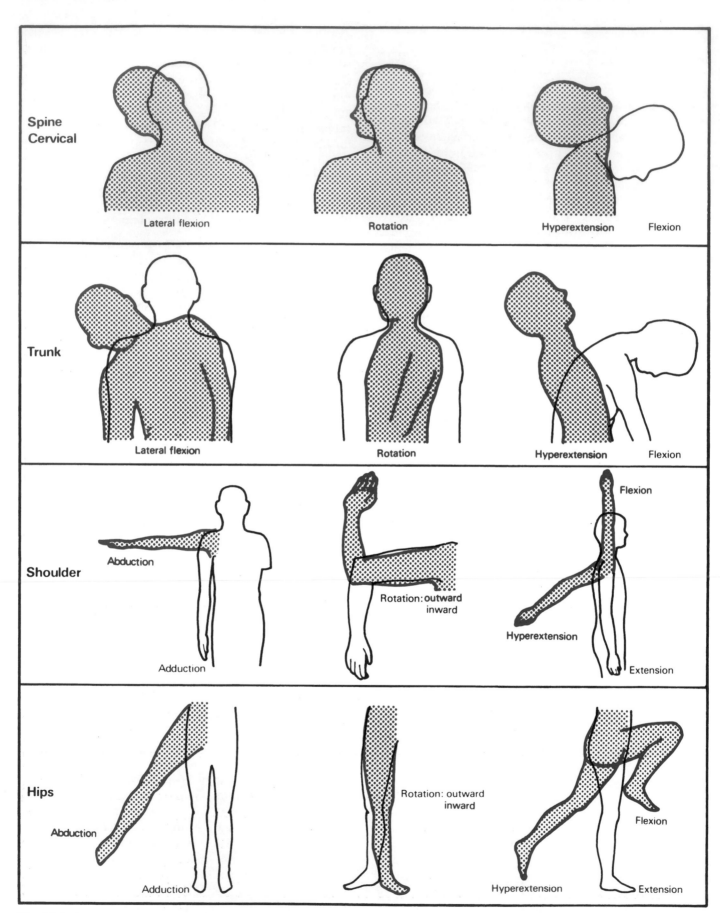

Fig. 11.6 Assisted (passive) exercises for bedfast patients

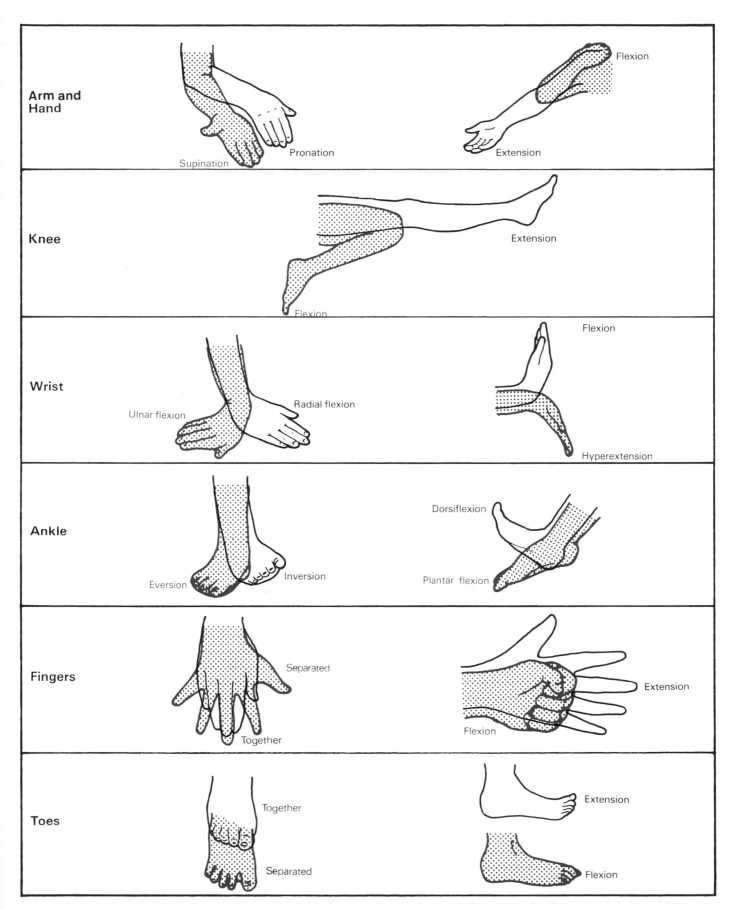

Fig. 11.6 (*contd*)

return to normal. However, osteoporosis is now regarded as a metabolic bone disease, which in the last few decades has become recognized in postmenopausal women in Western society (Box 11.1).

Understandably, if joints are left in one position due to immobilization over a prolonged period, they too become adversely affected. Muscle fibres around the joint shorten and loose connective tissue within the joint is gradually transformed into dense tissue, the combined processes leading to contracture. If allowed to progress without intervention, these processes are irreversible.

An increased interest is now being taken in people who have musculoskeletal mobilizing problems. The initial cause is often brain damage, which can occur at birth (cerebral palsy), or later in life when it is usually due to trauma or pathology causing paralysis of one or two upper and/or lower limbs according to the site of the damage in the brain. 'Conductive education' for these conditions was pioneered at the Peto Institute in Budapest following the Second World War. It approaches the person's problems, not as a medical condition which requires treatment, but as learning difficulties which require teaching.

At the Scottish Centre for Children with Motor Impairments, inspired by the Peto philosophy, conductive education is defined as:

'a system of education which aims to teach the child with cerebral palsy all aspects of daily life. It uses the normal activities of the day to develop the child's ability to learn, and it prepares the child for school. In so doing, it develops the child's personality, language, communication, mobility and hand function'.

There are three general principles:

* the child is introduced to skills and is active in the learning
* the child has opportunities to practise the skills
* the skills are developed and generalized at home and in the community.

The Centre considers that the cooperation of families is essential throughout the process and parents are enthusiastic about the results (Louden, 1993). It has to be remembered that, to each child, their own body is 'normal'. This is why the Peto philosophy considers that the problem is not medical but educational; an educational challenge to encourage these children to establish neuromuscular pathways which promote a mobilizing status acceptable to them. Pollock (1994) reports on a centre in Northern Ireland.

The Bobath technique is similar in some ways and is used for people who have had a CVA. The main principle is to move the damaged body symmetrically so that it is retrained in natural patterns of movement; it needs to be encouraged to develop new nerve pathways to accom-

plish the movements independently. Another principle is to break the automatic pattern of spasticity which is characterized by the clawed hand and the stiff bent elbow; the straightened knee and pointed foot. In a bid to become independent, patients who have had a CVA are often encouraged to learn ways 'around problems' by using the unaffected side of the body, so the affected side is not rehabilitated. Because nurses are with patients round the clock, their support and involvement is crucial to the success of rehabilitation using the Bobath technique (Holmes, 1988). An article by Woodrow et al (1993) emphasizes the role of research in beginning to improve the services for people who have had a CVA. The Barthel Disability Scale and the Rankin Handicap Scale are used to assess pre- and post-stroke activities of living status.

Apart from the initial acute episode, many people who have physical disabilities are not in hospital; they are living in the community. Sahai (1992) describes a community nursing programme set up to benefit clients and carers, and Dix (1992) describes a North American concept in rehabilitation where simulated environments help people to relearn everyday skills in realistic, yet controlled settings before they are discharged from hospital.

CHANGE IN MOBILIZING HABIT

Although it is difficult to describe, most people have some idea of what constitutes normal or average activity in relation to the human body and comment may be passed when a person's activity level changes from busy and bustling to lethargy and relative inactivity. There are gradations of activity/inactivity, but when appearing in an extreme form both over-activity and under-activity are pathological.

Hyperactivity and hypoactivity

A change to generalized hyperactivity and hypoactivity is found, for example, where there are defects in the function of the thyroid gland, part of the endocrine system. Hyperthyroidism occurs when there is oversecretion of the gland and the person has problems because of hyperactivity, breathlessness on exertion, increased pulse rate, and perhaps palpitations; there is tiredness yet constant restlessness. On the other hand hypothyroidism occurs when there is undersecretion of the gland and in extreme cases the patient's problem is that there is a gradual slowing down to a state of almost complete inertia. Due to the hormone deficiency, energy is not being produced in the body. Usually medications can be prescribed to achieve hormonal balance and counteract the hyperactivity/hypoactivity.

Muscular hyperactivity in the form of spasticity is a problem for some congenitally brain-damaged people. The sinuous, writhing, purposeless movements interfere with manual dexterity and if the muscles in the lower limbs are affected, they dictate the strange and uncoordinated movement of the legs, while walking. Writhing, purposeless movement along with a shuffling gait is characteristic also of Parkinson's disease (West, 1991), and muscular hyperactivity occurs too, though usually transiently, during an epileptic fit (p. 392).

Some psychiatric illnesses have physical manifestations which include change in the normal level of activity. The patient with a psychoneurotic disorder has a problem because of difficulty with emotional adaptation to circumstances. In a florid anxiety state, patients may be acutely distressed because they experience intense feelings of anxiety. One manifestation of the condition is an increased output of energy indicated by general restlessness and sometimes uncontrollable tremors. Some patients reduce the anxiety level by the use of a mechanism called a conversion reaction. The mechanism is always unconscious and it produces physical impairment in a part of the body which would normally be under voluntary control. Motor symptoms include paralysis of the limbs, twitchings, tics and fits and there may also be sensory symptoms including numbness and pain. A description of the symptoms is often a reflection of the person's own idea of anatomical structure and when examined medically, there is no indication of organic disease. But such people have an emotional and a physical problem and until effective psychiatric treatment is given, they will not part with this physical mobility/immobility impairment.

It is not sufficient to inform the individual that there is no evidence of organic pathology; it must be made clear that the distress and symptoms are recognized as genuine and in need of exploration. As an example it may emerge that the patient has a life-long pattern of minor phobias and proneness to worry, perhaps because of prolonged, emotionally disturbing experiences as a child, and some recent traumatic event — a disappointment in career plans, a bereavement — has precipitated extreme emotional distress along with an accompanying mobilizing problem. Behaviour therapy or explorative psychotherapy may be used, sometimes prefaced by medication therapy to reduce the distressing mood disturbance before embarking on psychiatric treatment.

Although a more unusual occurrence, Tourette's syndrome is characterized by abnormal body movement such as:

- facial tics
- complex, involuntary movements of the limbs e.g. jerking arms and shoulders, jumping, stamping
- obsessive compulsive actions
- vocalizations e.g. grunting, clicking sounds; repetitive shouting of obscenities.

Garoghan & Polczyk-Przybyla (1994) describe the

nursing interventions used in a psychiatric unit to treat a client who exhibited these features. In contrast to his initial destructive and aggressive behaviour he was able, eventually, to live successfully in a hostel in his local area.

Another example of a psychiatric condition which has motor manifestations is catatonic schizophrenia. Schizophrenia is characterized by a withdrawal of interest from everyday affairs and an emotional coldness. In extreme forms of catatonic schizophrenia, behaviour may range from stupor to excessive excitement and hyperactivity. In complete stupor, patients often lie in an unusual position in bed, completely rigid. They may passively allow the position to be altered or may resist and can maintain the unusual position for hours; some patients are known to have held their heads a few inches above the pillow for many hours or to have remained standing on one leg until their position is physically altered by one of the staff.

These are examples of mobilizing problems experienced by patients who have psychoneurotic and psychotic conditions involving physical hyperactivity or hypoactivity. As a result, apart from their emotional imbalance which requires expert psychiatric care, problems can arise related to almost any of the activities of everyday living, since mobilization is a part of most ALs.

Over the last few decades a problem of hyperactivity in certain children has assumed the title of 'hyperkinesis' or Attention Deficit Hyperactivity Disorder (ADHD). Many of these children have behaviour problems; mealtimes are difficult and there are usually learning disabilities. Parents seek help when home life becomes intolerable (Box 11.5). Health visitors and school nurses may encounter such children, and of course they can be admitted to hospital for a reason other than hyperkinesis.

However, when considering changes in mobilizing habit, some of the obvious examples are related to people who have a physical (locomotor) disability.

Physical disability

Where available, a multidisciplinary team including nurses is necessary to help to prevent diseases and accidents which can produce disability; and to intervene in such a manner as to diminish the impact of disability. Three levels of intervention are recognized:

- first level prevention: action to reduce the occurrence of impairment; for example, immunization against conditions such as poliomyelitis; health control of workers; provision of a safe environment in the home and at places of employment
- second level prevention: when impairment has occurred, emphasis is placed on prevention of

Box 11.5 Hyperactivity

Hyperactivity known formally as Attention Deficit Hyperactivity Disorder (ADHD) is the leading psychiatric diagnosis in American children, and clinicians are discovering that people deemed hyperactive in childhood may suffer lifelong consequences. Researchers in New York found that when these children reached adulthood, they are disproportionately uneducated, underemployed and plagued by mental problems. Experts estimate that ADHD affects 10 million Americans and that ¾ of the sufferers are male (Cowley & Cooper, 1993).

In the New York study, two groups of white, middle class adolescent boys — 103 hyperactive and 100 controls — were followed up and by late adolescence 16% of the hyperactives (3% of controls) were abusing drugs and 27% (8% of controls) had been diagnosed as having antisocial personalities. By their early twenties, the hyperactives were twice as likely to have arrest records, five times as likely to have felony convictions, and nine times as likely to have served in prison.

The cause of ADHD is not known. Children who cannot stifle their impulses are at an obvious disadvantage at school, and likely to live with constant rejection by teachers, parents and peers. Some experts believe these experiences foster a variety of emotional problems; others suspect ADHD is an hereditary defect.

However, all hyperactive children do not have adult problems, and specialists are striving to identify those at greatest risk so that they can be helped.

long-term functional limitations and this depends on:

— speedy diagnosis such as immediate detection of a fracture

— care in the acute stage such as intelligent first aid, effective care in the intensive care unit, the early use of exercise to assist in the return of muscle function

— care in the chronic stage such as establishment of a suitable regime in the Activities of Living for that individual

● third level prevention: the mobilization of available services — medical, social, vocational, educational — to prevent dependence, or in other words to encourage physical and economic independence.

Useful though this concept of physical disability is, nurses need further information about how they can help patients who are experiencing a reaction to the initial change in mobilizing routines, then how to help those who have to cope with long-term change.

Reaction to change: acute onset Physical disability, especially after sudden trauma, is a shattering experience for the person and the rehabilitation process may take many months. During the initial dramatic change and the attendant personal confusion and disorganization, the patient is aware only of deprivation. There may be loss of a limb and a sequence of painstaking stages may have to be worked through — grief for loss of the part, shock, denial, depression, aggression, regression — only then can the individual explore the reality of the situation and be helped to identify possibilities for social and emotional reorganization of life. It requires time and courage to adapt to a disfigured body image, (Price, 1993) an altered role image, loss of independence, loss of security, loss of self-esteem and loss of freedom.

Nurses, therefore, must learn to listen to patients and help them to work through the stages so that they can restore their image of personal worth and dignity. It may be necessary, also, to support the relatives by, among other things, encouraging them to express their feelings in response to behaviour of this type. Aggression or apathy might be quite atypical of the patient's usual behaviour and can cause extreme discomfort, distress and bewilderment to the family. When a child suffers such physical trauma, it is crucial to work with the parents who usually feel guilty about the accident which caused the trauma, and are often in despair about the child's future (Box 11.6).

Loss of even part of a limb can be worrying to a young person in terms of career and economic prospects, recreation choice and social acceptance. Much more so is the total limb and trunk paralysis (tetraplegia), a not uncommon result of diving accidents. But it must not be forgotten that impaired mobility for example, following a CVA (Box 11.7), is equally disrupting to an elderly person who is slower at re-learning to use injured muscles and slower at adapting to changed circumstances especially when other faculties such as sight and hearing may also be failing (Norton, 1993; Kyriazis, 1994).

Even in the protective environment of the hospital, patients keep on discovering just how much mobilizing impairment affects the other Activities of Living. After all, one can do very little without moving some part of the body. But if it is a long-term disability further adaptation is required to the harsh realities of modern living when faced with discharge and coping in the outside world.

Sometimes the person will progress through a rehabilitation unit (Jones, 1992; Williams, 1994) to ease the transition or may be referred to a Disabled Living Centre, but whether or not, a team of health and social service professionals is usually involved in the patient's assessment, care and adaptation — doctors, nurses, physiotherapists, occupational therapists, speech therapists, social workers, rehabilitation officers, educationists, employment officers, employers, housing officials — and the chaplain and voluntary agencies may also make an

Box 11.6 Loss of limbs in childhood: three glimpses of child and parent responses

Ferriman (1993) gives three examples of reactions when a child loses a limb or limbs:

(1) A 3-year-old had to have his left leg amputated after falling on an electrified railway line and his mother felt her world would collapse around her ... that it would be years before he could be well again ... that he would never lead a normal life. She was ridden with guilt. Now nine, the boy has learned to do everything other nine-year-olds do — he can ride a bike, swim, climb trees — although he does have to endure some name-calling at school!

(2) A joy-rider mounted a pavement and maimed a 9-year-old girl who required to have both legs amputated above the knee. Despite the seriousness of such a physical injury, experts say that the psychological trauma to the parents may be even worse. According to orthopaedic surgeons and specialists in rehabilitation, children who lose legs through accidents often bounce back quickly, but parents grieve for the healthy child they have lost and for the expectations that have been dashed ... the parents' reaction is one of despair ... you have to help them to be positive so that they can be positive with their child.

(3) A 27-year-old, married and working as a secretary, had a double above-knee amputation at the age of one year because at birth, the tibia was missing in both legs. She found the primary school years the worst because she was teased, and nobody in her peer group had an amputation. She relates my legs were made of wood until I was seventeen; they were heavy and ugly and I could never wear nice clothes. I now have suction-fitted limbs and can wear skirts and shorts with different coloured stockings ... I can also enjoy riding and have gone skiing'.

Box 11.7 Stroke rehabilitation

Stroke may have long-lasting physical, emotional and social consequences for patients and their families .... Developments in physiotherapy have emphasized the importance of ... facilitating normal movement ... and physical recovery has become the most important outcome measure of rehabilitation ... perhaps to the neglect of the emotional and social consequences say Forster and Young (1992).

Studies have shown that many patients, even some with good physical recovery, have high levels of psychological morbidity. The range of possible emotional disorders is wide and includes anxiety, agoraphobia and pathological emotionalism ... Some studies have highlighted the social inactivity of patients. One found that 90% of patients were able to walk indoors and climb stairs independently but ... were effectively housebound.

For the person's family, too, the psychological burden is heavy. It was found that many carers suffer from frustration, stress and frank depression which increased with time and became progressively unrelated to the patient's physical disability.

More attention should be paid, say the authors, to the social and psychological functioning of both patients and carers.

invaluable contribution. In fact there are now many agencies which provide information to the disabled and their carers, so much so that services may be fragmented. Mason (1993) reports on a Department of Health initiative to bring statutory and voluntary agencies together.

The most important members of the team however are the patients and their families. The patients' motivation to help is critical to successful rehabilitation, so it is imperative to include them in the planning process and the decision making about their future mode of living. Rehabilitation implies restoration to the fullest physical, mental and social capability for that individual.

Families, too, must be convinced that their efforts

are worthwhile and be helped to understand that it is not always in the interests of people who are disabled — whether due to learning difficulties, or to psychiatric disorders or to physical impairment — to have things done for them, because they find them difficult to do. For the nurse and the family, it is important to learn when to give assistance and when to withdraw.

Reactions to change: gradual onset Although not accompanied by the drama of the sudden physical accident, it is just as traumatic to be disabled by arthritis or rheumatism where the onset may be sudden, but more often can be gradual. According to the Arthritis and Rheumatism Council, more than one million people in the UK suffer from rheumatoid arthritis and five million from osteoarthritis. Again, the goal is integrated care by a range of health professionals as well as the carers at home. Nurses have a key role in assessing the circumstances and helping the individual and family members to achieve optimal independence (Cohen, 1994).

It should be remembered that juvenile chronic arthritis can occur at an early age. The nurse is part of a team to help the child and family to cope with, and adapt to the limitations which this disease imposes on their lives physically, psychologically and socially (Maycock, 1992).

CHANGE OF ENVIRONMENT AND ROUTINE

Some people who have both actual and potential problems related to the AL of mobilizing are cared for at home and problems may arise from either being chairbound for most of the day, or being totally bedbound. At home, the changed environment may involve confinement to one room of the house or a re-arrangement or removal of familiar furniture, or a modification of a bathroom or kitchen. A decreased capacity for mobilizing may also require the use of a special type of bed or specific handling and lifting equipment which are often provided on loan from the local health authority services.

The district nurse and occupational therapist usually assess the needs of the patient and, in collaboration with staff from the social work department, the suitability of the home facilities. The nurse uses the same principles for handling and moving which are discussed in the next section and the choice of equipment will be determined by the fact that the district nurse may have to handle the patient on her own, and/or may have to guide relations/ helpers regarding techniques which can be used during the times when a nurse is not available to assist.

Even when confined to bed at home, the individual is still in a familiar setting. Admission to any hospital however — paediatric, psychiatric, acute or long-stay — is an obvious change in environment and will be discussed as change in mobilizing routine, and lack of specific knowledge about mobilizing routine.

Change in mobilizing routine

In order to prepare an individualized plan related to a person's AL of mobilizing it is important to collect information about previous routines at the initial assessment. As mentioned previously, this AL is, for many people, so closely related to working and playing that it may be advisable to seek information about them, either together or in sequence. Knowledge about the previous pattern of the person's day will help the nurse to help the person to adapt accordingly. The help, of course, will be different according to whether the individual is mobile, bedfast or chairfast.

Mobile patients　Inevitably there is a degree of restriction in activities, even for mobile patients although some hospitals have amenities which permit them to exercise in the attractive grounds. Nowadays an increasing number of hospitals, particularly those providing long stay treatment for psychiatric and elderly people, acknowledge the important part mobilizing plays in daily living and make arrangements to ensure that they continue this AL.

As far as children are concerned, most are accustomed to playing out-of-doors for at least part of the day and nowadays, paediatric hospitals usually have excellent play facilities in the wards and garden, indeed in long-stay paediatric units, ambulant children may go daily to a local school in order to continue a normal activity in an otherwise unnatural and unusual routine. Research by Strachan (1993) about the emotional responses of children and their parents prior to, during, and after a hospital stay is a timely reminder of the stress involved. Much thought and effort has gone into minimizing the length of hospital stay and nowadays, day surgery is on the increase (Norris, 1992) and much more use is made of community paediatric services (Fradd, 1994).

Admission to hospital almost always causes a patient distress and anxiety of some sort. The anxiety may be exacerbated, however, for the person with a long-standing mobility impairment which has been present perhaps from birth and who may have learned to cope adequately in the privacy of home surroundings. Admission to hospital may be for some quite unrelated reason and disrupts an established daily mobilizing routine. Activities which were managed at home perhaps independently, perhaps with family help in the privacy of the bedroom or bathroom, may become a problem in an unfamiliar setting which does not have personal accustomed aids and fixtures.

A charter for Disabled People Using Hospitals (Royal College of Physicians and Prince of Wales Advisory Group on Disability, 1992) makes the point that personal wheelchairs and walking aids may be 'as individual as a pair of shoes and essential to independence'. The Report suggests that staff need more training programmes to increase their understanding of disability.

In these circumstances, the nurse must be sensitive to the person's need for privacy and appreciate that, for example, they may require a longer time for dressing/ undressing or for feeding. Help from the nurse may be interpreted as an intrusion and a threat to personal dignity and independence, so it is of paramount importance to assess what the patient can/cannot do, so that the individual can control the situation without having to struggle unnecessarily. Collaboration with other members of the health team, especially the physiotherapist and occupational therapist, is crucial so that positive coping mechanisms are recognized and reinforced while the current cause for admission is being investigated.

Bedfast and chairfast patients　Those patients who are confined to bed are deprived of many of their mobilizing routines and may well feel angry and distressed at their predicament. On the other hand they may be so ill that they are glad to regress and hand over control to the nursing staff. They may have difficulty maintaining the sitting position which (unless contraindicated) is desirable for eating purposes and to facilitate breathing, and is usually preferred by the patient during waking hours.

Bedfast patients may require assistance to maintain

the sitting position and there are specific techniques for moving and handling patients. There should always be careful assessment of the patient's ability to move (Box 11.8) and wherever possible, mechanical aids should be used (Box 11.9), in fact, Larcombe (1993) says 'most adult dependent patients are too heavy or too large to be lifted

manually'. The same moving and handling principles are used to help patients out of bed into a chair, to help a seated patient into the standing position and to help people with special needs (Box 11.10).

Oddy and Lodge (1993) outline a trial scheme, involving nursing and physiotherapy staff, to change patient-handling practices in a psychiatric hospital where patients required varying degrees of assistance to move from bed to chair to wheelchair; an 'Individual handling/mobility assessment' was devised for each person. Hempel (1993) states that in the community, nurses often have to overcome even more obstacles to enable them to handle patients safely; the nurse is in someone's home and is not able to demand that changes are made in the way that would be possible in hospital.

In the UK, legislation has been drawn up in relation to the EC Directive on manual handling of loads (Docker, 1993) which was implemented on 31 December 1992 and the content of the Directive is reflected in the policies of each health authority. It is mandatory that appropriate training in 'moving and handling' patients is included not only in the basic nursing curriculum, but also provided for existing staff, and that ongoing assessment of such skills is provided via regular inservice education programmes.

Many health authorities have appointed 'patient-handling teams' and readers are advised, when in doubt about moving and handling any particular patient, to

---

Box 11.8 Assessing a 'handling' episode

Prior to a moving and handling activity, Corlett et al (1993) place great emphasis on the need for careful assessment of the situation.

Assessing the patient
How dependent is the individual for mobilizing?
- weak and dependent people tend to forget their normal movement pattern and the nurse's task may be, simply, to remind them
- between being wholly dependent and fully independent, there are varying degrees of dependence

Allocating of functions
What is to be done for the patient?
What is the best way of doing it?
- a mechanical hoist should be used for dependent patients
- if this is not possible, how many handlers are needed and what handling equipment is required

Assessing the handling environment
Is it a safe environment?
- if the patient is in bed, is there adequate space around the bed, uncluttered by furniture?
- are there any spillages on the floor?
- are there constraints such as IV drips, drains, traction?
- has the bed height been adjusted?
- has the brake been applied to the wheelchair?

Assessing the handler
How knowledgeable is the handler about handling techniques? Criteria for assessing the suitability of the handler depend on:
- age
- height, weight and lean body mass
- history of back problems
- occupational experience of manual handling
- patient handling repertoire
- awareness of handling capacity.

(Reproduced by kind permission of the National Back Pain Association.)

Box 11.9 Equipment for patient 'handling' in bed

There are many different types of equipment for handling patients in bed, and specially designed beds, because of their construction, can minimize patient handling for example beds with adjustable head, leg and central hip sections operated either manually or electrically; water beds; and Stryker frames.

Apart from such special beds, Corlett et al (1993) consider that the following should be available and used as necessary:

- variable height beds with a foot pump mechanism
- monkey-poles, lifting blocks and rope-ladders to help the patient to move himself
- patient-handling slings, sliding devices (e.g. Easyslide, Patslide) to help the nurse to move the patient
- female urinals and a Charnley wedge to remove the need to lift
- overhead hoists for moving heavy patients in bed.

(Reproduced by kind permission of the National Back Pain Association.)

Box 11.10 'Handling' people with special needs

Although the principles of handling and moving are the same as already discussed, Corlett et al (1993) go into considerable detail about special needs when handling and carrying babies and children.

They also discuss what can be done when faced with a person who, for a variety of reasons, may be unduly excited or even obstreperous. Special handling skills may have to be used at certain times for certain people who have:

- learning disabilities
- acute mental health problems
- organic dementia and disorders characterized by disorientation
- violent, disoriented, disturbed behaviour due to excessive consumption of alcohol or drug/substance abuse
- personality problems.

(Reproduced by kind permission of the National Back Pain Association.)

Box 11.11 The nurse as a back pain victim

Professionally, a knowledge of ergonomics is important to the nurse when advising patients and their families about effective mobilization. On a personal level, however, this type of knowledge helps the nurse to acquire effective techniques when assisting partially dependent patients to mobilize in a variety of environments, and when mobilizing and handling equipment.

Lack of attention to ergonomic theory and practice may lead, particularly, to back injury. Not only physical agony is endured; psychological, social and economic stresses may also be involved. In the UK, when measured by time off work, back pain disability is more common than any other complaint; in 1990 almost 60 million working days were lost through back pain, costing industry about £3 billion in lost production.

Nurses in particular seem to end up as back pain 'victims' says Gillman (1992). The loss of trained nurses through back pain costs the NHS an estimated £50 million a year.

Undoubtedly employing authorities have a duty to provide appropriate instruction about ergonomics and make suitable equipment available for the handling of loads, but the employee also has a responsibility to keep fit, to use techniques which avoid stressing the spine, and to take reasonable care for health and safety.

consult one of the members of such a team. This is an area of nursing practice undergoing constant review because of changing legislation and ongoing research related to the safety of the patient but also to the safety of the nurse (Box 11.11).

Those patients who are chairfast for most of the day are frequently adapting to change in their mobilizing routines. They usually require the help of a nurse to rise from the chair and to walk whatever distance they are capable of walking, supported by another person; and usually the walking exercise is organized to include a visit to the toilet.

Whether in bed or seated in a chair, the person with reduced capacity for movement must be assisted to feel as independent as possible and it is the nurse's responsibility to ensure that a glass of water, the call-bell, and articles such as spectacles, paper tissues, books and newspapers are within reach; that an immobilized arm or leg is adequately supported by pads and pillows in a desirable position; that the person is not exposed to chill; that the person is not left in one position for too long a period. Even when there is loss of sensation in the impaired part, other parts of the body may be strained in maintaining that position.

Lack of specific knowledge about mobilizing routine

It is important for patients to know what they can, and what they should not do in relation to mobilizing. Newly

admitted but mobile patients may feel insecure about continuing the AL of mobilizing unless they are told where it is permissible for them to walk; whether or not there are specific times when they require to be in bed or at the bedside; whether it is customary for patients to leave the ward, for example, to go the hospital shop, the public telephone booths or for a walk in the grounds.

Those who are on 'early ambulation' programmes need to understand exactly how much and what type of activity they carry out each day; and the increasing activity should be clearly described in the patient's nursing plan.

Particularly for recently ambulant people, falls are a potential problem, and especially for those at the upper end of the lifespan. In an acute hospital, over a 6-month period, Gaebler (1993) studied 382 patients who were reported to have sustained 578 falls: 37% fell more than once and accounted for 52% of all falls. The mean age for single fallers was 74 years and for multiple fallers was 71 years. Gaebler classified the location of falls as:

- from the bed
- beside the bed
- from a chair
- from a commode/toilet

- when standing/walking
- miscellaneous.

Injuries included abrasions and lacerations but bone fractures were sustained by 8% of multiple fallers. The researcher suggests that potential multiple fallers may be identifiable at the time of their first fall. She had nine categories of contributing factors and of these, poor mobility was most frequently cited (86% of multiple fallers) and the second was altered mental state (68% of multiple fallers).

Research by Sutton et al (1994) about falls in hospital; an audit of falls by Sweeting (1994); and findings about the use of restraints to prevent falls have already been discussed in Maintaining a Safe Environment (p. 90).

All patients are exposed to potential problems because of their reduction in mobilizing. However they can, whether they are ambulant, chairfast or bedfast help to prevent the potential problems becoming actual ones if they are given adequate information, encouragement and supervision.

One important purpose in exercising and early ambulation is to assist return of blood against gravity to the heart by the 'massage' action of active muscle on blood vessels, particularly in the legs. This is further assisted when the increased 'suction' from deep breathing draws blood along the large vessels back to the heart. Both these actions help to prevent stagnation of blood in the leg vessels. With reduction in mobilizing there is a danger of stagnant blood clotting (deep venous thrombosis). A portion of the clot can become detached (embolus) and flow in the blood until it impacts in a vessel too narrow to permit its passage, usually in the lungs. The condition, pulmonary embolism, may be fatal and it was to help to prevent this condition that 'early ambulation' was introduced in the 1950s. Patients should therefore be taught to do deep breathing exercises (which also helps to prevent respiratory infections) and instructed about moving their feet and toes in a circular direction at regular times throughout waking hours. Effective circulation to the skin and associated tissues, helped by movement, also reduces the potential problem of pressure sores (p. 245).

PAIN ASSOCIATED WITH MOBILIZING

Pain is a subjective experience and for that reason was discussed in the AL of communicating on p. 130. However, because the prime purpose of the musculoskeletal system is to produce movement, it is not unnatural to expect that many of the dysfunctions produce pain specifically on movement, and information of this nature gained at the initial assessment can be documented at this AL.

Different kinds of pain can be experienced in relation to mobilizing for example:

- *Sudden severe pain.* The pain experienced by a person when a limb is fractured is certainly sudden and usually severe. It results from muscle spasm and tissue damage; it produces deformity and shortening of the limb, impaired mobility and loss of function. The immobility continues until the person can have specialist treatment usually in hospital, to align the bone ends and immobilize the limb.
- *Chronic pain.* Many people experience chronic pain associated with the musculoskeletal system variously referred to as rheumatism, low-back pain and joint pain. These dysfunctions are responsible for much temporary and permanent disablement and are the cause of much absenteeism from work.
- *Sharp shooting pain.* Even a tiny protrusion from a compromised intervertebral disc can touch a nerve root causing a sharp shooting pain which is experienced along the pathway of the nerve. The nurse needs to discover whether or not these people do heavy lifting at work or at home and what knowledge they have about safe handling methods.
- *Deep boring pain.* Pain in bone is often described as excruciating. Since bone is a relatively dense structure it has little space to accommodate the swelling caused by inflammation or the extra tissue from a new growth like a cancer.
- *Phantom pain.* A discomfort which is particularly disturbing to patients who have had an amputation is 'phantom limb pain'; it is peculiarly distressing to patients, because they can see that, physically, the amputated part is no longer there. Such patients require special care and attention from the nurse, to help them with this manifestation of pain which is very real to them (Davis, 1993).

As pain on mobilizing may be the main reason for seeking medical aid, much of the treatment is aimed at relieving this distressing symptom. The measures used include:

- rest of the involved joints
- physiotherapy
- medications, e.g. anti-inflammatory, analgesics, corticosteroids
- surgery to restructure affected joints with prostheses
- therapies complementary to medicine e.g. osteopathy (Waldman, 1993).

PLANNING AND IMPLEMENTING NURSING ACTIVITIES AND EVALUATING OUTCOMES

In the preceding section, some examples of clients' problems in the AL of mobilizing have been outlined and it will be apparent that the causes and effects of problems are diverse and often multifaceted. In fact, the entire chapter provides a background of general information about the AL of mobilizing which can be used as an aide-mémoire to assess the individual in the AL (Box 11.4) and help to identify some specific problems which any one person might experience.

Having identified the individual's problems, actual and potential, it is possible, in conjunction with the person, to agree on related goals to cope with or solve them, or to prevent potential problems from actualizing. For example, following surgery for a knee replacement, a goal might be 'will be able to bend the knee to an angle of 70° by postoperative day 5'. Or a discharge goal might be 'will achieve their preoperative level of independence in all ALs but with aided independence in mobilizing, i.e. use two rubber-tipped sticks'. Whenever possible the goals should be stated in measurable terms in order to help to establish at the evaluation stage, whether or not the desired outcomes are achieved.

Having identified the individual's problems and agreed on related goals, it is possible to devise a nursing plan. A plan is a prelude to implementation and all nursing staff have to be aware of the plan so that their activities can be coordinated. For people with physical mobilizing problems, these plans should state clearly how patients should be handled or moved, for example, moving in bed, out of bed, to the bathroom, walking and so on. And in most instances, there should be a planned withdrawal of support — a part of the nurse's role which is much more subtle than visible activities, especially in circumstances where a psychiatric disorder has been the cause of the mobilizing problem.

In order to implement the plan to achieve the goals, many kinds of nursing activities may be used with the aim of helping the individual to prevent, cope with or solve problems with the AL of mobilizing. They may be for example:

- hands-on nursing practices such as passive exercises (Fig. 11.6)
- using the nurse's skills as a listener, e.g. when a person has a conversion reaction manifested by a constantly clenched fist as a response to some deep emotional distress
- using the nurse's skills as an information-giver, e.g. facts about outside agencies which can assist a wheelchair user in everyday living including working and playing activities; and the availability of voluntary agencies such as special-interest groups
- using the nurse's skills as a health teacher, e.g. helping relatives/carers to learn about effective sitting, standing and moving techniques when a client who has had a CVA is living at home, and has residual motor and sensory deficits.

It is important to recognize, of course, that a number of nursing activities involve collaboration with other members of the health team, indeed this team input although desirable, contributes to the complexity of nursing evaluation!

Evaluating the outcome of nursing is an intricate matter but is integral to individualizing nursing. For example, pain while mobilizing could be evaluated using as a measure a painometer (p. 133) and then subsequent variations could be recorded over a period of days while an exercise programme is implemented, or a medication régime commenced. Or (over a series of weeks at predetermined dates) the progress might be evaluated when a teenage girl who has learning difficulties copes with walking from a hostel to a nearby shop to buy specific food items; initially with supervision but eventually unaided.

However goals related to the AL of mobilizing (and their evaluation) are not necessarily only about physical movement as such. For example, a goal, as indicated above, could be concerned with providing information to the client, and the client might be the evaluator – deciding whether or not the information was clear and relevant to the individual's circumstances; and whether or not the methods used were effective (e.g. oral, written, printed, pictorial, or demonstration). It is important for beginning students to learn to think about planning nursing in a way which makes the outcome explicit but it is acknowledged that more research is needed about evaluating. In the UK, the current pressure on the use of audit in the cause of efficiency and cost-effectiveness throughout the health service underscores the many facets of evaluation.

A more detailed discussion about individualizing nursing can be found in Chapter 3. As depicted in Figure 3.9, the four phases – assessing, planning, implementing, evaluating – are not linear: there is frequent feedback, re-assessment and adjustment as the person's problems are resolved or changed, or as new problems arise.

It is necessary to emphasize, however, that there are many instances when it may not be relevant to investigate or document a client's circumstances in relation to the AL of mobilizing and this is a matter for professional judgement. When it is necessary, the information would be combined with information about the person's other relevant ALs. It is only for the purposes of discussion that any AL can be considered on its own; in reality they are closely related and rarely have distinct boundaries.

REFERENCES

Boon E, Graham L 1992 Hip arthroplasty for osteoarthritis. British Journal of Nursing 1 (11): 562–566

Cohen P 1994 Joint efforts (arthritis and rheumatism). Nursing Times 90 (2) January 12: 18

Corlett E, Lloyd P, Tarling C, Troup J, Wright B 1993 The guide to the handling of patients. National Back Pain Association in collaboration with the Royal College of Nursing, Middlesex

Cowley G, Cooper J 1993 The not-young and the restless. Newsweek CXX11 (04) July 26: 44–45

Davis P 1993 Opening up the gate control theory. Nursing Standard 7 (45) July 28: 25–27

Department of Health 1992 The health of the nation. HMSO, London

Devlin R 1989 Helping disabled mothers. Community Outlook April: 4–10

Dix A 1992 Life on easy street (rehabilitation). Nursing Times 88 (43) October 21: 26–29

Docker S 1993 Effects of the European Community directive on lifting and handling practice. Professional Nurse July: 644–649

Ferriman A 1993 In mourning for a lost limb. The Independent, April 20

Fewster C 1990 Wheelchair apartheid. Nursing Times 86 (23) June 6: 49–51

Forster A, Young J 1992 Stroke rehabilitation: can we do better? British Medical Journal 305 (6857) December 12: 1446–1447

Fradd E 1994 Whose responsibility? (Community paediatric services). Nursing Times 90 (6) February 9: 34–36

Gaebler S 1993 Predicting which patient will fall again . . . . and again. Journal of Advanced Nursing 18: 1895–1902

Garoghan M, Polczyk-Przybyla M 1994 Saved from himself (Tourette's syndrome). Nursing Times 90 (17) April 27: 54–59

Gillman V 1992 Back pain and charity. Nursing Standard 6 (32) April 29: 50

Hempel S 1993 Home truths (handling patients at home). Nursing Times 89 (15) April 14: 40–41

Holmes P 1988 A world turned upside down. Nursing Times 84 (6) February 10: 42 (Bobath technique)

Jones L 1992 Positive progress (rehabilitation unit). Nursing Times 88 (5) January 29: 39–40

Kinsella C, Chaloner C, Brosnan C 1993 An alternative to seclusion? Nursing Times 89 (18) May 5: 62–64

Kyriazis M 1994 Developments in the treatment of stroke patients. Nursing Times 90 (29) July 20: 30–32

Larcombe J 1993 Too heavy to handle? Nursing Times 89 (40) October 6: 46–50

Law M, Wald N, Meade T 1991 Strategies for prevention of osteoporosis and hip fracture. British Medical Journal 303 (6800) August 24: 453–459

Louden D 1993 Skills for living life to the full. The Herald, August 25: 22

McHenry C 1991 Handy work (surgery for rheumatoid arthritis). Nursing Times 87 (45) November 6: 18–19

Martell R 1993 Disabled network. Nursing Standard 7 (48) August 18: 18–19

Mason S 1993 Providing a multi-agency approach. Nursing Standard 7 (25) March 10: 18–19

Maycock J 1992 Juvenile chronic arthritis. British Journal of Nursing 1 (5): 232–235

Murphy S, Khaw K, May H, Compston J 1994 Milk consumption and bone mineral density in middle-aged and elderly women. British Medical Journal 308 (6934) April 9: 939–941

National Osteoporosis Society 1993 PO Box 10, Radstock, Bath BA3 3YB

Nichol D 1993 Preventing infection (skeletal pins). Nursing Times 89 (13) March 31: 78–80

Norris E 1992 Care of the paediatric day-surgery patient. British Journal of Nursing 1 (11): 548–551

Norton I 1993 Altered circumstances. (CVA). Nursing Times 89 (30) July 28: 62–64

Oddy R, Lodge L 1993 Special support (patient handling: psychiatric hospital). Nursing Times 89 (3) January 20: 44–46

O'Neill G, Park S, Park A 1994 Why the bones break. Time 143 (5) January 31: 43

Partridge C 1994 Spinal cord injuries: aspects of psychological care. British Journal of Nursing 3 (1): 12–15

Pollock L 1994 Unorthodox conduct (conductive education). Nursing Times 90 (6) February 9: 14–15

Price B 1993 Profiling the high-risk altered body image patient. Senior Nurse 13 (4) July/August: 17–21

Raw M 1993 Personal view. British Medical Journal 306 (3873) January 30: 343–4

RCN Nursing Update 1993 Established osteoporosis: a time for action. Nursing Standard 7 (33) May 5: 5 14

Royal College of Physicians and Prince of Wales Advisory Group on Disability 1992 A Charter for Disabled People using Hospitals. RCP, London

Sahai I 1992 Setting an example to improve quality of life: care in the community for people with physical disabilities. Professional Nurse 8 (1) October: 62–64

Shinton R, Shagar G 1993 Lifelong exercise and stroke. British Medical Journal 307 (6898) July 24: 231–234

Spooner A 1995 A personal perspective: the psychological needs of spine-injured patients. Professional Nurse 10 (6) March: 359–362

Strachan A 1993 Emotional responses to paediatric hospitalisation. Nursing Times 89 (46) November 17: 45–49

Sutton J, Standen P, Wallace A 1994 Incidence and documentation of patient accidents in hospital. Nursing Times 90 (33) August 17: 29–35

Sweeting H 1994 Patient fall prevention — a structured approach. Journal of Nursing Management 2 (4) July: 187–192

Waldman P 1993 Osteopathy — an aid to the healing process. Professional Nurse April: 452–454

Waterlow J 1992 Positive attitude will aid treatment: a guide to rheumatoid arthritis. Professional Nurse 7 (4) January: 242–247

West R 1991 Parkinson's Disease. Office of Health Economics, London

Williams J 1994 The rehabilitation process for older people and their carers. Nursing Times 90 (29) July 20: 33–34

Wolman R 1994 Osteoporosis and exercise. British Medical Journal 309 (6951) August 6: 400–403

Woodrow J, Richardson L, Wolfe C 1993 Stroke registers: a way to improve care. Nursing Standard 8 (5) October 20: 36–39

World Health Organization 1993 Implementation of the Global Strategy for H2000. Vol. 1. WHO, Geneva

Young A, Dinan S 1994 Fitness for older people. British Medical Journal 309 (6950) July 30: 331–334

ADDITIONAL READING

Barnes M 1994 Switching devices and independence of disabled people. British Medical Journal 309 (6963) November 5: 1181–1182

Hardy R 1993 Hip replacement in the elderly. British Journal of Nursing 2 (1): 57–63

Kent E 1995 Information as and when required (multiple injuries). Nursing Times 91 (13) March 29: 29–30

Lauder W 1993 Preventive measures to maintain control: management and treatment of vertigo. Professional Nurse 8 (8) May: 506–509

Pollock A 1994 Carers' literature review. Nursing Times 90 (25) June 22: 31–33

Professional Development 1995 Lifting and handling: knowledge for practice (Unit No. 12 Part 1) Nursing Times 91 (1) January 4

12 Working and playing

The AL of working and playing

Broadly speaking, most people spend about one-third of the day sleeping. For the remainder, a major portion of the day is used for 'working' and the free time left over is available, ostensibly, for 'playing'. Work and play are complementary, and both are fundamental aspects of living. As the following discussion shows, the activities of working and playing have many dimensions and, particularly according to the different stages of the lifespan, their nature and purpose are open to various interpretations.

Working is the word most commonly used to describe an individual's main daily activity and tends to be thought of first in terms of gainful employment. People work to earn an income in order to provide for the necessities of living, for themselves and their dependants. Because work is necessary, it is often thought of in a rather negative way. However, it is worth remembering that a job not only provides an income: it is also an important part of a person's identity and provides a sense of purpose and accomplishment, a structure to each day and the year, a source of company (and this is still the case for most people although teleworking from home is becoming more common) and a certain status in the family and in society. In these times of high unemployment, it is vital to recognize that many people are being deprived of these benefits as well as being denied the right to earn their living. Nevertheless, they — like others, such as school-children, students, mothers at home, housewives, voluntary workers and retired people — would still describe much of their daily activity as 'work'. So, although discussion of the nature of the activity of 'working' inevitably focuses on gainful employment, the broader interpretation of the term should not be forgotten.

Even when work is for financial gain, remuneration is not the only consideration when choosing a job or career. For example, nursing is frequently chosen by those who wish to find a job which allows them 'to work with people'. Others pursue their jobs as an opportunity to use their hands or their intellect or particular qualifications; to be able to travel; or to become powerful. People who choose to do voluntary work see their purpose as giving service to the community. Women who choose to stay at home to look after children would describe their purpose in terms of their children's well-being. Whatever the job, be it paid or unpaid, prevention of boredom and meaningful use of time are basic reasons for working.

Playing is the term being used to describe what a person does in 'non-work' time. It is a convenient term because it emphasizes that, by nature, 'playing' is the opposite of 'working' and in the context of this book it is an all-inclusive term which covers many other words such as leisure, relaxation, recreation, hobby, exercise, sport and holiday. In recent years as unemployment has grown, as retirement has come at an earlier age and as working hours have become shorter, so there has been increased interest in the use of leisure. Enjoyment and occupation of time are prime objectives in all forms of playing. However, for children, playing is also essentially a means of learning and development.

There are many aspects to the enormous subjects of working and playing, and the possibility of accidents at work and at play has already been introduced in the AL of maintaining a safe environment (p. 77). Only a sample of topics has been selected to discuss within the concepts of our model — lifespan, dependence/independence, factors influencing the AL, individualizing nursing for the AL of working and playing (Fig. 12.1).

Lifespan: relationship to the AL of working and playing

The inclusion of the lifespan in the model serves as a reminder that the way an individual carries out any Activity of Living varies throughout life. This is certainly true of the AL of working and playing and there is a change in the balance between the two activities at different stages of the lifespan.

Childhood and adolescence

In infancy and early childhood it is the activity of playing which assumes priority; playing is a universal activity of children and is absent only in conditions of extreme deprivation. The importance of purposeful playing in the development of physical, intellectual, interpersonal and social skills is undisputed. Play begins spontaneously and there is general agreement that its satisfactory development depends on continuing adult encouragement and the provision of suitable toys and play equipment.

Four provisions are of primary importance — playthings, playspace, playtime and play fellows. There are many different types of play — ranging from the exploratory finger play of the young infant to imitative play, constructive play, make-believe play, games with rules, and hobbies. These different types of play emerge in sequence as the child first learns to use the five senses and body movement and then, later, the ability to communicate, interact with others and use creativity and imagination (Bateman, 1987).

Toys are the tools of play. They should be fun but

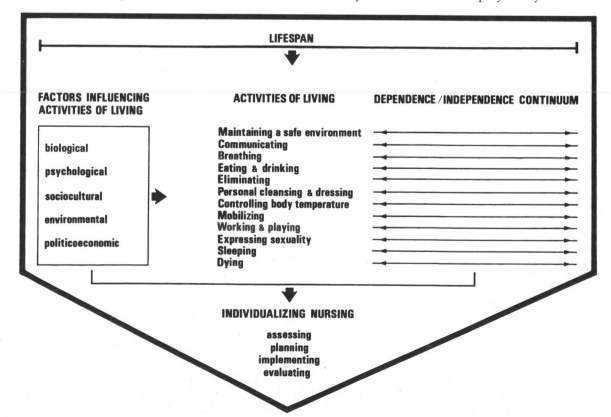

Fig. 12.1 The AL of working and playing within the model for nursing

should also present the child with some sort of challenge, while at the same time allowing a degree of success. Toys allow practice in object discrimination and exploration of shape and texture, and a balance can be found between visual manipulation and intellectual function. By means of imaginative play, the child transforms objects and people into entities which best fit the existing structures of their thinking, giving them a sense of mastery. Persistent day-dreaming and resort to a fantasy world, however, may be a form of escape from a stressful situation and may even be pathological.

Recognition of the importance of playing in early life has resulted in widespread provision of playgroups and nurseries for children of preschool age. Even in the early stages of primary school, there is little distinction nowadays between working and playing, for much of what is traditionally described as school 'work' is accomplished through 'play' activities. However, most people's perception of secondary school would include a clearer differentiation between 'working' and 'playing' activities. In the past, the emphasis was very much on preparation for work and acquiring qualifications for employment.

Nowadays, however, the process of choosing a career seems to have become much more stressful, so much so that in recent years, there have been increasing opportunities at school for what is termed work orientation; senior pupils spend time as observers in local factories, banks and other workplaces as part of the school curriculum. Indeed in the context of high unemployment and with an increasing awareness of the need for preparation for all aspects of adult life, school education has taken on a broader perspective.

A word of caution is sounded, however, about 'adolescent burnout' when parents try to fill every gap in a youngster's day with 'potted packages of stimulation'. Adolescent worries about performance at school — the stress, the competition, the pressure for success — is emerging as a cause of deliberate self-poisoning (McGibben et al, 1992) and even suicide (Deane, 1993).

Adulthood and retirement

The choice of, and establishment in, an occupation must be regarded as a central task of young adulthood although for a few people, what is usually considered a play activity actually becomes work: for example, there are sportsmen and women who earn their income as 'professionals'. Indeed, there are many examples of activities which can be one man's work and another man's play, illustrating that work and play are relative terms.

In both the activities of working and playing, peak performance is usually reached in the years of adulthood. However, whereas young athletes may be past their peak by their 30s, at the other extreme there are people, such as judges and politicians, who may not reach their peak until an age when many people are retiring from work. The effects of the process of ageing on working and playing vary greatly according to the nature of the work and play, and the person's health and psychological outlook. Certainly for playing, adults pursue different types of leisure activities with different purposes — outdoor activities to breathe fresh air; sporting activities for exercise, slimming or competition; group activities for company; reading, theatre or musical activities for relaxation and enlightenment. Whatever the choice, enjoyment, recreation and prevention of boredom are the basic purposes of playing.

With retirement from work, there is more time for activities which fall into the category of 'playing'. Society now recognizes the importance of providing suitable and varied leisure activities for older people so that mental and physical health is maintained. *Preparation for a healthy retirement* is now regarded as extremely important in view of the increased life expectancy — now 80 years for women and 75 for men (Central Statistical Office, 1993) — and it is accepted that people need to be educated about measures which can be taken to maintain health and prevent illness in retirement. Psychological readiness for retirement is also important and, increasingly, employers see it as a responsibility to provide pre-retirement courses so that people can prepare themselves to cope with the changes involved.

Although there is now an almost universal acceptance of the principle of retirement, in pre-industrial society the worker was expected to continue at his job just as long as he remained physically able. As long ago as 1983, Garret said that for working class men, retirement is often associated with four 'losses' — the loss of social status and role; of companionship; of income; and of a meaningful lifestyle. Seen this way, it is not surprising that retirement was viewed as a negative event, and for some people, this is still the case.

However, all 'work' is not necessarily linked to paid employment and there are many non-financial benefits of work which can be obtained in other ways in the post-retirement period.

So, it can be seen that the AL of working and playing undergoes considerable change as a person progresses through the stages of the lifespan. For most people, the lifespan is punctuated by significant work-related events — starting school, leaving school, starting work, changing jobs, gaining promotion and, ultimately, retiring. Though 'working' predominates in the adult years and 'playing' in the early years, both activities are an integral and important aspect at every stage of the lifespan, indeed especially in the working years, an imbalance can be detrimental to health.

Dependence/independence in the AL of working and playing

Childhood and adolescence

The inclusion of the dependence/independence continuum in our model draws attention to the fact that there are periods in life when 'dependence' is to be expected and, at other times, 'independence' is the expectation, and this principle applies to the AL of working and playing. Children are dependent on adults for the development of skills in playing and the provision of playthings and, at a later stage, they are dependent on the education system for the acquisition of skills to equip them for working.

There is even more dependence on adults if a child has learning difficulties or a chronic disabling disease, and although these children may join mainstream education, it is often necessary to provide special tuition, again with even more dependence on teachers and parents. For some of them, although optimum independence in everyday living is the aim, the goal of open employment may not be realistic.

Adulthood and retirement

The so-called 'independence' of adulthood is largely due to the adult's ability to be financially independent, a state which is possible through income from working. By definition, a 'dependant' is a person who is not financially self-sufficient: a child is dependent on parents and an unemployed person may be dependent on state aid. Independence in playing allows the adult to make choices about leisure activities, including the choice to give up previously compulsory school sport and perhaps thus to jeopardize health through lack of exercise!

To a great extent, independent control of working and playing activities continues throughout the rest of the lifespan. Whereas some people would say that there is a loss of independence on retirement from work, others might argue that independence is actually increased. However, frailty and ill-health in old age may cause some loss of independence and necessitate dependence on others or on aids.

There are a number of reasons why people, at any stage of the lifespan, might be unable to achieve or maintain independence in the activities of working and playing. The main reasons — physical disability, learning disability, mental illness and sensory loss/impairment — are discussed later in this chapter.

Factors influencing the AL of working and playing

The nature of the AL of working and playing is multifaceted, and as described earlier, there is variation in both of these activities in the course of the human lifespan. However, there is great variation in working and playing even among individuals of similar age because many factors can influence this AL. In keeping with the relevant component of our model, this section is subdivided into biological, psychological, sociocultural, environmental and politicoeconomic factors. The last of these is discussed in some detail in view of its importance to the subject of this chapter.

BIOLOGICAL

In infancy and childhood, the development of increasingly complex and varied play is closely related to physical growth and the maturation of the neuromuscular system.

Physique and health

Physique enters into the suitability of a person for some occupations, for example, a maximum weight for a jockey or a specific build for a model. Some jobs — such as those in heavy industry, those which are concerned with sport and others like nursing — require considerable physical fitness and energy while others do not, notably sedentary jobs such as working in a bank. People who work in the physically demanding occupations may experience considerable tiredness towards the end of their working lives, when physical fitness and energy decline in the process of ageing.

The capacity for both working and playing, at any stage of the lifespan, is obviously influenced by a person's state of physical health. Athletes and those who participate in physically demanding sport, either as professionals or amateurs, are considered to have reached a pinnacle of physical fitness, although it is a sad indictment on the concept of sport that so many instances are currently being identified where competitors are resorting to the use of steroids and hormones in an attempt to gain, for example, Olympic glory. Apart from the 'cheating element', continued use of such drugs can have substantial neuropsychiatric effects including euphoria . . . mood swings, hostility, violent feelings, and even hypomania and mania (Minerva, 1993).

However, it appears that a growing number of amateur sports people are also misusing these drugs. Petersen's article (1993) discusses the potential adverse effects on various body systems, not to mention the risks of hepatitis B and HIV if the drugs are injected. She urges nurses to be aware of the signs and symptoms of anabolic steroid misuse, and to be knowledgeable about contacts with agencies which specialize in the subject. In the UK, more severe measures are now being taken to halt the unscrupulous, illicit suppliers and traffickers who feed steroid misuse.

Physical dysfunction

Any physical dysfunction in the form of, for example, obesity, heart disease, respiratory problems, musculoskeletal disorders and certain specific conditions, such as diabetes mellitus, may dictate that certain types of work and play are impossible, or undesirable, or necessary to regulate within certain limits. For example, an international survey studied the licensing policies applied to professional lorry drivers who had diabetes mellitus treated by insulin. Responses from 24 countries indicated that regulations differ considerably ranging from a complete ban to no restriction at all. Obviously, it is necessary to balance the right to employment against the risk of potential accidents (Diamond Project Group, 1993).

Physical disability or impairment of the senses, too, are important factors which influence this AL. People who become physically disabled may need to be retrained for work within their altered physical capacity. Similarly people who are visually or hearing-impaired need to choose work which is compatible with their reduced sensory input. What disabled people choose to do in non-work time is influenced by the special facilities available to them. In recent years the scope of playing activities for the physically and visually disabled have increased, for example, riding, swimming, and cycling on tandem bicycles, though deaf people have fared less well and many are frustrated by inadequate leisure time activities.

Because of the many physical variables involved in the AL of working and playing, no specific biological system is aligned with this AL in the Roper, Logan and Tierney model.

PSYCHOLOGICAL

As described in the section on the lifespan, both purposeful playing in childhood and productive work in adulthood contribute to an individual's intellectual and emotional development and, indeed, to the development of their total personality. There are many different kinds of psychological factors which can influence a person's working and playing habits and preferences.

Level of intelligence and personality traits

Level of intelligence is usually one factor in the type of occupation which the individual can satisfactorily follow and this may be manifest by, for example, academic qualifications or dexterity tests or sophisticated computer tests or interview performance, or previous work experience. Inevitably, employment which demands a high level of intelligence is closed to people with major learning difficulties, although they can excel in jobs which demand other types of skills and competencies, and which are just as important to the life of a community.

Temperament and traits are also important. The many possible traits range from patience to impatience, from gregariousness to being a loner. No one is patient all the time but an impatient person is unlikely to enjoy working at intricate tasks or with ill people. Similarly a gregarious person usually enjoys being alone sometimes and a loner sometimes seeks the company of others, but a loner is unlikely to enjoy working with a number of people in the same room or constantly meeting new people as in nursing. It is hoped that career counselling will help people choose occupations suited to their particular attributes in fact, some occupations devise and use entrance tests in an attempt to reduce malplacement of new staff.

Level of intelligence, temperament and personality traits also play an important part in choosing leisure time activities. There is now a wide range of activities available, catering for the skills and tastes of most people including those with disabilities. If the desired choice is not available in the locality in which a person lives, it may be possible to travel to a nearby centre offering the facilities at weekends and in holiday periods.

Self-discipline

At work, lack of development in self-discipline can result in difficulties. Workers may fail to take adequate precautions in hazardous occupations, for instance construction staff not wearing safety helmets and nurses not using well-defined handling and moving techniques and not taking adequate preventive measures in relation to infection.

People who have a learning disability are usually not so mature emotionally and may find self-discipline more challenging, and those who have a depressive illness may be unable to initiate the relevant behaviour even when aware of the need.

Likewise in sport, self-discipline is important in team games or in group hobbies such as sailing and hillwalking where the safety of oneself and others may be at stake. However, self-discipline can be just as essential in individual activities such as writing or composing music.

Stress

Safety at work is a phrase which immediately conjures up

the idea of physical safety, but it also includes the less tangible but potentially harmful risk of working in an environment which is too demanding emotionally. Rogers & Salvage (1988) maintain that stress is a major occupational hazard, causing not only the obvious problems such as headache or depression; heart disease, asthma, diabetes, peptic ulcer and many other 'physical' illnesses have been linked to stress. The word stress, say Rogers & Salvage, is normally used to describe an unpleasant feeling of too much pressure and a subsequent inability to cope; although those who have studied the subject in depth are usually careful to distinguish between 'stress' and 'dis-stress' — the associated harmful effects when stress is in excess of the optimum. As a rule, stress is associated with excessive pressure and over-stimulation but it can also be caused by understimulation, and the experience of unpleasant over- or understimulation can, actually or potentially, lead to ill-health.

Stress can occur in any occupation but Rogers & Salvage (1988) suggest some issues which contribute to stress in nursing and categorize them as:

- *societal stressors* — domestic commitments, childcare, caring for dependants/relatives or neighbours, sexual harassment, racism, homophobia
- *employer-induced stressors* — workload, shift-work, home/work conflicts, pay and conditions
- *professional stressors* — daily contact with illness/death/disability/pain, lack of attention to individual development, inadequate role preparation, lack of professional autonomy, the speed of change socially and in the profession.

They go on to suggest how personal coping strategies can help and how peer group support as well as counselling and education can contribute to alleviation of stress. Learning how to manage stress is immediately important, but the long-term strategy, of course, is to deal with the cause. However, some of the stress at work may be induced by non-work causes — a family crisis or incipient disease. Whatever the cause, the personnel officer and the occupational health nurse can often identify people at risk, and if the occupational health service does not have the necessary facilities or expertise, individuals can be referred to a suitable resource or advised to consult their own general practitioner.

Discussing stress in organizations, O'Kell (1993) reviews the confusing variety of definitions and proposes a four-component conceptual model for understanding stress:

- stressors
- perceived stress
- general adaptation
- consequences of stress

and various methods used by a number of companies to deal with actual and potential stress in the workplace are discussed in an HMSO publication (1992). It is an increasingly recognised problem. Younger (1993) reports the use of an 89-item Likert-type questionnaire when developing and testing a 'Mastery of Stress' instrument.

Absence of work

So far, discussion of psychological factors has concentrated on people in work, but the absence of work has equally important psychological considerations. Unemployment can have severe consequences for the individual and the family. Not only is there the loss of financial independence, but also the loss of self-esteem and self-confidence; there are threatening and humiliating experiences when they apply for a job and are rejected, and there is a decline in social standing. The person is denied the opportunity to use existing skills and to develop new ones; and there is, too, the loss of social contacts. These losses can lead to feelings of frustration and anger, or to depression and a feeling of worthlessness, even to the point of contemplating suicide.

Reviewing a series of articles and research studies on unemployment, an OHE paper (1993) reveals there are strong indications that unemployed people die earlier, especially by suicide, and suffer more mental and physical ill-health than those in work. In most surveys, the unemployed reported a deterioration in mental health since losing jobs (more anxiety, insomnia, depression, irritability and so on) and the longer the unemployment lasts, the worse the health becomes.

Redundancy

Redundancy, too, or even the fear of it can have dramatic effects and, contrary to expectations, this is even happening to nurses (Makin, 1994). Beale & Nethercott (1988) found that workers fearing job loss reported more illness, and their periods of absence were significantly longer, especially for men who had previously consulted their general practitioner infrequently. Gillam (1993), a psychiatric nurse quotes a member of his therapeutic group who spoke of redundancy as 'the time when I finished' — a term of depressing finality — and discussing redundancy for over-55s, Laurance (1986) comments that for many, it seemed like an early death. When firms are forced into retrenchment and job losses — and this is not uncommon in today's economic climate — it is often those in the over-50 age group who are 'expected' to accept redundancy payments. But there is increasing pressure to denounce this discrimination in terms of age.

However, the scene is not totally negative because Laurance indicates that 5% of unemployed people said their health had improved — some because they said they had escaped from miserable jobs, but others because they found positive aspects to unemployment, revealing new areas of interest which may ultimately result in a new job. There is further discussion of unemployment and redundancy later in the Chapter (p. 332).

Retirement

Although a different situation, retirement from work may cause reactions which are similar to the 'worthlessness' of unemployment. The syndrome is now well recognized to the extent that pre- and post-retirement assistance is available from statutory and voluntary sources although industry also now contributes; and there are many pre-retirement courses, services, benefits, workshops, and social and leisure activities available. They are planned to help people disengage from work and re-engage in leisure. Retirement from work can, undoubtedly, offer opportunities for self-development and continuing happiness well into old age, but coming to terms with the absence of work requires considerable psychological adjustment and, in turn, a new attitude towards playing.

SOCIOCULTURAL

Structure of society

When the structure of society was less complex, both working and playing were centred round small, self-sufficient communities of families. For all members there was no differentiation between those people comprising the work, play and family groups; and those with disabilities were integrated. As society grew more complex, communities began to exchange different commodities and goods by the bartering method. Later money was used as the mode of exchange. The realization that the commodities produced by one community were 'desired' by another created supply and demand which encouraged more organized trading systems resulting in intercommunity dependence.

These changes had significant effects on the activity of working. It often became necessary to leave the community to pursue one's work, thus the work group was differentiated from the family and play groups. The long process of industrialization brought the gradual changeover from handmade to mass-produced goods, and from intercommunity to international trading systems, resulting in even further differentiation of the play, work and family groups; the basic groups from which a person obtains support and recognition.

In most cultures the sex of an individual affects choice of work. There are preconceived ideas about the kind of work which only men and only women can do, not just as an occupation but also in the home. However, these attitudes are changing rapidly in many countries, and in some, it is illegal for advertisements to state the sex of the person required for the work. Also the current trend for both wife and husband to follow their occupations and the gradual acceptance of shared parental responsibility is changing the expectations, especially of a man's 'work' in the home.

Similarly in many cultures there are games which are usually played by boys and others which are usually played by girls. However, it is likely that the currently changing attitudes toward adult work will have their effect on the games children (as opposed to boys and girls) will play in the future. Play is often an imitation of adult life and as the distinctions break down for adults so will they for children.

Religion and work/play

Religious factors can influence work and play; beliefs may preclude some activities in both. There are religions which do not permit drinking or gambling and adherents would not choose to work in industries associated with such pursuits. Followers of some religions, and some people because of secular beliefs, do not countenance abortion and would not therefore seek employment in agencies where this procedure might be performed. Some communities will not permit local factories to function on a Sunday. There are still some religious sects which forbid their members to dance, to visit cinemas and theatres, to listen to radio, to watch television and to read any book other than the Bible on Sundays.

Violence at work

In industrialized countries in general, there seems to be an increase in the incidence of violent crime and this was discussed in the chapter about Maintaining a Safe Environment. A feature which is relatively new to the social scene in the UK is the increase in the amount of violence at work. This issue is of major concern in the NHS (NHS Management Executive Report, 1993) and a Nursing Times Survey revealed the extent of the problem for nurses (Ryan & Poster, 1993).

Turnbull (1993) maintains that, among other things, violence towards staff is a health and safety problem which requires an organizational response including effective reporting, counselling and monitoring from the occupational health department, as well as staff training in methods to cope with violence. Holland and Leiba (1993) provide an educational approach to prevent, manage and resolve such situations, and Vanderslott (1994) shows how effective use of management and communication skills based on counselling techniques can defuse a potentially violent situation without alienating the individual.

Much of the published information on physical

assaults to nurses refers to incidents in psychiatric settings yet it is clear that assaults can occur in a variety of inpatient and outpatient settings and also, increasingly, in clients' homes (Morning, 1994; RCN, 1994). Poster and Ryan (1993) conducted a study to determine the effect on the nurse (Box 12.1) and Ravenscroft (1994) enlarges on the growing evidence of post-traumatic stress disorder (p. 75) when emergency health staff are assaulted.

Discussing workplace violence in general, in the USA, Solomon and King (1993) spoke of employees injuring and even killing fellow-workers on the job, indeed the National Institute for Occupational Safety and Health reported violence as the third leading cause of occupational death, and a significant public health problem.

For someone who feels deprived of material goods and feels consumed by helplessness, perhaps violence can become a way of taking things you need as well as avenging yourself on a society which has deprived you of work and money.

Sexual harassment at work could be interpreted as a form of violence, although its anti-social and unacceptable nature went largely unrecognized until about 15 years ago, quotes McMillan (1993). He goes on to say that evidence of its existence has prompted employers' organizations, trades unions and professional bodies to formulate policies to deal with the problem and he refers to the Whitley Council document which makes suggestions about the content of local policy statements (Box 12.2).

Finnis et al (1993) reinforce the need for all health authorities to have a formal policy, and they describe the results of their own pilot study where, in some instances, patients were the perpetrators.

Social class and occupation

The significance of work has come to be a crucial feature in industrialized countries and although it may seem a crude yardstick, the nature of the work contributed by each person is used by many governments to define social class. An example of this, as used in the UK, is given in Table 12.1; and children are categorized according to the father's occupation.

Box 12.2 Sexual harassment: local policy statements

McMillan (1993) refers to The Whitley Council agreement on harassment which suggests that all local policy statements should:

- clearly state what is considered to be inappropriate behaviour at work
- stress that the policy applies to all employees, regardless of their grade or level
- declare that harassment will be treated as a disciplinary offence
- explain that such behaviour may be unlawful in certain circumstances (it could contravene the Sex Discrimination Act)
- describe where to get help, and when necessary, complain about the harassment
- make clear that allegations of harassment will be treated seriously by managers at all levels and that no employee who makes a complaint or who helps someone else to do so, will be victimized
- emphasize that all staff members are responsible for their own behaviour.

Box 12.1 Violence at work: effect on the nurse

Nurses working in accident and emergency, paediatric units, and in acute and learning disability services may all be vulnerable to assault say Poster and Ryan (1993). They report on various studies and refer to one they conducted in the USA to determine the effect on the nurse.

Apparently, although a wide range of responses is experienced during the 6 weeks following an assault, the most commonly reported are:

anxiety	hyperalertness
helplessness	sadness
irritability	depression
soreness	shock

They go on to say that although most nurses have no symptoms 6 weeks later, a small number continue to report moderate to severe reactions at 6 months and one year following the assault, even in the absence of severe injury. The researchers suggest that such nursing staff could become victims of the recognized anxiety condition — post-traumatic stress disorder (PTSD).

Table 12.1 Social class by occupation

Social class	
I	Professional occupations
II	Managerial and technical occupations
III (N)	Skilled occupations: non-manual
III (M)	Skilled occupations: manual
IV	Partly skilled occupations
V	Unskilled occupations

Source: Registrar General's classification

ENVIRONMENTAL

An infinite variety of environmental, including climatic factors, can affect working conditions. In fact to ensure that the workplace is as healthy as possible, legal requirements place a duty on employers to protect the health and safety of the workforce (there are about 30 million people of employable age in England & Wales), and on employees to comply with the various regulations.

Health and safety at work

There are conditions which employers must provide and others which they are advised to provide for both indoor and outdoor workers. Examples are protective clothing for dirty work; pads for kneeling; gloves for handling hot materials; goggles to prevent not only strain from glare but also injury from sparks, hot metals and corrosive liquids; filters and masks in dusty industries and for the prevention of spread of infection; and the provision of a fluorescent garment wherever it is important for workers to be easily visible, for example on highways. And with the current heightened publicity about AIDS/HIV (p. 354), there are specific guidelines (UKCC 1994, Hart 1993, Department of Health, 1993) about maintaining a safe environment in the workplace, especially in relation to health care personnel.

Following the evidence of research, there are now also requirements to have 'no smoking' areas at work so that employees are not subjected to breathing smoke-laden air which, it has been proved, is injurious to health (US Environmental Protection Agency, 1992; He et al, 1994), and this topic is discussed in more detail in the chapter on the AL of breathing (p. 143). In relation to the use of specific hazardous substances in the workplace, there is also legislation (Control of Substances Hazardous to Health, 1988) which requires all employers to make, and usually record, a comprehensive assessment of all the risks of using such substances.

Noise control

The noise level, too, is subject to control, for example, noise associated with construction work, equipment and loudspeakers. Excessive noise in the workplace can be a source of mental and physical stress, annoyance, fatigue, loss of concentration; is a contributory factor in workplace accidents; and is also thought to be implicated in illnesses such as hypertension, stroke and ulcers. However the harmful effects depend on volume, frequency and length of exposure (Payling, 1994). At levels of 90 dB (A) or more (p. 90) employers must ensure that ear protectors are worn, and the provision of audiometric screening is recommended in the workplace; payment of compensation for loss of hearing may be enforced by law when an employer can be proved to have been negligent. Payling discusses the recent legislation to ensure employee protection and indicates how occupational health nurses can take steps to reduce exposure to noise at work.

Temperature control

Excessive heat, whether climatic or environmental, can also be a hazard at the workplace. Perspiration may be so considerable that salted, fruit drinks are needed to maintain the body's fluid balance. Researchers on a Healthy (non-alcoholic) Drinks project maintain that a loss of up to 4% body fluid can have significant effects such as headache, nausea, vomiting and cramps; and by the time 5% is lost, there is lack of concentration thus increasing the risk of accidents. The Royal College of Nursing adviser in occupational health reinforced the need for non-alcoholic drinks to be available, especially for people working in industrial settings (Seymour, 1993).

Outdoor weather conditions can from time to time adversely affect indoor working conditions. For example large expanses of window can cause excessive cold in winter and excessive heat in summer as well as glare from the sun, resulting in a slower pace of working and potentially less tolerance of irritation.

The 'sick building' syndrome

Noise and faulty temperature control may, among other factors, be the cause of a form of indoor pollution, now recognized as 'the sick building syndrome', featuring for example, headache, fatigue, difficulty in concentrating, cough, irritation of the eyes, nose and throat. It seems to occur in offices, schools, hospitals and other non-industrial environments; is most often reported in air-conditioned buildings; and symptoms are most common in the afternoon. O'Malley (1991) reports that it may be induced by heaters or the ventilation system; by lighting level; by VDU equipment; by noise; by low humidity; or by toxic, irritant or allergic substances, some of which may be produced by the occupants. Poor building design/construction and low staff morale have also been cited as being contributory. However, as yet, no specific cause has been identified despite considerable will and effort to do so.

Work environment legislation

Most of the above points are embodied in recent legislation related to health and safety in the workplace. Although Noise at Work Regulations (1989) and Control of Substances Hazardous to Health Regulations (1988) are retained, many piecemeal legal requirements were streamlined in 1992 to comply with EU Directives and implemented in 1993 — the Six-Pack (Box 12.3).

Regulations 1–5 virtually only update existing legisla-

Box 12.3 The six pack
Outline of a document prepared by the Health and Safety Executive (1993)

1. *Management of Health and Safety at Work Regulations 1992*

   Employers are required to:
   - assess risks to health and safety so that preventive and protective measures can be identified and implemented
   - provide appropriate health surveillance for employees when risk assessment shows it to be necessary
   - set up emergency measures
   - provide employees with information and training about health and safety measures.

2. *Provision and Use of Work Equipment Regulations 1992*

   Employers are required to:
   - ensure equipment is suitable for specific use, that it is used only for such operations, and maintained in an efficient state
   - provide equipment which conforms to EC product safety directives
   - provide employees with adequate information and training.

   Specific requirements are related to, for example, guarding dangerous machinery; protecting against hazards such as falling articles, overheating, explosion; providing control systems; providing suitable warnings and markings; ensuring adequate lighting.

3. *Manual Handling Regulations 1992*

   Particularly relevant to nursing in that it relates to lifting and handling of patients (p. 303).

   There are 3 key steps:
   - avoid hazardous manual handling operations; use mechanical methods if a load must be moved
   - assess hazardous operations that cannot be avoided using ergonomic assessment; not only the weight of the load but its size and shape, the handler's posture, the working environment, the individual's capability
   - reduce the risk of injury as far as reasonably practicable.

4. *Workplace (Health, Safety and Welfare) Regulations 1992*

   There are 4 broad areas:
   - *working environment:* temperature; ventilation; lighting; room dimensions; suitability of work stations and seating
   - *safety:* for pedestrians and vehicles; for opening/closing/cleaning windows; for construction and marking of transparent doors; safety devices for doors and escalators; slipping/tripping hazards on floors; safety against falling objects and falling into dangerous substances
   - *facilities:* toilets; washing, eating and changing amenities; clothing storage; drinking water; rest areas (protection from tobacco smoke); rest facilities for pregnant women and nursing mothers
   - *housekeeping:* maintenance of workplace and equipment; cleanliness; removal of waste materials.

5. *Personal Protective Equipment at Work (PPE) Regulations 1992*

   Includes all equipment to be worn or held to protect against risk to health and safety for example clothing; eye, foot, and head protection; safety harnesses; life jackets and high visibility clothing.

   Employers are required to assess risks and provide training.

6. *Health and Safety (Display Screen Equipment) Regulations 1992*

   Employers are required to:
   - assess display screen equipment and workstations, and reduce risks which are discovered
   - ensure workstations satisfy minimum requirements for the display screen, keyboard, desk and chair; working environment; task design and software
   - provide information and training for users
   - make available appropriate eye and eyesight tests and provide special spectacles if required.
   (Crown copyright: reproduced with the permission of the Controller of HMSO.)

---

tion, but number 6 covers a new area of work activity. Work with display screen equipment can lead to muscular and other problems such as eye fatigue and mental stress, much of which, it is maintained, can be alleviated by studying good ergonomic design of furniture; the working environment; and the tasks performed. It is interesting that the eyestrain caused by constant refocusing on a flickering screen (though perhaps more obvious) is being superseded as a problem by tenosynovitis and upper limb disorders collectively classified as Repetitive Strain Injury (Payling, 1993). RSI involving a constantly repeated muscle movement is thought to have been first identified among the leather beaters of Ancient Babylon, then again in the 18th century by washerwomen and more recently by hairdressers, supermarket checkout operators, and computer users (Gow, 1992).

In the UK, the Health and Safety Commission has responsibility for the oversight of work-related risks to health and safety. It proposes legislation, as well as codes and standards to ensure that action is taken to prevent accidents and disease, not just by inspection and enforcement but also by providing advice and guidance. The Commission also sponsors research to identify the nature, scale and severity of hazards.

Women and the work environment

The effect of the work environment on women in the reproductive age group merits particular mention in view of the fact that, more women spend more of their lives in paid employment than ever before. It is difficult to assess the proportion of reproductive problems caused by occupational hazards — agents such as chemicals and radiation, and working conditions such as stress and heavy manual work — say Rogers & Salvage (1988) but adverse effects can result in infertility, stillbirth, miscarriage, congenital abnormality and childhood cancer. Such environmental hazards may be relevant in a number of occupations, but they go on to say that health workers are at greater risk because the majority are women. However, men, too, are at risk and lowered sperm counts, damaged sperm, loss of libido, and impotence have all been ascribed to adverse environmental conditions in the workplace.

Leisure and the environment

Leisure time activities, too, reflect a region's climate and environment, sailing and hill walking being examples. However, swimming although traditionally associated with hot weather and the sea, is available nowadays in all weather conditions even thousands of miles from the sea. Similarly skiing was once dependent on the availability of snow-covered slopes but there are now artificial ski slopes in the environs of many large cities.

The importance of maintaining a safe environment for the activities of working and playing has been discussed in some detail in Chapter 4, particularly in the section on 'preventing accidents at work' (p. 79) and 'preventing accidents at play' (p. 79).

POLITICOECONOMIC

This section concentrates almost entirely on the 'working' aspect of this AL, with only a comparatively brief mention of 'playing'.

Work in an industrial society

Work is the means by which an individual earns an income and the level of that income is a very important factor which influences many aspects of living. Social class is determined by the nature of a person's occupation (Table 12.1) and this, in turn, determines economic status.

Collectively, work is the basis of a nation's wealth. All work involved in commercially producing goods or services represents the Gross National Product (GNP) of a country; and by implication, the more economically wealthy the nation, the more services it can provide, although which services and in what quantity and to whom is a political decision. In the Western world, the process of industrialization has been the main factor in creating wealth and currently contributes to the highly complex national and international economic systems. However, although industrialization has been conducive to economic improvement, it has also helped to create poor working conditions and numerous social problems.

In most industrialized countries therefore, over the course of many years, health and social systems have been developed to deal with the social ills, and employment legislation has been introduced to establish protective measures, for example:

- the minimum age at which a person can be gainfully employed
- the maximum number of hours to be worked per week in certain jobs
- alternative remuneration during unemployment or absence from work due to illness, injury or maternity leave
- the number of weeks of paid holiday
- the age at which there can be retirement from work on a pension.

Financing services in an industrial society

In any national economy which provides employment, as well as health and social services, the relative numbers of certain population groups are of critical importance: children, workers unemployed, workers absent because of illness/pregnancy and pensioners. These people are financially dependent, and the services have to be paid for by the earners.

For work a person receives remuneration in the form of a wage or salary, exceptions being voluntary work and the occupation of housewife/mother. In the UK, national insurance paid by the workers, and income tax paid by those with an income above a stipulated amount contribute to the total national income, part of which is used to finance services such as the National Health Service, unemployment and sickness benefit, and the retirement pension. There is great disparity, some would say inequity, in the level of income accorded to different occupations. The way in which income is determined is largely historical and any changes in pay structure, and any pay increases, are introduced by agreement of the employers, government and trades unions.

Contrary to the impression which may be created by the media, trades unions are not only interested in pay negotiations but, in various ways, act to safeguard the rights of employees. From a health and safety point of view unions are particularly interested in:

- identification of health hazards
- provision of a safe work environment
- provision of education for workers in an attempt to prevent accident and minimize risk
- surveillance of the worker's health
- collection of data to monitor the effect of health on work and vice versa.

Occupational health services

In the UK, important pieces of legislation aim to secure the health and safety of workers, and various applications are mentioned in Environmental Factors (p. 318) and in the chapter on the AL of maintaining a safe environment (p. 79). And in many countries, there is an occupational health service, employing nurses and doctors, which also plays a vital role in the promotion of health and safety at work. The nurses' role is essentially preventive and educational, though occupational health nurses deal with any accidents which occur and with certain treatment regimes; and they are also concerned with rehabilitation and resettlement at work after an extended absence due to injury or illness.

Absenteeism for short and long periods has become alarmingly high in several occupations. Following a report to the Royal College of Nursing by the Institute of Manpower Studies, there was great concern about absenteeism among nurses in the NHS (News, 1994). Nurses make up about half of the workforce, and the 1.5 million lost working days ran up a bill of £70 million a year. Appalled at the size of the problem, the NHS Chief Executive maintained:

'Our business is health and if we cannot be seen to look after our own staff, what impression must we give to our patients?'

Promoting health at work makes good business sense.

Disability and resettlement

Resettlement of disabled people in work is a subject discussed in more detail later in this chapter but it is appropriate here to mention the role of the government in relation to this matter. There is a wide range of facilities provided to help disabled people to find, train for and keep suitable work and, in the UK, these are mainly provided under Acts of Parliament. From the individual's point of view, a key figure in the complex system is the Disability Employment Adviser who works closely with members of the health professions and with voluntary agencies, some of which have financial assistance from central or local government. Another aspect of the Acts is the provision of a quota scheme whereby firms of a certain size are required to employ a percentage of disabled people.

Changing attitudes to job security

Help with deployment and re-employment is available, too, to the able bodied and in many countries advice on employment is offered by guidance units sponsored by the government. Technological advances may mean that some workers in future will need to be trained for a second and possibly a third type of employment in a lifetime. High unemployment in certain occupations, and mid-career redundancy, are other reasons why more people nowadays may need to retrain in the course of their working lives. The 'second industrial revolution' or 'technological revolution' involves a switch, even for high income earners, from traditional commerce and industry to processing information or technology-intensive manufacturing. There are no 'jobs for life'.

New attitudes towards working are becoming essential in these times. The age of retirement is reducing; the working week is shorter; more women are working outside the home than before; part-time work is becoming increasingly common; and the concept of job-sharing is gaining ground. Part-time work and job-sharing are ways of spreading the increasingly limited work available more equitably. As long ago as 1983, Tierney argued that nursing was one profession which appeared to have tremendous potential for a widescale introduction of job-sharing as already a substantial proportion of practising nurses worked part-time, a fact not surprising because the majority are married women.

There is no doubt that in much of the industrialized world, unemployment is a crucial politicoeconomic issue of our time. In the UK, the number of unemployed people is still high (over 2 million in 1995) and many other Western countries too have high levels of unemployment. The way in which governments attempt to deal with the problem, and the way societies react to it and cope with it, will determine the nature of the activity of working for future generations.

High unemployment and, for others, reduced working hours and longer retirement, means however that people increasingly have more time for the activity which complements working — playing.

Economics of leisure

All schools encourage physical education and sport and

the foundation for enjoying other leisure-time activities in adult life is often laid in various school classes, such as domestic science and music. Apart from school, other reforms have resulted in provision by local government for community recreation and this includes adventure playgrounds for children and a range of sports and arts facilities to cater for people of all ages.

Although in relative terms more people nowadays have more time for leisure and more money, many recreational pursuits are expensive and this can be a problem for the lowest paid workers, parents with several children, lone parents, students, the unemployed and pensioners. This fact is recognized for these groups who are often offered reduced rates for travelling, and for attendance at theatres and cinemas.

There is no doubt that, with less work, there will be greater emphasis on play. Education for leisure and the provision of adequate recreation facilities will therefore assume even greater political importance in the future since a bored society can so easily become a troubled and rebellious society.

However, in some developing countries, there is no question of seeking leisure; even the children cannot indulge in play.

A number of countries in Southern Asia are reputed to have millions of child labourers, many of them in bondage. They work in cigarette manufacturing, the glass industry, gem cutting, pottery, mining and the carpet industry. Theoretically a battery of laws protect them from exploitation, but apparently police and bureaucrats collaborate with employers to profit everybody except the children and their families (Thomas, 1992). A study by the Indian Social Institute in Delhi, says Thomas, showed that child labourers in the carpet trade worked at least 10 hours per day and had to sleep next to the looms, were unwell, often beaten and usually ill-fed. Various welfare groups cooperate to oppose such child slavery but so far, have had little impact. These children will never know school or the luxury of playing, but their family's survival often depends on their working.

Individualizing nursing for the AL of working and playing

The time at which the day's work — whatever kind of work it is — begins and ends, are the two points around which the rest of the day is organized. During waking hours, when people are not 'working', they can be said to be relaxing or 'playing'. These two activities then are an integral part of people's lives. However, the nature of the activities and their relation to one another varies espe-

cially at different stages of the lifespan and each person develops individuality in the AL of working and playing.

ASSESSING THE INDIVIDUAL IN THE AL

If individualized nursing is to take account of this aspect of a person's lifestyle, nurses need information about individual working and playing habits. Such information can be obtained in the course of nursing assessment by using as a mental framework, knowledge of the topics outlined in the preceding part of this Chapter (Box 12.4). While discussing relevant topics with the individual, the nurse might bear in mind the following questions:

- what kind of working/playing activities does the individual usually engage in?
- how much time does the individual spend working/playing, and when?
- where does the individual work/play, and with whom?
- what factors influence the individual's working/playing?
- what does the individual know about the relationship of working/playing to health?
- what is the individual's attitude to working/playing?
- has the individual any longstanding problems with working/playing and, if so, how have these been coped with?
- what problems, if any, does the individual have at present with working/playing or seem likely to develop?

Of course answers to these questions may be evident from medical/other records, and some may be revealed when there is discussion about the home environment and mobilizing, indeed the AL of mobilizing is so closely related to working and playing that it may be appropriate to collect information about these topics simultaneously.

The objective in collecting this information is to discover the person's usual working and playing routines; what can and cannot be done independently; previous coping mechanisms; and current problems. Some clients' problems with this AL, although identified from nursing assessment, may well lie outwith the scope of nursing intervention. In such cases, after discussion with the person, those problems may be referred to other members of the health care team, such as the doctor, or occupational therapist or social worker.

It is usual for nurses to know something about an individual's job and leisure interests. This knowledge is frequently used to initiate social conversation, thus indicating to patients an interest in them as individuals. The perceptive nurse is likely to realize too that events such as starting work, being made redundant and retiring from

---

Box 12.4 Assessing the individual in the AL of working and playing

Lifespan: effect on working and playing
- Infancy — type of play/playthings
- Childhood — play and work in school/out of school
- Adolescence — preparation for work
- Adulthood — type of occupation and recreation
- Old age — retirement

Dependence/independence in working and playing
- Dependence on others (e.g. children, disabled)
- Dependence on aids (e.g. disabled)
- Financial dependence (e.g. unemployed)

Factors influencing working and playing
- Biological — physique
  - physical fitness/energy level
  - state of health/ill-health
  - physical/sensory disability
- Psychological — intelligence
  - knowledge about legislation
  - self-discipline and attitude to safety
  - temperament and personality, reaction to stress
  - fulfilment/boredom/motivation
  - reaction to colleagues at work and play
  - reaction to unemployment/redundancy
  - reaction to retirement
  - balanced attitude to work/play
- Sociocultural — sex differences
  - cultural factors
  - religious factors, secular beliefs
  - social pressures at work
  - violence at work
  - sexual harassment at work
  - social class by occupation
- Environmental — climate and milieu for work/play
  - hazards to health and safety at work/play
- Politicoeconomic — personal economic status
  - health and safety at work legislation
  - employment of disabled people
  - job security
  - redundancy
  - government services
  - cost of leisure

---

work constitute significant life events. People who have recently experienced these events may well be anxious or depressed and welcome additional emotional support from the nursing staff and, if appropriate, reference to other agencies.

IDENTIFYING ACTUAL AND POTENTIAL PROBLEMS

Further discussion in the remainder of this Chapter by no means covers the entire range of an individual's potential and actual problems with working and playing, but should go some way towards helping readers to see how an understanding of these activities of everyday living can be applied in the context of nursing whether in a health setting or an illness setting.

The selected problems are considered under the following headings:

- change of dependence/independence status
- change in working and playing habit resulting from:
  (a) drug/substance abuse
  (b) unemployment
- change of environment and routine imposed by a hospital setting.

CHANGE OF DEPENDENCE/INDEPENDENCE STATUS

Independence in the activities of working and playing is regarded as the desirable norm for adults. Clearly, then, those who are unable to achieve or retain independence are disadvantaged members of society. In any country there are some people who are unable to work and, therefore, are financially dependent on their families and/or the state.

There are many different reasons for lack or loss of independence and here these are categorized as physical disability, mental disability, mental illness and sensory loss/impairment. An understanding of the causes and effects of dependence in the activities of working and playing is a relevant part of nursing knowledge. There are many different circumstances in which nurses can contribute to helping people to achieve their optimal level of independence in work and play activities, emphasizing their abilities rather than their disabilities. In most instances, however, the nurse achieves this in partnership with other members of the multidisciplinary team.

Physical disability

Obviously there will be a difference in the difficulties experienced in gaining or maintaining independence for working and playing depending on the nature of the disability and the body systems affected. Disease of the cardiopulmonary system can render a person so breathless and short of oxygen that 'work' is impossible and entertainment only of the passive variety is possible. On the other hand, many of the chronic disabling diseases affect the nervous system and the musculoskeletal system, and the patient's work and play problems are in fact mobilizing problems.

Depending on the person's previous working and playing activities, the degree of dependence caused by the disability will vary and there will need to be more or less adaptation. The outdoor worker and the active sports enthusiast may well find it difficult to settle for sedentary work and more passive leisure time activities. If the sedentary workers can be rehabilitated to an 'independent' wheelchair life, they are more likely to be able to resume their previous work.

Legislation   Prior to the 1970s there was legislation in the UK about people disabled when in the armed services or following industrial accidents, but legislation affecting the so-called 'civilian' population was extremely limited; the single factor which influenced provisions for improving their daily lives dramatically was the Chronically Sick & Disabled Persons Bill of 1970. Thereafter, in fact, all legislation affecting the general population has been scrutinized to ensure that equality of opportunity is provided for disabled people, for example in relation to education, housing, transport and employment.

Further publicity was given, worldwide, to the plight of disabled people when the United Nations Organization launched the International Year of Disabled People in 1981 and great emphasis was given to their rights including the right to secure and retain employment, and the right to enjoy recreation.

Many disabled people are additionally handicapped by prejudice, discrimination, lack of opportunity and sheer callousness. In fact, disabled people are only too well aware of their disability and will often prove far more conscientious and hard-working than their able-bodied counterparts. Various studies indicate that they are less likely to be absent from work, less likely to have accidents, and are just as productive or more so. The Chronically Sick & Disabled Persons (Amendment) Act 1976 and subsequent amendments further improved matters with regard to access to work (both to and within premises), parking facilities, toilet arrangements, and lifts with suitably placed control buttons reachable from a wheelchair.

An individual may be disabled from birth or may become disabled because of disease or injury, and for the latter, following a period of rehabilitation, various government services and voluntary agencies are now available to assist them to find suitable re-employment, and to provide financial support when needed. Two Acts (the Social Security Contributions and Benefits Act 1992, and the Social Security Administration Act 1992) establish the legal framework, but numerous leaflets are available from Social Security offices giving up-to-date details about the benefits and services which are provided.

Access to work   A programme called Access to Work was started in 1994 to extend and simplify the range of services available to people with disabilities and their employers. It is for unemployed, employed and self-employed disabled people who need to find a job, keep a job or make progress in their career.

To employers who want to recruit someone with a disability or to retain a recently disabled employee, the Access to Work scheme will pay for:

- a communicator for people who have a hearing impairment
- a part-time reader or assistant at work for someone who is visually impaired
- a support worker if someone needs practical help either at work or getting to work
- equipment for adaptations to existing equipment to suit individual needs
- alterations to premises or working environments
- adaptations to a car, or taxi fares, or other transport costs if needed because the person cannot use public transport.

Employers collaborating in this Scheme use a special symbol on their literature (Box 12.5).

Access to Work is run by Placing, Assessment and Counselling Teams (PACTs) and one of the team, the Disability Employment Adviser (DEA) works with disabled people who need extra help to assess their abilities and find the right job. They may need tuition to update existing skills or gain new ones and Career Development Loans are available which provide a percentage of training and related costs. The tuition is offered by Training and Enterprise Councils (TECs) or equivalent bodies, and they also offer information and support to people who wish to set up their own businesses.

With current advances in electronics and technology, it is possible to place even severely disabled people in open employment but some may be able to function only in Supported Employment Programmes or Sheltered Placement Schemes, and these may be operated by a voluntary organization, a local authority or a government-sponsored, non-profit-making company.

Even when work in open employment is not a reality, financial benefits provided by the government can help the disabled person — and thereby their carers — to cope with everyday living in the community, and to maximize home-based work possibilities as well as leisure time activities.

Play and recreation   Physical disablement not only changes a person's independence status for working, but better equipped to enable physically disabled people to make use of, and enjoy these facilities; indeed, new buildings are intentionally designed to allow easy physical access and to provide toilet accommodation.

Holidays, too, are much more accessible. Tour operators now offer many more facilities, and detailed information about suitable accommodation is published annually by, for example, the Royal Association for Disability and Rehabilitation, and the Automobile Association. Helpful guides are also produced by certain voluntary bodies some of which may provide financial help.

Mental disability/learning disability

By definition, mentally disabled people may be expected to be less independent in the AL of working and playing than others within society, but they too have the need for the satisfaction and occupation of time which are obtained from working and playing. In industralized societies, 'work' has become so complex that there has tended to be an almost unquestioned assumption that someone who has learning disabilities is incapable of working. However, this can be seen to be a false notion if a logical view is taken. All but the most severely disabled are quite capable of work which does not necessarily demand a high level of intellectual capacity. Contrary to many expectations, some have talent in areas such as writing and art which tend to be viewed as more intellectual than physical.

In the UK, where the emphasis has shifted from institutional care to community living, opportunities for work and leisure activities become even more important for people who have learning difficulties.

Access to work Working is part of normal adult life and the principle of 'normalization' for mentally disabled people is based on the argument that they, too, have the right and need to work. To cope with the demands of work in contemporary society, this means that they require education and training for work. Gilbert (1993) argues that because they are not socially valued, there is a lack of effort and resources for the development of skills and attitudes which promote their competence. He goes on to commend a 'materialist' paradigm rather than the 'normalization' principle, as a more realistic basis for understanding their social experience.

Certainly there are now increasing opportunities for the more able person to be employed under normal working conditions. Voluntary bodies do some excellent work in this respect, sometimes assisted by government funding. For example, the St. Aidan's Initiative, founded in 1983, is dedicated to placing people with learning disabilities into suitable employment (in collaboration with the person's wishes), backed by in-depth professional training, continued monitoring, and support where necessary. There is no cost to the employer during the

may effect playing. In fact, the only difference between them and able-bodied people is their *degree* of ability, and 'adventure' does not need to involve climbing mountains. Swimming, sailing, canoeing, fishing, riding, camping, and snow sports such as tobogganing, are all possible and all offer the excitement and stimulation which result from the challenge of adventure. Increasing awareness of the wishes of disabled people in this respect has led to the development of special sports facilities, and international sports events are now organized in just the same way as they are for able-bodied sportsmen and women.

The Paralympic Games, pioneered at Stoke Mandeville, England, and held to coincide with the London Olympic Games in 1948 is now arranged, like the Olympic Games, every 4 years. Representatives from various national sports organizations for the disabled compile the team to represent Great Britain; they include people with a visual impairment, people who have paraplegia, cerebral palsy, and amputations. In the 1992 Games at Barcelona, the UK team won 40 gold medals (data from British Sports Association for the Disabled, 1993). Other disabled people of course, may prefer to choose more passive indoor leisure pursuits such as card and board games, reading, writing and many other sedentary hobbies.

Entry to public places for re-creation is also becoming much more feasible. Theatres, cinemas, art galleries, restaurants, hotels and churches are becoming much training period, indeed a subsidy is provided. An outline of their plan of operation and findings is in Box 12.6.

For people who have more profound difficulties, there has been an increase in the provision of adult training centres. Courses at these centres emphasize:

- skills of self-reliance
    general appearance
    health
    travel
    care for others
- social skills
    satisfactory relationships in
    everyday settings e.g. shops,
    recreation, casual encounters,
    friendships
- basic education
    literacy
    numeracy
    environmental studies
- work practices
    handling materials
    use of utensils and tools
    awareness of the importance of
    punctuality and regularity
- leisure skills
    using available resources
    widening range of interests.

Box 12.6 Employment for people who have learning disabilities

The St. Aidan's literature (1993) outlines their plan of operation and findings.

- highly skilled Job Trainers work at the potential employer's premises, learn the potential job then find a suitable person (who has a learning disability) to fill it, and ensure that the person is trained to the required level of performance
- as the new employee learns to do parts of the job, the Job Trainer monitors performance and provides supplementary training if required
- selected people with learning disabilities have been shown to work safely around machinery and adhere to correct safety procedures
- research among companies who have employed people with learning disabilities shows that they are willing, hardworking, friendly, honest and loyal
- people with learning disabilities derive substantial benefit and satisfaction, apart from payment, from the opportunity to be part of the working community

---

Local initiatives to pick up on these skills include schemes where volunteers will accompany a person with learning difficulties to an evening class of choice, and Befriending Schemes where a pool of people take it in turn to share a hobby or attend a sports club thus providing opportunities for the person to develop friendships as well as enjoying the activity.

Barr (1993) maintains however that people with learning difficulties are decanted from long-stay hospitals to residential homes allowing 'institutionalization' to become relocated rather than resolved — 'they are in the community but not of it'. The public do not understand and do not want them as next-door neighbours!

An interesting local attempt to promote public awareness of the strengths and needs of individuals who have a learning disability is described by Moses (1993) a community mental health nurse, who devised Disability Awareness Packages for use with children in both primary and secondary schools — the next generation of carers, neighbours and potential employers! Feedback from pupils and teachers was positive, with many schools participating in the suggested follow-up work.

Despite enlightened initiatives the 'eternal child' adult image still prevails so people with learning difficulties become the victims of overprotection. For example, they are not allowed to take the normal risks involved in using machinery, working in a kitchen, and crossing roads. As a consequence, they are effectively denied many of the activities of normal living, made to feel more dependent than necessary, and segregated from the rest of society. Mental disability is a social handicap. However, even when employers adopt a more enlightened attitude, these people are unlikely to fare well in the competitiveness which a state of high unemployment has created in many industrialized countries.

For people who are so severely disabled as to be unable to achieve sufficient independence to live in the community, countries vary as to the type of residential provision which is made for them. Some utilize the model of a village with a group of houses, a workshop, shops and a village hall for sports and entertainment. Other countries care for them in hospitals, although the emphasis in the UK has changed to care in the community.

Play and recreation   For children who have learning disabilities, play as a means of communication can have considerable impact. Although for most children play is spontaneous, one of the features of mental disability is that the spontaneity is reduced or absent. So when playing with these children it is important to choose a topic which the individual can enjoy; ensure that the enjoyment span is not exceeded (it is shorter than the attention span); give the child the opportunity to join in the fun and interact with others; and allow play to involve small groups.

Children who have learning disabilities can enjoy the

same types of play as other children — exploratory, energetic, skilful, social, imaginative, puzzle-it-out play — although the last two may be reduced or absent in children who are severely disabled. Different media can be used such as water play, sand play, music, painting, rough and tumble play, large ball games, soft plastic playgrounds (with large cushions and hundreds of brightly coloured balls), adventure playgrounds, and short tricycle journeys under supervision. Some units for these children have a toy library although quite ingenious toys can be created often at low cost. Toys and games of course are only an aid to play; the impetus must come from staff to encourage and to demonstrate the use of the toy. Play fosters communication, intellectual development and social interaction, and toys are virtually tools to aid the enhancement of these skills.

However, routine activities such as bathing and dressing can often be made into games to provide learning opportunities, and the nurse should try to think of ways in which this extra dimension can be incorporated into the daily care of even the multiply disabled person. Potent reinforcement of play behaviours or a training programme or a combination of the two methods can be devised. These activities can be used not only for children, but for adults who have learning difficulties but the nurse has to judge the appropriateness of the type and age of play for each person (Shanley & Starrs, 1993).

In relation to adult mentally disabled people, nurses often seem to be uncertain as to the appropriateness of play as an activity. Play can help to overcome many of the secondary handicaps or problem areas projected by those with severe disabilities; lack of motivation, poor concentration, difficulties in hand-eye coordination, balance and movement problems, and general lack of physical coordination.

Nowadays the pleasure derived from play and recreation is recognized not only at local and national levels. Teams from several countries attend the Special Olympic Games; the games include track and field athletics, gymnastics, swimming, football, hockey and bowls. Participants derive exactly the same sort of enjoyment and sense of achievement as any other people involved in sport.

One of the attendant medical team (Heller, 1994) at The Sheffield Games commented:

'. . . . the coaching, training and regular build up of strength and stamina, and the development of new skills (there were 1000 athletes) had obviously had a beneficial influence on their lives . . . dynamic proof of the way in which concepts of positive health should involve both physical and mental health and wellbeing. These athletes were glowing; bursting with enthusiasm and pride . . . not only élite athletes can gain from the exploration of our physical limits.'

Apparently thousands of people in Sheffield became involved, in a true spirit of camaraderie, indeed an effective way of helping to overcome some of the prejudice about people with a mental disability.

Playing, then, is a means of increasing independence, and like working, it is an important dimension of the lives of people with learning difficulties.

However, it is considered that some people with learning disabilities are susceptible to developing mental health problems, owing to a reduced capability to withstand stress or to resolve mental and emotional instability; and Thiru (1994) reports a 1993 study where 41% of such referrals to a Community Specialist Psychiatric Service had a psychiatric diagnosis and a further 20% had behavioural problems. Indeed they used 'CPNs in learning disabilities' to cope with nursing assessment, planning and monitoring; and care of these people required close cooperation between mental health services, education services, social services departments, psychology services and general practitioners. Mental illness coupled with a learning difficulty provides staff with even more of a challenge when guiding such people to take advantage of working and playing opportunities.

Mental illness

Some people experience difficulty in gaining or maintaining independence for working and playing because of mental illness. Among the more commonly occurring features of mental illness are excessive anxiety, depression, phobias, obsessional thoughts or behaviour, delusions, confusion, overactivity or apathy, aggression, loss of confidence, forgetfulness, dependence on alcohol and disturbed personal relationships. It is not difficult to appreciate that these kinds of psychological difficulties can diminish a person's independence for the activities of working and playing.

The 'institutionalization' syndrome Reviewing the literature on the provision of mental health services McKenna (1993) recognizes a study which concluded that some patients do require the sanctuary and care provided by psychiatric hospitals. However, during the last three decades due to more enlightened therapeutic approaches as well as developments in chemotherapy, many of the older psychiatric institutions have been gradually reducing their bed complements or have been closed. They were often large, old buildings cut off from the local community — a most abnormal environment — and it was there that the adverse effects of 'institutionalization' were first noted. At first it was thought to be the result of the psychiatric illness itself, then it was considered to be the effect of the patient's resignation to the unchallenging and unchanging environment. The syndrome was described by Barton in 1966 as institutional neurosis characterized by a stooping gait, vacant facial expression, little interest in general appearance, and general inactivity. Such people were so uninterested that staff were unaware of the individual's abilities and mistakenly, answered and acted for them.

As Barton's doctrine became increasingly well-known, the approach to long-stay patients began to change and there was more focus on rehabilitation, including work and leisure activities.

More recently, community care began to be seen as the answer to institutionalization. However Bowers (1991) warns, the concept is confused. Patients who have not ever been in an institution, he says, can be as profoundly institutionalized as those who have spent many years in hospital. There are many similarities between poor institutional care and poor community care in other words — neglect. Socially, neglect triggers stigma, prejudice and vulnerability, and exacerbates the social disabilities produced by chronic mental illness.

Discussing community care in general, and describing a study he carried out, Barker (1994) mentions case management as one of the emerging forms of service delivery in the community. Case management stresses consumers' strengths, abilities and competencies rather than deficits, weaknesses or problems, and he quotes:

> 'The consumer is viewed as the director of the helping process within which the relationship is one of collaboration, mutuality and partnership; and the consumer's community is viewed as an oasis of potential resources rather than an obstacle to integration.'

These seem commendable goals, although Barker's study produced concerns about the divergence of perceptions between users (they all had enduring mental health problems) and professionals regarding diagnoses and the remedies which were on offer.

Even when a well-organized community mental health service exists, a minority of patients reject all help offered, refuse medication, and turn down day care and home support; indeed this may be interpreted by some as respecting the individual's independence and choice (and it may pose an ethical dilemma from a professional's point of view). Nevertheless many people with a mental illness who have been rehabilitated into the community thrive on their freedom and accept responsibility for a mutually agreed régime of treatment.

Recreation and work as therapeutic tools In any programme of rehabilitation from hospital, leisure activities can be used as a therapeutic tool. A recognized characteristic of mental illness is the inability to plan or enjoy leisure, and leisure activities which include social contacts are unsuccessful because the person is not at ease in the company of others.

Assisting individuals to recover an interest in leisure, however, is a considerable art, and the person should be involved at every stage of the planning and deciding. The degree of organization by staff and the degree of participation by the person can be graded starting with group activities rather than individual effort. And as recovery progresses, it is desirable to make provision for more 'unorganized' time involving activities such as reading, writing letters, talking with others — as occurs in everyday living.

The cooperation of the family is an important facet of rehabilitation and, especially for longer-stay hospital patients; going out with them to 'practise' living in the community is valuable to both parties — although it has to be recognized that some such patients may not have, or may no longer have, caring families or friends. Group homes, therefore are often used where, with some supervision, they can become accustomed to budgeting, housekeeping, cleaning, shopping, cooking and entertaining friends in a normal setting. Eventually some graduate from these group homes to live, unaided, in the community. Some may live outside but come back to the hospital occupational therapy unit to work, sometimes for payment; others acquire employment on their own merit; yet others may find work under the Disabled Persons (Employment) Act which makes it compulsory for certain employers to engage a percentage of registered disabled people.

Whatever method is used, the objective is to help the person to become as independent as possible. Doing this utilizes the concept of each individual having a dependence/independence continuum for each AL as described in our model.

An example of a successful leisure programme for people with a long-term mental problem but living in the community is summarized in Box 12.7. For employment of people with long-term mental health problems, Crichton (1993) commends the use of workers cooperatives, created and run by themselves but with back-up from a mental health unit. Crichton maintains that if groups who are marginalized or disadvantaged in the labour market form a cooperative, not only can they learn new skills; it can confer the benefits of increased independence, improved self-esteem, and the creation of new opportunities. Other spin-off advantages would be the reduction of stigma and the potential, through social education, of altering the values and attitudes of society at large.

Quite apart from the examples of programmes just mentioned, the treatment and care of people who are mentally ill has changed considerably in recent years especially for those newly diagnosed and for those who have acute episodes. The availability of antipsychotic medications has meant that many people can be helped, or at least the symptoms sufficiently controlled, without the necessity for admission to a psychiatric hospital or even much time off work.

Of course, medication is only one aspect of treatment.

Box 12.7 Beneficial effects of sport for a group using psychiatric services

Bell and Cooney (1993) describe how a group of community psychiatric nurses, working in a Community Support Team, was successful in encouraging clients to take part in team sport. The clients involved (mostly with a diagnosis of schizophrenia or manic depression) were encouraged to deal with their own mental health problems and to live in the community, but it was considered desirable to develop interaction skills in an environment other than a mental health setting.

After reviewing research studies which showed that exercise can benefit people using psychiatric services, the team collaborated with clients and their relatives, and with relevant health staff, to arrange a weekly sports session at a local leisure centre — initially for swimming and football — and followed it with a visit to the café.

An evaluation questionnaire conducted after 3 years, showed that offering a mixture of sport and social gathering promotes feelings of well-being, increases social interaction, improves mood, and alleviates stress and tension in a social environment. The findings pointed to client enjoyment and satisfaction, evidenced by the favourable attendance.

Psychological and social interventions with the person and family play important roles in preventing relapse (Pollard et al, 1994). Behaviour therapy can be provided on an out-patient basis, as can psychotherapy and counselling, and being encouraged to continue with regular working and recreational activities may in itself be therapeutic.

In fact, many community mental health agencies are devoting an increasing amount of time to identifying mental health problems as early as possible in order to prevent the onset and development of chronic mental illness.

Sensory loss/impairment

In the chapter dealing with the AL of communicating, some of the difficulties encountered by people who have dysfunctions related to speech, hearing and sight are discussed (p. 115). For most people so affected, these difficulties are reflected in their capacity for work and play.

Most people who become *partially sighted or blind* can be faced with changing their occupation. Some may take special training programmes, such as typing, computer use or physiotherapy. As far as leisure habits are concerned, some may be continued and others enjoyed in a modified form, for example, reading journals in Braille; listening to tape recordings of books and selected news-

papers; learning to use electronic reading aids; adjusting to adapted board and card games. Those keen on gardening need not be deterred; the Royal National Institute for the Blind (RNIB) produces a leaflet 'Gardening without Sight'. Children, too, can have special sound and tactile toys and take advantage of computer age games. A number of organizations, including the RNIB, provide practical information which utilizes the abilities and interests of the sight-impaired person in a wide range of leisure pursuits from music to football, and from museum visits to crosswords.

Gradual onset of *hearing impairment* may permit a person to learn to lip read and to make preparation for future working. Some can continue with their previous employment, but there are many types of work which require a person with adequate hearing. When it is possible, there should be preparation for enjoying leisure time when eventually all hearing is lost, although ongoing research with hearing aids promises some remarkable outcomes. Even now, church services, theatres and cinemas can be enjoyed by people with impaired hearing if the relevant facilities are installed in the building. There are adaptors to amplify sound on radio and television and also for the telephone, thus allowing the person to retain communication links with friends. Nurses can encourage people with hearing difficulties to develop suitable activities in which they are interested, and refer them to the relevant agencies specializing in providing information about work and leisure activities which take account of their altered capacity for hearing.

For the child who is hearing and visually impaired, there is multisensory deprivation, and McInnes and Treffry (1993) provide practical information about emotional, social and motor development as well as ways of dealing with communication and life skills.

Impairment of speech will cause considerable problems since for most people verbal communication is an essential part of working and playing. The problem of aphasia commonly results, in addition to paralysis, from a cerebrovascular accident. Whether it is mainly expressive or receptive (p. 116), or a mixture of the two, it will interfere with their ability to communicate. Nurses can be guided by speech therapists as to the ways in which they can help these people to improve or regain their ability to communicate while working and playing.

CHANGE IN WORKING AND PLAYING HABIT

A change in dependence/independence status for the activities of working and playing often results, as is apparent in the foregoing section, in a change in habit. For example, chronic disabling disease which causes physical disability is very likely to necessitate a change in both working and playing habits. In this section, the two problems discussed — drug/substance abuse and unemployment — do have links with the concept of dependence/independence. However, primarily they result in change of working and playing *habit* and for that reason are placed here.

Change due to drug/substance abuse

The seduction of drug use   Experimentation with drugs and various substances which can be abused often starts in relation to leisure time activities. In many countries it seems to be part of present day culture and indeed some people look on it as part of growing up (Box 12.8 and Box 12.9). Adolescents claim that the selected 'sub-

---

Box 12.8 Why do young people abuse drugs?

From various references, the following are given as reasons for taking drugs:

- they know their peer group use drugs and do not want to be excluded/considered cowards
- they want/already enjoy the excitement of risk-taking
- they want to shock parents
- they want to escape from personal problems
- they are curious about the reputed effects of drugs
- they enjoy the sensations experienced under the influence of drugs.

Box 12.9 Teenage drug abuse

Neustatter (1993) quotes various pieces of research about drug abuse among teenagers. Studies spanning a number of years are being conducted by two universities in England (using samples of 8000 and 25 000 schoolchildren); one found as many as 22%, and the other 40% of these teenagers had taken drugs. She quotes one of the researchers who, among other experts, points out that drug usage spans all classes, colours and types, including children from the most authoritarian to the most liberal homes, at state and private schools. It would appear, however, that drug use is more prevalent among children who dislike school, play truant, and wish to identify with an outside group.

She refers also to a young adult group featured in the Youth Lifestyles Report (1993) which used a sample of 15 to 24-year-olds; a third of the sample had taken drugs, and a quarter of these had used hard drugs.

Drugs, says Neustatter, are easily obtainable at inner city clubs, rural pubs, university campuses, on the street, and in friends' homes.

---

stance' makes them feel excited and allows them to experience heightened awareness. It could be argued that no one has the right to deprive another of experiences which are a precious part of living, but if use turns into abuse, problems can arise — physical, psychological, social and legal.

Caring for youngsters who are substance abusers has an added complication and is a highly emotive and sensitive responsibility. The Children Act 1989 gives children the right to refuse treatment, so health staff have to balance the child's right to confidentiality with the parent's need to know (Harding-Price, 1993). It is the nurse's responsibility to develop procedures which help even child and teenager clients to make informed choices about seeking help, and in this context, the school nurse can have an important role.

Rassool (1993a, 1993b) considers that primary health team workers such as health visitors, district nurses, domiciliary midwives, practice nurses and community psychiatric nurses are particularly well placed to deal with substance misusers and quotes the WHO/ICN document on substance abuse (1991) which defines the role of the nurse as a provider of care, educator, counsellor/therapist, advocate, health promoter, researcher, supervisor and consultant. However when Carroll (1993) studied the attitudes of various professionals (including nurses) working with IV drug abusers, he found that attitudes varied according to their professional socialisation so members of the health team would have to be aware of potential differences in approach.

Drugs/substances used   Substance abuse is not new. Cameron (1987) reminds us that down through the ages, man has experimented with a variety of substances. The Ancient Greeks used incense for religious ceremonies, for example, and chloroform has an interesting history of recreational usage. During this century, substances such as amyl-nitrate and transmission fluid have been abused in the USA, as has glue-butane gas in the UK, and coca leaves in some South American countries.

Nowadays, a staggering number of substances are being abused; they change according to fashion and availability. They include aspirin combined with Coca Cola; banana skins, generally grilled and smoked in a cigarette; table tennis balls, bin liners and plastic containers, often burned over a smoking fire and sniffed; and inhalation of fumes from substances such as hair lacquer and shoe polish. Over-the-counter medications, too, can be abused, for example cough expectorants, codeine, and travel sickness pills. When these or more potent drugs are not available, youngsters gravitate to the use of solvents and every shop, home, handbag and jacket is a source of solvents. Moreover, they are cheaper than drugs, so infinitely more accessible. To provide an overview of the problem, a few of the main groups of 'abused' substances are mentioned below.

• *Solvent abuse*   The term solvent abuse has come to be used in place of 'glue sniffing' or 'fume sniffing'. Cameron describes how a solvent intoxication session may last only an hour, although for chronic abusers it may extend over 48 hours, when they will inhale, then sleep, then resume inhaling. The method of inhalation varies according to the substance. Glue is usually put into an empty crisp bag, placed over the nose and mouth, then sniffed; butane gas is often inhaled from a gas lighter refill cannister, the nozzle of which is put against the teeth and pressed, thereby spraying the back of the throat; hair lacquers and sprays are inhaled after several cans have been sprayed into a small room, where gaps in windows and doors have been sealed.

Headache and nausea are two common complaints after a solvent intoxication session, but more serious complications can occur such as damage to cardiac muscle, respiratory failure, convulsive disorders, memory failure, renal failure and psychotic disorders. More immediate damage may occur, too, because while under the influence of the solvent, abusers can be asphyxiated; some have been known to indulge in bizarre and dangerous behaviour such as jumping out of windows or trying to climb high walls; and following a severe reaction, instances of sudden death have been recorded in a number of countries.

Pointers to solvent abuse include a lingering smell of solvent on hair and clothes and possession of glue and bags. Staggering walk, slurred speech, violent behaviour, dilated pupils, and spots around the mouth and nose are other signs of solvent abuse.

• *Marijuana*   Other terms used are cannabis, pot, dope, hash, joint, reefer, weed or grass and a super-strong strain called skunk (Bennetto, 1992). The source is the hemp plant which can be found in many parts of the world, and the cannabis can be eaten in the form of 'hash cookies', or can be smoked as a cigarette which can affect pulmonary function. In general marijuana can cause euphoria and hallucinations and is associated with mood swings, so its use can have an effect on both working and playing.

There is a possibility that the use of cannabis (a soft drug) can lead to a *life of dependence* on hard drugs so there are those who are for, and those who are against decriminalizing the use of cannabis. Currently, however, there are many countries in which the use of cannabis is illegal and possession of the drug is a punishable offence.

• *Amphetamines*   These are the much talked about 'pep' pills; they can be obtained in tablet or capsule form and have a variety of street names — black bombers, French blues, purple hearts, uppers, wake-ups, speed, jelly beans and copilots. After ingestion the pupils dilate and behaviour can be described as boisterous. When the effects wear off, there is usually lethargy, irritability and

unsociability. This psychological see-saw is an indication to members of the family, and to work and play groups that an individual 'might be using amphetamines for other than medicinal purposes. Loss of appetite with consequent loss of weight and sleeplessness can also result from taking this drug, and constant users may become mentally ill.

• *Ecstasy*   This is also a stimulant, made up in white or brown tablets or different coloured capsules and marketed as love hearts, Dennis the Menace, love doves, 'E', disco burgers and phase 4. Ecstasy raises body temperature and when used at 'raves', the dancers can develop heatstroke (they sometimes rest at 'chill-out' areas) or coagulopathy which on some occasions have even proved fatal (Preston, 1992).

Salt (1993) describes the work of a specialist Paratech Team who attend licensed 'rave parties' to help prevent insidious problems among the participants (in the instance quoted, a crowd of 7000 at an isolated outdoor venue) from becoming individual tragedies.

• *Ketamine* is another drug used at dances. This surgical anaesthetic is snorted; it magnifies dance sensations such as lights, music and rhythm and induces a state of numbed confusion (Rogers & Katel, 1993).

• *Heroin, cocaine and morphine*   Heroin is a narcotic derived from the opium poppy and has street names including skag, horse and smoke. It can be smoked (chasing the dragon) or injected. Cocaine comes from the leaves of the coca bush and has street names such as coke, snow, toot and blow. *Crack* is cocaine heated with bicarbonate of soda to remove impurities and 'rocks' or 'stones' of pure cystallized cocaine are produced which are then smoked — free-basing. Hutchings (1991) quotes a user who maintains:

'it would be difficult to sustain a crack lifestyle for very long: you get so manic . . . most people use heroin and crack together — they need the heroin to bring them down.'

Heroin, cocaine and morphine all have a useful though small part to play in medical therapy. 'Hard drugs' is the term used when they are peddled for illicit purposes and they are often introduced in a social setting when the uninitiated are invited to experiment with 'just one injection'. Unfortunately for some personalities however, even after just one injection, abstinence is not possible. Such people find themselves on the road to a gradual decline in health and loss of independence which eventually rules their lives (McLennan, 1986). They become 'dropouts' from work because obtaining the next dose ('fix') takes precedence over any other activity. Eventually they may have to be injected up to several times daily, the dose getting higher and higher to satisfy the craving. In addition there is always the danger that infected syringes will cause hepatitis B, AIDS, local sepsis or fatal septicaemia. Other common accompaniments of drug taking are loss of interest in personal appearance and lack of appetite to the extent of causing malnutrition with a consequent lowered resistance to infection.

- *LSD/Lysergic acid diethylamide* LSD is a hallucinogen which has street names including acid strawberries, Chinese dragon, and pearly gates. It is a transparent liquid, effective in minute quantities so can be dropped on to sugar cubes or the back of postage stamps both of which are common means of distribution. It can also be made in tablet form and is usually taken orally but may be injected. It has the effect of raising the blood pressure and increasing the heart rate and may also cause insomnia, convulsions and hallucinations (false perceptions occurring without any sensory stimulus). Coping with the torrent of psychological experience released by the drug can be difficult and dangerous.

Preventing and 'managing' drug abuse For some time now, in order to prevent the problem of drug abuse from arising, schools and youth organizations, sometimes in collaboration with parents, have conducted health education sessions to inform youngsters about drugs, their misuse and the sequelae. And of course, many youngsters who sample drugs on one or two occasions, do not go on to become drug abusers. At the other extreme, for those people who have become drug-dependent, some do decide to stop taking drugs, while others make a positive choice to continue taking them. Others feel unable to face life without drugs.

Previously, health workers advocated abstention, but gradually it has come to be accepted that this is not the only answer; a more flexible approach may yield better results. Sheehan (1990) writing about the problem of illicit drug-taking as viewed in Amsterdam — a city perceived as liberal in its attitude to hard drug users — advocates a model of intervention which aims to *manage* the problem rather than always struggling to *cure* (Box 12.10).

Currently, although amid considerable controversy, these ideas are being used in certain states of the USA and in blackspots in Europe. In one scheme, a doctor in the UK considers that a controlled dose given at his surgery — and with accompanying counselling — is better than pushing abusers towards risky behaviour such as committing crime to obtain cash for the purchase of drugs (for example '£100 per day for dodgy stuff from a dealer') and it safeguards them against the AIDS virus which is speedily transmitted when shared needles are used (Bellos, 1993).

Similar positive effects are claimed when methadone maintenance is employed as a form of 'management' for drug abuse, although the use of methadone continues to arouse professional and political controversy (Farrell et al, 1994).

> **Box 12.10 Managing versus curing drug abuse: a model of intervention**
>
> Sheehan (1990) advocates *managing* the problem of drug abuse rather than always struggling to *cure*. The model suggested has 3 levels:
>
> - low level maintenance
> - detoxification
> - treatment and rehabilitation.
>
> The general aim is to support individuals to reach their own goals when they feel ready to do so; only the most highly motivated and those ready to relinquish addiction are guided to Level 3, thereby reducing the number of inappropriate referrals. Although helping agencies, involving a multidisciplinary team, provide support and assistance at all levels, individual drug users are allowed to advance towards *cure* at their own pace. The intense therapy at Level 3, aimed at giving back power and control to the individual is followed by ongoing support to develop a new and satisfying lifestyle, usually through education and work opportunities.

Public health dimensions of drug abuse Illicit drug use, in itself, is a problem but has assumed new public health dimensions since the advent of the HIV/AIDS pandemic (see p. 354). The transmission of HIV infection in Europe is firmly linked to infected intravenous users and one aspect of what is termed 'harm reduction' is to keep drug injectors safe from HIV infection. Faugier (1994) refers to the UK Report of the Advisory Council on the Misuse of Drugs (DoH, 1993) and comments that the availability of clean injecting equipment, the increased prescribing of substitute drugs and the use of outreach methods have 'contained' HIV prevalence figures. But, he continues, there is a new generation of drug users for whom the threat of HIV is no longer novel, and there are now additional public health concerns such as high rates of hepatitis C and increasing rates of tuberculosis in the drug-using population.

Many local initiatives to contain the problem of drug abuse have proved successful. But in order to promote systematic collection and analysis of data on a trans-Europe level, and put drug policy on a sound, scientific basis, the European Union has established a Monitoring Centre for Drugs and Drug Addiction. Of course, concern is international.

International dimensions of drug abuse Around the world the problem of the illicit use of drugs is increasing dramatically says the International Narcotics Control Board. In areas which were considered to be producers rather than consumers of drugs such as Latin America, the drugs barons are now seeking new outlets and marketing the products among their own people. What was previously considered to be a 'gringo' problem is now spreading throughout the continent and for example, Panama is having its first 'crack' babies (Padgett, 1993).

A certain degree of drama seems to surround drug smuggling itself, but it can be fatal; international drug smuggling receives considerable publicity in the media when couriers die following rupture of the packages they carry. The drug may be wrapped in condoms, toy balloons, plastic bags or aluminium foil and may be swallowed or concealed in the vagina or rectum. In spite of such coverings, the drug may leach out and the smuggler can present at a casualty department with fever, cardiovascular manifestations, euphoria, disorientation, acute toxic psychosis or coma; it is not always easy to recognize the cause. The signs may be indicative of 'body-packing' (Ramrakha & Barton, 1993).

As already mentioned, substance abuse often arises in relation to leisure time activities. When addiction develops, however, the adverse effects are so pervasive that not only the enjoyment of playing is reduced, work is also affected perhaps causing absenteeism, accidents and poor performance. And this deterioration of the self spills over to affect many other activities of living.

Of course, some people would maintain that smoking and alcohol consumption are also drug addictions!

Change due to unemployment

Change in lifestyle It is not difficult to appreciate that having been part of the workforce, becoming unemployed necessitates tremendous change in a person's established working and playing habits. Loss of work is a problem in its own right, denying the person a whole range of benefits: personal, social and financial. But having no job to go to also obviates the purpose of many daily living habits which are primarily work-related, for example, habitual time of rising; usual daily dress; regular exercise obtained getting to and from work; and the type and timing of meals. Although written in 1969, Greenwood sums up the frustration and helplessness of unemployment in a quote from 'Love on the Dole':

'. . . . nothing to do with time; nothing to spend; nothing to do tomorrow nor the day after; nothing to wear; can't get married; a living corpse . . . .'

Being without work, of course, means that potentially, there is unlimited time for playing. For some resourceful people this may not pose a problem, but for most it does. Almost all leisure activities cost money. Deprived of income from work, established playing habits may be impossible to continue. Apart from that, the person's motivation to seek enjoyment and diversion may be lost

and the inevitable stress and gloom which unemployment brings may cause such apathy and depression of mood that there is no enthusiasm or energy for playing. There is little incentive to get up in the morning and sleeping longer is one way of passing the time and obliterating worries. Watching television, smoking and drinking are other ways of coping with boredom and anxiety. None of these habits in excess is conducive to health (they are a form of negative coping) and some can lead to further financial difficulties.

Change in health status There is increasing concern that unemployment has deleterious effects on health and it seems reasonable to conjecture that the enforced change in working and playing habits contributes to this. Stress-related health problems, such as high blood pressure and heart disease, have been cited in discussion linking ill-health and unemployment, as have psychiatric illness, alcohol-related problems and parasuicide (OHE, 1993).

In 1987, Smith updated his previous intensive review of data, still seeking for the links, and concluded that the evidence linking unemployment with poor mental health was stronger than links with poor physical health. Studies which have measured the mental health of the unemployed, using standardized questionnaires countenanced in psychological and psychiatric research, show consistently that the mental health of those out of work is poorer than that of the employed. The unemployed tend to be more anxious, depressed, unhappy, dissatisfied, neurotic and worried; they have lower confidence and self-esteem; and they sleep worse than the employed. A study by Kammerling and O'Connor (1993) confirmed these findings regarding unemployment as a predictor of psychiatric admission. However, Smith maintains the evidence does not prove that unemployment, on its own, is the cause of deterioration; it may be that people with poorer mental health are more likely to become unemployed.

As far as physical health is concerned, there were also pointers to associate unemployment with deteriorating health but, again, there were no conclusive data. He quotes studies in the UK, USA and Canada.

Families suffer too. Unemployment is associated with high divorce rates, child abuse and neglect, wife battering, unwanted pregnancies, abortion, reduced birth weights of babies, increased prenatal and infant mortality rates, reduced growth in children, and increased morbidity in wives and children. Yet from his research, Smith concluded that it was not possible to be confident that only unemployment was the cause.

More than anything else, quotes Smith, poverty may be the link between unemployment and poor health, and he goes on to suggest that raising the living standards of the unemployed may be one of the most effective ways of improving their health.

Of course unemployment is not equally distributed

among the population, for example, the young, the old, the disabled, and the socially disadvantaged are all over-represented among long-term unemployed. Another important group over-represented among unemployed is that of men aged 50–59; they are more likely to be made redundant and also find it more difficult to find another job (OHE, 1993).

Initiatives to reduce unemployment   Various schemes have been introduced by the UK government to provide work and training for the unemployed, particularly the young. Youth training schemes have many critics, but undeniably they have provided work experience, as well as training, for thousands of young people. There are also various enterprise schemes to help unemployed people to start their own businesses; community programmes for long-term unemployed; and at Job Centres there is in-depth counselling especially for long-term unemployed people. However, community psychiatric nurses are concerned about the rise in mental illness referrals, which in some instances are coming direct from Job Centres (Gillam, 1993). He says:

'. . . it is as if the state is admitting, "we cannot find you a job but we understand this causes you a lot of stress. Perhaps you need psychiatric help." '

The OHE Paper (1993) suggests some measures to help alleviate the stress (Box 12.11).

Black (1993) discusses the negative relationship between the experience (or threat) of unemployment and the maintenance of health. However she emphasizes that there are a few protective factors related mainly to intrinsic personality and income, which can be used to devise a strategy to deal with potential problems. She exhorts community nurses to use preventive and educational approaches to promote positive behavioural change.

Of course, the unemployment problem is not peculiar to the UK; it is affecting many countries. Burger (1993) gives a worldwide view of the situation in Europe, USA and Japan and describes how the EU has launched an economic initiative to attack what it calls an unacceptable level of joblessness. The concern is well founded. High unemployment, Burger goes on to say, burdens government social programmes, reduces tax revenue, wastes human capital, increases income disparities, and deprives people of their sense of self-worth.

However, not only governments are attempting to grapple with the problem; industry, trades unions, employers, voluntary organizations and individuals all have a part to play. The provision of work is not the only goal for the unemployed; there are many examples of free or subsidized entry to entertainment, sport and leisure facilities; free travel; and free entry to educational facilities. Thus recognition is being given to the importance of working and playing habits in the lives of people who have the misfortune to be unemployed.

Box 12.11 Unemployment: measures to alleviate the stress

The OHE Paper (1993) suggests some measures which might be taken to alleviate the stress caused by unemployment:

- general practitioners should be encouraged to provide 'well unemployed' sessions addressing the mental, dietary and lifestyle pressures faced by those out of work
- the government should recognize that training courses, 'job clubs' and other initiatives to help people to get employment will have important intrinsic benefits by, for example, providing a time structure to their day and enabling them to develop contacts and share experiences with people outside their immediate family
- employers should be offering counselling to newly unemployed regarding the potential impact of job loss on their mental and physical health — in addition to providing financial advice and advice on seeking alternative work
- the Department of Social Security should recognize the health value that voluntary work and education can provide and ensure that its 'available for work' criteria do not prevent unemployed people from undertaking activities which improve their mental well-being and social skills.

Nursing and unemployment   Like many aspects of the AL of working and playing, it is not easy to be precise about the nature of nursing activities which are directly related to the problem of unemployment. After all, the problem of a person's joblessness cannot be solved by nurses. On the other hand, an understanding of this problem — especially its links with ill-health — is relevant in nursing. So, too, is a sympathetic attitude to those who have the misfortune to be unemployed, for many suffer from feelings of shame and desolation.

Thinking in more specific terms, the knowledge that unemployment can affect the health of the whole family is obviously of particular relevance to those nurses who are concerned with health surveillance and health promotion in the community. Families in which there are young children, and one or both parents are unemployed, might be visited more frequently, thus allowing them an opportunity to discuss their problems and feelings. Assessment of what changes have been made to compensate for lack of working, and to fill the unlimited time available for playing, might reveal some actual and potential health problems. The unemployed member of the family might welcome the opportunity to review their changed lifestyle in this way and to be helped to plan activities which would maintain, rather than endanger, their health.

This might also be very relevant in the context of hospital nursing and, indeed in that setting, patients might be highly receptive to education about health problems to which they may be vulnerable because they are unemployed. Actual and potential problems might be identified from nursing assessment on admission and the fact that the person is unemployed should be borne in mind when assessing all the Activities of Living. When finding out about usual habits and routines, it might be revealing to find out whether these have changed since unemployment. If problems identified, such as excessive alcohol intake or insomnia, do appear to have resulted from unemployment then planning to deal with them would have to take that into account. Indeed, the fact of a person's joblessness is relevant to much of the nursing plan which, after all, is geared towards rehabilitation and discharge. The needs of a person who is returning to work are different from those of the person who has no job to go back to. This would certainly be a major pre-occupation of treatment and rehabilitation of clients in the context of psychiatric nursing.

There are, therefore, implications of unemployment for individualized nursing, both in hospitals and in the community. In direct contact with families and sick people, the nurse may be able to help constructively with some of the adverse consequences of joblessness.

Some would say that nurses have another responsibility too — to become involved politically in the matter of unemployment. The nursing profession are uniquely placed, in their privileged access to people's lives, to make sense of some of the remorseless pressures and to raise their voice against them. Of course nurses themselves may become unemployed, and Cohen (1994) reports that unemployment is on the increase, yet many are unaware of the help they could have from the Nursing Employment Service (NES) which comes under the Department of Employment and operates from Job Centres.

CHANGE OF ENVIRONMENT AND ROUTINE

A hospital is a very different environment from the surroundings in which people normally spend their day, working and playing. Although it may be true for some elderly or disabled people, it is unusual to spend all day in one place and people seldom sleep in the same place as they spend the day. So, it is not surprising that patients who are confined to a hospital ward for days, and sometimes weeks, may become tired by the monotony of their surroundings and bored by the lack of stimulation and variety. It is no wonder that they often

take an intense interest in the goings on around them, for they have little else by way of distraction. Another problem for patients in hospital, or indeed for people who are ill in bed at home, is that they are confined indoors.

Confinement to indoor environment

Most children are accustomed to playing out of doors for at least part of the time, and for them it is unnatural to be indoors all day in a confined space in hospital. Similarly those adults whose working and playing activities take them outside for much of the time are likely to find confinement to a hospital ward particularly irksome. Whatever their occupation, there are few people who do not go outdoors for some part of each day, even if it is just travelling to and from work or going to the local shops or collecting children from school. Such outings have a specific purpose, but they also provide diversion, fresh air, physical exercise and the opportunity to meet and talk to people.

If nurses are to help patients to cope with the change of environment which results from hospitalization, they must have information about the patient's usual working and playing habits in order to appreciate the results of deprivation and if appropriate, to plan suitable alternative activities. The day room is intended to provide an alternative and a more relaxing environment than the bedside area and is often equipped with television, books and games. In some wards, nurses and/or physiotherapists organize daily exercise sessions to compensate to some extent for the sedentary lifestyle which patients lead.

Sometimes patients are able to walk about the hospital and if there are facilities such as a café or shop or library, nurses should make sure that they know about them and where they are situated. Some hospitals have attractive grounds in which, health and weather permitting, patients can walk and sit at leisure and enjoy a change from the environment of the ward; hospitals and residences for psychiatric, mentally disabled and elderly people, and also those for children, tend to have more spacious grounds.

Altered daily routine: the child

For children in hospital, an altered daily routine can be disturbing. However, arrangements can be made for children of school age to have homework brought in so that the effects of absence from school are minimized, and also to provide purposeful occupation. In fact in long-stay paediatric units, school lessons may be available within the hospital and links with local schools for ambulant patients can also be organized. The value of schooling as one of the normal activities should be encouraged in an otherwise unusual and unnatural routine.

The value of play to the sick child has long been recognized. However, children do not play with concentration or enjoyment when left to their own devices. Without assistance, many young children may become increasingly passive, or helpless in play. They may even stop playing altogether or do tasks well below their developmental level — a clear sign of an inability to cope.

Recognizing the significance of these findings, play coordinators and play therapists are now employed by many paediatric units, but this does not mean that nurses have abdicated that part of their role; indeed, experience has shown that they become more skilled at helping children to play purposefully when a therapist is available.

The child's feelings of fear, anger, hope and love can often be safely expressed in play. In special circumstances even a visiting pet may have a part to play in assisting the child to keep in touch with normality.

Nevertheless, says Thomas (1994) children should be discharged from hospital as soon as socially and clinically appropriate, and full support should be provided for subsequent home or day care. She refers to a study (Thornes, 1993) investigating the interface between hospital and community services for children with special needs (for example those who have asthma, diabetes mellitus and cystic fibrosis) which highlights the value of paediatric community nurses. A study available from the Cancer Relief Macmillan Fund (1994) shows that by being available throughout the illness, POONS (Paediatric Oncology Outreach Nurse Specialists) play a vital part in helping to reduce the sense of isolation felt by families of children who have cancer.

Altered daily routine: the adult

For adults, too, an altered daily routine can be disturbing. It has already been mentioned that the activities of working and playing are important in that they provide a structure to each person's day. According to a person's occupation, the time at which work begins and ends each day determines the time of rising and going to bed, and the amount of time left for pursuing leisure interests. Hospital routine has become more flexible in recent years, but in some health care settings there could be good practical reasons for patients being expected to conform to regular times for example for rising, going to bed, and having meals. For the majority of patients this routine, even though different from their norm, is unlikely to cause undue upset, indeed for children and some elderly people, it may provide a reassuring framework for their day.

Nevertheless, everyone becomes anxious when faced with uncertainty so nurses should inform patients and relatives about the ward routine — other patients will doubtless inform newcomers about the flexibility or otherwise of the 'official' routine!

Altered control over decision-making

In their everyday lives, adults make decisions and exercise choice as an integral part of working and playing. How difficult then, if, as patients, they are treated by nurses as though incapable of making decisions and taking initiatives. Nurses who have been patients may well have experienced the loss of self-esteem which results from such insensitivity. Male patients, especially those whose job gives them authority over others, may resent being dominated by young female nurses. Female patients who, as mothers, are accustomed to running a home and attending to the ceaseless demands of a family, might equally well be demoralized by being made to feel incapable of continuing to do as much as possible for themselves.

Nurses not only create unnecessary distress by failing to recognize that patients have a need to cling to their accustomed roles and routines, but they do them a disservice. After all, their established working and playing routines will hopefully be resumed and so, the less disruption there is, the easier rehabilitation will be.

How can patients be helped to incorporate their work and play interests into the daily routine of the hospital ward? For many people, having a daily newspaper, reading, watching the news or a favourite programme on television, listening to the radio or making telephone calls are regular daily activities. In hospital, the sale of daily papers, a trolley library service, television facilities, radio earphones and portable telephones are provided to help people to continue with these activities.

There is no reason either, providing it is not detrimental to health and does not interfere with treatment, why patients should not continue with work activities if that is possible. Students might keep up with reading and writing essays; teachers might do marking; businessmen and women might be able to keep abreast with correspondence; and mothers might want to make shopping lists and menus, or continue to help with homework when children visit.

Not all patients would be able to continue with work in this way, either because of the nature of their job or the severity of their illness. Some may need to be convinced that doing work or even worrying about it may jeopardize their recovery, and others may welcome the opportunity of 'doing nothing' for a change. Encouraging patients to do something to occupy the time may not always be in their best interest; skilled judgement is needed to assess when patients are ready to start occupying their time and Sutch (1993) while commending the therapeutic effects of recreation for people with mental health problems, warns that such activities can have a negative effect if inappropriate for the individual. Thoughtful yet simple acts can be helpful, such as introducing those patients with similar interests. Patients do appreciate the nurse who conveys a concern to prevent their day from being long and boring.

Being encouraged and enabled to exercise control over their own lives is important to patients and Gardner and Thompson (1994) explain how people with schizophrenia can be helped to take an active part in the management of their problems. Children too, have rights, and Peace (1994) writing about youngsters with serious chronic diseases, emphasizes that they, as well as parents and staff, should be helped to exercise self-determination in matters affecting their quality of life.

Absence from work and play groups

It is not only the loss of a familiar working and playing *routine* which patients find difficult but, equally, their absence from the *people* with whom they work and play. Apart from the family group (which is discussed separately below), work and play groups make up a major part of an adult's network of social relationships.

Absence from work and play groups may cause emotional problems in that there is a lack of the day-to-day feedback which is so important as a source of feelings of acceptance and belonging. Since membership of one's play groups is from choice, they are probably chosen by most people to enhance self-esteem and self-confidence. Membership of the work group may result less from choice than necessity, and may be more or less rewarding. Furthermore when things are going badly in the work group, a person may rely more on the play group for reinforcement of self-esteem, and vice versa. The person in hospital is thus denied the usual sources of company and emotional support and has to rely on staff and fellow patients instead. It is important that new patients are helped to feel a part of the ward group so that feelings of insecurity and isolation are decreased, and those of acceptance and support are increased.

Absence from family group

The child Play is certainly important in the child's life, but even more so is the family. An understanding of the adverse effects of separation of children from their parents has resulted in open visiting being the norm, with parent care much in evidence.

Working with parents (and also siblings) is described by Robbins (1991), a sister in a ward with special interests in oncology and endocrinology. Some parents, she says, may simply be present as a reassuring and familiar figure, giving their child a sense of security in a strange environment; others may wish to be involved in procedures such as taking a temperature; some have access to their child's medicines (in a locked cabinet); others may take on more complex procedures involving nasogastric feeding or parenteral nutrition. The child, too, can help,

for example, clamping or unclamping a catheter, thus allowing some element of autonomy, and making the activity seem less invasive.

This family-centred approach has many advantages (Box 12.12) but is not without difficulties, says Robbins. For example, the whole ward team must develop and agree to a philosophy of shared care; considerable time is required to prepare, teach, assess and support parents in these skills; and respective responsibilities must be clarified and coordinated. An obvious element is open and continuing communication between staff and parents; and staff must expect and accept constructive criticism:

'Nurses must respect the fact that parents have the intimate knowledge of their child through the nature of their relationship and shared, previous experiences . . . . and face the fact that parents may be more skilled at delivering care to their child than the nurse . . . .'

Box 12.12 Children in hospital: advantages of a family-centred approach

There are several advantages of a family-centred approach to nursing children, says Robbins (1991):

- Children often find nursing procedures that are strange and frightening much easier to accept when they are carried out by a familiar and reassuring figure
- At diagnosis and on admission to hospital, parents — who were previously the prime care-givers for their child and had ultimate control over events in their child's life — may find themselves overwhelmed by a situation that is out of their control and experience. They often feel de-skilled, inadequate and, consequently, isolated from their child. By allowing parents to participate in their child's care, an element of control is returned and they regain their confidence and self-respect
- Involving parents helps staff adopt a more personal and individualized approach. Parents can fit nursing care into their child's normal routine more easily. A nurse is often busy with commitments to other children in the ward and is less able to be as flexible
- Promoting self-care within the family unit in hospital encourages early discharge. It helps to teach parents how to manage new nursing interventions while they are in hospital and have direct and immediate access to supervision and help. This is one of the biggest incentives for many of the parents who become involved in complicated nursing care.

The importance of visits from siblings should not be forgotten. The separation can sometimes inflict on them as much anxiety as it causes the patient and Byrne's research (1994) reveals the emotional trauma among well siblings when a child has cancer.

Children can also be very distressed when an adult member of the family is being taken to hospital. This is now recognized and it is government policy in the UK that children should be allowed to visit adults and relieve the nagging fear that the person has gone away and left them. As long ago as 1859 Florence Nightingale wrote:

'There is no better society than babies and sick people for one another. Of course you must manage this so that neither shall suffer from it which is perfectly possible. If you think the "air of the sick room" bad for baby, why it is bad for the invalid too, and therefore, you will of course correct it for both. It freshens up a sick person's whole mind to see "the baby". And a very young child, if unspoiled, will generally adapt itself wonderfully to the ways of the sick person, if the time they spend together is not too long.'

Notes on Nursing

The adult Visiting, and being visited, is very important in the case of children and so it is for adults. For anyone who belongs to a family, absence from it on account of being in hospital can be a distressing and traumatic experience. Though using the term 'family' here, it needs to be remembered that not all patients have a family and, even if they have, it should not be assumed that members of the family are necessarily the most important people to the patient.

For these reasons, the nurses should find out who are the 'significant others' for each individual patient and it may be a pet (Gilbert, 1994). It is also important for nurses to appreciate that the separation not only affects the patient, but equally those who have been left at home. Sometimes they may experience considerable difficulties while a family member is in hospital: for example, the young husband who has to take over running the house and looking after the children when his wife is admitted; or the elderly woman in poor health who, deprived of her husband's help, is trying to cope on her own. These are just two examples but serve to illustrate the general point that absence from the family group during hospitalization does affect the patient, but also affects the rest of the family.

The value of visiting Hospital visiting is, therefore, a facility which is important to both parties — the person being visited and the family members and others who are the visitors. Being visited in hospital can, however, be a rather strange experience. At home, the person has some control over who visits, when and for how long. When in hospital, this control is usually forfeited. The visitors can also find the experience somewhat strange because, after all, a hospital ward does not afford either privacy or comfort; it is busy and often noisy; and to some people it is an intimidating, even frightening environment. For both parties then, hospital visiting may be somewhat stressful but it is an important means of minimizing the effects of the patient's absence from the family group.

Separating patients from their families is a feature of our culture; in many parts of the world, it would be considered a strange practice. The authority of the hospital to exclude visitors has, of course, been more stridently questioned with the growth of consumerism, and current concepts of health care are moving closer to accepting the basic notion of patient autonomy and empowerment, about visiting as in several other issues. Nevertheless, Gilbert (1994) expresses surprise that so many wards do not yet favour open visiting.

For a flexible policy to succeed, however, there has to be adequate extensive preparation of the staff and the public. Certainly, with visitors spread over a longer period it can afford both visitors and staff a much better opportunity to communicate with each other. For each ill person there are anxious relatives and friends who need information, not only to keep their anxiety within reasonable limits, but also to teach them how they can help their ill relative to recover or to die peacefully. Each dying patient has special visiting needs; if conscious the patient's wishes should be granted; if unconscious, it is the relatives who need information and consideration about whether or not to stay at the bedside.

There are a few occasions when a patient may need to be 'protected' from large numbers of visitors, for example a patient who is breathless and distressed, but while acknowledging that there can be problems associated with liberal hospital visiting, 'significant others' are part of the patient's care. Beggs (1991) describes a small research study conducted to investigate and evaluate the effect of a change in visiting arrangements, and while patients and visitors showed preference for extended visiting, the staff had doubts.

There are, of course, some patients whose family may not be able to visit and for them, communication by phone and letter may help to compensate. Others may have lost contact with family and friends, for example, the elderly or those who are long-term residents in hospitals for those who are mentally ill or who have a learning disability. Nurses can help by discussing with them whether they would like to take advantage of any of the voluntary visitors' schemes, should these be available in the area.

In conclusion, the objectives of hospital visiting are to enable contact to be maintained between members of the family group; to make the patient's day more meaningful; and to provide mutual benefit and pleasure for both patients and their visitors. Nurses are in a strategic position to help in the achievement of these objectives, whatever visiting policy is adopted by the institution.

PLANNING AND IMPLEMENTING NURSING ACTIVITIES AND EVALUATING OUTCOMES

In the preceding section, some examples of clients' problems in the AL of working and playing have been outlined; the causes and effects of problems are obviously varied and complex. In fact, the entire chapter provides a background of *general* information about the AL of working and playing which can be used as a mental framework, making it possible for the beginning student to identify via assessment (Box 12.4) some *specific* problems which any one client may experience.

Having identified the individual's problems, actual and potential, it is possible, in conjunction with the person, to agree about goals. For example, for a person recovering from a depressive illness, one of the agreed goals might be to become independent in planning for and enjoying a game of golf or football, or going to a concert. Or for a person who has a paraplegia following a driving accident, a planned outcome might be independence in getting to work when he has learned to use a mechanized wheelchair, safely, out-of-doors. Goals should be stated in terms of outcomes which can be observed, measured or tested so that subsequent evaluation can be undertaken.

Having identified the individual's problems and agreed on related goals, it is possible to devise a nursing plan which can be recorded (Appendix 1 is a guideline) and used by all staff in order to provide continuity of care.

In order to implement the plan to achieve the goals, many kinds of nursing activities may be used with the aim of helping the person to prevent, cope with or solve problems with the AL of working and playing. It may be that the skills of the nurse as a listener are paramount (e.g. a community nurse in the home may detect family health problems which it is known can arise when the income earner has been unemployed over a lengthy period); or as an information-giver or health teacher (e.g. a CPN in contact with a teenager who has committed a minor offence while indulging in the abuse of drugs); or it may be an Occupational Health Nurse collaborating with management to reduce the noise level in a working environment when an employee has exhibited restlessness, lack of concentration and reduced output because of an irritating noise level; or it may involve collaborating with other members of the health team or with voluntary agencies.

Evaluating the outcome of nursing interventions is a complex matter but is integral to individualizing nursing.

For someone who is unemployed, an obvious measure of success might be procuring paid employment which a client had aspired to during a training programme following discharge from a psychiatric unit. Or for someone who had been abusing drugs but had been attending sessions attached at a mental health clinic, evaluation of success might be the person's voluntary adoption of other interests over a sustained period which made the abuse of drugs unnecessary to the person's lifestyle.

Of course evaluation success is not always immediate or so clearcut. Moreover, like the AL of maintaining a safe environment, working and playing is an obvious example of an AL where the nurse, although identifying problems, does not necessarily work alone in helping to solve them, for example, unemployment. However, as far as unemployment is concerned although the government, local employers, trades unions and voluntary organizations may have a more obvious input, people may be particularly receptive to education about health problems to which they are vulnerable (OHE, 1993; Smith, 1987) because they are unemployed — and to which their families may be vulnerable. The community health nurse, and the nurse in hospital, can make an effective contribution to promoting health and preventing ill-health in such circumstances.

A more detailed discussion about individualizing nursing — assessing, planning, implementing and evaluating — can be found in Chapter 3. Figure 3.9 depicts the four phases but indicates that they are not linear and not rigid; there is frequent feedback, re-assessment and adjustment as the client's problems are resolved or changed, or as new problems arise.

It is necessary to emphasize, however, that there are many instances when it may not be relevant to investigate or document a client's circumstances in relation to the AL of working and playing and this is a matter for professional judgement. When it is necessary, the information would be combined with information about the person's other relevant ALs. It is only for the purposes of discussion that any AL can be considered on its own; in reality they are closely related and frequently overlap.

REFERENCES

Barker P 1994 Point of view. Nursing Times 90(8) February 23: 66–68
Barr O 1993 Community homes: institutions in waiting? Nursing Standard 7(41) June 30: 34–37
Bateman H 1987 Fun and games. Community Outlook in Nursing Times 83(14) April: 12–17
Beale N, Nethercott S 1988 Certified sickness absence in individual employees threatened with redundancy. British Medical Journal 296(6635) May 28: 1508–1510
Beggs H 1991 Extended visiting in a surgical ward. Nursing Standard 5(33) May 8: 29–31
Bell R, Cooney M 1993 Sporting chances. Nursing Times 89(43) October 3: 62–63

Bellos A 1993 Prescription for a fall in crime. Sunday Telegraph October 3: 22

Bennetto J 1992 Fears over design cannabis. Independent on Sunday November 8: 2

Black P 1993 Bringing purpose to life: the relationship between unemployment and health. Professional Nurse August: 748–752

Bowers L 1991 Don't blame the institution. Nursing Times 87(22) May 29: 32–34

Burger W 1993 Jobs. Newsweek CXX1(24) June 14: 10–12

Byrne D 1994 Out in the cold. Nursing Times 90(11) March 16: 38–40

Cameron J 1987 Hidden dangers. Nursing Times 83(11) March 18: 59–60

Cancer Relief Macmillan Fund 1994 The experience of families with cancer and the work of Specialist Paediatric Oncology Outreach Nurses (SPOONS). CRMF, London

Carroll J 1993 Attitudes of professionals to drug abusers. British Journal of Nursing 2(14): 705–711

Central Statistical Office 1993 Social Trends 23. HMSO, London

Cohen P 1994 Job finders. Nursing Times 90(7) February 16: 18

Crichton J 1993 The cooperative dividend. Nursing Times 89(43) October 27: 66–67

Deane D 1993 Why end it all at 14? Newsweek CXX1(8) February 22: 37

Department of Health 1993 Aids and Drug Misuse. Update Report by the Advisory Council on the Misuse of Drugs. HMSO, London

Diamond Project Group 1993 Global regulations on diabetics treated with insulin and their operation of commercial motor vehicles. British Medical Journal 307 (6898) July 24: 250–253

Employment Department Group 1994 The disability symbol. EDG, London

Farrell M, Ward J, Mattick R et al 1994 Methadone maintenance treatment in opiate dependence: a review. British Medical Journal 309(6960): 997–1001

Faugier J 1994 Dual purpose. Nursing Times 90(11) March 16: 18

Finnis S, Robbins I, Bender M 1993 A pilot study of the prevalence and psychological sequelae of sexual harassment of nursing staff. Journal of Clinical Nursing 2: 23–27

Gardner B, Thompson S 1994 Strategic thinking. Nursing Times 90(1) January 5: 32–34

Gilbert T 1993 Learning disability nursing: from normalisation to materialism — towards a new paradigm. Journal of Advanced Nursing 18: 1604–1609

Gilbert V 1994 Visitors welcome. Nursing Times 90(6) February 9: 52

Gillam T 1993 Unemployment links with mental illness. Nursing Standard 7(34) May 12: 20–21

Gow N 1992 New checks on the health risks from computers. The Herald, June 24

Greenwood W 1969 Love on the dole. Penguin, Harmondsworth (original publication 1933)

Harding-Price D 1993 A sensitive response without discrimination: drug misuse in children and adolescents. Professional Nurse 8(7) April: 419–422

Hart S 1993 HIV and the health care worker, Part 1. Nursing Standard 7(45) July 28: 38–39

He Y, Lam T, Li L, Du R, Jia G, Huang J, Zheng J 1994 Passive smoking at work as a risk factor for coronary heart disease in Chinese women who have never smoked. British Medical Journal 308(6925) February 5: 380–384

Health and Safety Executive 1993 New Health and Safety at Work Regulations. HSE, Sheffield

Heller T 1994 Who's got learning disabilities? British Medical Journal 308 March 5: 664–665

Her Majesty's Stationery Office 1992 Prevention of mental ill-health at work. HMSO, London

Holland S, Leiba T 1993 Approaching with care: violence at work. Nursing Standard 7(52) September 15: 3–8

Hutchings V 1991 A paler shade of white. New Statesman and Society July 19: 17–19

Kammerling R, O'Connor S 1993 Unemployment rate as predictor of rate of psychiatric admission. British Medical Journal 307(6918) December 11: 1536–1539

Laurance J 1986 Unemployment: health hazards. New Society 75(1212) March 21: 492–493

McGibben L, Ballard C, Handy S, Silviera W 1992 School attendance as a factor in deliberate self-poisoning. British Medical Journal 304(6818) January 4: 28

McInnes J, Treffry J 1993 Deaf-blind infants and children. University of Toronto Press, Toronto

McKenna H 1993 A long-term view. Nursing Times 89(41) October 13: 50–53

McLennan A 1986 Taken over by heroin. Nursing Times 82(7) February 12: 45–47

McMillan I 1993 A practical response. Nursing Times 39(13) March 31: 48–49

Makin R 1994 A bitter blow. Nursing Times 90(9) March 2: 26–28

Minerva 1993 British Medical Journal 306(6892) June 12: 1624

Morning D 1994 Coping with violence; workshops for CPNs. Nursing Standard 8(23) March 2: 30–33

Moses S 1993 Working for awareness. Nursing Standard 8(5) October 20: 18–20

NHS Management Executive 1993 Preventing crime in the NHS: the management challenge. Department of Health, London

Neustatter A 1993 Parental agony and the ecstasy. The Independent on Sunday April 11: 65

News 1994 Nursing Times 90(5) February 2: 7

Office of Health Economics 1993 The impact of unemployment on health. OHE, London

O'Kell S 1993 Managing organisational stress, Part 1. Senior Nurse 13(3) May/June: 9–13

O'Malley P 1991 Sick building syndrome. Nursing Standard 5(50) September 4–10: 37–39

Padgett T 1993 Latin America. Newsweek CXX1(13) March 29: 23–25

Payling K 1994 A hazard we can no longer ignore: effects of excessive noise on well-being. Professional Nurse 9(6) March: 418–421

Payling K 1993 Take the strain out of repetitive movement. Professional Nurse October: 64–67

Peace G 1994 Sensitive choices. Nursing Times 90(8) February 23: 35–36

Petersen T 1993 Strong medicine. Nursing Times 89(43) October 27: 50–52

Pollard A, Friedman T, Aslam M 1994 Tranquilising actions. Nursing Times 90(11) March 16: 34–36

Poster E, Ryan J 1993 At risk of assault. Nursing Times 89(23) June 9: 30–33

Preston A 1992 Pointing out the risk (substance abuse). Nursing Times 88(13) March 25: 24–26

Ramrakha P, Barton I 1993 Drug smuggler's delirium. British Medical Journal 306(6876) February 20: 470–471

Rassool G 1993a Prime movers. Nursing Times 89(17) April 28: 40–42

Rassool G 1993b Nursing and substance abuse: responding to the challenge. Journal of Advanced Nursing 18: 1401–1407

Ravenscroft T 1994 After the crisis (PTSD). Nursing Times 90(12) March 3: 26-28

Robbins M 1991 Sharing the care. Nursing Times 87(8) February 20: 36–38

Rogers P, Katel P 1993 The new view from on high. Newsweek CXX11: 23 December 6: 48

Rogers R, Salvage J 1988 Nurses at risk. Heinemann, London p 48–56, 132–133

Royal College of Nursing 1994 Violence and community nursing staff. RCN, London

Ryan J, Poster E 1993 Workplace violence. Nursing Times 89(48) December 1: 38–41

St. Aidan's 1993 Initiative into employment service. St. Aidan's, Dundee

Salt P 1993 Rave review. Nursing Times 89(50) December 15: 36–38

Seymour J 1993 Drink problem. Nursing Times 89(10) March 10: 25

Shanley E, Starrs T 1993 Learning disabilities; a handbook of care. Churchill Livingstone, Edinburgh

Sheehan A 1990 HIV and drug users — a three level intervention model. Nursing Standard 4(27) March 28: 36–38

Smith R 1987 Unemployment and health. Oxford University Press, Oxford

Solomon J, King P 1993 Waging war in the workplace. Newsweek CXX11(03) July 19: 30–32

Sutch L 1993 Working at play. Professional Nurse. August: 745–747

Thiru S 1994 Focal point. Nursing Times 90(12) March 23: 62–64

Thomas C 1992 Southern Asia fights bonded labour. British Medical Journal 305(6852) August 29: 493

Thomas S 1994 Child's play? Nursing Times 90(3) January 19: 42–44

Thornes J 1993 Bridging the gap: an exploratory study of the interfaces between primary and specialist care for children within the health service. Caring for Children in the Health Services, London

Turnbull J 1993 Victim support. Nursing Times 89(23) June 9: 33–34

United Kingdom Central Council 1994 AIDS and HIV Infection: The Council's Position Statement. UKCC, London

US Environmental Protection Agency 1992 Respiratory health effects of passive smoking. USEPA, Washington

Vanderslott J 1992 A supportive therapy that undermines violence: counselling to prevent ward violence. Professional Nurse 7(7) April: 427–430

World Health Organization/International Council of Nurses 1991 Nurses responding to substance abuse. WHO/ICN, Geneva

Younger J 1993 Development and testing of the Mastery of Stress Instrument. Nursing Research 42(2) March/April: 68–73

ADDITIONAL READING

Allen D 1989 The effects of de-institutionalisation on people with mental handicaps: a review. Mental Handicap Research 2(1): 18–37

Barr O 1995 Normalisation: What it means in practice. British Journal of Nursing 4(2): 90–94

Cole A, Ezelle L, Lloyd A, Moore M 1994 Investing in people. Nursing Times 90(7) February 16: 26–30

Department of Health 1993 AIDS/HIV — Infected health care workers: guidance on the management of infected health care workers. DoH, London

Farnsworth B, Cox T, Cox S, Ferguson E 1994 Managing health and safety in hospitals. British Journal of Nursing 3(16) September 8–21: 831–836

Kinsella C, Chaloner C, Brosnan C 1993 An alternative to seclusion. Nursing Times 89(18) May 5: 62–64

Naish J 1993 The soft drug approaches. Nursing Standard 8(8) November 10: 18–21

Sines D 1994 Positive partnerships (learning disability nursing). Nursing Times 90(23) June 8: 55–57

Usherwood V 1995 Depression: lifting the cloud. Nursing Standard (RCN Nursing Update Unit 027) 9(17) January 18: 3–8

Walker Z, Seifert R 1994 Violent incidents in a psychiatric intensive care unit. British Journal of Psychiatry 164(6): 826–828

13

Expressing sexuality

The AL of expressing sexuality

'It's a boy' or 'It's a girl' is almost always the very first thing which parents are told about their newly-delivered baby. As the basic body structure of males and females is distinctly different even at birth, identification of the baby's sex is almost instantaneous. Interestingly, scientists have long been puzzled by exactly what determines whether a baby is a boy or a girl. Geneticists now think that sex seems to be fixed by a single gene called testis determining factor (TDF) on the Y chromosome; this triggers male sexual development, and without this gene the embryo becomes female (Lemonick, 1988). Whatever the mechanism, a person's sex is determined at conception and, throughout the entire lifespan, sexuality is a significant dimension of personality and interpersonal behaviour.

Each human being is a 'sexual' human being and has a sexual identity: that is, there is a perception of 'self' as boy or girl, then as man or woman. The ways in which sexuality is expressed vary according to culture but, in any given society, males and females tend to show differentiation in a variety of ways other than simply those determined by biological difference. Invariably, men and women adopt different styles of dress; and, traditionally, males and females have tended to occupy different roles, both domestically and socially.

In many parts of the Western world, however, long-established differences between the sexes are fast disappearing. There is generally a more egalitarian view and, at the same time, social mores have become more liberal in terms of the ways in which sexuality may be expressed. There is a less rigid interpretation of activities, attitudes, beliefs and values associated with expressing sexuality as being 'good' or 'bad', 'normal' or 'abnormal'. The subject of sex is no longer taboo: it is aired by the media and discussed in school and at home and, as a result, people are becoming more aware of the many dimensions of the AL of expressing sexuality, not least in terms of its relationship to health and illness.

Perhaps this relationship has never been more to the fore than it is now as a result of the AIDS epidemic which is recognized as a major health threat throughout the world. The virus responsible for AIDS (i.e. acquired immunodeficiency syndrome) was isolated in 1983 and named the human immunodeficiency virus (HIV). Towards the end of the 1980s it was estimated that between 5 and 10 million people throughout the world were infected with HIV and the World Health Organization has predicted that by the year 2000 there will be a cumulative prevalence of 30 million cases of AIDS (Blaxter, 1991). Not everyone with the HIV infection appears necessarily to develop AIDS. But for those who do, there is as yet no cure and despite optimism about vaccine development, there are many hurdles still to be overcome by the scientists (Carr & Hawkins, 1992). Therefore preventing the further spread of HIV infection is vital.

There is no means of HIV/AIDS prevention other than education aimed at modifying risk behaviour and reducing the risk of exposure and transmission. Since sexual transmission of HIV is the most important mode of spread of the virus, the target of education is sexual behaviour. So, the AL of expressing sexuality has to be considered in a new light and the subject of HIV/AIDS will be touched on time and again throughout this chapter. Although references are up to date at the time of writing, it will be appreciated that the literature on HIV/AIDS is continually expanding as new knowledge about the disease is acquired.

This chapter, as for all of the ALs, is presented within the framework of the model for nursing. It begins, therefore, with discussion of the relationship of the lifespan to the AL of expressing sexuality; then describes dependence/independence in the AL and factors influencing the AL; and, finally, individualizing nursing for the AL of expressing sexuality is discussed (see Fig. 13.1).

Lifespan: relationship to the AL of expressing sexuality

The lifespan component of the model of living is intimately connected with the AL of expressing sexuality. Through infancy, childhood, adolescence, adulthood and old age there is a continual adjustment in terms of the ways in which sexuality is expressed. Table 13.1 provides a summary of aspects of sexual development throughout the lifespan.

Infancy and childhood

Human beings have an innate sensuality; being cuddled, rocked and stroked are pleasurable experiences for even the very young infant. It is not long before children discover how to create enjoyable sensations themselves by, for example, mouthing objects, body rocking and touching particular parts of the body, including the genitals and, indeed, baby boys can have penile erections. From the child's point of view there is nothing explicitly sexual about these activities at this stage.

However, a little later on, the child's increasing curios-

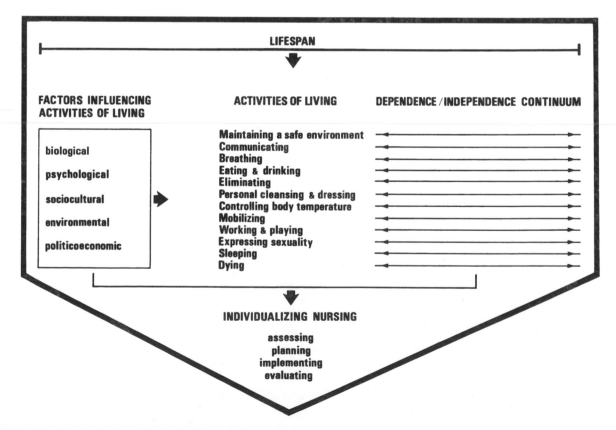

Fig. 13.1 The AL of expressing sexuality within the model for nursing

Table 13.1 Summary of aspects of the development of sexuality throughout the lifespan

	Pre-natal	INFANCY (0–5 years)	CHILDHOOD (6–12 years)	ADOLESCENCE (13–18 years)	YOUNG ADULTHOOD (19–30 years)	MIDDLE YEARS (31–44 years)	LATE ADULTHOOD (45–64 years)	OLD AGE (65+)
PHYSICAL SEXUAL DEVELOPMENT	DETERMINATION OF SEX	Growth of sex organs		♂ PUBERTY / ♀ MENARCHE	Continuing sex differences in body build and strength / Completion of development of secondary sex characteristics	Changes of pregnancy ♀	MENOPAUSE ♀	Physical and hormonal changes may cause decline in libido and potency
PSYCHOSEXUAL DEVELOPMENT		Establishment of sexual orientation (masculine/feminine)		Consolidation of sexual self-image	Development and modification of sexual self-image and attitudes towards sex, sexual relationships, sexual behaviour and sex-related roles and functions			
SEXUALITY AND SOCIAL ROLES		Sex differences in roles and functions within family, school and community settings		Problem of unwanted teenage pregnancy	Sex differences in family roles: / Sex differences in social roles / Sex differences in occupational roles	♂ as FATHER / ♀ as MOTHER		Decreasing differentiation of role and function according to sex
INTERPERSONAL/ SEXUAL RELATIONSHIPS		Mainly confined to FAMILY relationships / Friendships with same and opposite sex		Homosexual liaisons / Heterosexual friendship and partnerships	ESTABLISHMENT AND DEVELOPMENT OF ADULT SEXUAL PARTNERSHIPS- Temporary liaisons or long-term mateship/marriage (heterosexual or homosexual)			Possible loss of sexual partner through death
SEXUAL BEHAVIOUR		EARLY SELF-STIMULATORY SEX PLAY		MASTURBATION / Various forms of non-coital behaviour with same and opposite sex	ADULT SEXUAL BEHAVIOUR PATTERNS Attracting/courting behaviours / Self-stimulatory activities / Sexual intercourse			Possible decline in sexual behaviour and in libido
SEXUAL REPRODUCTION				CAPABILITY FOR EJACULATION AND FERTILIZATION ♂ / CAPABILITY TO CONCEIVE ♀	♂ EJACULATION AND FERTILIZATION OF FEMALE / ♀ CAPABILITY FOR CONCEPTION AND REPRODUCTION (i.e. FERTILE)			♀ Incapable of conception after menopause

ity about body structure and function manifests itself in constant questioning of the parents, not least of all, the age-old questions about sex and reproduction. All of this is quite natural and normal; the child is expressing an interest in sex in general and, in particular, about his/her sexuality.

Children experiment with the concept of sexuality in their everyday play and in their private fantasy world. They act out the ways in which masculinity and femininity can be conveyed in gait, mode of dress, make-up and choice of working and playing activities. Children's play characters can be the stereotype of the strong, aggressive male or the seductive, submissive female. Inevitably, families feature prominently in children's play and this allows them to act out their view of the roles of men and women as fathers and mothers. From these learning opportunities, the growing child becomes increasingly aware of the complexities of human sexuality and the different ways in which men and women express their masculinity and femininity.

There are, of course, also problems with sex even in childhood. Sexual abuse of children is an apparently growing problem in many countries, including the UK, and the trauma of such an experience may seriously affect the personality and sexual development of the child (Gillespie, 1993). The problem of HIV/AIDS is equally serious. HIV infection may be transmitted from an infected mother to her infant before, during or after birth and it is estimated that, by the year 2000, AIDS will affect as many as 10 million children worldwide (Blaxter, 1991).

Adolescence

Adolescence is heralded by the onset of puberty (in males) and the menarche (in females) resulting in the capability for fertilization/conception. With the onset of the menarche, around 12 years of age, female menstruation occurs periodically (the 'normal' menstrual cycle described as a 28-day cycle, from the first day of one period to the first day of the next) until ceasing, usually only except with pregnancy, with the menopause. Learning to cope with menstruation, and any mood fluctuations which result from the hormonal variations, is an important developmental task for girls.

For both girls and boys adolescence is a critical period of emotional as well as physical development; and it is a time of experimentation in friendships and partnerships. In private, masturbation enables the youngster to try out and enjoy the physical pleasure of sex in preparation for subsequent sexual relationships. Added to all the usual anxieties and uncertainties which accompany sexual development, today's adolescents have to cope with the very serious threat of HIV/AIDS. 'Safe sex' and only safe sex is the message now, and this requires a degree of thought and care about sexual partners and

sexual behaviour which, in past times of sexual permissiveness, has not been considered necessary (whether or not it was desirable).

Sound sex education for adolescents is certainly needed because of the problem of HIV/AIDS, but also in order to prevent unwanted teenage pregnancies. The increase in teenage pregnancies was highlighted as a problem in the UK Government's 'Health of the Nation' report (DoH, 1992) and a target was set to reduce the rate of conception among the under 16s by at least 50% by the year 2000 (i.e. from 9.5 per 1000 girls aged 13–15 in 1989 to no more than 4.8 in 2000). Thompson (1993) notes that teenage pregnancies are not just a 'social problem': teenagers are often ill-prepared for pregnancy, childbirth and parenthood, and they have higher than average rates of obstetric and postnatal complications.

Adulthood

Relating to each other in an explicitly sexual way is central to intimate adult relationships and especially in marriage or other forms of long-term partnership. Many different ways of expressing sexuality are involved in adult sexual relationships in addition to sexual intercourse although this is, of course, the ultimate form of sexual behaviour. It is interesting that in most lower mammals, sexual behaviour tends to occur only when fertilization can take place and courting and mating activities are inextricably linked to reproduction. In contrast, human sexual behaviour serves both reproductive and non-reproductive functions and, indeed, is much more frequently performed for non-reproductive reasons than for the purpose of procreation.

For adults, as for adolescents, the threat of HIV/AIDS has altered sexual behaviour. All forms of intercourse carry a risk of transmission of HIV infection, the highest risk being for men and women who engage in anal intercourse with an infected partner; and, in general, important variables are the number of sexual partners a person has, the type and number of sexual acts and the disease stage of an infected partner (Blaxter, 1991).

That apart, adulthood can be a particularly satisfying stage of the lifespan in terms of sex and reproduction before the onset of the menopause which, although technically a female condition, also affects males.

The literal meaning of the word menopause is cessation of menstruation which can occur at any time from the late thirties to early sixties, 50 being the average age (Kelly, 1993). That event, however, as well as marking the end of natural childbearing potential, is part of a transitional phase in a woman's life. The menopause is often viewed negatively on account of society's apparent preoccupation with youth and physical attractiveness although feminist writers such as Germaine Greer (Greer, 1991) have encouraged women to see the positive benefits of freedom from periods and the demands of child-bearing. For many women, however, the time of the menopause is a stressful one on account of readjustments and demands associated with children leaving home and the needs of ageing parents.

Old age

There has been a tendency for older people to be ignored in matters related to sexuality. Although sexual activity generally decreases with age, many older adults continue to be sexually active and human beings do not cease to be sexual beings in old age. Studies which have solicited the views of older people themselves have shown that they do indeed remain interested in sexual enjoyment, even in declining health and regardless of living circumstances (i.e. whether they live at home or in a nursing home), and many wish to be better informed about the impact of illness on sexuality (Steinke, 1994).

The tendency for older people to be a neglected target group for sex information/education is certainly true in relation to HIV/AIDS. The virus, of course, can be transmitted and contracted by an older adult in just the same ways as in a younger adult. Jones (1993) suggests, however, that there has been insufficient attention to the prevention, diagnosis and treatment of HIV/AIDS in the elderly population because the risk of older people has not been properly recognized as a result of the continuing tendency to misassociate sex with youth.

Dependence/ independence in the AL of expressing sexuality

In relation to all of the Activities of Living, the lifespan is closely linked with another component of the model — the dependence/independence continuum.

DEPENDENCE ON EDUCATION

Children's dependence is for guidance in development; for knowledge, not only to understand their current individual development but also to anticipate what they can expect will happen in their development at later stages of the lifespan. They are dependent on protection from sexual abuse and exploitation and need to be taught the undesirability of going with strangers without impeding the development of friendliness.

Independence can only be achieved by having adequate knowledge and experience; only then can people behave independently and responsibly in relation to aspects of the AL of expressing sexuality according to the

attitudes, knowledge and beliefs acquired in the early years. For these reasons, the importance of effective sex education is increasingly recognized. There is plenty of evidence which shows that sex and health education is not as effective as it must be if, for example, teenage pregnancies are to be prevented and young people are to grow up well informed and confident about sexual matters. Even myths about menstruation still exist: in a survey conducted with girls aged between 11 and 17 years, Smithson (1992) found that many lacked knowledge and confidence, in particular about sanitary protection, and some had been given inappropriate advice, such as not to run about a lot or do sport while menstruating.

However, sex education is not something on which only the young depend. Ignorance about the menopause, for example, is still common among older women: in a survey conducted by Mendham & Rees (1992), over one-third of the women stated that they required more information about the menopause than they had received or obtained.

Older people, too, as already mentioned, continue to need information and education about sexual matters; and, in this sense, they are dependent on others (notably health professionals) in relation to the AL of expressing sexuality.

DEPENDENCE OF DISABLED PEOPLE

By definition, people with learning disabilities are slow to learn and therefore, although they have the same basic rights as other people (see Box 13.1), they may not be able to achieve independence in some aspects of this AL, as one would expect of people with greater intellectual ability. For example, adolescent girls with learning disabilities may not be able to be independent in relation to coping with menstruation, and young adults may be

---

Box 13.1 Sexuality: rights of people with learning disabilities

- The right to 'grow up' — to be treated with the respect and dignity accorded to adults
- The right to 'know' — to have access to as much information about themselves and their bodies as others do
- The right to be sexual and to make and break relationships
- The right not to be at the mercy of the sexual attitudes of care givers
- The right not to be sexually abused
- The right to humane and dignified environments

(Moore, 1991)

unable to make independent decisions about the appropriateness of a sexual relationship or about the need for, and type of, contraception. More is said later in this chapter about ways in which people with learning disabilities can be helped to achieve optimal independence in these and other aspects of this AL.

For different reasons, some people who are physically disabled may not achieve independence for all aspects of this AL. They have the intellectual ability to understand their sexuality, but may lack the physical ability to carry out what they wish to do: for example, to manage a date or accomplish sexual intercourse or use contraceptives in the way able-bodied people can. Again, further discussion of problems which physically disabled people may experience comes later, along with suggestions about ways in which they can be helped to enjoy the AL of expressing sexuality.

Factors influencing the AL of expressing sexuality

In the introductory account of the model (Ch. 2), factors which influence each AL were considered and they are particularly applicable to expressing sexuality. The five factors — biological, psychological, sociocultural, environmental and politicoeconomic — will now be considered.

BIOLOGICAL

The stage on the lifespan is obviously important in terms of the influence which biological factors exert on the AL of expressing sexuality. The main features of physical sexual development were outlined in the preceding section concerned with the lifespan component of the model in relation to this AL, and are highlighted in the summary provided in Table 13.1.

Following puberty and the menarche, the reproductive system is fully developed and the physical capability established for sexual function and reproduction. Although the reproductive system is the body structure and function most obviously associated with sex and reproduction, equally important is a fully functioning nervous system, sensory system and musculoskeletal system for the carrying out of the many activities which are encompassed in the AL of expressing sexuality. A detailed knowledge of the human reproductive system is, of course, particularly important for an informed understanding of the processes and problems of sexual function and reproduction. Knowledge of the differences between the male and female reproductive systems is especially relevant to an understanding of how biological and physical factors influence the AL of expressing sexuality.

Gender differences

The male and female reproductive systems differ, both in terms of structure and function. The organs which comprise the male reproductive system are the testes (glands which produce the spermatozoa capable of fertilizing the female ova and the male sex hormone testosterone, responsible for the secondary sex characteristics); the mechanisms for transfer of semen, containing the spermatozoa, to the exterior (i.e. the epididymis, vas deferens, seminal vesicle, ejaculatory duct, prostate gland and urethra); and the penis, the most sensitive part being the glans which is covered by the prepuce or foreskin (which is not present if the man has been circumcized). This brief mention of the names of the organs of the male reproductive system will remind readers of this knowledge, covered fully in the biology course in the nursing curriculum.

A reminder of the fact that the reproductive system is linked with other systems of the body, a point made a little earlier, is evident in relation to male erection and ejaculation. Penile erection is the male's response to sexual excitement; it results from a spinal reflex, but is also influenced by impulses from higher centres in the brain. Ejaculation (by which the male achieves orgasm) occurs as a spinal reflex, triggered by friction which, in penetrative sexual intercourse, can make considerable demands on the musculoskeletal and cardiopulmonary systems of the body.

Sexual intercourse can be just as physically energetic for women although the form of activity and orgasm is different, for reasons determined by the body structure and function of the female reproductive system. Again, by way of reminder — and because these anatomical terms will be used later in the text without definition — mention is made here of the female sex organs. These are the external genitalia (the mons veneris, labia majora, labia minora, clitoris, vaginal orifice, Skene's and Bartholin's lubricating glands and the hymen); the internal genitalia which are contained within the pelvic cavity (and consist of the vagina, cervix, uterus, uterine tubes and ovaries); and the breasts (which are accessory organs). The vagina, which is penetrated by the penis in heterosexual intercourse, lies between the bladder and urethra in front, and the rectum and anus behind.

The close physical proximity of the female reproductive organs and those of the urinary/defaecatory systems means that either system can be readily affected by dysfunction or infection of the other. Vaginal fluid, being acid, inhibits the growth of invading pathogenic microorganisms. However, before puberty and after the menopause, this mechanism is not so effective and the vagina is more susceptible to infection at these stages of the life-span, as well as during pregnancy.

Pregnancy

Pregnancy is most often suspected on the basis of a missed menstrual period. Although some 350 ripened ova are produced during a woman's fertile years, only two or three on average become fertilized to result in pregnancy. Pregnancy lasts about 40 weeks and the expected date of delivery is calculated as 9 calendar months and 1 week from the first day of the last normal menstrual period.

In the early weeks of pregnancy, breast tenderness and enlargement, nausea and vomiting, and fatigue are commonly experienced by the woman. Pregnancy tests can be done to confirm the diagnosis of pregnancy. These are based on the fact that human chorionic gonadotrophin (HCG) is produced by the placenta and excreted in the mother's urine.

Later, positive signs of pregnancy become established. Fetal heart sounds can be heard on auscultation and fetal parts felt by examination from about the 24th week and are visible much earlier by the use of ultrasound.

After the 12th week the enlarging uterus becomes palpable abdominally. The growth of the uterus is the most overt sign of pregnancy, along with changes which occur in the breasts. The nipples and areolae darken in colour and the sebaceous glands (Montgomery's tubercles) become more noticeable. From the 16th week or so, small amounts of colostrum can be expressed from the breasts.

In addition to changes within the reproductive organs, many other systems of the body alter in adaptation to pregnancy.

- The cardiovascular system increases its capacity, a 30% increase in blood volume occurring by the 30th week. With this the haemoglobin concentration may fall and iron may be prescribed to prevent anaemia.
- Due to the action of progesterone the veins become relaxed and varicose veins and haemorrhoids may develop.
- Extra oxygen is needed for the fetus and pregnant women breathe more deeply to obtain this.
- It is now established that cigarette smoking can diminish the oxygen supply to the fetus via the placenta and so smoking is strongly discouraged (see Box 13.2).
- The urinary system has to cope with the increased volume of fluid and so the rate of glomerular filtration rises. Increased frequency of micturition is common in the first and last trimester of pregnancy. Progesterone acts on the digestive tract to relax smooth muscle and this can cause the

discomforts of heart-burn, indigestion, nausea and constipation.
- As the body shape alters during pregnancy, posture and gait change and the tendency to exaggerate the lumbar curve often results in backache.
- The skin also shows changes with pigmentation occurring on the areola of the breasts, the linea nigra (midline of the lower abdomen) and sometimes the face (called chloasma, 'the mask of pregnancy'). The skin of the abdomen and breasts becomes stretched and marks (striae gravidarum) appear on these areas.

There is no need to increase greatly the amount of food taken during pregnancy but a balanced diet is essential for the health of the mother and the growth of the fetus. Protein, calcium and vitamins are important constituents of the diet at this time. All pregnant women are now advised to take enough folic acid: an increased consumption of folates (found in dark-green leafy vegetables) and a 400 mcg daily tablet of folic acid is recommended, ideally from at least a month before conception until the third month of pregnancy (Cassidy, 1993). This is now

---

Box 13.2 Smoking and pregnancy

KEY POINTS

1. It is now well-established that smoking in pregnancy is harmful to the fetus.
2. The most common harmful effect is the reduced birth weight of babies and retarded physical and mental development in young children has been linked to smoking in pregnancy.
3. There are conflicting views about what stage of pregnancy smoking needs to be reduced to prevent the damage but, ideally, women should stop smoking (or reduce their consumption) before they conceive if possible.
4. There are various reasons which prevent pregnant women from giving up smoking, including addiction, ingrained habit and fear of gaining weight.
5. Individual expert health education should be provided to help pregnant women give up or, at least, cut down on, smoking.
6. Postnatal smoking is also harmful: adverse effects of passive smoking on young children have been demonstrated. Therefore, women who have given up smoking, or cut down, during pregnancy should be advised to maintain this achievement.

Based on Satterthwaite (1993)

known to be important in the prevention of neural tube defects, including spina bifida.

Alcohol is discouraged. Excessive alcohol during pregnancy may lead to birth defects related to the condition known as 'fetal alcohol syndrome'. There is, however, considerable disagreement on what constitutes a 'safe' level of alcohol intake in pregnancy and Thompson (1993) advises abstinence or a limit of one unit of alcohol per day.

All pregnant women are advised to have regular prenatal care to help them maintain good health and to enable the early detection and treatment of complications. Perhaps, however, it should be noted that sexual intercourse (including orgasm) has no ill-effects during pregnancy. Thompson (1987) considered that this, and other advice on sexuality during pregnancy, is something which many couples would welcome. Equally, there is a need for advice on postnatal sexuality; Yates (1987) explains some of the changes and problems which occur (such as pain during intercourse) and suggests ways in which couples can be better informed to cope with and prevent such difficulties.

After pregnancy the reproductive organs gradually return to their non-pregnant state and regular menstruation recommences within 3 months or so of delivery. Because the time of the first ovulation cannot be predicted, contraception should be practised whenever sexual relations are resumed as a further early pregnancy is undesirable.

Control of fertility

The availability of contraceptive techniques — which are mainly by physical or chemical control of fertility — is considered to be an important advance of modern times. Contraception allows women to exercise control over their lives as well as making it possible for the problem of overpopulation to be dealt with. This, for some countries, poses a major threat to economic and social survival. In many developing and/or densely populated countries, governments are active in promoting family planning services and educating people about the importance of birth control.

A wide variety of contraceptive methods is available and some of the most commonly used are described below. Contraception prevents pregnancy by inhibiting ovulation, fertilisation or implantation. Many factors enter into the choice of a particular method of contraception for a particular couple at a particular time. Dobree (1991), Urwin (1994) and Wootton (1994) discuss the factors involved, along with a brief description of common contraceptive methods, similar to the following account.

- *The pill* is a hormonal method of contraception. The 'combined pill' (oestrogen and progesterone) works by inhibiting ovulation. It is taken orally and is the most reliable method of contraception available today. There is the small risk of thrombosis associated with prolonged use, and it is now thought that the degree of risk increases with age and in women who smoke. Lower levels of oestrogen and use of specific progestogens in combined pills have reduced potential complications.

The progestogen only pill (sometimes called the minipill) carries less risk of cardiovascular complications and, therefore, is useful for older women although it has disadvantages (i.e. requires to be taken at precisely the same time each day, and irregular periods and breakthrough bleeding can occur).

- *A morning-after pill* (post-coital hormonal contraception) can be used by those who have had unprotected sexual intercourse but this form of contraception must be supervised by a doctor or a family planning clinic. One pill is taken as soon as possible and the other 12 hours later and they must be taken within 72 hours of the intercourse before the fertilized ovum has had a chance to implant in the uterus. Such treatment is useful in cases of rape.

- *The male pill* went on trial in the UK in 1994 (Nursing Standard, 1994). This contains a progestogen, is taken daily and a weekly injection of testosterone is also required. It remains to be seen whether the male pill becomes an established method of contraception.

- *An injectable long-term contraceptive*, Depo-Provera, is one of the long-acting progestins and is given by intramuscular injection at 12 week intervals. It has been the cause of much controversy about its safeness. Wigington (1981) reviewed the early research findings on its action, side-effects, and use in 65 countries — many of them in the Third World. Dobree (1991) notes that the use of Depo-Provera (or Noristerat, given at 8 week intervals) remains controversial on account of potential abuse with women who may not have been given the opportunity to make an informed choice. However, Dobree commends the effectiveness and convenience of this contraception and suggests it remains useful for women unsuited to other methods.

- *A contraceptive implant* which lasts up to 5 years has been introduced more recently. The implant (Norplant) is a set of small capsules inserted under local anaesthetic into the arm. It is claimed to be a significant advance for women who want continuous, reliable and reversible birth control, and it already is in use in 29 countries (Nursing Times, 1993).

- *The diaphragm* is a barrier method used by the woman and is a latex cap which covers the cervix and thereby creates a mechanical barrier between ova and spermatozoa. It is inserted into the vagina before intercourse and removed not less than 6 hours afterwards (but should not be left longer than 24 hours without being removed and cleaned). There are no harmful side-effects to consider, although some women find the diaphragm a distasteful and bothersome method and it is not highly reliable. Even with careful use, 4–8 users in every 100 will get pregnant in the first year of use (Wootton, 1994). However, it has become more popular again since other methods of contraception (notably the pill and the IUD) have been associated with hazards.

• *The male condom* is a barrier method and is a cover fitted over the penis to prevent the semen entering the vagina. Nowadays condoms are available in all sorts of colours and textures, the idea being to give 'new life' to an old product and make it an attractive form of contraception for people of all ages. It is a reliable method if the sheath is put on prior to any genital contact and if care is taken to prevent leakage on removal. Reliability can be improved if used in conjunction with a spermicide and the sheath may give some protection to the partner if one of them suffers from a sexually transmitted disease. Use of a condom is currently being promoted as the most effective protection against HIV infection and AIDS Wootton (1994). Its valuable protective effect against the spread of HIV has led to the recommendation that a condom be used in conjunction with the pill, this serving to combine maximum contraceptive efficacy with high protection from infection.

However, as Wootton also notes, it is often wrongly assumed that everyone knows how to use a condom properly. Since incorrect use is one of the commonest causes of failure of condoms, she provides guidance and advice which can be given by nurses to both male and female clients (see Box 13.3).

• *A female condom* was first reported in the late 1980s (Ernsberger & Jones, 1988), one advantage of this, in terms of protection against AIDS and other sexually-transmitted diseases, being that women would not need to depend on their partner's prudency. The female condom (Femidom) can be put in before lovemaking and,

being made of very thin material, it gives the sensation for both partners of barrier-free safe sex (Agnew, 1992).

• *The intra-uterine device (IUD)* is a device inserted (by a doctor) into the uterine cavity through the cervix. In situ it prevents the successful implantation of a fertilized ovum in the endometrium. It is a reliable method and requires no special preparation by either partner prior to intercourse, although for a variety of reasons it may not be the most suitable method for some women to use. There can be complications such as bleeding, pain, infection and uterine perforation. But these have steadily been reduced with improvements in the shape of IUDs and in techniques of insertion (Biescher & Mackay, 1986).

• *The 'rhythm' method*, also called the calendar method, involves abstinence from intercourse during the female's fertile time of the menstrual cycle. The time of ovulation is estimated from records of the woman's menstrual cycle or, more accurately, from recordings of body temperature. The temperature rises after ovulation and there should be abstention from intercourse for 7 days prior to the earliest recorded temperature rise and for 5 days afterwards. The method requires high motivation on the part of both partners and is not reliable because the time of ovulation can vary unpredictably and as Torrance & Milligan (1986) point out, there is the relative imprecision inherent in both the use of thermometers and the detection of the small temperature shifts.

• *Sterilization* is a permanent method of contraception, completely reliable in the majority of cases, and often the ideal method after a couple have completed their family or do not wish to have any children.

• *Male sterilization* is called *vasectomy* and involves the division of the vas deferens to prevent spermatozoa reaching the urethra. The operation is performed under local anaesthetic and has no adverse effects on the production of semen or on sexual sensation and performance. It takes some time for the semen to become completely void of spermatozoa and another contraceptive method must always be used until tests of the ejaculate indicate that it is clear.

• *Female sterilization*, tubal occlusion, is usually performed under general anaesthetic via laparoscopy and is effective immediately. It involves the closing of the uterine tubes to prevent ova reaching the uterus.

More men and women each year choose sterilization as their preferred method of controlling fertility; Dobree (1991) emphasizes the importance of counselling because sterilization must be assumed to be irreversible and, therefore, is only performed if the couple are certain that they do not want to conceive in the future.

The effectiveness of a particular method, apart from the IUD and sterilization, depends largely on the correctness of its use. Choice of method must be based not only on the degree of reliability ensured but also on the couple's preference about which method is most appropriate to

---

Box 13.3 Advice to give on the use of condoms

1. Use approved products (BSI standard) from a reliable source and check expiry date.
2. Avoid genital contact before the condom is in place.
3. Expel air from the teat (or plain end) before condom is unrolled over the full length of the erect penis.
4. Avoid damage to the latex by fingernails, jewellery or oil-based products.
5. Hold the condom on the base of the penis while withdrawing after ejaculation.
6. Avoid further genital contact once the condom has been removed.

(Wootton, 1994)

them and their needs. People's feelings about contraception can be very complex indeed. Their decision to use contraception and which method to choose is influenced by the nature of their relationship, attitude to sex, desire to have or not to have children, knowledge about sex and contraception, family upbringing and religion.

Abortion is the termination of a pregnancy and it can be accidental or induced. Many pregnancies terminate spontaneously during the first trimester, most of these due to fetal malformation or some abnormality in the mother. Vaginal bleeding during pregnancy is the cardinal sign of a threatened abortion.

In the UK the 1967 Abortion Act permitted termination of pregnancy up to the 28th week but, in 1990, in spite of controversy, the law was changed, reducing the time limit for legal termination of pregnancy from 28 to 24 weeks (and the new Abortion Regulations came into effect on April 1st 1991). Due to improved neonatal intensive care, some infants born before even this date have survived so, if possible, induced abortion is carried out before the 12th week of pregnancy. As well as medical reasons for carrying out abortion, there may be social and psychological reasons. There is concern, however, about the high number of abortions: in Britain in the 1980s one in every five pregnancies was terminated (Smith, 1990).

The 1991 amendments to the 1967 Abortion Act do not affect nurses' responsibilities in relation to abortion (RCN, 1992), and the 'conscience clause' of the Act still applies (i.e. providing protection to conscientious objectors).

Infertility

The growing problem of infertility, exacerbated by a generation of would-be parents who put off starting a family until their 30s and 40s, has stimulated revolutionary developments in reproductive technology. Following the success of in vitro ('test tube') fertilization, many new techniques have been developed to help childless couples, even after the female menopause. Southern (1991) outlines some of the most common causes of male and female infertility (notably sperm defects and dysfunction in males and tubal disease in females) and describes available treatments.

The menopause

The menopause most commonly happens around the 50th year of life, but can occur at any time between the late thirties and early sixties. The menopause marks the cessation of ovarian function and the loss of the capability to conceive and reproduce naturally. Discontinuation of the monthly periods is sometimes sudden but more often is gradual with a lengthening of the intervals between periods.

Like puberty, this is a time of hormonal change and

imbalance and there are often temporary emotional and physical disturbances. Symptoms can be experienced such as hot flushes, insomnia, palpitations, sweating, vertigo, headache, depression and fatigue; these result from the decrease in the levels of the sex hormones. Loss of libido at the menopause is not uncommon, but the physical changes which occur do not in fact reduce a woman's potential to experience normal sexual feelings and to achieve orgasm and sexual satisfaction.

The symptoms experienced by menopausal women are listed in Box 13.4. Although 75% of women will experience at least some of the symptoms, their severity differs between individuals. It is not only physical changes and problems which make the menopause a tiresome phase for women, but also the accompanying emotional and psychological stresses; these are mentioned in the next section which discusses 'psychological factors'.

There has been growing concern to provide menopausal women with helpful advice and with treatment of symptoms. There are many symptoms which can be relieved (e.g. vaginal lubricating gels alleviate vaginal dryness and dyspareunia, and homeopathic remedies or other complementary therapies may be helpful in relation to psychological symptoms). The therapeutic use of hormone replacement (HRT) in maintaining health during

---

Box 13.4 Symptoms and effects of the menopause

Duration	System	Symptoms/effects
Acute	Vasomotor	Hot flushes, night sweats, insomnia
	Neuroendocrine	Mood changes, anxiety, irritability, poor memory and concentration, loss of self esteem
Intermediate	Lower urogenital tract	Genital tract atrophy, dyspareunia, urethral syndrome, loss of libido
Long-term	Connective tissue	Skin thinning, joint aches/pains, prolapse, incontinence
	Arterial	CVA, coronary heart disease, osteoporosis

(Hillard, 1992)

and after the menopause is increasingly being viewed positively (see Hillard 1994 for an account of HRT, its uses and risks). Apart from providing symptom relief, HRT has proven benefits in terms of reducing the risk of both osteoporosis and arterial disease in older women.

PSYCHOLOGICAL

Although sex and reproduction are inextricably bound up with human biology, the AL of expressing sexuality is clearly influenced in many ways by psychological factors.

Intelligence

It is self-evident that a certain level of intelligence is necessary for learning about sex and reproduction; the changes that can be expected at puberty and how to cope with them; what is involved in close relationships with people of the same and opposite sex; the social norms concerning expressing sexuality; and how to cope with contraception, pregnancy, childbirth and rearing a family.

For people of lesser intelligence, especially those with a significant learning disability, all of these demands associated with the AL of expressing sexuality can present difficulties. Moore (1991) notes that parents of children with learning difficulties can find it particularly difficult to acknowledge the onset of puberty in their child and, as a result, support and education may be lacking.

Attitudes to expressing sexuality are established during the early years. Children who are reprimanded, for example for touching the genital area or masturbating, may develop a negative attitude to this aspect of expressing sexuality. As Deakin (1988) pointed out, as learning is so central to the development of an individual's sexuality, maladaptive learning can occur relatively easily. Preferences for unusual or inappropriate sexual behaviour are not uncommon, he says, appearing to result from reinforced learning in the course of development. The development of male sexuality is, according to Deakin, particularly complicated by the multiple pressures of contemporary society through changes in the role of women, employment and media pressure.

Attitudes

However, it could be argued that everyone is subjected to the pressures of social change and prejudice, and attitudes to sexuality and sexual behaviour are continually shifting. Over the past decade, there is no doubt that everyone's attitude to 'sex' has been challenged by the threat of HIV/AIDS and the 'coming out' of gay men and lesbian women.

Sexual orientation

Modes of sexual behaviour are shaped as well as re-stricted by social pressure. However, individuals have always exercised considerable control over the ways in which they wish to express their sexuality and nowadays are doing so more publicly.

Heterosexuality Preference for heterosexuality is still the norm for the majority of adults. For those who are involved in a heterosexual relationship, various factors influence how the partners express their sexual drives and achieve a mutually satisfying sexual relationship. There is now much greater understanding of the nature of sexual relationships as a result of research investigation, in particular the work of Masters & Johnson (1966, 1970). Such work has helped to clarify what constitutes 'normal' sexual behaviour. For example, it was learned that married couples engage in intercourse about two or three times a week on average, although individual variation is great. It has been found that the age of the husband tends to influence the frequency, a decrease being common from several times a week in the early 20s to once a week in the 60s.

With advancing age there is a progressive increase in the length of time and amount of stimulation necessary to produce an erection, a decrease in the duration of complete erection and in the capacity for multiple orgasms. Sexual responsiveness varies with changes in physiological condition and, for example, extreme physical tiredness inhibits libido and potency. Many women experience cycles of increased sexual desire according to their pattern of menstruation. There may be decreased libido during the menopause and in later life.

However, as more information is produced from studies of adult heterosexual behaviour, the more it seems that these 'rules' are broken and the picture is one of great variation, both among couples as well as within couples at different stages and phases of their relationship.

Homosexuality Sexual attraction to a person of the same sex — homosexuality — has existed through the ages and is found in all societies. It has been treated in different ways at different times, ranging from acceptance and understanding to hostility, ignorance and sometimes imprisonment. In Western countries today there is an accelerating trend towards a greater enlightenment and acceptance of the right of consenting adults to have homosexual relationships if that is their wish.

Preference for homosexuality is much more common than many people imagine. Even in the late seventies Fong (1978) drew attention to the fact that the Kinsey Report indicated that as many as 37% of men and 13% of women had had a homosexual experience leading to orgasm by the age of 45, that probably up to 10% of the adult population remain exclusively homosexual and that about half of all unmarried men over the age of 35 are homosexual. Many homosexuals are also heterosexual (i.e. *bisexual*) and often marry and have children; homosexuality is not an absolute state but a sexual orientation on the continuum which ranges from exclusively hetero-sexual to exclusively homosexual.

People at either extreme often have difficulty in understanding the sexuality of others and homophobia was a not uncommon feature of early reactions to the outbreak of HIV/AIDS, first recognized through a cluster of cases among homosexual men in the United States in the early 1980s. Although HIV/AIDS is no longer an exclusively 'homosexual problem', it has brought to the fore the need for health care workers and health services to be more sensitive to the needs of gay men and lesbian women; and, indeed, for a better understanding of the difficulties of staff who are homosexual and working in hostile environments (Rose & Plater, 1993).

Transsexuality There are a few people who, even in childhood, feel that they have been mysteriously born into the sex opposite their actual body structure, a condition described as transsexuality. Transsexualism has as its central feature altered gender identity and the transsexual not only dresses and acts like a person of the opposite sex, but usually wants to have surgery and treatment to make the body like that of the opposite sex, although this may not be possible. Transvestites, on the other hand, although they dress in clothes of the opposite sex for sexual gratification, do not generally wish to belong to the opposite sex.

As Thomas (1993) points out, transexualism remains a much misunderstood condition and continues to be sensationalized by the media. They often experience almost intolerable pressure, not only because of lack of sexual well-being, but also because of the insensitivity of others and, sometimes, victimization and ridicule. Thomas urges nurses to become more aware of the needs of transsexuals so that they are cared for sensitively by health professionals.

Sexual dysfunction

Whereas unconventional forms of sexual behaviour need not be viewed as 'problems', there is another group of conditions called sexual dysfunctions which are problems as such. Deakin & Kirkpatrick (1987) state: 'A sexual problem where impairment of pleasure, both giving or receiving, and the inability to participate in and perform adequately with another person in sexual activity is reduced, is termed a sexual dysfunction'. Deakin and Kirkpatrick comment that these difficulties are common and a significant factor in marital breakdown. Treatment of sexual dysfunction has developed rapidly in recent years and the main approaches of sex therapy/counselling are described in their article.

Sexual abuse

Among adults who experience sexual problems are those who experienced sexual abuse in childhood, or in adulthood are the victims of rape or other forms of sexual assault.

Child sexual abuse It was estimated in the early 1990s that over 6000 children under the age of 16 years are sexually abused each year in England and Wales; of these incidents, 78% involve female children and 22% male children; most abusers are known to the child (most are male, boys in one-third of cases and adult males in the rest: see Bentovim, 1993); and the effects on the child range from self-mutilating behaviour and dissociative disorders to suicide (Gillespie, 1993).

The true incidence of child sexual abuse is difficult to ascertain but, in recent years, the number of reported incidents has been steadily increasing. This must be, in part at least, the result of greater public and professional awareness and concern about this problem in view of its recognized trauma and the potentially serious effects on the child's subsequent psychosexual development. Nurses who work in schools and other community health settings, and in A&E (accident and emergency) departments (Saines, 1992), have a role to play in the detection and prevention of child sexual abuse.

Rape and sexual assault The psychological trauma which is suffered by a woman who is raped (i.e. penetrated without true consent) or otherwise sexually assaulted (e.g. forced oral sex or the forceable insertion of an object into the vagina) is now much better recognized. As a result, there is continuing improvement in the way medical and police investigations are conducted, and in the care and counselling provided for women who have been raped (RCN, 1992; Holloway, 1993). The trauma to a woman who has been raped can affect her physically, socially and sexually as well as psychologically.

Male rape (i.e. when a man rapes a man) is much less often reported and even less well understood, but similarly traumatic. Forced penetrative sexual assault of men has many parallels with rape of women in terms of the circumstances of the assault and the reactions of the victims (King, 1990). Laurent (1993) suggests that the care they require is very similar to the care now given to women who have been raped.

Psychological aspects of pregnancy and childbirth

As well as the physical changes which occur in pregnancy (which have been described), pregnancy is also a time of emotional and psychological adaptation. Increasingly, prenatal education and support is taking account of this fact and includes the emotional preparation of the mother and her partner for the birth and the postnatal period too.

This appreciation of the support which the partner needs, as well as provides, is reflected in the positive encouragement which is now given for partners to be involved in prenatal classes and to be present at the birth.

The presence of the father at the birth was something almost unheard of in the UK 30 years ago and is just one of the indications of major changes which have occurred in the fatherhood role. It also heralded an era of more liberal approaches in midwifery and, nowadays, women and their partners are actively encouraged to choose how they would like the delivery of their baby to be conducted so that their psychological needs are being met as well as the health and safety needs of the mother and baby.

The special needs of single mothers are also better understood these days. Teenage mothers have particular need of support with the emotional aspects of pregnancy, and parentcraft classes and postnatal support groups especially designed for these young, usually single, mothers have been set up (Thompson, 1993).

Irrespective of age and circumstances, the emotional stresses of parenting and family life are also increasingly being better recognized. An example of this is the growing awareness of the problem of postnatal depression. It is thought that at least 10% of women are affected. There are numerous theories of the causes: some argue that postnatal depression is a 'medical' condition and others that it is, rather, a 'social' disease (Mclntosh, 1993). Either way, early detection is stressed since, untreated, the depression can have profound effects, not only on the new mother but the family as a whole. Research has shown that health visitors can successfully intervene in the treatment of mothers with postnatal depression, using non-directive counselling techniques (Gerrald et al, 1993).

Psychological distress of miscarriage and infertility

Both miscarriage and infertility have been likened to bereavement in terms of the psychological distress they can cause. The true incidence of miscarriage is unknown; it can occur at different stages of pregnancy; there are various causes (e.g. fetal abnormality); and couples differ in their reactions and length of grieving (Stewart et al, 1992).

Similarly, childlessness due to infertility (i.e inability to conceive after at least a year of unprotected, unlimited intercourse) causes a variety of reactions, ranging from mild depression to severe marital and sexual difficulties. For many couples the process of diagnosis and treatment is a traumatic one and, if unsuccessfully treated, the process of coming to terms with childlessness can be a long and emotionally difficult one (Pearson, 1992).

Psychological difficulties at the menopause

As was noted earlier, it is not only the physical effects of the menopause which women find difficult, but also the emotional and psychological difficulties which seem to characterize these 'middle years'. Although menopausal

women tended to be dealt with somewhat unsympathetically in the past by doctors, it is clear that there is an increasing concern to help women with menopausal problems and a growing range of treatments available (Hillard 1992, 1993). There is little objective evidence, however, of the extent to which these new treatments work, but research is beginning to be done and, for example, Daly et al (1993) report on a study which did show that perceived improvements in quality of life were substantial among women using hormone replacement therapy.

It may be, too, that women's perceptions of the menopause as a 'difficult phase' of life may gradually change as writers, such as Germaine Greer, publicize a more positive image of female ageing (Greer, 1991).

SOCIOCULTURAL

Like all of the Activities of Living, the AL of expressing sexuality is universal and it is both interesting and important to understand the way in which this AL is influenced by sociocultural factors.

Socialization

Individuals learn to adopt the norms and mores of their society through the process of socialization. Parents influence the child's sexual development from an early age; femininity or masculinity can be encouraged by the particular choice of clothes and games, and by the sexual behaviour of the parents themselves. Nowadays, because of varied forms of 'family' (i.e. more lone parent families and more children reared by homosexual couples) and through exposure to more liberal television, children must be growing up with a more realistic view of the variety in adult relationships than they did in the past.

School education further shapes the child's developing concept of sexuality by reinforcing societal attitudes towards sex and the respective roles and functions of men and women. Gradually the child begins to learn society's expectations of how men and women should behave and what overt expressions of sexuality are permissible. With sex education in schools being taken ever more seriously and interpreted more broadly, children of today are given much more opportunity than in the past to learn about — and debate — social norms and mores associated with the AL of expressing sexuality.

Sociocultural similarities and differences

While forms of sexual expression vary considerably from one society to another, similar forms of behaviour to attract a sexual partner are universal. Physical appearance is of considerable importance in this, although there are no uniform standards of sexual attractiveness.

Some religious rites and some cultural customs reinforce in members a positive perception of themselves as man/woman. To give but a few examples, all orthodox male Jews are circumcized shortly after birth; female circumcision is still practised in some parts of the world (although the adverse effects of this are increasingly being recognized: see Robson, 1994); and some cultures have a rite-de-passage to demarcate childhood from adulthood, this usually coinciding with the time when the individual becomes physically capable of reproduction. In many societies, however, rites and customs tend to reinforce the status of men (e.g. traditions which perpetrate the preferential treatment of sons) and to devalue the status of women. This point is made in Trevelyan's (1994) article which takes a closer look at how a society's traditions can adversely affect the status and health of its female members. Whatever view may be taken of it, each society has its own code of sexual behaviour based on cultural values, norms, attitudes, morals and laws.

In most societies there is a taboo on touching certain areas of the body which are regarded as connotations of a sexual relationship. Jourard (1966) outlined the different patterns of physical contact which are 'permitted' between individuals in different kinds of relationships in Western society. He showed that the amount of bodily contact is closely related to the degree to which the relationship involves sexual affiliation.

While universal regulations prohibit some particularly undesirable sexual relationships such as incest and adult sexual intercourse with children, most societies have their own laws delineating the forms of sexual partnerships which are acceptable. In Western civilization the monogamous marriage (or long-term partnership) is still the norm whereas in other parts of the world, polygamy (two or more females married to one male) is practised.

However, gradually some of these long-established norms are disappearing and there is almost more variety than there is uniformity in the so-called 'social permissiveness' of modern times.

Social permissiveness and its problems

Social permissiveness has brought about a so-called 'sexual revolution' in this century; and, while there are no doubt real benefits, it is also clear that there are many problems as a result. Never before has Western society, at least, seen in such large numbers people suffering from dissatisfaction about sexual adequacy, from marital stress, from the difficulties which follow separation and divorce, from the strains of single-parenting and from the perpetration of sexual abuse in the form of incest, rape and sexual assault. The growing invasion of pornography is another unsavoury trend, an issue particularly commented on in relation to children by Tate (1990).

Social permissiveness towards sex has removed the stigma which used to be attached to multiple sexual partnerships and such behaviour, made more possible by more available and reliable contraception and by free travel around the world, has resulted in the ever-increasing problem of sexually-transmitted disease (STD) although this is by no means a new problem (Evans, 1994).

According to Panja (1988), over the previous decade in the UK, the number of patients attending STD clinics had increased at the rate of 10% annually. Data collected by that author at one clinic over a year on 1000 consecutive female patients showed that the majority were young (61% below the age of 25) and single (72%); 28% of these women had regular sexual contact before the legal consent age of 16; and 86% had casual partners within the last 12 months (while 38% had 1–5 sexual partners during that time, the remainder had more and some 17% had 16 or above). Of the group, 92% were regular alcohol drinkers and drugs were very frequently used.

Although these data cannot necessarily be generalized, they do support a general picture (and one which has changed little in recent years) which is one of young people in society today as being sexually active and, as a result — compounded by the effects of alcohol and drugs — at risk of contracting sexually-transmitted diseases. Added to the problem of infection with chlamydia, warts and herpes is the even more serious risk of HIV infection and AIDS.

Society threatened by HIV/AIDS

Virtually no sector of society is immune from the threat of HIV/AIDS. Although the problem of HIV infection first affected the homosexual community, it was not long before a quite unrelated group became involved — those haemophiliacs and others who had received infected blood by transfusion — and, since then, the disease has spread more and more widely throughout society. More babies are being born with AIDS than ever before (Hicks, 1987; Snell, 1988; Francis, 1994); intravenous drug users were recognized early on as a group in which the prevalence of HIV/AIDS was (and still is) high (Gafoor, 1988); and, increasingly, the disease has spread into the heterosexual population. The pattern of heterosexual spread, however, is still somewhat unclear (Johnson, 1992) and, as a result, it has been difficult for epidemiologists to predict with any certainty the possible future scale of the HIV/AIDS epidemic.

It is clear, however, that the distribution of HIV infection shows sociocultural variations and, even in any one country, there are differences; and, as the epidemic continues, its spread and patterns continue to change. Its rise has been less steep in recent years in countries first affected (i.e. N. America and Europe) compared with other regions now showing much greater proportional rises from year to year, notably in sub-Saharan Africa

(Blaxter, 1991). Within countries, changes have also been occurring: for example, in the UK, while the problem was largely one affecting the homosexual community in England, in parts of Scotland the initial picture was quite different. Greenwood (1988) provided statistics for Lothian Region which includes Scotland's capital city, Edinburgh; here, there was the highest known rate of HIV infection in the UK, the majority of those affected being young (average age 24), in a ratio of 2:1 male/ female and past or current drug abusers who had not changed their lifestyles.

Changes in sexual behaviour, however, have certainly taken place as a result of the relentless campaigning for 'safe sex'. While the disease has no cure, the only hope lies in prevention arising from behavioural change.

ENVIRONMENTAL

Environmental factors which influence the AL of expressing sexuality can be considered in terms of the home, school and work environments.

Influences at home

The provision of toys and games, for example, in the child's environment will exert some influence on how sexuality is expressed in the early years. Even although there is a move away from 'sexist' toys in many cultures, toys and games provide opportunities for expression of femininity and masculinity. An unnecessary degree of gender stereotyping, however, is unhelpful.

Such criticism might be made of the mass media; certainly, the dominance of the TV in some homes means that children (and adults) are greatly influenced through this medium, and particularly its advertising. There has been increasing criticism of the way in which sexuality is expressed, often portraying unrealistic and unhelpful images of women. Concern continues to grow about the increasing amount of explicit sexual material shown on TV and in videos which, some argue, is unsuitable for children and potentially damaging when it is associated with violence.

The home is also important to the AL of expressing sexuality in terms of being the place where adults can be sexually intimate in private.

Conduciveness of surroundings is certainly important in relation to sexual intimacy. It is usually the case that sexual intercourse is expected to take place in privacy, usually in a bedroom, at least in the Western world. When the parents and children have separate bedrooms, children can become curious about what goes on in their parents' bedroom. Whether or not they voice this curiosity, and if they do, how the parents deal with it may well influence developing attitudes to expressing sexuality.

However, sometimes from choice and sometimes

because there is no alternative, all members of the family may sleep in one room, either separately or huddled together. It has been suggested that huddling together can predispose to incest (Young, 1981). However, McMahon (1992) indicates that children are almost always abused when alone with the perpetrator and, indeed, that poor supervision arrangements and a general milieu of abandonment are common in families in which incest occurs.

The home environment, therefore, exerts both positive and negative influences on the AL of expressing sexuality: on the one hand it can provide a safe and loving environment in which children and adults thrive sexually but, on the other, it can be a hostile and even dangerous place in which sexual conflict and abuse can occur.

Influences at school

Similarly, school can exert both negative and positive influences on a child's sexual development and attitudes towards sex. School should provide an opportunity for children to be given sound information on sex and sexual health and opportunities for open, intelligent discussion of surrounding, often complex, issues. As Cohen (1994) notes, however, there is continuing controversy about how sex education is best 'dealt with' and, as a result, teachers and school nurses often feel confused in the current political and moral climate of divided opinion.

Influences at work

Sexual harassment at work has long been a not unusual experience, particularly for women, but it only relatively recently has been publicly acknowledged as an important industrial relations and legal issue. Sexual harassment can take various forms (verbal as well as physical) and its essential characteristic is that it is unwanted and unwelcome (i.e. as opposed to mutually enjoyable flirtation). For a fuller discussion of the nature and consequences of sexual harassment, and details of the European Commission code of practice see Forster (1992). For comment on a *Nursing Times* survey which revealed that sexual harassment at work is a common experience for nurses, see McMillan (1993).

For some people, however, sex is their work and those who earn their living in the 'sex industry' are vulnerable to HIV/AIDS (and other sexually transmitted diseases) and to violence. Jaquet (1992) describes a mobile health clinic set up to address the problems of spread of HIV infection and drug abuse among prostitutes in Edinburgh (Scotland).

Indeed, employers in all sectors are now recognizing that HIV/AIDS is a 'workplace issue': Hussey (1994) outlines the areas in which employers need assistance in this regard, including information about HIV/AIDS, for policy guidelines (e.g. regarding employment of HIV positive workers) and for resources (e.g. posters and leaflets). Safety precautions aimed at preventing the transmission of HIV infection at work (e.g. in hospitals and other health care settings) have been outlined earlier in the book (Ch. 4).

POLITICOECONOMIC

At first thought, it may seem strange to accept that the AL of expressing sexuality is influenced by politicoeconomic factors. But, it certainly is the case that even sex is subject to the influence of politics, economics (both personal and national), the law and ethics. The case of HIV/AIDS, essentially a sexually-transmitted disease, perhaps provides the most obvious confirmation of this. However, there are other examples of politicoeconomic influence on the AL of expressing sexuality.

Economic factors

Taking economic factors first, there are obvious examples in relation to personal finances (such as being able to afford fashionable clothes and other adornments which enhance sexuality) and also others on the level of national economy. Contraceptives are subsidized in many countries, and in some are provided free; and, in some of those countries where overpopulation is a problem, surgical sterilization is offered free. Even something as basic as sanitary protection can be a problem for women in poor countries, as Milligan (1987) pointed out, advocating the need for assistance and health education about menstruation. On a larger scale, and affecting all countries, is the economic cost of AIDS; this not only in terms of the cost of education and care, but also the loss of a vital sector of a nation's workforce. As Blaxter (1991) points out, the economic implications of the HIV/AIDS epidemic are 'infinitely more menacing' for developing countries.

The ever-increasing population has to be regarded as the single most important environmental and economic issue facing the world (see Box 13.5).

Legal factors

Now considering legal factors, again there are obvious examples of the influence of the law (and, often, inextricably linked ethical issues) on aspects of the AL of expressing sexuality. In many countries there are laws regarding permissible sexual relations. Homosexuality has been mentioned: in many countries it is no longer a criminal offence to have a sexual relationship with a consenting adult of the same sex and in some European countries prostitution has also been decriminalized. Incest on the other hand is usually a criminal offence which may well be a reason for the under-reporting of its occurrence. Rape is also deemed a criminal offence but, like incest, the

---

Box 13.5 World population

The world's population is approaching 6 billion

By the year 2050 it will reach 10, possibly 12, billion

Every year there are 100 million more people, 95% of them in developing countries

The crisis is most acute in Africa: the population of Nigeria, for example, is set to rise *eight*-fold to 900 m by 2060 yet the continent's food production has fallen by 5% in the past decade

Scientists have suggested that, to avoid environmental and economic catastrophe, we must achieve zero population growth within the lifetime of today's children

In 1994 the UN Population Fund called for a tripling of western aid for family planning services by the end of the century, and for more support for women's education programmes which, all experts agree, is crucial to reducing family size worldwide

(Ghazi, 1994)

---

number of victims who report the occurrence to the police is thought to be many less than the number of offences.

Legislation also exists in relation to termination of pregnancy; the term 'legal abortion' is used in contrast to 'illegal abortion' which is still a punishable offence in many countries. In the UK, as has been mentioned, the abortion law was amended in the early 1990s to reduce the time limit for legal terminating of pregnancy to 24 weeks. This is an example, therefore, of the fact that legal dimensions of the AL of expressing sexuality change as opinion alters and medical technology advances. It is likely that further changes in the law will occur in relation to, for example, the age of consent in homosexual relationships; and advances in reproductive technology will also require continual review of the legalities and, again, this is an area marked by controversy.

The 'politics' of AIDS

Controversy has also raged about some aspects of what has been called 'the politics of AIDS', although Warden (1987) argued that 'the politics of AIDS is not primarily about either money or law ... it is to do with morals, ethics, individual freedom, and communication'. The controversies, such as the issue of HIV testing (see Dimond, 1994), are an inevitable consequence of a worldwide disease epidemic which, without a cure, raises questions of the balance between the public health and personal freedom.

On one point at least, all governments are agreed; namely, that the way forward is through health education. WHO's strategy world-wide through the WHO Special Programme on AIDS had been discussed in Chapter 4 on maintaining a safe environment. According to Blaxter (1991), however, what has been learned from evaluations of national campaigns is that, although knowledge about HIV/AIDS and its prevention may be improved, the causal links between education, knowledge and behaviour are too complex to suppose that simple exposure to knowledge will lead directly to behavioural change.

Reflecting on the brief history of global AIDS, it is said there have been three periods — of silence, of discovery and of mobilization. The question now is whether 'mobilization' can halt the pandemic spread of this deadly disease. The cost already is enormous in terms of death and suffering. On the 1988 World AIDS Day (1st December), the total number of AIDS cases reported to the WHO from 142 countries (since 1979) stood at 129 385. As of 1st June 1991, a total of 366 455 cases of AIDS had been reported from 162 countries (WHO, 1992).

Although there is controversy about predictions (Illman, 1993; Stewart, 1993), WHO's estimate that by the year 2000 there will be a cumulative prevalence of 30 million cases of AIDS worldwide (Blaxter, 1991) is sufficient reason for all governments to continue to work, individually and collectively, with the aim of making a sustained impact on slowing the spread of this deadly disease. For a summary of some of the main points relating to discussion of HIV/AIDS in this chapter so far, see Box 13.6.

Individualizing nursing for the AL of expressing sexuality

It can be seen from the discussion so far that there are many dimensions to each of the components of the model of living which can influence individuality in expressing sexuality.

When this book was published in 1980, it was one of the first British nursing texts to take account of the dimension of expressing sexuality as an integral aspect of

---

Box 13.6 HIV/AIDS – Information summary

History
HIV (human immunodeficiency virus), the virus responsible for AIDS (acquired immunodeficiency syndrome), was isolated in 1983 following medical reports in 1981 of a cluster of cases among homosexual men in the United States.

Spread
Within 10 years (i.e. by 1991) over 300 000 cases of AIDS had been reported to WHO. Almost every country in the world has been touched by the epidemic and no sector of society is immune from risk now that the disease has spread into the heterosexual population. WHO has predicted there will be 30 million cases of AIDS worldwide by the year 2000.

No vaccine, no cure
In spite of costly research, a vaccine has still not been developed. It has been estimated that 50% of HIV+ve people will develop AIDS within 10 years and 75% by 15 years, but the incubation period is still unclear and the latency period may be longer.
There is no cure for AIDS: once diagnosed, life expectancy is short (approx 18 months).

Transmission
There are only three common methods of transmission:-

— by sexual intercourse, from a person with HIV to his or her sexual partner, through exposure to blood, semen or vaginal and cervical secretions
— from exposure to HIV-infected blood (or blood products) through transfusion or other means (e.g. contaminated syringes, hence the risk for drug users who share needles)
— from an infected mother to her foetus or infant before, during or shortly after birth (including the possibility of transmission in infected breast milk).

Blood-to-blood transmission is the most effective mode of transfer of the virus. The greatest risk of sexual transmission is for individuals (male or female) who engage in receptive anal intercourse with an infected partner.

Prevention
Public education, in the attempt to alter the behaviour which puts individuals at risk, is the main means of prevention. 'Safe sex' (especially through the use of condoms) and a reduction in the rate of partner exchange are, therefore, the main goals.

(Blaxter, 1991; Illman, 1993)

individualized nursing. Webb (1985, 1988) later did much to promote the importance and relevance of this topic, recognizing from her research in gynaecological nursing that both patients and nurses had low levels of knowledge about sexual matters, which included misinformation and folk-myths. The subject of human sexuality is at last being incorporated in the core curriculum of education programmes for nurses, doctors and other health care workers.

Talking with patients about sexual problems requires tact, sensitivity, tolerance and knowledge. Perhaps most important, it requires a nurse to be comfortable about his/her own sexuality and at ease when discussing sex-related topics with others. Certainly, it is important that the nurse is tolerant of a patient's sexuality, whether or not it is akin to her/his own sexual orientation (Allen, 1992). There is evidence that a significant number of doctors and nurses are prejudiced towards, even fearful of, gays and lesbians; and, concerned about this, the UK's Royal College of Nursing has been working to improve nurses' understanding of the issues and the needs of these groups (Platzer, 1993).

Eradicating prejudice and improving factual knowledge are especially important in relation to HIV/AIDS. The surveys which were conducted in the early years of the epidemic revealed that nurses (and other health care professionals) were fearful of AIDS, ill-informed and discriminatory in their attitudes towards sufferers and high-risk groups; and several large-scale surveys conducted by nurse-researchers in the UK in the late 1980s showed that, even then, many nurses had low levels of knowledge about HIV/AIDS and held judgemental or negative attitudes (Tierney, 1994). Much still needs to be done to improve this situation for as already discussed, by all predictions, there will be many more people with HIV/AIDS in years to come and the nurse's concern with the AL of expressing sexuality will assume even greater significance than it has in the past.

Most Activities of Living continue to be performed even if in a modified way during illness, whether at home or involving admission to hospital. The patient continues breathing, and eating and drinking; and perhaps with more emphasis than usual he performs personal cleansing activities. Communicating, a two-way process between nurse and patient, becomes a most important activity in orientation to the new and unfamiliar environment; the AL of maintaining a safe environment becomes crucial. But what happens to the AL of expressing sexuality? A patient does not cease to be 'male' or 'female' but the significance of sexuality has not always been adequately acknowledged in the context of a hospital ward or other health care setting.

Little is actually known about whether this seriously disadvantages patients. However, it certainly means that opportunities for sex-related health education are being missed and important information about the effects of illness and treatment on sexual functioning is not being adequately provided. Waterhouse and Metcalfe (1991) explored the attitudes of a sample of healthy people (i.e. representing the general public) and found that 92% of them thought that nurses *should* discuss sexual concerns with patients/clients. However, Lewis and Bor's (1994) study suggests that nurses' knowledge of and attitudes towards sexuality do not appear to be matching the increased public awareness and consequent expectations of patients.

ASSESSING THE INDIVIDUAL IN THE AL

If patients' expectations are to be understood, and their problems (whether actual or potential) with this AL are to be addressed, then assessment must be undertaken. A resumé of topics addressed in relation to each of the components of the model is provided in Box 13.7 and will serve as a reminder of the many dimensions of the AL of expressing sexuality which underpin nursing assessment. As for all ALs, assessment involves collecting biographical and health details; observing the patient; and asking relevant questions. From the information gathered the nurse will become aware of the patient's previous routines in the many activities which make up the AL of expressing sexuality; what can and cannot be done independently in expressing sexuality, and if there is a longstanding problem such as physical disability, how expressing sexuality has been coped with; and what worries the patient may have about the effects of his/her present illness on sexuality and sexual functioning. The extent to which this AL needs to be assessed depends on the circumstances of the individual: sexual matters may be of minimal concern to some patients whereas for others, they may be of considerable importance.

While collecting information it may be helpful to bear in mind the following questions:

- what factors influence the way in which the individual expresses sexuality?
- what does the individual know about expressing sexuality?
- what is the individual's attitude to expressing sexuality?
- has the individual any longstanding problems with expressing sexuality and, if so, how have these been coped with?
- what current problems (if any) does the individual have with expressing sexuality, and are any likely to develop?

For many nurses and doctors, even the most experienced, talking about sex with patients is not easy. Bor and

---

Box 13.7 Assessing the individual for the AL of expressing sexuality

Lifespan: effect on expressing sexuality
- Development of sexual self-image in childhood
- Puberty/menarche in adolescence
- Sexual/reproductive roles in adulthood
- Menopause in middle years
- Continuing importance of sexuality in old age

Dependence/independence status in expressing sexuality
- Knowledge/guidance needed in childhood
- Dependence for protection from sexual abuse
- Dependence arising from mental/physical handicap

Factors influencing expressing sexuality
- Biological
  - stage of physical sexual development
  - gender differences in body structure and function
  - changes in pregnancy
  - control of fertility
  - changes with the menopause
- Psychological
  - intellectual/emotional development
  - attitudes to sexuality
  - sexual orientation
  - aspects of pregnancy/childbirth
  - difficulties at the menopause
- Sociocultural
  - socialization process
  - sociocultural similarities/ differences
  - social permissiveness and resultant problems
  - society threatened by AIDS
- Environmental
  - influences at home
  - influences at school
  - influences at work
- Politicoeconomic
  - economic factors
  - legal factors
  - the 'politics' of AIDS

Box 13.8 Advice on talking to patients about sexual matters

Dos and don'ts:-
- Be purposeful
- Don't make assumptions
- Don't stereotype
- Ask questions; don't judge people
- Use the patient's words and language
- Remain professional
- Address relationships
- Ask when you don't understand
- Ask questions about sexual activities rather than lifestyle
- Address confidentiality, secrecy and privacy

(Bor & Watts, 1993)

Watts (1993) provide useful advice in their article on 'talking to patients about sexual matters' (see Box 13.8).

IDENTIFYING ACTUAL AND POTENTIAL PROBLEMS

On the basis of information obtained in the course of assessing the individual in relation to the AL of expressing sexuality, the nurse will, in discussion with the patient (and partner where appropriate), identify and agree about the nature of any actual and potential problems and their priority.

In order to think about individualized nursing a nurse needs to have a generalized idea of the sort of problems which can be experienced by patients with regard to the AL of expressing sexuality. These, as already mentioned, are likely to be more or less significant according to whether or not the patient's reason for admission is directly related to this AL. Bor and Watts (1993) classify problems into three groups:

- primary problems (i.e. primarily sexual in nature, such as sexually transmitted disease)
- secondary problems (i.e. arising from a non-sexual medical condition, such as impotence associated with diabetes)
- tertiary problems (i.e. not relating to illness but with implications for patient care, such as restrictions on sexual activity imposed by hospitalization or past experiences which may affect relationships, e.g. sexual abuse in childhood).

These different kinds of problems will be mentioned in the course of the discussion of patients' problems with the AL of expressing sexuality, this being organized under the following headings:-

- disability
- disease
- discomfort
- disfigurement
- difficulties of hospitalization
- difficulties of people with HIV/AIDS.

DISABILITY

People who are disabled, whether mentally or physically, are particularly vulnerable to problems with the AL of expressing sexuality. Nurses who are involved with disabled people, therefore, need to understand the kinds of problems which are common so that, whenever possible, they can assist those who are disabled with this AL, whether in community settings or (for the more disabled) in long-term care facilities.

Physical disability

It is probably true to say that most people's perception of physical disability is associated with musculoskeletal conditions, or people who are chairfast from whatever cause. However, there are many other forms of disability too. Here, disability will be discussed under the headings, sexuality and disablement; attitudes to sexuality and disablement; and helping disabled people who have sexual difficulties.

Sexuality and disablement   Attention was drawn to the range of issues in a book by Bullard & Knight (1982) in which disabled people expressed their views on their sexual needs, the problems which they have in satisfying these because of disability, and how they have achieved satisfaction by physical and psychological adaptation. Contributors included a blind person, a deaf person, an arthritic person, a young nurse who had a radical vaginectomy; and people with spinal cord injuries, cerebral palsy, head injuries, stoma formation and many other conditions.

All the contributors to the book viewed themselves not only as human beings but as sexual human beings with the same needs as those who are not disabled. They describe their struggle to maintain or achieve a sexual identity; and emphasize that the issue of a normal sex life is much more complex than erection, penetration and orgasm. These aspects of sexual function assume secondary importance to touch, closeness, alternative methods of satisfying a partner and establishing a lasting relationship thus making it clear that sexual intercourse is only a small part of the whole AL of expressing sexuality. The book states emphatically that society has no right to 'desexualize' individuals just because they are disabled, and that it has a duty to think in terms of 'sexualization' for those with disabilities from birth, and of 're-sexualization, for those whose disabilities occur after satisfactory sexualization has been achieved. There is advice on how to make sexual intimacy a meaningful part of the lovemaking ritual, for example removal of a leg caliper, or the clothes of a paraplegic person, by the partner.

With such information available about first-hand experience of problems encountered by people with very diverse physical disabilities, nurses can see how to be creative in helping patients to understand how to achieve alternative ways of participating in relationships so that they not only express their love, but also feel loved.

Attitudes to sexuality and disablement   Sometimes, however, able-bodied people feel repulsed by the idea of physically disabled people wanting to have sexual relations and even wishing to have children, or by the notion that unconventional modes of sexual activity may need to be used for sexual satisfaction. Anyone with such thoughts would do well to read the book so aptly called *Entitled to Love* (Greengross, 1976), and still of relevance today, in which the sexual needs and problems of disabled people are discussed with frankness and sympathy, making it clear that many of the problems would be alleviated by a more humane and informed attitude of society.

Helping disabled people who have sexual difficulties   A child disabled from birth needs the help of his parents and the encouragement of others to allow sexuality to develop as naturally as possible and to find ways of sexual expression compatible with the handicap. Difficulties will almost certainly arise if the child's sexuality is ignored and, in the course of answering questions and giving information about sex and reproduction, it may be helpful for the special difficulties and needs of the child to be acknowledged and openly discussed. A girl who has to wear an artificial limb may be helped to feel feminine despite this if special attention is paid to her personal appearance; and once she begins to menstruate, she may need advice to help her cope realistically with anxieties about the effect of her disability on relationships and reproductive function.

For an adolescent boy confined to a wheelchair, masturbation will provide an outlet for sexual frustration and he should be reassured, if anxious, that this is an absolutely normal activity. Throughout adolescence it is essential for girls and boys who are physically disabled to have opportunities to mix with able-bodied people of the opposite sex and as far as possible, like them, learn to enjoy and come to terms with their own sexuality.

People who become physically disabled in adulthood may have major readjustments to make in the sphere of sexuality depending on their previous level of sexual activity and feelings about how physical disability may affect sexual function. The disability may be the result of a sudden event, such as a road traffic accident causing the loss of a leg, or the result of a stroke causing paralysis or it may signify the onset of a chronic disabling illness such as multiple sclerosis or rheumatoid arthritis. The person's sexual difficulty may be the direct result of the physical disablement, perhaps difficulty in coping physically with sexual intercourse, or it may be predominantly psychological, for example a feeling of worthlessness or fear of rejection by the partner.

The disability does affect both the person and the

partner, sometimes drastically altering their relationship if, for example, the person affected is forced to give up work. Many people find it difficult to be both nurse and lover to a disabled spouse. A man may, as a result of direct damage to the central nervous system, have difficulties associated with erection or ejaculation or both. If the disability is accompanied by recurring or persistent pain this can cause loss of libido for a person of either sex.

If pain is a cause of difficulty, as for example the pain affecting joints in rheumatoid arthritis, the person could be advised to take analgesics prior to attempting intercourse. Sometimes, too, a warm bath in advance may add to relief of pain. Adopting a comfortable position is essential. The conventional 'man-on-top' position may not be the most comfortable or effective and very practical help can be given to couples about alternative positions for intercourse. A complete erection and full vaginal penetration of the penis are not essential for ejaculation and orgasm and a great deal of exertion is not necessary for the achievement of sexual satisfaction. If erection is impossible, a man may wish to try using a penile prosthesis, one of the many available sex aids. There is nothing weird or wrong about people trying out any of these possibilities. The important thing is that the solution to difficulties must be acceptable to both partners.

Mental disability

Attitudes towards the sexual needs of the mentally ill and the mentally disabled in the past have been most restrictive and, in institutions for those people, the practice was to deny patients any opportunity for expressing sexuality. Somehow it was thought that 'madness' and 'imbecility' rendered a person 'sexless' or sexually dangerous. Gradually it has been realized that it is desirable to allow sexual expression and that mental impairment does not preclude achieving enjoyment from sexuality. Indeed, it is now accepted that expressing sexuality is a right for people with learning disabilities, just as it is for anyone else, and the nature of their rights has already been outlined (Box 13.1, p. 345).

Helping individuals to cope with their sexuality and behave in a socially acceptable way is, therefore, an important aspect of care of people with learning disabilities. They need to be helped to understand how their bodies work and that changes in their bodies and emotions are a normal part of sexual development. Now that most young people with learning difficulties are no longer admitted to institutions but are looked after by their parents at home or in residential centres in the community, the role of nurses in community care is increasingly important. Parents may need advice on how to help their disabled child to cope with sexual development. For example, instead of being punitive towards

masturbation, the child needs to be taught that this is a normal form of sexual behaviour, but should be done in private. Teaching is certainly needed to help mentally disabled young women to learn to cope with the practical aspects of menstruation, as Fraser & Ross (1986) pointed out in their article which describes a health education programme with this purpose.

Like all human beings, mentally disabled people are capable of forming and maintaining intimate relationships with others. Hospitals now encourage male and female patients to mix together in occupational and recreational activities. This requires nurses to help them to learn about normal social patterns of interaction and it is obvious that the patients enjoy opportunities to behave as adult males and females do in everyday life. It is becoming common practice in hospitals for the mentally disabled to ensure that female patients are protected from unwanted pregnancy by teaching them about sex and, if appropriate, providing contraception. This removes the anxiety that social integration of patients may have undesirable consequences and encourages the patients themselves to appreciate that adult sexual behaviour carries with it serious responsibilities. While there is no reason to single out people with learning difficulties as a special group when considering HIV/AIDS, and there may be disadvantages in doing so, there is obvious need for education about HIV/AIDS to be provided for this group and their carers (Kay, 1990; Landman, 1994).

Mental illness

There is a similar need for people with long-term mental illness to be adequately educated about the dangers of HIV/AIDS. This is especially important in the current era in which integration into the community of mentally ill people who previously were cared for in institutions is taking place. Walker and Fraser (1994) refer to research studies which suggest that many people with long-term illness living in the community are sexually active but not engaging in 'safe sex' practices.

Firn (1994) believes that there is an urgent need for nurses to address the sexual health needs of people with mental health problems. Baguley and Brooker (1990) illustrate the nature of these people's sexual needs and problems in relation to the specific illness of schizophrenia: people who suffer from this illness often experience difficulties in establishing a sexual identity, and their sexual problems are often compounded by the drugs they require to take.

DISEASE

For those people leading a sexually active life, any one of the wide variety of diseases is likely to be accompanied by a temporary loss of interest in sex. Should the disease be acute and temporary in nature it is highly likely that libido will be restored as the illness subsides and the patient's previous sex life will be able to return to normal.

However, there are diseases, like those affecting the heart, which are associated in patients' minds with the prospect of sexual difficulties even although this is frequently unjustified and due simply to lack of knowledge. Other diseases, for example diabetes, can affect body function in such a way that sexual function becomes impaired. Disorders, such as incontinence, can have similar effects. And, understandably, patients undergoing surgery or treatment related to the sex organs, or women with menstrual or menopausal problems, may anticipate encountering sexual difficulties. These are some examples of patients' perceived and actual problems associated with physical disease and they have been selected for discussion here.

Heart disease and sex

Most people are aware that intercourse makes considerable demands on the cardiopulmonary system and so patients who have suffered a heart attack or have a chronic cardiac condition such as hypertension (high blood pressure), not surprisingly are fearful about the possible harmful effects of resuming normal sexual relations. It is true that sexual intercourse involves considerable activity and exertion. The pulse rate may rise from around 70 to as high as 180 beats per minute, the blood pressure by 20–100 mmHg systolic and 20–40 mmHg diastolic, and the respiratory rate from 16 to more than 40 per minute. These rates and pressures fall rapidly to pre-coital levels after orgasm.

However, there is general agreement among cardiologists that sexual activity is compatible with heart disease as long as the patients know how to assess their ability and identify warning signs of heart strain. The risk of reinfarction is low and death during sexual activity is rare. Intercourse can usually be resumed within a few weeks, readiness for this assessed on the patient's ability to perform exercises of comparable physical exertion. For example, the 'stair-climbing test' (two flights of stairs at a brisk rate) is a good form of assessment. The patient needs to be advised of warning signs of heart strain: a rapid pulse and respiration rate persisting 30 minutes after intercourse; palpitations 15 minutes after; chest pain during or after; exhaustion following intercourse or extreme fatigue on the next day.

Advice to avoid intercourse under the following conditions can also be given (Thompson 1990):-

- after heavy meals
- wearing restrictive clothing
- in extreme temperatures

- in unfamiliar/unusual surroundings
- after emotional outbursts
- after excessive alcohol
- during fatigue
- during illicit affairs.

Some patients may be advised to take additional medication before intercourse, and this would be on the advice of the doctor.

Nurses and doctors see fit to give heart patients every sort of advice — from dietary needs to whether gardening will be too strenuous for a while — but advice about sex is still given less frequently. This is probably thought to be the least of the patient's many concerns; and the patient probably feels too embarrassed to ask, thinking it trivial if the subject has not been raised for him. Much of this misunderstanding and anxiety could be avoided if advice and discussion about sexual activity were given to patients as routinely as other subjects concerning rehabilitation and this is becoming more common, particularly in specialist coronary care units.

Chronic respiratory disease and sex

A person suffering from a chronic respiratory disease such as emphysema (alveolar distension resulting in oxygen insufficiency) is likely to experience difficulty with sexual intercourse due to dyspnoea (p. 155). It is not easy to alleviate this problem due to destruction of the lung tissue and the person may be advised to consider finding alternative ways of obtaining sexual satisfaction which do not involve physical exertion with which the cardiopulmonary system cannot cope. Female-superior or lateral positions facilitate easier breathing during intercourse (Thompson, 1990).

Impotence in diabetes

Men who have had diabetes for a number of years, particularly those whose condition has not been kept well stabilized, may experience impairment of sexual function. Erectile impotence affects over one third of diabetic men (Price, 1993).

Poor or absent erectile capacity occurs because the diabetic condition affects the autonomic nerves, especially the parasympathetic supply. There is no cure, as such, for physical diabetic impotence but psychosexual therapy, the use of penile prostheses and mechanical methods of producing an erection (i.e. vacuum tumescence) can be employed to combat the problem.

MacDonald (1992) discussed his own personal experiences of diabetic impotence and describes techniques which can be used to produce an erection, as well as drawing attention to the nurse's role as adviser.

Less is known about the degree to which female

diabetics experience a loss of sexual interest or strength of orgasm.

Incontinence and sex

Urinary incontinence is a common problem, particularly in women, and appears to have a profound effect on sexual function (Cardozo, 1988). Cardozo mentions a study of 103 women attending an incontinence clinic; 46% reported that their urinary disorder had adversely affected sexual relations. Incontinence during sexual intercourse was reported by 24% of women referred to a gynaecological urology clinic in another study. Cardozo recommends that more attention should be paid to the subject of 'sex and the bladder' so that people with bladder problems can be helped to enjoy their sex lives despite their disability.

Wheeler (1990) suggests that nurses should not try to play the role of psychosexual counsellor but, rather, refer patients to such specialists if necessary and concentrate their own advice on practical issues which incontinent patients may have concerns about, namely:

- odour (best eliminated by careful hygiene and proper care of appliances)
- pants and pads (select closer-fitting, more feminine designs)
- male devices (conceal during the day and remove at night)
- leakage during intercourse (protect the bed, empty the bladder beforehand, choose positions which minimize pressure on the abdomen)
- dyspareunia (use a lubricant)
- embarrassment (encourage couples to discuss their feelings with each other).

Wheeler advises that both partners should be present when discussion of sexual matters takes place and she believes it is important that nurses impress on them that incontinence need not rule out a satisfactory sexual relationship.

Conditions affecting the sex organs

Prostate cancer Men in the middle and older age groups sometimes require to have a prostatectomy (removal of the prostate gland) and it is not surprising that many of them have anxieties about the effect on sexual functioning. Painful ejaculation is one of the symptoms of prostate cancer, the most common ones being difficulty in passing urine and increased frequency. Patients can be reassured that impotence is rare in men who were previously sexually active.

Testicular cancer For younger men, a more likely reason for treatment involving the sex organs is testicular cancer. Although relatively uncommon, naturally it is a

distressing disease but treatment at an early stage is successful and without long-term impairment of sexual function or fertility. For that reason, early detection is now emphasized and it is recommended that, from puberty onwards, men should practise testicular self-examination (see Box 13.9).

Gynaecological cancer The female sex organs are also susceptible to cancer and, for women who undergo

---

Box 13.9 Preventing testicular cancer

Facts about testicular cancer
- It's the most common form of cancer in young men
- Occurs mostly in men aged between 19 and 44
- It's rare (about 1400 new cases and 130 deaths per annum in UK) but the risk has doubled in the past 20 years

Prevention
- If caught at an early stage it is nearly always curable
- *But* more than 50% of sufferers consult their doctors *after* the disease has begun to spread
- A simple, regular self-check can detect early warning signs (*but* few men apparently do this)

When and how to check
- Check regularly from puberty onwards
- Do this in or after a bath or shower (the muscle in the scrotal sac is more relaxed)
- Hold the scrotum in the palms of the hands so that the fingers and thumb of both hands can examine the testicles (note: it's common for one to be larger or hang lower than the other)
- The testicles should feel smooth with no lumps or swellings

Signs and symptoms
- It's unusual for cancer to develop in both testicles at once
- The first sign is usually a swelling of one testicle or a pea-sized hard lump on the front or side
- There may be a dull ache; acute pain is rare

Diagnosis and treatment
- Don't wait to see if the signs and symptoms go away, but go to the doctor
- Most lumps found by self-examination are benign but, if cancerous, immediate treatment is essential
- Treatment (by surgical removal of the affected testicle) is now almost 100% effective in early stage disease

(Imperial Cancer Research Fund, 1994)

major surgery for carcinoma of the cervix or vulva, temporary or permanent loss of sexual function can be a traumatic concern. Among women who had undergone major gynaecological surgery for these conditions, Corney et al (1992) found that a high proportion remained depressed and anxious even years after treatment, and the majority reported sexual problems. Most indicated that they would have liked more information than they had been given on the physical, sexual and emotional after-effects of surgery. Although this study was conducted in one hospital, the need for improved advice and support following gynaecological surgery is likely to apply widely.

It is certainly now recognized that improved information-giving to women is essential if better uptake of cervical screening is to be achieved. Cervical cancer is a curable disease yet despite the introduction of a nationwide cervical screening programme in the UK in 1964, the number of cases registered has fallen only slightly. Reasons why women do not go for screening include fear of the procedure, anxiety about a disease which was portrayed in the past as a 'promiscuous' condition, the practical difficulties of making time to attend screening and fear of a positive result (Hurley, 1993).

Hysterectomy (removal of the uterus)   This may be undertaken for a number of reasons including fibroids, dysfunctional or heavy bleeding, pelvic inflammatory disease or cancer (Haslett, 1992). Because hysterectomy is usually performed to alleviate unpleasant symptoms (rather than treat life-threatening disease), for many women, it marks a positive turning point in sexual function with relief from problems such as heavy bleeding and the final removal of fear of pregnancy.

Some women however experience symptoms known as the 'post-hysterectomy syndrome' even when the ovaries have been conserved. The ovaries have an endocrine function and, among other substances, secrete androgen which is thought to be the basic hormone of libido. The symptoms are similar to those of the menopause and they can cause difficulty with some aspects of expressing sexuality. Nurses should be especially observant for any signs of undue fatigue and depression in women recovering from a hysterectomy. If the patient reports loss of libido and dyspareunia it should be reported to the doctor. Couch-Hockedy (1989) recommended that counselling should be offered to women undergoing hysterectomy, and to their partners, so that they are informed about problems which may arise and what might be done about them.

DISFIGUREMENT

Being and feeling physically attractive is a fundamental feature of any person's sexuality and an important aspect of sexual relationships. Western society places great emphasis on beauty and physical perfection. Indeed, numerous studies have demonstrated that physically attractive people fare better in all sorts of ways than those who are less attractive; and Darbyshire (1986) drew attention to the need for nurses to be aware of this since interactions with patients will be affected.

Altered body image of any kind inevitably affects self-image. Facial disfigurement is particularly devastating (Griffiths, 1989) but any disfigurement such as a burn, operation scar, physical malformation or loss of a limb, can alter a person's sexual self-image. This may cause a man or woman to fear that they may be unable to attract a partner, be regarded by others as sexually unattractive or even be rejected by their spouse. In considering the AL of expressing sexuality, nurses need to be aware of how they can help patients to cope with such problems resulting from disfigurement and altered body image. Two examples of radical, but not uncommon, disfigurement resulting from surgery are discussed here: stoma surgery and mastectomy.

Stoma surgery

Stoma surgery results in a form of permanent physical disfigurement. There is usually no physical reason for a loss of interest in sex or in the capacity to enjoy sexual intercourse. However, there is the need to come to terms with an altered body image and difficulty in accepting the stoma may lead to psychological difficulties about sex and even to impotence.

Couples may simply need reassurance that sexual relations can be resumed without harming the stoma or they may need very practical advice on how to conceal the bag, prevent leakage and odour, and perhaps an alternative position for intercourse. Conception, pregnancy and childbirth are all possible for women who have had stoma surgery, but good counselling support is essential.

As Taylor (1994) points out, a person who has had stoma surgery may be in a heterosexual *or* homosexual relationship and, therefore, counselling must be appropriately focused and non-judgemental.

Breast removal

Mastectomy (the removal of a breast) results in a form of physical disfigurement which causes tremendous anxiety to a woman. The procedure is usually performed as treatment for cancer and fear about this adds to the patient's anxieties. Although mastectomy was believed to be the necessary form of treatment for most breast cancers, it is now generally reserved only for larger tumors. Women with a single, small (less than 4 cm) breast tumour now usually have only the lump removed (i.e. lumpectomy) and chemotherapy and radiotherapy are more and more widely employed in the treatment of breast cancer (Hollinworth, 1992).

For women who do require (or choose) to have a mastectomy, cosmetic breast reconstruction is increasingly being made available. Reconstruction can be achieved by three methods: simple implant, reshaping by muscle and skin flap surgery or tissue expansion (Priestley, 1992).

Alternatively, a breast prosthesis can be worn. There are many types of prosthesis available and Horsfield (1994) reports on favourable reactions of women to a new self-supporting adhesive breast prosthesis. Whatever type is chosen, it is now agreed that women should be offered expert advice about prostheses which are available and how they are worn and cared for.

Although breast reconstruction and externally worn prostheses provide ways of minimizing the visibility of breast surgery, they do not necessarily remove the 'feeling' of disfigurement which a woman inevitably experiences after mastectomy. Many women fear that their partner will be repulsed by the scar and/or their changed sexual appearance and expert counselling is a crucial aspect of the care provided for women who require to undergo mastectomy.

Although it is not directly relevant to discussion of disfigurement, it is important for all nurses to know about *prevention* of breast cancer; therefore, information about early detection through self-examination and screening is provided in Box 13.10 and Figure 13.2.

DISCOMFORT

So far, patients' problems with the AL of expressing sexuality have been discussed under the headings of 'disability', 'disease' and 'disfigurement'. Some other types of problems are now described in terms of 'discomfort'.

Dysmenorrhoea

This is pain associated with menstruation, either coinciding with the onset of a period (primary dysmenorrhoea) or persisting throughout it (secondary dysmenorrhoea). Until relatively recently, dysmenorrhoea was largely ignored as a medical problem, being considered as mainly psychological and simply 'the woman's lot' (O'Brien, 1988). A greater understanding of the pathophysiological mechanisms of dysmenorrhoea now means that more effective treatment can be offered, and medical advice should be sought in the case of severe and persistent difficulties.

Although comfort measures (such as taking a warm, relaxing bath) are helpful, Gould (1994) exphasizes that modern treatment of dysmenorrhoea is essentially pharmacological: either involving the use of oral contraceptives (to prevent ovulation) or anti-inflammatory drugs

---

> **Box 13.10** Breast cancer
>
> **Some facts**
> - Breast cancer is among the commonest causes of death of women in the Western world
> - The UK has the worst record in the world: in 1992 alone more than 15 000 women died from breast cancer
> - One in every 12 women in the UK develops breast cancer
> - Breast cancer is most common in older women (i.e. 50 years+)
> - The smaller the tumour (i.e. the earlier it is found), the more amenable it is to successful treatment
> - A lump in the breast (even although it is almost always not malignant) should be reported without delay to the doctor
> - Women are now being encouraged to demand prompt referral by the GP for diagnosis by a breast cancer *specialist* (Macmillan Breast Cancer Campaign, 1994)
>
> **Early detection**
> - Although there remains controversy over the value of breast self-examination, Hill et al's (1988) meta-analysis of 12 studies of women with breast cancer indicated a favourable prognosis for women who had practised BSE
> - Women need to become confident and competent about BSE as do those (e.g. nurses) who teach it: Agars and McMurray's 1993 study suggests benefits of film and discussion in addition to learning from a booklet [see Figure 13.2 for BSE instructions]
> - In the UK there is now a systematic breast screening programme (using the technique of mammography) for women between 50 and 64 years of age. The 70% uptake target set for the early 1990s was achieved, but it is recognized (Reid, 1994) that continuing efforts are needed to maintain and further improve uptake of screening.

(e.g. aspirin or mefenamic acid/Ponstan). She draws attention to the fact that although menstruation is a normal physiological event, the experience of severe pain should *not* be regarded as normal.

Premenstrual syndrome

Some women experience before each period a feeling of tiredness and irritability. There is little concensus still about either the aetiology or treatment of premenstrual syndrome (O'Brien, 1993). The increased secretion of the ovarian hormones causes an increased blood supply to

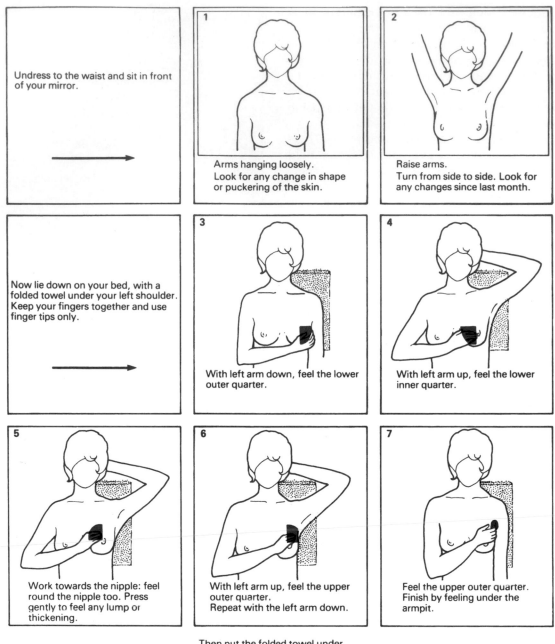

Undress to the waist and sit in front of your mirror.

1. Arms hanging loosely. Look for any change in shape or puckering of the skin.

2. Raise arms. Turn from side to side. Look for any changes since last month.

Now lie down on your bed, with a folded towel under your left shoulder. Keep your fingers together and use finger tips only.

3. With left arm down, feel the lower outer quarter.

4. With left arm up, feel the lower inner quarter.

5. Work towards the nipple: feel round the nipple too. Press gently to feel any lump or thickening.

6. With left arm up, feel the upper outer quarter. Repeat with the left arm down.

7. Feel the upper outer quarter. Finish by feeling under the armpit.

Then put the folded towel under your right shoulder and use your left hand to feel your right breast in the same way.

Fig. 13.2 Self-examination of the breasts (based on an illustration kindly supplied by the Family Planning Association, 27/35 Mortimer Street, London W1A 4QW)

the pelvic organs and this produces a feeling of weight and distension. Other physical symptoms include severe mastalgia (breast tenderness) and headache or migraine. Psychological features include depression, loss of concentration, accident proneness, and outbursts of irrational and possibly violent behaviour.

Andrews (1994) recommends that women with mild to moderate symptoms may benefit from simple advice aimed at stress avoidance and healthy eating (i.e. adequate fibre to avoid constipation and frequent small meals to prevent lowering of blood sugar). Medical advice, she recommends, should be sought by those who suffer more severe symptoms and medications may be helpful (e.g. diuretics if there is demonstrable fluid retention or hormone therapy to suppress the ovarian cycle).

Menorrhagia

This is heavy and/or prolonged bleeding during menstruation. According to Lui (1988), bleeding in excess of

80 ml is considered heavy, and prolonged as more than 7 days. Some women suffer this discomfort habitually but, for others, menorrhagia may be a sign of physical disease. The excessive blood loss may cause anaemia and patients should be advised to include adequate amounts of iron-containing foods (red meat, eggs, green vegetables) in their diet. One of the problems caused by anaemia is lethargy and there may be loss of libido. Menorrhagia may put a woman (or her partner) off sexual intercourse during menstruation and this may be a source of discontent. Treatment of menorrhagia can be classified as general, medical or surgical; hysterectomy should be regarded as a last resort (Lui, 1988).

Itchiness

Pruritus vulvae (vulval itchiness) is distressing and embarrassing and can be severe enough to interfere with sleep and aspects of expressing sexuality. Frequent washing of the genital area, using only bland soap, should be undertaken. Itching can be associated with diabetes, genital herpes or an abnormal urethral or vaginal discharge and the discomfort should always be medically investigated.

Abnormal discharges

Normally there is a discharge of clear or white mucus from the vagina and this thickens and increases in amount just before and after a period and throughout pregnancy. However, there may develop an excessive discharge which causes the woman's underclothes to be permanently wet or one which, when it dries, leaves a green or brown stain. Sometimes the discharge may have an offensive smell.

An abnormal discharge may result from infection (e.g. bacterial vaginosis: see Goodman, 1993) or perhaps from the presence of a foreign body, such as an unremoved tampon. A discharge which contains blood may indicate a more serious condition, such as cancer in the reproductive tract. Any abnormal vaginal discharge should be medically investigated.

A discharge from the penis may indicate infection and the possibility of venereal disease must be considered. As these are usually contracted during intercourse with an already infected person, they are referred to as 'sexually transmitted diseases'. Gonorrhoea is common in the UK but syphilis is relatively rare. A white or yellow discharge from the urethra, accompanied by an increased frequency of micturition and dysuria, is characteristic of gonorrhoea in the male. Immediate treatment is essential and it is necessary for contacts to be traced and treated in order to prevent spread of the infection.

Dysuria

Sexual intercourse may aggravate dysuria associated with recurrent urinary tract infection and, in addition, the woman's persistent discomfort may be worsened by the act of intercourse. Either reason may mean she is unable to maintain an enjoyable sexual relationship and, indeed, the discomfort may be sufficiently severe as to cause her to abstain from sexual activity altogether.

In addition to advice mentioned previously, the woman should be advised that she and her partner should both wash the genital area prior to intercourse and apply a lubricant jelly before penetration. After intercourse the woman should empty her bladder to help flush away any pathogens in the area of the urinary orifice and take a drink to assist further flushing of the bladder.

Dyspareunia

This is pain actually during sexual intercourse, felt either on penetration or during subsequent movement of the penis in the vagina. The former problem may occur at first intercourse, especially if the hymen is still intact; it may be due to soreness from tissue scarring following an episiotomy performed at childbirth, or from tightness of the vagina resulting from inadequate relaxation or dryness due to insufficient lubrication.

Vaginal dryness is a very common problem. Although it is most frequently referred to in connection with sexual intercourse, Key & Smith (1991) point out that it is also a discomfort when using tampons and even during walking or sitting. Lubricating creams or jellies do help, but prescribed medication (topical oestrogen creams or hormone replacement therapy) may be required.

Pain felt during intercourse usually means that nearby tissue is receiving pressure, directly or indirectly, and this may occur if the uterus is misplaced (retroverted uterus), or an ovary is enlarged or the rectum distended. People suffering from dyspareunia should therefore seek medical advice, because most of its causes are amenable to medical or psychological treatment, thus enabling the person to resume enjoyable intercourse.

DIFFICULTIES OF HOSPITALIZATION

Admission to hospital needs to be appreciated as an event which, in its own right, creates difficulties in relation to the AL of expressing sexuality even if the person's illness has no direct or indirect impact on sexual function. By far the biggest problem for most patients is embarrassment concerning aspects of sexuality and there are many ways in which, if the patient's individuality is appreciated, nurses can help to prevent or minimize embarrassment.

Violation of normal social taboos

Minimizing embarrassment is particularly important in instances where there is violation of the normal social taboos on touching which are closely associated with patterns of sexual affiliation. The intimate nature of many medical and nursing procedures can cause much embarrassment and confusion for both patients and staff. In helping patients with the ALs of personal cleansing and dressing, and eliminating, nurses see patients' bodies exposed, and they handle body parts normally kept discreetly covered. If, for example, a young female nurse is bedbathing a middle-aged man both parties may experience a sense of embarrassment.

Understanding that embarrassment is a natural reaction to being in a relationship which disregards normal social taboos can help to ease the uncomfortable feelings experienced. The patient will be reassured if the nurse deals with such situations tactfully and sensibly, acknowledging the mutual embarrassment and helping the patient to maintain dignity and privacy. Nurses soon become accustomed to this aspect of their professional role, but should never forget that patients may find intimate procedures disarming and embarrassing.

Embarrassment of intimate procedures

The vaginal examination is an example of an intimate medical procedure which few women manage to undergo without some anxiety and embarrassment. The woman is exposed and handled in a way which totally violates the usual codes of allowed physical contact. She may be confused by the sexual overtones of the examination and Moyes (1977), in a still pertinent article discussing women's reactions to the internal examination given at the prenatal booking clinic, emphasizes that such confusion need not arise if the encounter is not seen in sexual terms. However, as she points out, this means that the medical reason for the procedure must be explained clearly to the patient.

Sometimes the anxiety is because the woman is afraid she may be unable to allow entry of the speculum (the instrument used to open the vagina) or that the procedure may be painful or damaging. Recognizing these natural fears should help the doctor and nurse to prevent undue embarrassment. In preparation for the procedure nurses should appreciate the importance of an explicit explanation concerning its nature and the reason for it being done.

During the procedure nurses can convey their empathy by such acts as keeping the patient covered as much as possible. Couch-Hockedy (1989) provides a very apt description of the nurse's role in this context as 'to support the doctor by providing a running explanation of what is being done and to encourage the patient to ask any questions and express any fears'. She outlines the reasons why women 'dread pelvic examinations and smears' in terms of the following:

- Exposure and manipulation of the genitals is

intimate and usually in a relationship of mutual trust and closeness
- Violation of body privacy
- Fear of showing signs of sexual arousal
- Physical discomfort
- Fear of finding some pathology.

It is important for nurses to recognize these fears and help women to overcome them so that pelvic examinations and smears are not dreaded. The need for women to have smear tests regularly is of increasing importance as the problem of cervical cancer becomes worse and, therefore, early detection all the more important.

Restriction on normal sexual expression

Hospitalization also poses a problem for patients in terms of the restriction which this places on normal sexual expression, a matter which must be seriously considered in long-term care. A child in hospital for a considerable length of time will be less able to master sexual development if not given opportunities to express normal sexual feelings of childhood and to engage in the usual sex-related games and roles. An adolescent may experience frustration at being cut off from peers and unable to satisfy sexual desires by normal self-stimulatory activities such as masturbation, unless given opportunities for privacy. Wall-Haas (1991) found that the majority of nurses caring for adolescents in a large American hospital did not discuss issues of sexuality with their patients, and she argues that nurses should be better prepared for this aspect of adolescent care.

Long-term hospitalization for an adult can seriously disrupt the continuity of a sexual relationship. The patient and partner may suffer from loneliness and, if abstinence from sexual intercourse is prolonged, loss of libido and even severe dysfunction may result. If appropriate, such patients should be given opportunities to go home from time to time so that social and sexual relationships can be resumed and sustained. For elderly patients this may be particularly important, bearing in mind that long-term care (whether in a hospital or a nursing home) may bring separation for the first time to a couple who have lived intimately together for 50 years or more. Parke (1991) argues that attitudes and facilities need to change so that older people are enabled to express their sexuality even although they are denied the freedom of living independently in the community.

DIFFICULTIES OF PEOPLE WITH HIV AND AIDS

Before closing this section of the chapter which has been concerned with various groups of problems associated with the AL of expressing sexuality, note requires to be made of the very special difficulties of people who are HIV seropositive or who have AIDS or who, quite simply, are worried about this new and frightening epidemic. This book is not the place for a detailed discussion of the many problems which confront these people and the health and social services which have been developed to meet their needs. Indeed, despite the relatively short life of 'the AIDS problem', many books solely concerned with this topic have been published already and the literature continues to expand.

Much has been mentioned in this chapter about HIV and AIDS. Most of that has been about the nature and extent of the infection and disease and, importantly, about strategies for its prevention. Comparatively little has been mentioned about the effects of HIV and AIDS on the individual affected or about the nursing needs of those individuals. Yet, assuming the infection continues to spread and the number of people with AIDS continues to rise, the implications for nursing will be considerable.

Clinical features The clinical features of HIV infection are complex and include opportunistic diseases (such as infections and parasitic diseases which the body's damaged immune defence cannot fight; e.g. pneumonia, toxoplasmosis and tuberculosis) as well as those caused directly by the virus itself. Impairment of the immune system may also result in the development of unusual tumours, such as Kaposi's sarcomas and non-Hodgkins lymphomas. The progress of HIV infection has been described as having four stages — an acute phase, an asymptomatic stage, the stage known as ARC (AIDS-related complex) and then AIDS itself (WHO, 1988).

Treatment The development of treatments for people with HIV/AIDS is still evolving and there is still (as of now) no clear consensus regarding the right time to start a patient on anti-retroviral treatment, or about which drug or drugs to use. During episodes of acute illness, admission to hospital may be required for expert medical treatment and nursing care.

Specialist 'AIDS units' have been established for this purpose: they also provide respite care and hospice-type terminal care in an environment where staff are knowledgeable about, and sympathetic to, the special problems of people who are dying of AIDS.

It is well recognized that HIV/AIDS creates complex emotional and psychological problems and, therefore, counselling (and, when necessary, specialist psychiatric help) is an important aspect of the treatment and support of AIDS patients and their partners/families.

And, all of the time, the type of treatment and support which is appropriate is having to adjust to the changing patterns in the affected population. Although most AIDS victims to date have been young people, mainly homosexual men and youngsters with a history of intravenous drug abuse, the numbers of HIV-infected women (many of them mothers) are increasing; the incidence among children is rising (Francis, 1994); and more and more older people are living with AIDS (Marr, 1994).

Emphasis on care in the community In the development of services for HIV/AIDS patients, even although specialist in-patient facilities are recognized as being crucial, there has also been emphasis placed on the development of community-based health and social services for sufferers and, importantly, for their families and friends.

Community liaison support teams have been established in some cities with high numbers of HIV/AIDS victims (e.g. Edinburgh, Scotland) to bridge hospital and community care, their role described by Arkell (1993) as providing the following:-

- 24 hour on-call service
- counselling for patients and carers
- symptom control
- education
- nursing and terminal care
- bereavement follow-up
- help and advice with social problems.

Although nurses have played a key role in the development of liaison schemes for people with HIV/AIDS, and the co-ordinator is often a community nurse, the provision of community care has to be multidisciplinary. Indeed, the 'HIV/AIDS problem' has stimulated the development of multidisciplinary, integrated hospital-community services which can be seen as exemplars of the new style of service which the UK Government is seeking to achieve through its nationwide reform of health and social care.

PLANNING AND IMPLEMENTING NURSING ACTIVITIES AND EVALUATING OUTCOMES

In the preceding section, patients' problems with the AL of expressing sexuality were described in terms of:-

- disability
- disease
- disfigurement
- discomfort
- difficulties of hospitalization
- difficulties of people with HIV/AIDS.

It will be apparent that the causes and the effects of problems with this AL are many and varied. This is not surprising given the diverse and complex nature of the AL of expressing sexuality. Its many dimensions were described earlier in the Chapter in keeping with the components of the model: i.e. the relationship of the lifespan to the AL, dependence/independence in the AL and factors influencing the AL (biological, psychological, sociocultural, environmental and politicioeconomic). With this background of general information about the AL, the specific problems with the AL which patients may experience (or be at risk of), and which have been discussed, should have been easier to understand and to appreciate in context.

With such variation in the problems which patients and clients may experience with this AL, it is not surprising that there is enormous variety in the kinds of nursing activities which may be implemented with the aim of helping patients/clients to prevent, alleviate, cope with or solve problems with the AL of expressing sexuality. Various nursing activities have been mentioned in the course of the discussion of patients' problems — some of the problems being *actual* ones with which nurses can assist directly, even if often mainly in the form of providing informed advice rather than 'hands-on' nursing, and others being *potential* ones which draw on the nurse's skills as a health educator.

Indeed, the contribution of nurses to the promotion of sexual health cannot be overemphasized when considering nursing activities which are particularly relevant to the AL of expressing sexuality. Nurses who work in the community — and especially those whose work takes them into the home, school or workplace — are in an ideal position to exploit opportunities for sexual health education. Of course, nurses who work in family planning clinics, out-patient clinics for people with sexually transmitted diseases and out-reach centres for drug addicts and prostitutes must see sexual health education as an integral aspect of their nursing role. There is, in fact, virtually no sphere of nursing in which information-giving and education about sex and sexuality is *not* a relevant function. Certainly every nurse has a role to play in contributing to the public education about HIV/AIDS, and especially so now that the disease has spread into the population at large.

Individualizing nursing for the AL of expressing sexuality, as for all other ALs, requires that nursing activities which are implemented are appropriate to the individual's particular circumstances and problems. Some guidelines have already been given about assessing individuality in the AL of expressing sexuality. This information provides the basis on which the patient's problems with the AL are identified and, in collaboration with the patient (and partner), a nursing plan is devised.

Evaluating the outcomes of nursing activities which have been implemented can only be attempted if the goals (or expected outcomes) have been agreed in advance. In the case of this AL, many of the goals of nursing will be in the form of 'educational objectives' (e.g. for a diabetic patient to learn about what causes impotence and what methods can be used to achieve erection, or for a girl with learning disabilities to learn basic facts about menstruation and coping with periods, or for an HIV-positive woman who is pregnant to learn about the implications of her condition for her baby). In other cases, the patient's goal may be 'skill acquisition' (e.g. a woman who has had a mastectomy needs to learn the skills involved in wearing and caring for her breast prosthesis). Alternatively, 'attitude change' may be the goal (e.g. when the patient's problem is one of being confronted with the need for altered sexual self-image).

Whenever possible, whatever their type, the goals of nursing should be stated in measurable terms: i.e. in such a way that it will be possible to establish whether or not the desired outcomes have been achieved. When there are educational objectives, it may be appropriate to measure outcomes by administering an established knowledge test or it may be sufficient for the nurse to judge the patient's knowledge gain in conversation or, alternatively, the patient's own satisfaction with the information provided may be deemed to be the most relevant outcome measure.

Evaluating the outcomes of nursing is a complex matter and it is a 'science' which is still at an early stage of development. It is increasingly necessary, however, given the new emphasis in the health service on efficiency, effectiveness and consumer satisfaction, that nurses do develop the means of evaluating the outcomes of nursing. For beginning nursing students, however, the important task is simply in terms of learning to think about planning nursing care for (and with) each individual patient, and in relation to each of the ALs, in a way in which the purpose of nursing (i.e. the intended outcomes) is made explicit.

This view is integral to the notion of the 'process of nursing'. Although there has been growing criticism of this approach in some nursing circles, it remains useful (if interpreted sensibly and set in the context of a conceptual framework, such as our Activities of Living model) for purposes of individualizing nursing in a systematic way. Its four phases (see Fig. 3.9, p. 60) — assessing, planning, implementing and evaluating — should not be doggedly followed in linear fashion but, rather, seen as stages which run into each other and which are continually reviewed as the patient's circumstances alter and his/her problems with the Activities of Living continue to change or are resolved.

This Chapter has been concerned specifically with the AL of expressing sexuality. However, as has been emphasized previously, it is only for purposes of discussion and learning that the twelve ALs can be separated. In the course of assessing the individual, planning his/her nursing care, implementing the appropriate nursing activities and, finally, evaluating the outcomes, the AL of expressing sexuality must be seen as just one of the interlinked activities of living.

REFERENCES

Agars J, McMurray A 1993 An evaluation of comparative strategies for teaching breast self examination. Journal of Advanced Nursing 18: 1595–1603

Agnew T 1992 Women in charge (female condom). Nursing Times 88 (39): 21

Allen C 1992 Sexuality matters. Nursing Times 88 (33): 22

Andrews G 1994 Constructive advice for a poorly understood problem: Treatment and management of premenstrual syndrome. Professional Nurse 9 (6): 366–368, 370

Arkell S 1993 Health care delivery for people with HIV infection and AIDS. British Journal of Nursing 2 (21): 1065–1069

Baguley I, Brooker C 1990 Schizophrenia and sexual functioning. Nursing Standard 4 (39): 34–35

Behi R, Edwards-Behi E 1987 Sexuality and mental handicap. Nursing Times 83 (43) October 28: 50–53

Beischer N, Mackay E 1986 Obstetrics and the newborn. Bailliére Tindall, London, p 530

Bentovim A 1993 Why do adults sexually abuse children? British Medical Journal 307 (6897): 144–145

Blaxter M 1991 AIDS: Worldwide Policies and Problems. Office of Health Economics, London

Bor R, Watts M 1993 Talking to patients about sexual matters. British Journal of Nursing 2 (13): 657–661

Bullard D G, Knight S E (eds) 1982 Sexuality and physical disability, personal perspectives. Mosby, St Louis

Bunyan S, Clark N, Herranz A, Kaur S, Morley S, Morgan K, Owen S 1986 Mental handicap: human rights and relationships. The Professional Nurse 2 (2) November: 41–43

Cardozo L 1988 Sex and the bladder. British Medical Journal 296 (6622) 27 February: 587–588

Carr G, Hawkins P 1992 Developing a vaccine for HIV. Nursing Standard 6 (52): 53–55

Cassidy J 1993 Acid test (folic acid in pregnancy). Nursing Times 89 (50): 21

Cohen P 1994 The role of the school nurse in providing sex education. Nursing Times 90 (23): 36–38

Corney R, Everett H, Howells A, Crowther M 1992 The care of patients undergoing surgery for gynaecological cancer: the need for information, emotional support and counselling. Journal of Advanced Nursing 17: 667–671

Couch-Hockedy S 1989 Women's experiences of gynaecology. The Professional Nurse 4 (4) January: 173–175

Daly E, Gray A, Barlow D, McPherson K, Roche M, Vessey M 1993 Measuring the impact of menopausal symptoms on quality of life. British Medical Journal 307 (6908): 836–840

Darbyshire P 1986 Body image: when the face doesn't fit. Nursing Times 82 (40) October 1: 28–30

Deakin G 1988 Male sexuality. Nursing 26: 961–962

Deakin G, Kirkpatrick L 1987 Sexual problems and their treatment. Nursing 3 (19): 709–714

Dignan K 1993 Testing times (cervical screening). Nursing Times 89 (44): 28–30

Dobree L 1991 An informed choice ensures peace of mind: Contraceptive counselling in the community. Professional Nurse 6 (10): 616–621

DoH 1992 The Health of the Nation. Department of Health: HMSO, London

Ellis H 1981 Time is of the essence. Nursing Mirror 152 (26) June 24: 43–44

Ernsberger R, Jones E 1988 Femshield (a female condom). Newsweek CX1 (22) May 30: 3

Evans G 1994 A history of sexually transmitted diseases. Nursing Times 90 (18): 29–31

Faulkner A 1985 Mastectomy: reclaiming a body image. Nursing Times Community Outlook May: 11–13

Firn S 1994 No sex, please. Nursing Times 90 (14): 57

Fong R 1978 Sexual abnormalities 1. Harmless variations. Nursing Times 74 (24) June 15: 1015–1016

Forster P 1992 Sexual harrassment at work. British Medical Journal 305 (6859): 944–946

Francis B R 1994 The incidence of HIV / AIDS in children and their care needs. Nursing Times 90 (26): 47–49

Fraser J, Ross C 1986 Time of the month. Nursing Times 82 (30) July 23: 56–58

Gerrard J, Holden J M, Elliott S A, McKenzie P, McKenzie J, Cox J L M 1993 A trainer's perspective of an innovative programme teaching health visitors about the detection, treatment and prevention of postnatal depression. Journal of Advanced Nursing 18: 1825–1832

Ghazi P 1994 Too many kids. The Observer. Sunday 4 September: p 11

Gillespie F 1992 HIV / AIDS; the ethical and legal dilemmas. British Journal of Nursing 1 (4): 197–200

Gillespie F J 1993 Child sexual abuse: definitions, incidence and consequences. British Journal of Nursing 2 (5): 267–273

Goodman M 1993 A growing concern: Bacterial vaginosis. Nursing Standard (RCN Nursing Update) 7 (50): 3–8

Gould D 1994 Facing the pain of dysmenorrhoea. Nursing Standard 8 (42): 25–28

Graham S 1984 The unkindest cut. Nursing Times 80 (3) January 18: 8–10

Greengross W 1976 Entitled to love: the sexual and emotional needs of the handicapped. Malaby Press, London

Greenwood J 1988 Or die of ignorance. Editorial. Edinburgh Medicine 52: 3

Greer G 1991 The Change: Women, Ageing and the Menopause. Hamish Hamilton, London

Griffiths E 1989 More than skin deep (facial disfigurement). Nursing Times 85 (40): 34–36

Haslett S 1992 Reviewing the options to hysterectomy. Nursing Standard 6 (39): 33–36

Hicks C 1987 AIDS: Innocent victims. Nursing Times 83(6) February 18: 19

Hill D, White V, Jolley D, Mapperson K 1988 Self-examination of the breast: is it beneficial? Meta-analysis of studies investigating breast self-examination and extent of disease in patients with breast cancer. British Medical Journal 297 (6643): 271–275

Hillard A 1992 The menopause and beyond. Nursing Standard (RCN Nursing Update) 7 (8): 3–8

Hillard A 1994 Hormone replacement therapy (HRT). Nursing Standard 8 (18): 31–34

Hollinworth H 1992 Choice without fear (mastectomy and alternatives). Nursing Times 88 (50): 27–29

Holloway M, Swan A 1993 A & E management of sexual assault. Nursing Standard 7 (45): 31–35

Horsfield S 1994 Adhesive prosthesis. Nursing Times 90 (8): 44–46

Hussey J 1994 HIV and AIDS at work: positive reactions. Nursing Standard 8 (43): 46–47

Illman J 1993 AIDS/HIV: History lesson. Nursing Times 89 (26): 26–29

Imperial Cancer Research Fund 1994 Testicular Cancer Fact Sheet and Booklet ('A whole new ball game'). ICRF, PO Box 123, Lincoln's Inn Fields, London WC2A 3PX

Jaquet C 1992 Help on the streets (A mobile health care facility for prostitutes). Nursing Times 88 (39): 24–26

Johnson A M 1992 Home grown heterosexually acquired HIV infection: Still difficult to predict. British Medical Journal 304 (6835): 1125–1126

Jones H 1993 HIV mistreatment: policy, resources and practice. Senior Nurse 13 (6): 19–22

Jourard S M 1966 An exploratory study of body accessibility. British Journal of Social and Clinical Psychology 5: 221–231

Kay B 1990 Mental handicap and HIV: the issues. Nursing Standard 4 (23): 30–34

Kelly J 1993 Effects and treatment of the menopause. British Journal of Nursing 2 (2): 123–125

Key E, Smith S 1991 Management of vaginal dryness. Nursing Standard 5 (31): 24–27

King M B 1990 Male rape: Victims need sensitive management. British Medical Journal 301 (6765): 1345

Landman R 1994 Making sex safer for people with learning disabilities. Nursing Times 90 (28): 35–37

Laurent C 1993 Male rape. Nursing Times 89 (6): 18–19

Lemonick 1988 It's a boy, and here's why. Time 131 (1) January 4: 45

Lewis S, Bor R 1994 Nurses' knowledge of and attitudes towards sexuality and the relationship of these with nursing practice. Journal of Advanced Nursing 20: 251–259

Lui D 1988 Management approaches in menorrhagia. British Journal of Sexual Medicine July: 10–13

MacDonald R 1992 A sensitive issue (diabetic impotence). Nursing 5 (6): 23–25

Macmillan Breast Cancer Campaign 1994 Breast cancer: how to help yourself. Cancer Relief Macmillan Fund, Anchor House, 15/19 Britten Street, London SW3 3TZ

Marr J 1994 The impact of HIV on older people. Nursing Standard 8 (46): 28–31 and 8, 47, 25–27

Masters W H, Johnson V E 1966 Human sexual response. Little Brown, Boston

Masters W H, Johnson V E 1970 Human sexual inadequacy. Little Brown, Boston

McIntosh J 1993 The experience of motherhood and the development of depression in the postnatal period. Journal of Clinical Nursing 2: 243–249

McMahon B 1992 Incest: the family context – Understanding and detecting childhood sexual abuse. Professional Nurse 7 (11): 701–705

McMillan I 1993 A disturbing picture (Sexual harrassment at work). Nursing Times 89 (8): 30–34

Mendham C, Rees C 1992 Menopause: A positive change. Nursing Times 88 (12): 34–35

Milligan A 1987 Lifting the curse. Nursing Times 83 (18) May 6: 50–51

Moore K 1991 Confronting taboo (Helping people with learning disabilities to understand their own sexuality). Nursing Times 87 (42): 46–47

Moyes B 1977 A doctor is a doctor. New Society November 10: 289–291

Nichols S 1983 The Southampton breast study — implications for nurses. Nursing Times 79 (50) December 14: 24–27

Nursing Standard 1994 Male contraceptive pill to undergo trials. Nursing Standard News 8 (49): 14

Nursing Times 1993 Contraceptive implant launched. Nursing Times News 89: 41, 9

O'Brien P M S 1993 Helping women with premenstrual syndrome. British Medical Journal 307 (6917): 1471–1475

O'Brien P M S 1988 Management approaches in dysmenorrhoea. British Journal of Sexual Medicine July: 6–10

Panja S K 1988 Behavioural profile of females attending sexually transmitted diseases (STD) clinics. British Journal of Sexual Medicine 15 (2) February: 50–52

Parke F 1991 Sexuality in later life. Nursing Times 87 (50): 40–42

Pearson L H 1992 The stigma of infertility. Nursing Times 88 (1): 36–38

Platzer H 1993 Nursing care of gay and lesbian patients. Nursing Standard 7 (17): 34–37

Power D 1981 Children in danger. Nursing Mirror 152 (5) January 29: 29–32

Price B 1986 Body image: keeping up appearances. Nursing Times 82 (40) October 1: 58–61

Price D E 1993 Managing impotence in diabetes. British Medical Journal 307 (6899): 275–276

Priestley M 1992 Breast reconstruction following mastectomy. British Journal of Nursing 1 (3): 118–121

RCN 1992 Responding to rape and sexual assault. (Issues in Nursing and Health Care Series) Nursing Standard 6 (18): 31

Reid T 1994 Women's health: Screened out? Nursing Times 90 (18): 48–50

Robson R 1994 The issue of unspoken abuse (female genital mutilation). Nursing Standard 8 (32): 16–17

Rose P, Platzer H 1993 Confronting prejudice: gay and lesbian issues. Nursing Times 89 (31): 52–54

RCN 1992 Abortion: the nurse's responsibilities. Nursing Standard (RCN 'Issues in Nursing and Health') 7 (3): 35

Saines J 1992 A & E nurses' role in detecting child sexual abuse. Professional Nurse 8 (3): 148–152

Satterthwaite S J 1993 The right time to give up: Advising women on smoking in pregnancy. Professional Nurse 8 (4): 244–248

Schäufele B 1988 Teaching testicular self-examination. The Professional Nurse 3 (10) July: 409–411

Smith T 1990 Unwanted pregnancies. British Medical Journal 300 (6733): 1154

Smithson A 1992 Girls will be women. Nursing Times 88 (6): 46–48

Snell J 1988 AIDS and the risk to infants. Nursing Times 84 (9) March 2: 20

Southern C 1991 Causes and treatment of infertility. Nursing 4 (37): 13–19

Spencer B 1986 If the cap fits . . . Nursing Times 82 (5) January 29: 22–24

Stanford J 1986 Testicular self-examination. The Professional Nurse 1 (5) February: 132–133

Steinke E E 1994 Knowledge and attitudes of older adults about sexuality in ageing: a comparison of two studies. Journal of Advanced Nursing 19: 477–485

Stewart G 1993 AIDS/HIV: Predictable and preventable? Nursing Times 89 (26): 29–33

Stewart A, Harker L, Ford J 1992 An unfinished story: Helping people come to terms with miscarriage. Professional Nurse 7 (10): 656–659

Swaffield L 1988 Mastectomy — and more . . . Nursing Standard 2 April 30: 36

Tate T 1990 Web of deceit (child pornography). Nursing Times 86 (32): 16–17

Taylor P 1994 Beating the taboo (stoma and sex). Nursing Times 90 (13): 51–53

Thomas B 1993 Gender loving care. Nursing Times 89 (10): 50–51

Thompson D 1990 Intercourse after myocardial infarction. Nursing Standard 4 (43): 32–33

Thompson J 1993 Nutrition in pregnancy. Nursing Times 89 (2): 38–40

Thompson J 1993 Supporting young mothers. Nursing Times 89 (51): 64–67

Thompson V 1987 Sexuality in pregnancy. Nursing Times 83 (7) February 18: 63

Tierney A J 1995 HIV/AIDS – Knowledge, attitudes and education of nurses: A research review. Journal of Clinical Nursing 4: 13–21

Torrance C, Milligan S 1986 How safe is the 'safe' period? Nursing Times 82 (26) June 25: 37–38

Trevelyan J 1994 Women's health: A woman's lot . . . Nursing Times 90 (15): 49–50

Urwin J 1944 Choice advice (contraception). Nursing Times 90 (26): 56–59

Walker S, Fraiser D 1994 HIV and the long-term mentally ill. Nursing Standard 8 (16): 51–53

Wall-Haas C L 1991 Nurses' attitudes towards sexuality in adolescent patients. Pediatric Nursing 17 (6): 549–555

Warden J 1987 The politics of AIDS. British Medical Journal 294 (6569): 455

Waterhouse J, Metcalfe M 1991 Attitudes towards discussing sexual concerns with patients. Journal of Advanced Nursing 16: 1048–1054

Webb C 1985 Teaching sexuality in the curriculum. Senior Nurse 3 (5) November: 10–12

Webb C 1986 Sexuality, nursing and health. John Wiley, Bristol

Westgate B 1981 Facts and figures. Nursing Mirror 152 (1) January 1: 30–32

Wheeler V 1990 A new kind of loving? The effect of continence problems on sexuality. Professional Nurse 5 (9): 492–496

WHO 1992 AIDS in Europe: the challenge for today and tomorrow. Journal of Advanced Nursing 17: 888–891

Wigington S 1981 Depo-Provera: an injectable contraceptive. Nursing Times 77 (42) October 14: 1794–1798

Wootton G 1994 Risk cover: Barrier methods. Nursing Times 90 (26): 58–59

Yates A 1987 Sexuality: And baby makes three . . . Nursing Times 83 (32) August 12: 31–33

Young M 1981 Incest victims and offenders: myths and realities. Journal of Psychosocial Nursing 9 (10) October: 37–39

14

Sleeping

The AL of sleeping

All parents are familiar with their children asking 'Why do we have to go to bed?' Most parents believe that because children are growing, they need relatively more sleep than adults. Scientists have now produced evidence to support this idea and have unravelled many other mysteries about sleep, although some still remain. Adults vary considerably in the amount of sleep they require but, on average, spend about one-quarter to one-third of their lives sleeping. In terms of time alone then, sleeping is for everyone an important Activity of Living.

It appears that all living creatures have periods of activity alternating with periods of inactivity and these are governed by the sleep-wakefulness cycle controlled largely by the hypothalamus. Human beings do not seem to be born with a 24-hour rhythm of sleeping and waking. The recurrence of sleep every 24 hours constitutes a rhythm which the human body has 'learned' through experience. The word circadian describes this learned rhythm, and the term 'biological clock' refers to the mechanism which produces the rhythm. The old idea that all babies slept for most of the 24 hours is now refuted; each baby is different. In acquiring their rhythm most babies sleep for about 16 hours, at first spread round the clock but by the time they are 3 months old the amount of night sleep has usually doubled.

To include sleeping as an 'activity' is not paradoxical, for although sleep provides the greatest degree of rest, the body systems are still functioning albeit at a reduced level. Sleep has been described as a recurrent state of inertia and unresponsiveness; a state in which a person does not respond overtly to what is going on in the surrounding environment. Although consciousness is lost temporarily, a sufficient new stimulus, such as an alarm clock going off, will rouse the person. In this respect sleeping differs from the states of coma and anaesthesia which are also discussed in this chapter.

THE NATURE AND FUNCTION OF SLEEP

How does one know that a person is asleep? Most people sleep with closed eyes; they lie still for part of the time, but they move at intervals throughout the sleep periods; sometimes there is relaxation in the muscles of the face and neck so that the jaw is unsupported and the mouth open; breathing is slower and usually deeper; flaccid muscles in the upper respiratory tract are thought to be responsible for snoring. But what is the nature of this phenomenon called sleep?

For many years, this very question has been exercising the minds of experts in various parts of the world who specialize in research on sleep. Although complete answers have not yet been found to all the mysteries about sleep, a great deal of information has been collected, much of it by recording tracings of the electrical waves from the brains of people who are sleeping — electroencephalographs (EEGs). The information which has accumulated from the work in sleep laboratories, particularly about sleep occurring in cycles, has been vital to understanding the nature and function of sleep.

The sleep cycle

Each sleep cycle is approximately 90–100 minutes in duration and there are usually four to six cycles in a person's normal sleep period (Oswald & Adam, 1983). Each sleep cycle can be described as having five stages which were defined by Rechtshaffen & Kales in 1968. The pattern which these stages tend to follow in young healthy adults is shown in Figure 14.1. The first four stages are what is described as non-REM (rapid eye movement) sleep (NREM) and the fifth is REM sleep. These are two distinct physiological states, described by Shapiro and Flanigan (1993) as being 'as different from each other as each one is from wakefulness'. Characteristics of the stages of sleep are described in Box 14.1.

There is a cycle of NREM and REM sleep throughout

Box 14.1 Stages of sleep

Stage 1. This is the transition from wakefulness to sleep. The sleeper has just 'dropped off'. There is a general relaxation; there are fleeting thoughts, and the sleeper can be wakened by any slight stimulus. If awakened, the stage is remembered merely as one of drowsiness; it is not described as sleep. But if not interrupted, the next stage is entered after about 15 minutes.

Stage 2. There is greater relaxation, and thoughts have a dream-like quality. The sleeper is unmistakedly asleep but can be wakened easily.

Stage 3. This stage usually occurs after 30 minutes of sleep. There is complete relaxation and the pulse rate slows as do most other bodily functions. Familiar noises such as a flushing toilet do not usually waken the sleeper. If undisturbed, the next stage follows.

Stage 4. The sleeper is relaxed, rarely moves, is difficult to waken, and is in a 'deep sleep'. If sleepwalking occurs, or if there is enuresis, it occurs at this stage. (Stages 3 and 4 collectively are known as 'slow wave sleep' because, on an electrocephalograph, they show as low frequency, synchronized waves.)

Stage 5. This is the stage of sleep during which most dreaming occurs. The eyes move rapidly back and forth giving the name Rapid Eye Movement (REM) sleep to this stage. Physiologically, REM sleep is remarkably similar to wakefulness.

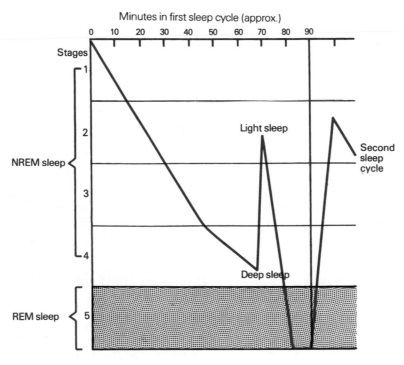

Fig. 14.1 A sleep cycle

the night and, as time passes, the episodes of NREM sleep become shorter and the periods of REM sleep become longer. A baby's sleep has more REM than NREM stages; with increasing age there is less REM sleep. Overall, young healthy adults tend to have sleep in the proportion of Stage 1, 4%; Stage 2, 50%; Stage 3, 10%; Stage 4, 13%; and Stage 5 — REM — 23% (Johns, 1984). If awakened during the REM stages people may report vivid dreams full of action. It is thought that dreams may promote psychological integration; it is as if they update memory and integrate emotionally meaningful experiences with those of the past. Since REM sleep is also observed in fetuses, perhaps its function could be described more simply as organising electrical circuits within the brain.

Although everyone's sleep has cycles, there is considerable variation in the length of time which people will spend sleeping and in what is considered 'sufficient' sleep.

The sufficiency of sleep

It is difficult to say what constitutes sufficient sleep; according to Johns (1984) the range of normal for adults is 3–12 hours, with an average sleep time of 7.25 hours per night. It would seem, however, that a sleep debt can be built up over time which can be compensated by a longer than usual sleep period. After deprivation, Stages 3 and 4 deficit is made up before REM sleep deficit, and for this reason some writers refer to NREM sleep as 'obligatory'.

In one study, in an attempt to discover the effects of sleep loss, experimental volunteers were kept awake for over a week at a time. As well as having difficulty in performing certain tasks it was found that they had a strong tendency to fall asleep yet seemed to be able to maintain semi-automatic activity such as walking while they slept; a point which highlights the danger of continuing to work while short of sleep at jobs which carry risk for the worker and for others. In some instances bizarre hallucinations also occurred after extreme sleep deprivation. It would seem, however, that the 'effects of sleep loss are not only evident after extreme deficits; fine effects can be detected after as little as 2 hours deprivation' (Wedderburn & Smith, 1980). To go to the other extreme, 'extra' sleep has not been shown to improve performance. A researcher, quoted by Wedderburn & Smith, gave people extra sleep after they already had a long night's sleep, and found that their performance on some tasks was worse after 'excessive' sleep.

It is difficult to say what 'lack of sleep' and 'extra sleep' mean because people have been identified who claim to require only about 2 hours of sleep each night and these healthy non-somniacs appear to enjoy a happy and constructive lifestyle (Meddis, 1977). It would seem that each person learns a circadian rhythm of sleep which there-

after is governed by an inbuilt 'biological clock'. During the day, however, there is a related cycle — the ultradian cycle — which appears to be related to restlessness.

Restlessness and resting

Even in non-sleep, alertness and drowsiness can come and go according to a 100-minute ultradian rhythm. Generally people are so involved in what they are doing that they are unaware of the rhythm; but on their own, in a dull or boring situation, it appears that individuals 'become more restless and less restless about every 100 minutes' (Oswald & Adam, 1983). It is interesting to consider the states of restlessness and resting.

The state of resting incorporates the art of relaxation, both physical and mental, although it is now a common belief that as the pace of living has greatly increased, there is less time for relaxation, and people have become less skilled in the art. In recent years, a growing interest in, for example, yoga and transcendental meditation may be indicative of a renewed public awareness of the value of relaxation and rest. Often the term relaxation is used to describe pleasurable activities such as sport or reading or art, usually as a change from the daily work routine but sometimes involving a great deal of activity. The relaxation of yoga however is claimed to be not a change but a resting period, a cessation of activity, a complete 'letting go' permitting refreshment of body and mind. Authorities on yoga believe that 20 minutes of yoga can bring greater benefits than hours of sleep (Lathlean, 1980).

So, the benefits of long, sound sleep are not entirely clear and even sleep researchers are by no means in agreement about the purpose of sleeping.

The function of sleep

In spite of all the information produced by sleep research over the years, the function of sleep is still not fully understood. Shapiro & Flanigan (1993) discuss the two most strongly supported theories:

- theories of restoration
- theories of conservation.

Restoration: Oswald & Adam (1983) support the theory of 'total restoration': i.e. that sleep promotes the restoration and growth of all body cells. It is slow wave sleep (Stages 3 and 4) which appears to be crucial in this regard and, being associated with recovery of the cerebrum (and possibly other tissues), it is the most indispensable part of our sleep.

The restorative theory of sleep is based on the knowledge that the adrenal gland releases adrenaline, noradrenaline and corticosteroids in large amounts during wakefulness but only in small quantities during sleep and, among other things, these hormones inhibit the formation of new protein in tissues. When asleep, the relative absence of adrenocorticosteroids, and the presence of other hormones, especially the growth hormone and testosterone, promote renewal of body tissue. Of course these activities are only part of a complex chemical and enzymatic system controlling the body's renewal and restoration. The processes involved, however, are not yet fully understood and it could even be that these restorative processes occur simply because the body is resting, rather than that the person is actually sleeping.

Some researchers, according to Shapiro & Flanigan (1993), have argued that it is the brain not the body which recuperates during sleep. Various hypotheses have been put forward to support the 'neurological restoration' theory of sleep.

Conservation: The other main theoretical stance is that the primary function of sleep is energy conservation: i.e. the energy expended during the day must be balanced by a recuperative period. The decreasing amount of sleep taken in old age might therefore be due to the decreasing metabolic rate and energy usage associated with advancing years (Canavan, 1984). Horne (1983) suggests that only specific portions of sleep (Stage 4 and about 50% of REM) are obligatory. Further, he suggests that this portion of sleep is essential only to brain functioning, while the rest of the body needs only

> **Box 14.2** Function of sleep
>
> 'In summary there are two main theories about the function of sleep—conservation of energy and restoration of energy . . . no one hypothesis completely explains the complexities and vagaries of sleep, but taken together they may form the foundation of the explanation for the indisputable need for sleep.'
>
> Shapiro & Flanigan (1993)

physical rest and feeding for restoration to take place. (See Box 14.2 for summary.)

Lifespan: relationship to the AL of sleeping

The lifespan component of the model (see Figure 14.2) is certainly relevant when considering sleeping. This AL is affected by age both in terms of duration and quality. The 'chronology of sleep', showing shifts in sleep patterns over the course of a lifetime, is outlined by Wardle (1986).

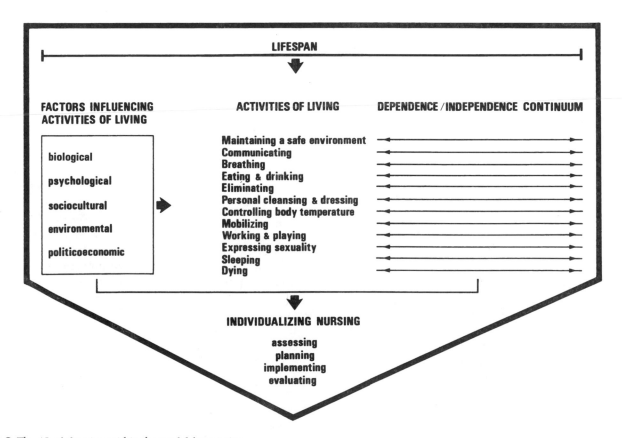

Fig. 14.2 The AL of sleeping within the model for nursing

Infancy and childhood

Not only do the young require more sleep than adults, as already stated, but their sleep has relatively more Stages 3 and 4 sleep in which the growth hormones are secreted, and this is not surprising in view of their rapid physical growth. They also have relatively more REM sleep presumably because of the vast amount of brain development and learning in the early years of life.

The sleep of the neonate is composed of almost equal amounts of REM and NREM sleep. Babies sleep for about 16 hours each day split into 6 to 8 sleep periods, but gradually there are longer periods of sleep, mostly at night, and longer periods awake.

Because sudden death in infancy (sudden infant death syndrome) usually occurs at night, the sleeping patterns of babies have been studied extensively in recent years. Retrospective studies in the UK and other countries revealed that there had been significantly fewer 'cot deaths' among babies who did not sleep in the prone position. Following a public campaign to instruct parents to put their babies to sleep lying on their back or side, the number of cot deaths decreased remarkably. Exactly how the sleeping position prevents or increases risk of sudden death is not clear, but the evidence is an important breakthrough in efforts to reduce cot deaths (Jaffa et al, 1993).

This threat of death during sleep is rare after the first year of life. By then, the infant's sleep electroencephalogram resembles an adult's. By the age of 4, the average child sleeps for 11 hours each night, perhaps with an additional short day-time nap. However, although babies and toddlers seem to spend quite a lot of time asleep, waking problems in young children are not uncommon. Richman (1983) found that about 20% of children in their second year waken regularly at night. The wakefulness can be related to factors within the child, or stress and tension within the family, but sometimes it is due to parental over-responsiveness to wakefulness which, in fact, reinforces the pattern. A useful discussion of the problems of sleeping difficulties among young children, and ways in which parents can prevent them, is provided by Keys (1988) on the basis of her experience as a health visitor.

Adolescence and adulthood

By the age of 15 years, most people have a sleep period which, on average, is of 7–8 hours' duration. However, during the 'growth spurt' in adolescence, there is a temporary increase in sleeping time. Not recognizing that this extra sleep is needed, parents may mistakenly accuse teenage children of laziness (Jaffa et al, 1993).

From adolescence onwards, REM averages about 20% of the time spent asleep, though the absolute amount of time spent sleeping tends to diminish gradually with age.

Healthy adolescents and young adults usually sleep so well that little will disturb them. However as these same sound sleepers become middle-aged they may complain of insufficient or broken sleep, especially the women (Oswald, 1980).

Old age

In general, the older person, according to Adam (1980) sleeps for a shorter period than the young and it is more broken by periods of wakefulness; it also contains relatively less REM sleep. Adam describes an interesting study of 212 healthy people aged 65–93, carried out in the USA, which found that by the age of 75, the older person (and no difference was found between males and females) spends more time in bed, though not necessarily asleep, and had more naps than younger people; and that by age 85, there was an increasing use of sedatives probably indicating more difficulty in falling asleep. In this study, 92% of these healthy elderly people believed that they got the right amount of sleep.

Swift & Shapiro (1993), however, emphasize that the overall pattern of research evidence indicates that dissatisfaction with the quality of sleep is common in the elderly age group and they contend that there is a need for a more circumspect and thoughtful approach to sleep problems in later life. More will be said on this later in the chapter.

Dependence/ independence in the AL of sleeping

Unlike some of the other ALs already discussed, each individual is independent for the actual activity of sleeping. Like the majority of the other ALs too, this component has a direct relationship with the lifespan component of the model. Babies, although helpless for many ALs, spend most of their time sleeping; and the elderly, at the opposite end of the lifespan and sometimes dependent for other ALs, also spend more time in bed, although not necessarily asleep, than younger adults. However, while the activity itself is independent, the provision of suitable environmental conditions for sleep may involve dependence on others.

The infant is dependent on others for maintaining a suitable temperature conducive to sleep, at least by use of clothing if not by control of atmospheric temperature. The safety of the environment is also controlled by others and there can be accidents, for example, because the bed is not safe, risking a fall, or because of the risk of smothering or because of danger from pets or hazardous toys.

Children and adolescents can also be dependent on others for sleep. If there is prolonged stress or tension in the family they may develop disturbed sleeping patterns (Richman, 1983) and when there is noise, for whatever reason, there may be difficulty in getting to sleep and the problem of getting back to sleep, once wakened. Jaffa et al (1993) identify a range of sleep problems in childhood which require parental or professional support, including problems provoked by anxiety (e.g. nightmares and night terrors) and disturbed sleep provoked by somatic symptoms (e.g. abdominal pain, irritation caused by eczema and cough or breathlessness due to asthma).

Adults may also be dependent on others, especially in relation to minimizing disturbance by excessive noise and particularly if on shiftwork. Perhaps the major concern about dependence in adulthood, however, is related to the use of hypnotic drugs (sleeping pills). A considerable number of adults, especially in industrialized countries, are anxious about difficulties with falling asleep and staying asleep for what they believe to be an insufficient period, and they resort to medications to enhance their sleep. Their widespread use creates problems not only in terms of cost (particularly if there is a national health service where they are free or heavily subsidized) but also in terms of creating long-term dependence. Many hypnotics, anyway, become less effective with regular use; studies of people who have taken sleep medications for months or years have found few beneficial effects in terms of either falling asleep or staying asleep (Canavan, 1984). Nonetheless, people taking these medications long-term often express satisfaction with the results despite undesirable side-effects, such as impaired day-time performance and lowered cognition (Swift & Shapiro, 1993). On the whole, however, long-term dependence on sleeping pills is not a satisfactory solution to a person's sleep problem, whatever its nature.

Factors influencing the AL of sleeping

Like all other ALs, sleeping is influenced by a variety of factors. In keeping with the relevant component of the model, these are described under the following headings — biological, psychological, sociocultural, environmental and politicoeconomic factors.

BIOLOGICAL

Sleeping is influenced by a variety of biological factors and, in turn, sleep/wake rhythms affect the physiology and biochemistry of the human body.

Circadian rhythms

The 24-hourly cycle is one to which most species synchronize their bodily rhythms. During a 24-hour period there is a cycle of many physiological functions such as heart rate, metabolic rate, respiratory rate and body temperature all tending to reach maximum values during the late afternoon and early evening, and minimum values in the early hours of the morning (Hawkins & Armstrong-Esther, 1978).

Perhaps this would be expected. Most people are active during the day and asleep at night. There is evidence that these internally controlled rhythms are timed to synchronize with external cues and when the harmony is upset, for example by travelling rapidly across time zones, there is desynchronization which manifests itself as fatigue, malaise, lassitude and inability to make effective decisions — the syndrome known as jet-lag. The period varies with the individual, but it usually takes about 3 to 7 days to correct jet-lag and get body time and sleep time back in harmony (Smith & Wedderburn, 1980).

Waterhouse (1993) points out that the constant association which usually exists between sleep/wake rhythms is 'biologically adaptive', with 'rhythmic humans' integrating with a 'rhythmic environment' (i.e. active during the day and partially 'shut down' during the night).

While in tune with this general rhythm, the population as a whole tends to be divided between early risers ('larks') and late bedders ('owls'). In noting this, Brugne (1994) refers to the example of an opinion poll taken in a monastery in Southern France: it showed that exactly 50% of the monks would prefer a longer morning service and the other 50% a longer evening service!

Physical exercise

Children enjoy a great deal of exercise during their waking hours, and although overstimulation may, on occasion, prevent them from falling asleep quickly, exercise can raise body temperature which, in turn, may contribute to their sleep having relatively longer periods of Stages 3 and 4 sleep when the growth hormones are secreted in large amounts.

It has been shown too that after exercise athletes have more Stages 3 and 4 sleep, and even adults taking more exercise than usual will secrete more growth hormone from the pituitary gland during the succeeding sleep period, thus facilitating maximal protein synthesis and restoration of the body cells (Oswald & Adam, 1983).

Food and drink

Eating certain foods and drinking certain beverages is also said to affect sleep. There is a popular belief, for example, that cheese and coffee cause disturbed sleep.

Although there does not seem to be much evidence about cheese perhaps there is some justification for advocating decaffeinated coffee. It is now well-known that caffeine is an alerting chemical and, because it has a long half life (5 hours), it is not just coffee taken in the evening that is the problem but also the accumulated intake, hence six cups a day is advised as the maximum (Stradling, 1993). Indeed, two cupfuls of coffee (300 mg caffeine) were found to cause disturbed sleep in old people whereas a milk and cereal drink, Horlicks, led to less wakefulness when compared with nights when a placebo pill was taken by those who participated in this research (Brezinova & Oswald, 1972). However Oswald & Adam (1983) subsequently concluded that although milk and proprietary food drinks, being easily digestible sources of nourishment, probably are helpful in inducing sleep their effect should not be exaggerated.

The effect of a change in usual food and fluid intake at bedtime may be more important than the actual type of food/drink taken. Again, the notion of rhythmicity (or regularity) is apparently linked with promoting sleep. Indeed, although still an untested hypothesis, it has been suggested that regular timing of meals will help to promote readjustment of the body clock after disruption, such as jet lag (Waterhouse, 1993).

Some people consider that alcohol helps them to sleep and, indeed, alcohol is a brain sedative. This belief may be true if alcohol is taken in moderation, especially if related to a pattern of fluid intake as a bedtime beverage, but some years ago it was shown that alcohol produces a lighter sleep pattern with more awakenings (Whitfield, 1982). As with other short-acting sedatives, the effect of the alcohol wears off and 'rebound arousal' occurs and the amount of REM sleep increases, resulting (at least for some people) in recurrent awakening with tachycardia, sweating and headache (Stradling, 1993). Probably for similar reasons, it has been found that change in weight affects sleep. As obese people lose weight, they sleep less; and when patients with anorexia nervosa are regaining weight, they sleep longer and REM sleep is increased (Adam, 1980).

Snoring

Snoring may affect sleep, although it is the listener who is kept awake. Snoring may be indicative of a number of pathological conditions so should not be dismissed lightly but it may have no known cause or cure. Usually any mention of snoring is greeted with hilarity but in fact, as recognized many years ago, it can disrupt a sleeping partnership and become a justification for divorce (Felstein, 1979). Later research suggested that one type of snoring — sleep apnoea — can also be dangerous (Dopson, 1988).

In sleep apnoea, there is loud snoring and 'breathing pauses'. In view of the potential danger (an association with increased risk of myocardial infarction and stroke has been reported: Shapiro & Dement, 1993), it is recommended that the condition should be recognized and treated. Night nurses are in a position to diagnose the condition and should let the doctor know if a patient snores loudly or has breathing difficulties at night. Douglas (1993) warns that failure to diagnose the sleep apnoea/hypopnoea syndrome leads to unnecessary impairment of the quality of life and to avoidable deaths.

PSYCHOLOGICAL

The individual's psychological status is linked to sleeping in a number of ways.

Mood

Mood can be considered as a continuum with excitement at one pole and depression at the other. Transient insomnia caused by excitement has been experienced by most people and may not cause undue distress. The sleeplessness associated with depression may however be severe, and continue over time.

The depressed person can lie awake for hours dwelling on unhappy themes of hopelessness, and when sleep does come, is easily wakened, only to resume thoughts of rejection and failure, or even suicide. The primary characteristic of sleep change in depression is early morning wakening; indeed, it is a major diagnostic feature. Depression is common in old age and, often undetected, insomnia should be considered as a possible indicator. Dementia, also largely a condition of old age, is also known to cause sleep problems (Swift & Shapiro, 1993). With reductions in slow wave and REM sleep, dementia brings increased wakefulness during the night; and, indeed, in the late stages of dementia there may be breakdown in the circadian rhythm altogether.

Anxiety

Perhaps worry and anxiety rather than excitement and depression are the most common disturbers of sleep. It would seem that people who are worried or dissatisfied with their daytime lives are often worried and dissatisfied with their sleep. Almost everyone has had periods of anxiety and apprehension at some point in their lives, over examinations or employment interviews, for example. However Oswald (1980) contended that the individual should be 'protected from over-treatment'. After all, a certain amount of anxiety is inevitable in the process of living.

With children, however, sleep problems which appear to be caused by anxiety should not be ignored. Night terrors, which occur in about 3% of children, apparently increase at times of stress and difficulty in getting to sleep or frequent wakening may be signs of anxiety about marital/domestic disharmony or sexual abuse or problems at school (Jaffa et al, 1993).

Dreams

Dreams are believed by some people to have enormous psychological significance (Hearne, 1986). Dreams certainly have a strange fascination for man. At one time it was thought that the soul departed from the body during sleep in order to mingle with supernatural beings who would provide guidance about the future. The possible symbolism of dreams has also been given considerable credence and reinforced by writers such as Freud and Jung. Cohen (1979) maintains that 'the heart (and soul) of classic sleep research was to attempt to ... establish correlations between specific physiological events and dream characteristics'.

It is now known that dreaming occurs mainly, although not exclusively, during REM sleep. The researchers assure us that everyone dreams but most are not remembered. The rate of forgetting is remarkably fast. Subjects in the Sleep Research Laboratory in Edinburgh who were wakened during REM sleep recalled a dream in about 80% of cases; wakened 5 minutes after REM sleep, there was only fragmentary recall; aroused 10 minutes later, there was scarcely any recall. So anyone who wakens up recalling a vivid dream, has probably surfaced out of REM sleep. Dreams themselves can be frightening, some are bizarre, some are amusing; most are interesting to recount; indeed not uncommonly, dreams are the substance of art, music, drama, and literature.

More recently, interest has increased in the relationship between dreams and illness; and Katz & Shapiro (1993) note that current research is indicating that dreams may reflect the presence of organic disease, even cause or precipitate organic disease (e.g. migraine, cardiac arrhythmias, nocturnal asthma), and serve as a marker for the potential of an individual to develop psychosomatic illness.

Beliefs

Whatever the 'science' of sleep, and whatever the quantity or quality of sleep, the psychological effect of wakening up refreshed or unrefreshed determines a person's belief about being a good or bad sleeper; in other words, assessment of sleep is largely subjective.

SOCIOCULTURAL

Sociocultural factors also influence sleeping. For example they will determine where a person sleeps and with whom. In Western cultures, it is usual to sleep in a bed which is raised up from the floor but in Japan the bedroll on the floor is traditional; and in some nomadic, ethnic groups it is usual to sleep on the ground in the open, or in a tent or in a hammock.

In Western cultures, it is usual for a husband and wife or a co-habiting couple to sleep together in one bed, but most other people sleep alone. However in other cultures it is not uncommon for several members of the family (or extended family) to sleep in the same 'sleeping-space' and if they do sleep singly or in couples, it may not be in a segregated personal bedroom; it could be in a room common to the entire family.

Cultural differences can also be identified with regard to what is worn for sleeping. Nomadic Eskimos, for example, wear the same clothes during the day and at night; in other cultures, nightdresses or pyjamas are worn, and for some people are a means of expressing sexuality; for other people the accepted norm is to sleep in the nude.

Differences across the globe are also to be found in relation to use of medication for sleeping. Hypnotics are among the most widely prescribed drugs in Western society. The impact of sleep disorders on society also appears to vary across the world, the cost in the US having been calculated as billions of dollars a year as a result of medical care, loss of productivity due to absence from work and admission of elderly people to hospital when sleep problems become too much for carers (Shapiro & Dement, 1993).

Some of these sociocultural differences related to sleeping may seem strange but with the ease of international travel and the popularity of television-viewing, most people now know much more about the effect that social and cultural characteristics have on the AL of sleeping.

ENVIRONMENTAL

Sleep can be affected by a number of environmental factors. Sleep tends to come more easily in a familiar environment — a cool, quiet dark room in surroundings which are well known, with personal belongings at hand and so on.

Safety

The safety of the environment is also important. A high bed, where there is difficulty getting in and out and anxiety of falling, may disturb the sleep of an elderly or disabled person; and the sleep of parents temporarily may be affected when a child changes from sleeping in a cot to sleeping in a bed. People who know they are sleep-walkers may not be able to fall asleep unless they are reassured that windows have been closed, and that objects which potentially could cause accidents have been removed from the immediate environment; indeed some sleep-walkers find some means of attaching themselves to the bed so that they will wake up rather than sleep walk. People affected by unfamiliar surroundings, such as a hotel or hospital ward, may have to reassure themselves by checking the fire precautions and the siting of fire escape doors.

Noise

Environmental noise may or may not affect sleep. Again familiarity with the environment allows many people to sleep despite, for example, the noise of a nearby factory or a busy thoroughfare or an aircraft flight path. Yet these same people may have difficulty falling asleep in a strange environment perhaps because of the sound of the waves on a beach or even by the excessive quietness of a rural setting. Night shift workers may have major complaints about noise when they are attempting to sleep during the day; although if habitually on night shift, many seem to learn to ignore background noise.

Ambient temperature

Room temperature may affect the ability to fall asleep and to remain asleep. The body temperature falls during sleep; there is a slight normal lowering between the hours of 0200 and 0600 which is not surprising because, during sleep, there is minimal functioning of the various body systems. However, any further lowering of temperature usually wakens the sleeper, as indeed does any increase.

Perhaps to be expected, the climate has an influence, and where there are extremes of climate, attempts are made to control and modify the indoor temperature. In hot climates, bedrooms increasingly are equipped with air-conditioning systems; some are sophisticated and expensive; others primitive, although sometimes amazingly effective. Likewise in cold climates, insulation and central heating systems are used or some other means of providing heat and warmth.

As detailed in Chapter 10, the physiological control of body temperature is less efficient in children and the elderly so it is recommended that bedroom temperatures should not fall below 18°C during the night. For elderly people who cannot afford to heat a bedroom during winter, having the bed moved into the heated livingroom is suggested; wearing socks and a hat in bed is further advice given to the elderly in order to prevent hypothermia. A more detailed account of measures which elderly people can take to stay warm, thus avoiding hypothermia, was given in the chapter on the AL of controlling body temperature (Ch. 10).

It is interesting that latitude does not seem to alter sleeping. Within the Arctic Circle, the inhabitants sleep similar hours to us despite experiencing unending day-light in the summer and months of darkness during the winter. In countries where an afternoon siesta is the norm, the people sleep again at night.

Space

The effect of space and weightlessness on sleep is still being researched. During the last two decades there have been spectacular advances in space exploration and data are being collected about the effect of this somewhat novel environment on human sleeping patterns.

POLITICOECONOMIC

It may not strike one immediately that the AL of sleeping is influenced by politicoeconomic factors. However any consideration of where people sleep will usually involve housing or a shelter of some kind and, certainly in Western culture, this will be related to economic status.

Housing and overcrowding

The size of the house will influence whether family members have their own bedroom or a shared one, their own bed or a shared one. Some people, however, because of low earning power (for whatever reason), may have to cope with a living space which is grossly overcrowded and the family may have to sleep in the room in which they have lived and cooked all day; there is no choice. For children in particular, unfavourable housing conditions which necessitate sharing a bed or, at least, a room with siblings of varying ages will exacerbate if not directly cause sleep disturbances in childhood (Jaffa et al, 1993).

Homelessness

In the UK, as in many other countries, the number of homeless people has increased in recent times. For the homeless, even in a cold climate, sleeping 'rough', exposed to unfavourable weather conditions which endanger health, is certainly not conducive to satisfactory sleep. Where the government or voluntary agencies make provision for such people, it is usually in the form of communal sleeping accommodation at low cost and, although better than nothing, it is not the ideal sleeping environment for adults.

Shift work

It is necessary to any country's economy that some people work shifts in order to ensure continuity in factories and service industries which must operate 'around the clock'. During the last few decades, there have been numerous studies about shift work and its effect on sleep. As a rule the 24-hour biological clock makes man fall asleep at night and awaken in the morning, and this reflects the individual's normal body rhythms, with their characteristic low level of arousal at night and higher level during the day. However night shift removes sleeping from the night sequence and out of harmony with body time.

Much of the early research on sleep and nightshift work concluded that the body clock would gradually be reset over a period of about 7 nights and then, following a spell of night work, there would be a delayed return to normal. However results of later studies quoted in Smith & Wedderburn (1980) and covering a wide range of variables (including deep body temperature, potassium excretion, adrenalin excretion, blood pressure and reaction time) all show that experienced shift workers demonstrate a flatter than normal night shift curve of these readings on the first night, and that this is retained without much deviation over subsequent consecutive night shifts. It is replaced by a typical day curve on the first full day without night work. So the body clocks of shift workers remain set to 'real' time. Smith & Wedderburn suggest that these findings became available because the researchers were able to collect more data; instead of using one or two readings each night, as in the older studies, they used body-worn microchip recorders which collected continuous readings of several variables. They conclude that although shift workers get used to night work, this is because they 'become better at handling the contradiction of being biologically geared to day activity while being required to work at night, and not because they reset their body clocks!'

Typically the duration of daytime sleeps after night shifts are short and often, although feeling fatigued, it is difficult to fall asleep. So a sleep debt builds up. Although it is well recognized that shift workers often suffer from chronic fatigue and disturbed sleep, not to forget the inconvenience to family and social life, no clear solutions have been found to ease the problems. Recent research, however, as noted by Waterhouse (1993) has suggested that a short sleep period in the middle of a night shift increases later performance and apparently helps to stabilize the circadian rhythms, thus easing adaptation to normal daily routines on rest days.

Does this evidence suggest that night nurses of the future will be encouraged to retire to bed after 'lunch'?! The problem of shift work in nursing continues to be an issue of concern and controversy. Brown (1988) examined various shift patterns in nursing. She notes recommendations made by an Australian scientist who, on the basis of research which revealed a high error and accident rate among people who worked an early morning shift which followed a late afternoon/evening shift, considers this combination should be avoided and, instead, the shift rotas should move forwards (i.e. earlies, lates, nights, off) in sympathy with the body's 'running clock'.

By the time this book is published, the outcome of research commissioned by the UK Department of Health into shift systems should be available. Barton (1994) reports on the preliminary work to date. The survey conducted in England and Wales found 122 different shift systems operating in 182 hospitals. There was, however, not as much actual variation in shift hours and patterns as this implies and Barton commends the trend towards flexibility and the licence given to individual nurses to choose shift hours best suited to their domestic lives.

Excessive working hours

The problems of shift work are also of concern to doctors but, in medicine, the greater concern is with interruptions of sleep and lack of sleep due to their long working week. In a study of young hospital doctors in Cambridge, UK and New York, and reported by Oswald & Adam (1983), it was shown that sleep loss caused them to be more easily irritated; they could not react to complexity and could only think of one thing at a time. Such impairment of functioning can affect the safety of patients as well as the doctors themselves.

More recently, the issue of junior doctors' working hours has become a matter of public as well as professional debate in the UK. Junior hospital doctors pressed for a reduction in working hours and the Government agreed that this should happen. There was concern, however, that a reduction even to 72 hours per week, although substantial, would not be adequate. Wilkie (1989) reported that, although junior doctors in the United States only work 36-hour shifts, a leading sleep researcher considers this to be overlong for safety. He emphasizes the need for reduction in the length of time continuously without sleep, rather than overall reduction in hours.

Such rules apply to pilots as Durnford (1988) outlines, arguing that the reasoning pertains equally to the situation of doctors. Like pilots, there are certain occupational groups — another example being long-distance lorry drivers — which have to comply with rules and regulations which limit working hours. The International Labour Organisation has recommendations regarding working hours, but they are not always implemented.

Whether long working hours actually adversely affect health remains a matter of debate (Harrington, 1994). There is clear evidence, however, that circadian rhythms are disrupted by night shifts and extended work schedules, with fatigue and sleep problems occurring as a result.

Sleep-related vehicle accidents

Tiredness certainly increases the risk of an accident while driving, and recent research (Horne & Reyner,

1995) has provided evidence from the UK which fits with the trends worldwide. Sleep-related accidents (for example, the driver falling asleep at the wheel or admitting inattention due to tiredness) were found to account for a considerable proportion of vehicle accidents (over 20% on midland motorways). Further, it was found that a 'surge' occurred between two and three o'clock in the morning, one of the periods of lowest density traffic. The researchers point out that, because of the profound influence of the circadian rhythm, sleepiness or sleep-related vehicle accidents can occur after even a short period of driving; and they call for more public awareness of the dangers of driving while sleepy.

Individualizing nursing for the AL of sleeping

Individualizing nursing is the final component of the model. From the foregoing discussion, it is evident that there are many dimensions in each component of the model which help one to describe how a particular person develops individuality in the AL of sleeping (see Box 14.3).

Sleeping is such a complex activity and highly sensitive to disturbance, so perhaps it is to be expected that when a person is ill, some problems will be encountered, even transiently, in relation to this AL. However, as refreshing sleep is considered to be therapeutic, it is important for the nurse to know about the person's usual habits in relation to sleeping so that this knowledge can be used to ensure that everything possible is done to promote normal sleep. As Carter (1985) commented, 'assisting patients to fulfil their individual sleep requirements would seem to be an important aspect of patient care for nurses'.

ASSESSING THE INDIVIDUAL IN THE AL

In order to individualize nursing, it is necessary to assess the AL of sleeping in so far as it is relevant to the particular person's circumstances. For a patient in hospital, assessing involves observing the patient; acquiring information about the patient's sleeping habits (partly by asking appropriate questions, partly by listening to the patient and/or relatives); and using relevant information from the patient's records. The nurse would be seeking answers to the following questions:

- when does the individual usually sleep?
- what factors influence the individual's sleep?
- how well does the individual sleep?
- has the individual any long-standing difficulties

Box 14.3 Assessing the individual in the AL of sleeping

Lifespan: effect on sleeping
- Length/frequency/type of sleep
  - in infancy and childhood
  - in adolescence and adulthood
  - in old age

Dependence/independence in sleeping
- Infants
- Children and adolescents
- Adults and elderly people

Factors influencing sleeping
- Biological
  - circadian rhythms
  - physical exercise
  - food and drink
  - snoring
- Psychological
  - mood (especially depression)
  - anxiety
  - dreams
  - knowledge about sleep
  - beliefs about sleep
- Sociocultural
  - sleeping space
  - type of bed/bedding
  - own/shared bed
  - use of hypnotic drugs
- Environmental
  - safety
  - noise
  - ambient temperature
- Politicoeconomic
  - housing and overcrowding
  - homelessness
  - shift work
  - excessive working hours

with sleeping and if so, how have these been coped with?
- what problems, if any, does the individual have at present with sleeping or seems likely to develop?

Of course, the nurse does not necessarily ask these actual questions because much of the information can be acquired in the course of discussing other topics included in an admission assessment interview and, later, in a less formal way by conversing with the patient. However it is achieved, Manian (1988) advocates proper assessment of a patient's sleep within the framework of the nursing process. There may be benefits in incorporating a 'sleep history' since, as Clapin-French (1986) pointed out in relation to long-term elderly patients, this tends to be a neglected aspect of history-taking in nursing assessment. A sleep diary is a particularly useful way of obtaining information about a child's sleeping and waking pattern, and the parents' responses (Jaffa et al, 1993).

IDENTIFYING ACTUAL AND POTENTIAL PROBLEMS

The collected information can then be examined to identify any actual and potential problems with the AL of sleeping. Realistic goals can then be set in conjunction with the patient (or the parents, in the case of a child) to prevent potential problems from becoming actual ones; to alleviate or solve the actual problems; or to help the patient cope with those which cannot be alleviated or solved.

Keeping in mind what the patient can and cannot do independently, the nursing interventions to achieve the set goals can then be selected according to circumstances and available resources. These interventions should be written on the nursing plan along with the date on which evaluation will be carried out in order to discern whether or not the stated goals are achieved.

Of course, other professional groups such as doctors, physiotherapists and dietitians are usually also involved in the patient's care and it is important to ensure that the total care of the patient is discussed and mutually agreed. On the Nursing Plan proforma suggested for use with the model (Appendix 1), there is a page for appropriate entries of this type in order to indicate the relationship between nursing interventions derived from medical/other prescription and nurse-initiated interventions. In relation to the AL of sleeping, one area of medically-prescribed nursing intervention relates to the administration of hypnotic drugs, if prescribed by the doctor.

There are various circumstances and conditions which can be responsible for changing a person's dependence/ independence status for the AL of sleeping and for creating problems with sleep. As far as nursing is concerned, the problems of sleep in hospital are of particular relevance and these are discussed mainly in terms of problems arising from the change of environment and routine which hospitalization precipitates. Then, under the heading of 'change of dependence/independence status', the problems of sleeplessness and restlessness are discussed; and the problem of dependence on drugs for sleeping is addressed. Finally, although not strictly a 'sleep' problem, altered consciousness is discussed. Patients' problems with this AL are grouped, therefore, under three headings:

- Change of environment and routine
- Change of dependence/independence status
- Altered consciousness.

CHANGE OF ENVIRONMENT AND ROUTINE

Admission to hospital

It is well recognized that hospitalization is disruptive to sleep. While this may not cause any lasting problems, lack of sleep is not helpful to recovery from illness or surgery and, furthermore, it can add to the misery of being unwell and in hospital. An appreciation of the causes of sleep disruption in hospital will help nurses to minimize these and to promote optimal conditions for each patient's usual sleeping habits and routines to be maintained.

There are many reasons for a newly-admitted patient to experience sleep problems. One major reason may be the strange environment of a hospital ward. Whatever their previous sleeping arrangements, many patients are still admitted into an open 'Nightingale-type' ward; some into two-, four- or six-bedded bays, recesses or rooms; and only a minority may have single rooms. In many instances a patient has no choice about sleeping in the presence of others. Other forced changes in routine and other factors which may cause sleep problems for hospital patients are discussed below, including:

- hospital beds and mattresses
- hospital bedding and nightwear
- pre-sleep routine
- sleeping posture
- ward temperature and light
- noise at night
- disorientation
- disturbance of circadian rhythm
- pain
- medical illness.

Hospital beds and mattresses

The hospital bed Compared with home, the hospital bed itself may be very different. All patients are admitted into a single bed, yet many will have been used to sleeping in a double bed. The majority of hospital beds are higher than the divan type of bed used in most homes although new models can be mechanically adjusted. If the height cannot be adjusted, this can be anxiety-producing for those who are accustomed to getting up to go to the toilet during the night; the nurse can help by establishing whether the patient would prefer to summon assistance or to have at hand a commode, bedpan or urinal. This information would be written on the nursing plan so that all staff would be informed. Where adjustable height beds are in use, it is important for nurses to remember to lower them before the patient goes to sleep.

Some beds are specially designed, for example some are adjustable so that the sitting position can be maintained during sleep. If it is necessary for the patient to adopt this position because of severe dyspnoea, it is often a relief to be so well supported, and although not a natural position for sleeping, the patient usually adapts reasonably well. Other special beds which may be used by patients include: air, low air loss, water, sand, fluidized sand, mud, bead, net suspension, Ko-Ro, Stryker and flotation beds. Sleeping on these types of beds is 'different' and initially there is a period of adaptation until the patient becomes gradually used to the change. The objective in using them is dispersal of body weight over a greater surface area for the prevention of pressure sores (p. 245). The patient needs to understand why such a bed is necessary and should be encouraged to report any problems with it.

Hospital mattresses Most people's ideal bed includes careful selection of a mattress and the choice can be very personal. Hospital mattresses can be sufficiently different to interfere with sleep, particularly on the first few nights. Horsehair mattresses continued to be used in hospitals long after most people no longer had these at home, and they were found to be a particular cause of sleep disturbance in a study of patients' sleep on surgical wards (Closs, 1988). Plastic covers on mattresses and/or pillows were also a source of complaint among patients involved in that research; Closs recommended that favourable consideration be given to the waterproof, but vapour-permeable, materials which are now available.

That study's findings about patients' dissatisfaction with hospital beds, however, were not novel; a Royal Commission on the National Health Service (1978) reported that one in eight patients found their hospital beds uncomfortable.

Hospital bedding and nightwear Hospital bedding, too, can differ from that used at home and patients who experience such a difference may require some time for adjustment. Nowadays many people favour one single cover for ease of bed-making, such as a quilt or a duvet. However some people like to feel the weight of bedclothes and therefore choose to use conventional sheets and blankets. Wherever possible, arrangements should be made to interfere as little as possible with patients' preferences and thereby provide the greatest possibility of continuance of good sleeping habits. To this end an increasing number of hospitals offer patients the choice between a duvet and conventional bedding.

Nightwear provided by the hospital for all patients is no longer considered to be good practice because, just as day clothes are personal and important to one's self-image, so are night clothes and any change can therefore interfere with sleep. In some cases where night clothes might become soiled with excreta or vomit, it may be helpful for the patient to be offered hospital nightwear. In the interests of maintaining morale, it is important that the garments provided are attractive as well as comfortable.

Pre-sleep routine

Each patient has acquired a pre-sleep routine with an individualized sequence which is necessary for comfort and conducive to relaxation and getting to sleep. Many patients continue to be capable of carrying out that routine while in hospital and they should be encouraged to do so. Information from dependent patients, or their relatives if patients are not able to give it, will help nurses develop a nursing plan which includes pre-sleep routines along lines with which the patient is familiar.

Obviously, in a hospital ward, the routines of individual patients have to be compatible with communal living and care requirements but, sometimes perhaps, nursing routines unnecessarily compromise those of importance to individual patients. The inevitable hospital routine which dictates that patients retire early to bed (and wake up earlier) does seem to have detrimental consequences, in particular contributing to the increased time which patients take to get to sleep in hospital compared with home (Closs, 1988).

Sleeping posture

Depending on the cause for admission to hospital, and the patient's treatment, a changed sleeping posture may be necessary, and help may be required to adapt to the change. For example, in the absence of a special bed when a patient has to be nursed sitting up it may be more comfortable to use an adjustable height bed-table with a pillow on it, on which to rest with flexed arms, thus ensuring the best conditions for breathing and sleeping.

Lying supine over a length of time for any reason can cause a feeling of fullness in the abdomen; this can be due to the upper abdominal organs resting against the diaphragm, so slight raising of the head of the bed may allow the organs to slide down a little, relieving the pressure and permitting sleep.

Patients with a lower limb on traction are usually nursed in a high bed with the bedclothes arranged in two sections around the elevated limb; such patients may feel more comfortable if a pillow is placed close to each side of the body on which they can rest their arms.

Research has shown that both snoring and sleep apnoea (temporary cessation of breathing during sleep) occur more commonly among people who sleep flat on their backs (Koskenvuo et al, 1985). Nurses could help alleviate these problems by encouraging patients to adopt alternative positions for sleeping.

Whatever recommendation is made regarding posture during sleep, it should be written on the nursing plan so that all staff are informed of these measures.

Ward temperature and light

Temperature People who have sleeping problems are

often highly sensitive to the environmental temperature. Sometimes however, it is difficult for the nurse to exert any control over local conditions. For example, for safety reasons in high-rise hospitals, the windows on the upper floors may not be able to be opened, so natural ventilation is not possible. Also the heating or cooling system is often controlled centrally and not all radiators, if there are radiators, have individual heat control mechanisms. In such circumstances, an immediate solution is to make adjustments to night attire and to bedding if patients feel they are too hot or too cold; or to use cooling fans, or adequately covered hot water bottles or an electric blanket.

Increased body temperature (pyrexia) also leads to disturbed sleep. Active management of pyrexial patients, perhaps by administering an anti-pyrexial agent, might assist in promoting sleep along with other temperature-reducing interventions (p. 276).

Light Many people are very sensitive to and disturbed by even a low intensity of light for sleeping. Night lighting in the newer hospitals is well dimmed and arranged near floor level so that it is below the eye level of patients in bed. If a nurse decides to help a patient to sleep by shading a nearby light, fire safety factors should be complied with; otherwise drawing bed curtains or using a mobile screen may help to intercept the disturbing light.

Noise at night

In the last few decades, almost everyone has had to become more tolerant to an increase in the noise level from a variety of environmental sources; the term 'noise pollution' is now used and was discussed in Chapter 4 in relation to maintaining a safe environment. But even people who appear to enjoy bombardment by noise when well, can rarely tolerate it when they are ill. Certainly, nurses should be aware of the fact that noise is one of the most important causes of sleep disturbance for hospital patients, a fact reinforced by the findings of the research study conducted by Closs (1988); noise emerged as the most frequent of all causes of night-time awakening in patients' reports of sleep problems in hospital.

The night nurse's work should be pre-planned so that noisy trolleys are not needed in the ward after patients have settled for the night, and any procedures which must be performed during the night should be carried out as quietly as possible. Empty beds for possible new admissions can be near the ward entrance so that their occupation will cause as little disturbance to as few patients as possible. The same applies if the death of a patient is expected during the night. These are just some of the feasible ways in which nurses can attempt to minimize noise at night in the interests of patients' sleep.

It may be sensible, however, to accept that a certain level of noise is inevitable in hospitals. Perhaps patients should be provided with earplugs. Haddock (1994)

reports promising results from a small-scale study: patients found the earplugs comfortable and there were indications that earplugs reduced their perceptions of noise.

Disorientation

When a patient becomes disorientated at night transfer to a single room may be helpful. This allows adequate lighting to be put on (this simulates daytime and lessens shadows which may be the cause of distress); and staff can speak normally (as opposed to whispering which is thought to increase the patient's confusion). On the other hand, the patient may be more confused by the move, in which case re-orientation in the ward may be more practical; a short period of disturbance there being preferable for all concerned to a longer one in a side ward.

In an intensive care unit (ICU), however, it is much more difficult to prevent, and to manage, disturbance during the night. Disorientation appears to be a common problem in ICUs and Briggs (1991) outlines some practical steps which nursing staff can take to reduce patient's risk of perceptual deprivation and sensory overload.

Disturbance of circadian rhythm

It is useful to remember that there are some people admitted to hospital who have been working on night shift and they may have problems with sleeping because of their altered sleeping pattern. Also travellers who have passed through time zones can become ill or have an accident and may arrive in hospital with altered circadian rhythms due to jet lag.

A study done by Armstrong-Esther & Hawkins (1982) tentatively suggested that some elderly people may have lost their physical responsiveness to light and dark and come to rely more on social synchronizers. Once these are disturbed by admission to hospital, the elderly patient may have no reliable cues and goes into a state of internal desynchronization. This state in which the body's rhythms are out of synchrony may be the cause of sleep disturbance, as well as confusion and incontinence, which indeed are often observed in the elderly after admission to hospital.

Nurses should be alert to these possible variants when gathering information about a patient's sleeping habits in order to assist adaptation to the change in environment and routine which occurs on admission to hospital.

Pain

Of the many factors which may interfere with sleep and rest in hospital, pain is a particular source of sleep disturbance. Closs (1988) found, in her study of sleep in surgical wards, that pain was cited along with noise as being the

Box 14.4 Hospitalization disrupts sleep

Closs J (1988) Patients' sleep-wake rhythms in hospital. *Nursing Times* (Occasional Paper), 84, 1, 48–50 and 84, 2, 54–55.

Summary
'It is evident from the available literature that, for a considerable proportion of patients, hospital admission causes disruption of the normal sleep-wake cycle, and the functions of sleep should be understood (by nurses) in order to comprehend the adverse effects of this disruption. Although REM (rapid eye movement) sleep has no clear function, SWS (slow wave sleep) appears to be associated with restorative processes such as secretion of growth hormone, and peak rate of mitosis and cell replacement. Total sleep deprivation results in psychological disturbances such as reduced motivation, irritability, confusion and paranoia. All of these are detrimental to recovery from illness or surgery. . . . . In view of the increasing evidence which suggests that sleep enhances healing processes, it may be of considerably greater importance than is generally appreciated, that certain patients receive an optimum quantity and quality of sleep, preferably following as closely as possible their normal 'home sleep' patterns.'

main factors perceived as disturbing to sleep in hospital. Pain was mentioned by 127 patients of the 200 questioned, with a further 45 who reported other kinds of discomfort (such as cramp, nausea and indigestion). Closs recommended that closer attention should be paid to night-time pain management, both in terms of administration of analgesia as well as the use of non-medical methods of pain control and sleep promotion. (See Box 14.4.)

One type of pain which, rightly or wrongly, is sometimes associated with sleep is cramp. The patient wakens during a sleep period complaining of intense pain in the foot or calf. The surrounding muscles are tense and rigid and when the foot is affected there is inability to move, usually the big toe. It is thought to be due to interference with the blood supply; alternate raising of the leg above the level of the bed, and letting it dangle at the side below the level of the bed helps to drain the blood from, and take fresh blood into the area, giving relief. Some people find that pressing the foot on a cold surface relieves the spasm, but there does not appear to be any documented evidence that this is so. It is best for the nurse to find out whether or not the patient has had cramp previously and if so, how it was coped with. Medical management of night cramps may include prescription of oral quinine.

Medical illness

Certain medical conditions can impair sleep and nurses must be aware of this when assessing patients, identifying problems and individualizing nursing. An account of sleep problems in patients with medical illness is provided by Shapiro et al (1993). Among the medical conditions which significantly alter sleep are end stage renal disease (causing profound sleep disturbance due to periodic involuntary limb movements), rheumatoid arthritis (characterized by fragmented sleep during exacerbations of illness) and neuromuscular conditions (e.g. Parkinson's disease in which there is activation of muscle tone).

CHANGE OF DEPENDENCE/INDEPENDENCE STATUS

It is clear from the above discussion that even people who would normally be considered 'good' sleepers, may require some assistance to sleep when in hospital. But there are also people who suffer from chronic sleep problems and, whether in hospital or at home, they may be dependent on others (including nurses) for understanding, assistance and advice. The problems of sleeplessness and restlessness are discussed below. Then the problem of dependence on drugs for sleeping is also addressed in this section.

Sleeplessness

Inability to get to sleep Some people habitually take as long as 90 minutes to get to sleep. Provided that they are not unduly anxious about it and that it is not interfering with their health, there is no need for treatment. As Berrios & Shapiro (1993) point out, there are many factors which can disrupt the initiation of sleep: for example, changes in diet, anxiety, high levels of arousal, obsessive thoughts and environmental disturbances. Helping a person to identify the cause(s) of delayed sleep may be sufficient 'treatment' and, in many cases, the problem may be a transitory one and nothing more. In the hospital situation, however, should patients remain wakeful for a long period, they may need help from the nurse. Among the 'delayed onset' sleepers are a group who could be termed 'worriers'; having ensured that they are physically comfortable, an opportunity to talk about the cause of the worry may leave them feeling less anxious which, in itself, can encourage sleep. Whenever possible such patients should be left to sleep until they awaken naturally in the morning.

Excessive wakefulness There are people, on the other hand, who fall asleep quickly but report that they waken frequently and stay awake for longer or shorter periods. When this information appears in the nursing notes, the night nurse should be alerted to observing the patient frequently throughout the night in an attempt to verify the sleep pattern. It is well-known that a few minutes awake during the night can seem much longer. It should also be recognized that, for elderly people, an increase in the number and amount of wake times after sleep onset is a normal phenomenon (Hayter, 1983), and perhaps they simply require reassurance that this is so.

The patient who stays awake for longer periods may fall asleep again quite naturally after voiding and having a hot drink. Being dismissive of patients who state that they have had a poor night, but to the nurse appear to have been asleep, is unrealistic; if the patient feels that he has had a poor night, then the quality of sleep has not been sufficient to produce a feeling of refreshment. Sleep researchers acknowledge that the EEG does not record the 'quality' of sleep. A sympathetic understanding of these patients', expressed by attending to their pre-sleep routine, may help them to relax and fall into a refreshing sleep. The nurse should attempt to identify any change in the patient's daytime activities and note if, because of lack of sleep, they are more easily fatigued. Appetite should also be observed; tired people seldom eat well.

For community nurses, it may be the carers as much as the patients whose fatigue from frequent wakening merits attention. Hodgson (1991) draws attention to the possible consequences of sleep disruption and deprivation over time for carers of patients with long-term or advanced disease at home: namely, increased anxiety, lessened motivation and consequent decreasing ability to cope as carer. Depression may follow.

People who suffer from depression already may be troubled by excessive wakefulness. Depression is an illness which can now be treated successfully and if patients showing signs of depression have not already sought medical help, they can be encouraged to do so.

Early morning waking Depression is often characterized by early morning waking, but the age group most commonly reporting regular early waking, as early as 0500 hours, is the elderly. If elderly hospital patients awaken early feeling refreshed, they can be offered a morning beverage; those in single rooms may wish to read or occupy themselves in some way; those in large wards can be encouraged to continue resting in bed to avoid disturbing the other patients.

Restlessness

Restlessness is a feature found in many patients with insomnia. After an extensive literature survey and many observations of restlessness in patients, Norris (1975) wrote:

> 'Restlessness is a universal, discontinuous, animal behaviour evidenced by nonspecific, repetitive, unorganized, diffuse, apparently nonpurposeful motor activity that is subject to limited control.'

Nowadays, tape-recordings are available which teach pre-sleep relaxation, the intention being to reduce restlessness and promote sleep and some people find them effective. The use of rhythmic sound on tape recordings has also proved helpful, such as the noise of waves on a seashore, but more research would be required before making generalizations about the desirability of nurses introducing such methods of reducing restlessness and thus inducing sleep.

Although certain forms of restlessness may be nonspecific the nurse must realise that some medications prescribed for purposes other than sleeping, are disturbers of sleep and promote restlessness. A commonly used medication in this category is the diuretic group. As well as relieving oedema for example, they promote frequent elimination of urine, and although these drugs are normally administered in the early part of the day to preclude disturbance of sleep, their effect may persist into the night. Drugs given to relieve constipation may also cause minor abdominal discomfort and disturbed sleep, or even promote defaecation during the night unless administered at a time which will produce the desired effect during the day. Some anti-depressant medications may cause not only disturbance of sleep but actually induce wakefulness because they act in a manner similar to caffeine. When assessing a patient's sleeping pattern, it is therefore important that the nurse is aware of the effect of other currently prescribed medications which may in fact be the cause of restlessness.

It is worth noting too, that restlessness may occur because some people admitted to hospital do not mention, initially, that they have been accustomed to taking sedatives at home.

Medication dependence

In a survey of over 2000 people undertaken in the early 1980s in the UK (Whitfield, 1982) it was found that 15% of men and 25% of women who went to see the family doctor attended because of insomnia and many of these people would have been prescribed 'sleeping pills'. Over the past decade, however, doctors have become less willing to resort to medication and more interested in the use of behavioural, cognitive and educative techniques in helping patients to cope with insomnia (Espie, 1993).

There are some people, however, who do not respond to such approaches and require to have sleeping pills prescribed by the doctor. For people admitted to hospital already taking such medication, and for patients prescribed it on a short-term basis, administration of these drugs is undertaken or supervised by the nurse. When hypnotic drugs have been ordered to induce sleep, they should be given a few minutes before lights are turned out. If analgesics are also required to relieve pain they should be administered sufficiently early for them to take effect before the hypnotic is given thus enhancing the effect of the hypnotic. The name of the drug, and the dose and time at which it is given are recorded, and also the time at which the patient fell asleep, the time of waking, and mood on waking. The nurse's understanding of the desired action of prescribed sleeping medication is obviously increased by knowledge of the types of drugs which may be used. While hypnotic drugs are recommended for short-term treatment of acute, stress-induced insomnia, their value in the treatment of chronic insomnia is now questioned (Eisen et al, 1993).

Almost paradoxically, hypnotic drugs, although given to induce sleep, can have a detrimental effect on the individual's sleeping pattern due to the development of tolerance. From experiments carried out many years ago at the Edinburgh Sleep Research Laboratory, it was found that after taking sleeping pills for several nights, the person slept badly when the pills were discontinued; indeed, return to a natural sleeping pattern could take up to 6–8 weeks (Oswald & Adam, 1983). Nowadays, therefore, hypnotics are prescribed much more carefully and patients (and their carers) need to be fully-informed about the effects and side-effects of these medications. The main problem after withdrawal from sedative/ hypnotic pills is 'rebound insomnia' and, although this normally lasts for 1–3 weeks, it can persist for as long as two months (Tyrer, 1993).

In general, the use of hypnotics to treat sleep problems is often unsatisfactory and, knowing this, nurses have exploited non-pharmacological methods of promoting sleep for patients, whether in hospital or home. Gournay (1988) explained how a drug-free strategy can work by reporting on the successful management of two patients. In one case, a general practitioner with long-standing difficulty in sleeping was helped to 'learn' a new regime; and in the other case, an active and anxious working mother was taught relaxation techniques. The sleep diary completed by the patients from assessment to end of treatment is outlined in Box 14.5.

Clearly sleep is a state of altered consciousness but it is a normal Activity of Living. Other altered states of consciousness are found in a range of disease conditions which must be differentiated from sleep.

ALTERED CONSCIOUSNESS

Although not strictly a 'sleep' problem, there is good reason to discuss altered consciousness in the context of an account of patients' problems with the AL of sleeping.

In an article discussing altered states of consciousness, Findley (1984) first of all suggests a pragmatic definition of consciousness as 'a state of wakefulness, alertness and awareness of personal identity and environmental events, that is awareness of self and surroundings'. Consciousness refers to both arousal (requiring intact func-

---

Box 14.5 A sleep diary

A sleep diary is a useful way of collecting information from a person/patient who wishes help to improve the quantity and quality of their sleep.

Example of items in a sleep diary (Gournay 1988):
    Date
    Time to bed
    Length of sleep
    Approx time to fall asleep
    Number of awakenings
    Period of time up during night
    Quantity of sleep (hours and minutes)
    Quality of sleep (rated 0/worst – 8/best)

---

tioning of the ascending reticular formation of the brain stem) and the content of consciousness (requiring the intact functioning of the cerebral hemispheres). Altered consciousness, then, can be considered in terms of a gradual change from a normal conscious level through impaired attention, loss of alertness, drowsiness, sleep, stupor and finally coma. Clearly drowsiness and sleep are normal phenomena whereas stupor and coma are abnormal states.

Coma

The ability to assess accurately a patient's level of consciousness is one of the responsibilities of the nurse. The Glasgow Coma Scale, introduced in 1974 by Teasdale and Jennett, has been widely used as a means of assessing the level of consciousness of patients with head injury. The scale enables observation and description of the patient's behaviour in terms of three key responses:

- eye opening
- motor response
- verbal response.

Each of the three responses is assessed independently. The following account of their assessment follows the wording of the 15 point version of the Glasgow Coma Scale (Teasdale & Jennett, 1976) shown in Figure 14.3 (note: variations are discussed later).

- **Eye opening response**
Spontaneous eye opening   When the patient's eyes open on the approach of someone to his bedside, it is recorded as spontaneous. This observation will not be expected when the patient is asleep but nurses should be alert to the fact that in some brain-damaged patients the diurnal rhythm is reversed. Observation must therefore be made for any patient who can respond with spontaneous eye opening during the night and not during the day.

	Eye opening *Score*	Motor response *Score*	Verbal response *Score*
high *score*		**6** If command such as 'lift up your hands' is obeyed	
		5 If purposeful movement to remove painful stimulus such as pressure over eyebrow	**5** If oriented to person, place and time
	4 If eyes open spontaneously to approach of nurse to bedside	**4** If finger withdrawn after application of painful stimulus to it	**4** If conversation confused
	3 If eyes open in response to speech	**3** If painful stimulation at finger tip flexes the elbow	**3** If inappropriate words are used
	2 If eyes open in response to pain at finger tip	**2** If the patient's arms are flexed and finger tip stimulation results in extension of elbow	**2** If only incomprehensible sounds are uttered
low *score*	**1** If eyes do not open in response to pain at finger tip	**1** If there is no detectable response to repeated and various stimuli	**1** If no verbal response

A normal person would score 15 on the scale; the lowest possible score is 3 which is compatible with, but does not necessarily indicate, brain death. A score of 7 is used as a definition of coma.

Fig. 14.3 Glasgow coma scale (15 point version: Teasdale and Jennett, 1976)

Eye opening to speech If the patient's eyes do not open spontaneously he should be addressed in a normal voice by name and asked to open his eyes. If he does not do so repetition in a loud voice is used, avoiding a commanding tone because it is response to stimulation by sound which is being tested.

Eye opening to pain Lack of response to verbal stimulation is followed by testing for response to physical stimulation, such as exerting pressure on the patient's finger nail-bed as shown in Figure 14.4.

● **Motor response**

Obeys commands The patient is required to perform the specific movements requested. Should the relatives have informed the nurse (in the initial assessment phase) that the patient was deaf before the brain damage, then the request will be made by gesture or even in writing. It is preferable to ask the patient to raise an arm or a leg rather than to squeeze the tester's fingers which can trigger off a reflex contraction; if the latter test is used, it is wise to test that the patient will also release and squeeze again several times before recording this score.

Localizes pain Pressure applied over say the eyebrows (supra-orbital ridge) should stimulate the patient to move his arm thus showing that he has located the pain and is attempting to remove the stimulus.

Withdraws from painful stimulus Pressure as in Figure 14.4 causes withdrawal of the finger.

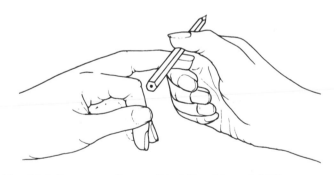

Fig. 14.4 Pressure on finger nail-bed (Teasdale et al, 1975)

Flexion response Painful stimulation at the finger tip (Fig. 14.4) flexes the elbow, but the patient does not achieve a localizing response when stimulus is applied at other sites.

Extension response The patient's arms are flexed and finger tip stimulation (Fig. 14.4) produces straightening at the elbow.

No response to pain This is scored when there is no detectable response to repeated and various stimuli.

● **Verbal response**

Orientated After arousal, the patient is asked who he is, where he is and what year and month it is; he is not expected to give the exact day of the month. If accurate answers are given it is recorded that he is orientated.

Confused conversation A patient can sometimes produce language, even phrases, but if he cannot give the correct answers to questions about orientation then it is recorded that his conversation is confused.

Inappropriate words   When a patient only utters one or two words, more often in response to physical stimulation than to speech, it is recorded that he is using inappropriate words.

Incomprehensible sounds   The utterance of groans, moans or indistinct mumbling without any intelligible words is recorded on this score.

No verbal response   If prolonged and repeated stimulation does not produce phonation then the nil score is recorded.

Use of some type of chart for factual information renders obsolete such terms as deeply unconscious, and semi-conscious; deeply comatose, and semi-comatose — all terms which can mean different things to different people. The chart can be marked and kept at the bedside so that any member of the team caring for the patient can see by glancing at the chart whether or not there has been any change on any item in the scale. When using this scale it should be remembered that the score obtained could be affected when the patient cannot speak due to the presence of an endotracheal tube, or if the patient is deaf or speaks a different language.

Scoring   The Glasgow Coma Scale provides an indication of over-all brain dysfunction when scored out of 15. As noted in Figure 14.3, a score of 7 is used as a definition of coma in the 15 point version of the scale.

Variations and use of the GCS   The 15 point version of the GCS (Glasgow Coma Scale), described above (after Teasdale & Jennett, 1976), was a later adaptation of the original version (Teasdale & Jennett, 1974) which has 14 points. As Watson et al (1992) point out, confusion can arise because both versions remain in use and, in addition, the GCS is sometimes incorporated in a multipurpose observation record chart (see e.g. Teasdale et al, 1975; Allan, 1984) which also covers other vital signs: i.e. temperature, pulse, respiration and blood pressure. It is essential, therefore, that nurses are clear which version of the GCS they are using and that they clearly record whether the scores relate to a 14- or 15-point scale. Watson et al favour the 14-point version with simple descriptors of the items (see Figure 14.5). Their article provides a clear account of proper use and interpretation of the GCS: the key points covered in their article are listed in Box 14.6.

Nurses' knowledge of coma assessment   In spite of an abundance of literature and long use of the Glasgow Coma Scale (GCS) in practice, there is evidence to suggest that nurses' knowledge of coma assessment remains poor. Crewe (1990) assessed the knowledge of 10 nurses who worked in a district general hospital with ready access to a neurosurgical centre. Eight were student nurses and three had never heard of any form of coma

G L A S G O W C O M A S C A L E	Eyes open	spontaneously to speech to pain none
	Best verbal response	orientated disorientated monosyllabic response incomprehensible sounds none
	Best motor response	obey commands local pain flexion to pain extension to pain

Fig. 14.5 The 14 point version of the Glasgow Coma Scale (For further details see Watson et al (1992).)

Box 14.6   The Glasgow Coma Scale

Watson M, Horn S, Curl J 1992 Searching for signs of revival: Uses and abuses of the Glasgow coma scale. *Professional Nurse*, 7, 10, 670–673

Key Points
1. The Glasgow coma scale is a simple method for monitoring patients' conscious levels.
2. Despite its inherent simplicity, it is often misused and misunderstood.
3. Consciousness is regained when a patient is consistently obeying commands.
4. The GCS should ideally be used until the patient has fully regained consciousness.

---

scale; seven of the whole group claimed not to have received any teaching on coma assessment; and five did not feel competent to undertake one. As Crewe herself notes, this was a very small sample and the findings cannot be generalized; nevertheless, they are worrying.

The need for experience as well as knowledge is underlined by Rowley and Fielding (1991): their study investigated whether the Glasgow Coma Scale could be reliably and accurately used by inexperienced observers. The results of this carefully conducted study showed that inexperienced users of the GCS made consistent and sometimes substantial errors, especially at the intermediate levels of consciousness where detection of changes is so crucial. The study did confirm, however, that the GCS was used accurately by experienced and highly trained users.

Care of the unconscious patient   As well as assessing responsiveness level it will be necessary for members of the ward team to accept responsibility for managing several of the unresponding comatose patient's other activities of living. These are breathing, eating and drinking, eliminating, personal cleansing and dressing (prevention of pressure sores), controlling body temperature, mobilizing passively and maintaining a safe environment. All practices associated with these ALs should be carried out by the nurse in such a way that not only life is maintained but also the patient's dignity is safeguarded.

Convulsions (fits)

A form of transient unconsciousness sometimes occurs as a feature of what is termed a convulsion. When a baby has a convulsion or seizure it often heralds a febrile illness. In other age groups, there may be a variety of causes, including cerebral anoxaemia, hypoglycaemia, disturbance of calcium balance, electrolyte imbalance, excessive hydration, the injection of certain drugs and poisons, infections which produce high temperature elevations, and a number of metabolic disorders.

Convulsions are also a feature of epilepsy but nowadays, good control, and indeed prevention of seizures, can be achieved by means of anticonvulsant medications. Around one third of people who have epilepsy have seizures less than once a year but, at the other extreme, one third of sufferers have more than one seizure a month (Nursing Times, 1994). The nurse has an important role to play in educating sufferers and their families about the treatment regime and the benefits of a regular and moderate routine in lifestyle, diet and exercise. Nevertheless, coping with epilepsy is not easy; some of the difficulties and stresses are described in an article called 'Facing up to my epilepsy', written by a district nurse who suffers from the condition (Cobell, 1989).

All nurses should know how to act when a person/ patient has a fit, for whatever reason, and guidelines are given in Box 14.7 (after Castledine, 1993).

Anaesthesia

It is possible to alter deliberately the level of human consciousness. This occurs when a patient is given a general anaesthetic. The anaesthetized person appears to be in a state of induced unconsciousness although there is increasing evidence that appearances are misleading; the patient on the operating table may actually hear what is being said and may be 'aware' of the inability to move. These findings certainly have implications for staff in the operating suite both prior to surgery and in the recovery room. Nowadays, for many operations, light anaesthetics are used so patients recover consciousness quite quickly after surgery.

Dependency in altered consciousness

In circumstances where there is altered consciousness —

Box 14.7 When a person has a fit
Key Points
Protect the person from further injury: • by removing dangerous objects nearby   • by carefully restraining and controlling the person's movements   A clear airway must be maintained   The person should be placed in the recovery position   Details of the fit should be observed   Castledine (1993)

---

coma, convulsions, general anaesthetic — the skill and adaptability of the nurse are of paramount importance. In these states, even when transient in nature, the person is dependent for all Activities of Living, indeed for survival.

Like sleep, as might be expected, these states of altered consciousness are characterized by changes in the electrical activity of the cerebral cortex when recorded by EEG. Every advance in the research centres provides more information about the 'how' and 'why' of altered consciousness, including sleep. Perhaps in the not too distant future, it will be possible to refute Dr Johnson's observation some decades ago:

> '. . . no searcher . . . can tell by what power the mind and body are thus chained down in irresistible stupefaction . . . the witty and the dull, the clamerous and the silent, the busy and the idle, are all overpowered by the gentle tyrant, and all lie down in the equality of sleep.'

PLANNING AND IMPLEMENTING NURSING ACTIVITIES AND EVALUATING OUTCOMES

In the course of discussing patients' problems with the AL of sleeping, various nursing activities have been mentioned. Unlike most of the other ALs, nursing activities in relation to this AL are mostly confined to the hospital setting. For that reason, problems which hospital patients commonly experience with sleeping were discussed at some length (pp. 384–387) and the kinds of nursing activities which can be implemented to prevent or alleviate these problems were identified. Increasingly, the nursing literature shows a growing awareness of the need to *prevent* disturbed sleep in hospital (see e.g. Duxbury, 1994).

These nursing activities need to be planned and the basis of planning is sound assessment followed by careful identification of the patient's problems (both actual and potential). A reminder of these stages of the process of nursing is provided in Figure 3.9 (p. 60).

Assessing individual patients in relation to the AL of sleeping (and in relation to altered consciousness) is quite a complex activity. It requires sound background knowledge of the nature of sleep (as outlined pp. 373–376) and the variations in sleep patterns at different stages of the lifespan.

Assessing a patient's sleeping is something which nurses working in the community may well do, even if they are less directly involved than hospital nurses in actually implementing sleep-related nursing activities. Good sleep is just as important for the patient who is being nursed at home rather than in hospital. And after discharge from hospital, which is ever quicker for most patients, adequate sleep is very important in the recovery period. In addition, community nurses will come into contact with many patients and carers whose sleep is perpetually poor; and, following assessment, there may be useful advice (or simply reassurance) which the nurse can offer.

Irrespective of whether the setting is an acute hospital ward, a long-stay facility or the patient's home, the effectiveness of any nursing activities which are implemented with the purpose of preventing or alleviating problems with sleeping should be evaluated. In order to do this, specific goals should be set in conjunction with the patient at the time of drawing up the nursing plan. Evaluating whether or not the set goals are achieved will almost always have to rely largely on the patient's own reports and estimation. This is certainly so in relation to evaluating outcomes in terms of the quality of sleep and, although the quantity of sleep is more amenable to objective measurement, again the nurse has to rely on the patient's own evaluation of the amount of improvement (or otherwise).

Sleep is a fascinating subject and there are still many mysteries about sleep which scientists have yet to explain. What we do know, however, is that sleep deprivation and sleep disruption are likely to hamper recovery from illness (or, at least, not to assist the process). In any case, poor sleep adds to the misery of being ill or anxious or in hospital. It is important, therefore, that nurses do whatever they can to assist patients to get the best possible sleep.

REFERENCES

Adam K 1980 A time for rest and a time for play. Nursing Mirror 150(10) March 6: 17–18
Allan D 1984 Glasgow coma scale. Nursing Mirror 158(23) June 13: 32–34
Armstrong-Esther C, Hawkins L 1982 Day for night: circadian rhythms in the elderly. Nursing Times 78(3) July 28: 1263–1265

Barton J 1994 Shift systems in England and Wales. Nursing Times 90: 21, 12
Berrios G E, Shapiro C M 1993 'I don't get enough sleep, doctor'. British Medical Journal 306(6881): 843–846
Brezinova V, Oswald I 1972 Sleep after a bedtime beverage. British Medical Journal 2 May 20: 431–433
Briggs D 1991 Preventing ICU psychosis. Nursing Times 87 (19): 30–31
Brown P 1988 Shift work: punching the body clock. Nursing Times 84(44) November 2: 26–28
Brugne J-F 1994 Sleep, wakefulness and the nurse. British Journal of Nursing 3(2): 68–71
Canavan T 1984 The psychobiology of sleep. Nursing 2(23) March: 682–683
Carter D 1985 In need of a good night's sleep. Nursing Times 81(46): 24–26
Castledine G 1993 Neurological emergencies: nurse-aid management of fits. British Journal of Nursing 2(6): 336–337
Clapin-French E 1986 Sleep patterns of aged persons in long-term care facilities. Journal of Advanced Nursing 11: 57–66
Closs S J 1988 A nursing study of sleep on surgical wards. Nursing Research Unit Research Report, Dept of Nursing Studies, University of Edinburgh, Scotland, UK
Closs S J 1988 Assessment of sleep in hospital patients. Journal of Advanced Nursing 13: 501–510
Closs S J 1988 Patients' sleep-wake rhythms in hospital. Nursing Times Occasional Papers 84(1 & 2): 48–50, 54–55
Cobell R 1989 Facing up to my epilepsy. Nursing Times 85(2) January 11: 27–29
Cohen D 1979 Sleep and dreaming. Pergamon Press, Oxford
Crewe H 1990 Nurses' knowledge of coma assessment. Nursing Times 86(41): 52–53
Dopson L 1988 When the snoring has to stop. Nursing Times 84(42) October 19: 22–23
Douglas N J 1993 The sleep apnoea/hypopnoea syndrome and snoring. British Medical Journal, 306(6884): 1057–1060
Durnford S 1988 Junior hospital doctors: tired and tested. British Medical Journal 297(6654) October 15: 931–932
Duxbury J 1994 Avoiding disturbed sleep in hospital. Nursing Standard 9(10): 31–34
Eisen J, MacFarlane J, Shapiro C M 1993 Psychotropic drugs and sleep. British Medical Journal 306(6888): 1331–1334
Espie C A 1993 Practical management of insomnia: behavioural and cognitive techniques. British Medical Journal 306(6876): 509–511
Felstein I 1979 The sufferer who doesn't suffer. Nursing Mirror 146 April 12: 42–43
Findley L 1984 Altered consciousness. Nursing 2(23) March: 663–666
Gournay K 1988 Sleeping without drugs. Nursing Times 84(11): 46–49
Haddock J 1994 Reducing the effects of noise in hospital. Nursing Times 8(43): 25–18
Harrington J M 1994 Working long hours and health. British Medical Journal 308(6984): 1581–1582
Hawkins L, Armstrong-Esther C 1978 Circadian rhythms and night shift working in nurses. Nursing Times Occasional Paper 74(13) May 4: 49–52
Hayter J 1983 Sleep behaviors of older persons. Nursing Research 32(4) July/August: 242–246
Hearne K 1986 Dream sense. Nursing Times 1(82): 28–31
Hodgson L A 1991 Why do we need sleep? Relating theory to nursing practice. Journal of Advanced Nursing 16: 1503–1510
Horne J A 1983 Human sleep and tissue restitution: some qualifications and doubts. Clinical Science 65: 569–578
Horne J A, Reyner L A 1995 Sleep related vehicle accidents. British Medical Journal 310: 565–568
Jaffa T, Scott S, Hendriks J H, Shapiro C M 1993 Sleep disorders in children. British Medical Journal 306(6878): 640–643
Johns M W 1984 Normal sleep. In: Priest R G (ed) Sleep: an international monograph, Update Books ch 1, p 13–17
Katz M, Shapiro C M 1993 Dreams and medical illness. British Medical Journal 306(6883): 993–995
Keys M 1988 Silent nights. Professional Nurse 3(9): 353–357
Koskenvuo M, Partinen M, Kaprio J 1985 Snoring and disease. Annals of Clinical Research 17(5): 247–251

Lathlean J 1980 Relaxation using yoga. Nursing 1(20) December: 882–884

Manian R 1988 Can I sleep now, nurse? Nursing Standard 12(3) December 17: 22–23

Norris C 1975 Restlessness: a nursing phenomenon in search of a meaning. Nursing Outlook 23: 103–107

Nursing Times 1994 Epilepsy — Revision notes. Nursing Times 90(20): 9–12

Oswald I 1980 No peace for the worried. Nursing Times 150(11) March 13: 34–35

Oswald I, Adam K 1983 Get a better night's sleep. Martin Dunitz, London

Professional Nurse 1986 Hypothermia nursing intervention — practice check. Professional Nurse 1(5): 136–138

Rechtshaffen A, Kales A 1968 A manual of standardised terminology, techniques and scoring system for sleep stages of human subjects. National Institutes of Health, Bethesda, Maryland, USA

Richman N 1983 Management of sleep problems. Maternal and Child Health 8(6) June: 227–233

Rowley G, Fielding K 1991 Reliability and accuracy of the Glasgow Coma Scale with experienced and inexperienced users. Lancet 337(8740): 535–538

Royal Commission on the National Health Service 1978 Patients' attitudes to the hospital service. Research paper No. 5. HMSO, London

Shapiro C M, Dement W C 1993 Impact and epidemiology of sleep disorders. British Medical Journal 306(6892): 1604–1607

Shapiro C M, Devins G M, Hussain M R G 1993 Sleep problems in patients with medical illness. British Medical Journal 306: 1532–1535

Shapiro C M, Flanigan M J 1993 Functions of sleep. British Medical Journal 306(6874): 383–385

Smith P, Wedderburn Z 1980 Sleep, body rhythms and night-work. Nursing 1(20) December: 889–892

Stradling J R 1993 Recreational drugs and sleep. British Medical Journal 306(6887): 573–575

Swift C G, Shapiro C M 1993 Sleep and sleep problems in elderly people. British Medical Journal 306: 1468–1471

Teasdale G, Galbraith S, Clarke K 1975 Observation record chart. Nursing Times 71(25) June 19: 972–973

Teasdale G, Jennett B 1974 Assessment of coma and impaired consciousness: a practical scale. Lancet, 2, 81–84

Teasdale G, Jennett B 1976 Assessment and prognosis of coma after head injury. Acta Neurochir., 34, 45–55

Tyrer P 1993 Withdrawal from hypnotic drugs. British Medical Journal 306(6879): 706–708

Wardle J 1986 The chronology of sleep. Nursing 3(9): 325–326

Waterhouse J 1993 Circadian rhythms. British Medical Journal 306(6875): 448–451

Watson M, Horn S, Curl J 1992 Searching for signs of revival: Uses and abuses of the Glasgow coma scale. Professional Nurse 7(10): 672–674

Wedderburn Z, Smith P 1980 Sleep: its function and measurement. Nursing 1(20) December: 852–855

Whitfield W 1982 Breaking the habit. Nursing Mirror 155(10) September 8: 59–60

Wilkie T 1989 Doctors working 36-hour shifts in US 'error-prone'. The Independent 709 January 18: 7

15

Dying

The AL of dying

Dying is the final act of living. Death is what marks the end of life on earth, just as the event of birth marks its beginning. Unlike the event of birth, however, death — unless it is sudden and unexpected — is preceded by a process (i.e. the process of dying) in which the individual actively participates: it is for this reason that dying is included as an Activity of Living in the model for nursing.

The only certain thing in our lives is that we will one day die; but there are many uncertainties as to why, when, where and how. It is probably these uncertainties about dying which provoke uneasy feelings when people think about the prospect of their own death and the death of those they love. Life would not be worth living if death became a preoccupation but, if the subject is ignored, how can people develop the resources needed to prepare themselves for their own death, comfort the bereaved, bear the sorrow of grieving and, finally, face death with dignity?

An understanding of death, dying and bereavement is certainly important for all health care professionals, and especially for nurses, if sympathetic and skilled care is to be provided for the dying and the bereaved.

DEATH AND DYING

To die suddenly from natural causes, in old age, and without loss of dignity is what most people would regard as a 'good death'.

Death from natural causes

Death may be sudden as occurs, for example, following a massive coronary attack or a major accident; or it may be preceded by a process of dying. Following an acute terminal illness or complicated surgery, dying may take only a few days or a few weeks. On the other hand, when there is chronic illness with a poor prognosis or only partial recovery from an acute illness, such as a stroke, the process of dying may span several months or even longer. The period of survival in a state of terminal illness, therefore, is very variable. Terminal illness is, by definition, an illness which has progressed beyond the possibility of cure or remission, and death is certain.

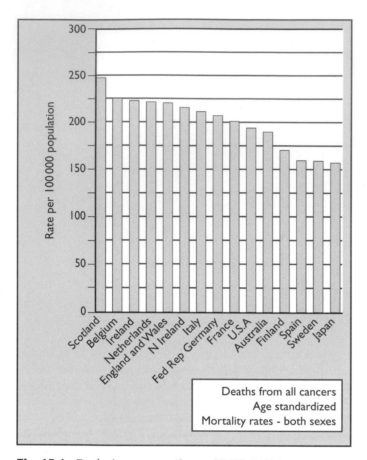

Fig. 15.1 Deaths from cancers (Source: HMSO (1992))

Throughout the Western world the major causes of death are:-
- heart disease
- cancer
- stroke.

Accidents and suicide (see below) are major causes of death in the younger age groups, as is cancer. Although more effective treatments are now available for some cancers, the incidence of cancer as a cause of premature death remains high. In some countries it is much higher than in others. Scotland has the worst record for deaths from cancer in the whole of the Western developed world (see Figure 15.1: Source HMSO, 1992).

Death by accident, violence or suicide

In contrast to death from natural causes, some people die as a result of accident, violence or suicide.

Accidental death In most countries of the Western world, road accidents are a major cause of death in young adults, normally a particularly healthy group. Other types of accident may cause mass death: international publicity is given to serious aircraft accidents which, although rare, almost always have a high mortality rate; industrial accidents, for example in mines, often cause mass deaths in large numbers; and in areas of the world where natural disasters such as floods, earthquakes, and hurricanes occur with relative frequency, there may be a heavy death toll. Every country has its major tragedies when whole families or even communities can be wiped out by such events.

Violent death Sudden violent death may not be accidental, however, but deliberate. Murder is not common but the incidence is rising in most industrialized nations. Most countries are aware of the increasing violence and terrorism in the modern world and of the corresponding need to protect individuals from undesirable and preventable acts of homicide. For many obvious reasons, the relatives' grief may be complicated by feelings of lust for revenge and fear for their own personal safety, and such circumstances may precipitate yet more deaths.

Violent death on a large scale as a result of war seems to be a constant feature in modern society. Following the Second World War, when the waste of human life on an international scale was recognized, the United Nations Organization was created to provide a forum for discussion about disputes in order to preclude the waging of war. Unfortunately, as evident in recent history, even in Europe there has been failure to reach negotiated settlements and the death toll among armed forces and civilians continues in countries still at war.

The possibility of a nuclear holocaust and the prospect of mass annihilation loomed large in the era of the 'cold war'. Although the nuclear threat has lessened, there is still need for efforts at international level to ensure that it will never return.

Suicide There are some individuals who, for a variety of reasons, want to die and intentionally take their own lives by committing suicide. Ritual suicide was once practised, for example, when a Hindu woman perished on the funeral pyre of her husband (Suttie); or when a Japanese Samurai, who for some reason felt dishonoured, committed Hari-Kari with a ceremonial sword. Nowadays these practices are rarely used, indeed Suttie is now illegal.

Suicide is no longer a crime in the UK and has not been since the Suicide Act in 1961, but there is still a stigma attached to suicide, and this may serve to increase the already great amount of distress and guilt suffered by the relatives. There has been growing concern about the incidence of suicide in the UK. Throughout the seventies and eighties, over 4000 suicides were registered each year (Palmer, 1993). The Government's 'Health of the Nation' report published in 1991 (DoH, 1991) set a target for a 15% reduction in the suicide rate by the end of the decade.

Although people often associate suicide with the younger age groups, in fact it is older people who have the highest suicide rates of any age group in the UK (see Figure 15.2).

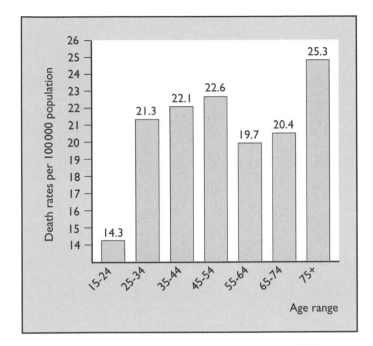

Fig. 15.2 Deaths from suicide by age, UK 1990 (Source: WHO (1991), taken from Bowles (1993))

Euthanasia

'Bringing about an easy death' is the actual meaning of the term euthanasia, although mercy killing is a phrase often used as a synonym. It is a topic which evokes strong emotions and heated debate. Those with particular religious or personal convictions argue that it is morally wrong to end life deliberately (active euthanasia). Others consider that euthanasia is not a deliberate act of killing but merely allows death to occur, for example by withholding antibiotics at the onset of a respiratory infection in an old, incapacitated person although providing care and comfort in every other way (passive euthanasia).

In a number of countries, proponents of euthanasia have formed societies — the first was in the UK in 1935 — to discuss and propagate their beliefs, and to provide information to people who wish assistance in reducing the distress of dying. In some instances, an even more positive stance has been taken and attempts have been made to introduce legislation making voluntary euthanasia permissible.

Active euthanasia remains illegal in the UK and many other countries. However, as a survey of doctors revealed, it is not uncommon for patients to request euthanasia and for doctors to comply with such a request in spite of the legal position (Ward & Tate, 1994: see Box 15.1).

Policy on euthanasia was reviewed by the British Medical Association in its 1988 Euthanasia Report. It did not support legalization of euthanasia and declared that active intervention to terminate life should remain illegal. It did, however, agree that the concept of patient

Box 15.1 Euthanasia: A survey of doctors' attitudes

Study method: Survey by anonymous questionnaire to 424 doctors (half GPs, half hospital consultants) in one area of England. Response rate of 73.6% (i.e. 312 returns).

Findings: Doctors were asked whether, in the course of their medical practice, a patient had ever asked them to hasten his or her death. Of those who answered (*n* = 273), 60% said 'yes' and 40% said 'no'. More GPs (64%) than consultants (52%) had received such a request. Of those who had received a request to take active steps to end a patient's life (i.e. active euthanasia), 32% reported that they had complied. A higher proportion (46%) indicated that they would do so *if* this were legal.

Implications: The authors conclude that British law on euthanasia is not satisfactory for either patients or doctors, and they suggest that there should be more open debate.

(Ward & Tate, 1994)

autonomy is a crucial aspect of sensitive and informed care and, therefore, suggested that doctors should heed 'living wills' (while cautioning that these are not binding in law). A 'living will' is usually taken to be a special kind of advance directive concerned with refusing life-prolonging treatment (Hope, 1992). In the United States, where the idea originated, a Patient Self Determination Act is now in force which requires health care institutions to advise all patients, on admission, of their right to execute advance directives. In his article, Hope argues that proper debate of the topic should take place in the UK and, as shown above (Box 15.1), there is evidence that doctors would welcome this. Since then the British Medical Association has declared its strong support for the principle of acting on an advance directive, but a House of Lords Select Commitee concluded that *legislation* for their use is generally unnecessary (Robertson, 1995).

There has been little research on nurses' feelings about euthanasia although the subject is frequently debated in the nursing press (see, for example, Ellis, 1991 and Johnson, 1993). It is also a subject which provokes heated public debate as happened, for example, in the UK in 1993 when the House of Lords upheld an appeal to allow Tony Bland, a young football fan, crushed and rendered to a permanent vegetative state in the Hillsborough disaster, to die (by the withdrawal of feeding): see Alderman (1993).

The 'euthanasia debate' is not new and history records

examples of group euthanasia practices in the Greek island of Cos in the 1st century BC. It has gone on down through the centuries but the debate has currently re-emerged with some force because of procedures made possible by technological advances which have seen the development of complex multi-system life support for critically ill patients. The medico-ethic and legal issue of withdrawing life support is, therefore, a relatively recent phenomenon (Fulbrook, 1992).

GRIEF AND BEREAVEMENT

It is difficult to discuss the nature of death and dying without considering the nature of grieving and bereavement. Most adults have some experience of these emotions following the death of a relative or friend; indeed grieving and bereavement are a part of the process of living although related to the process of dying and death.

Grief

Following the death of someone significant to them, those who are left behind almost inevitably suffer a deep sense of desolation. Grief is the emotional reaction which follows and is one of the most intense emotional experiences. Murray Parkes (1972) in his classic book, *Bereavement,* maintains that grief is 'the cost of commitment' in our lives.

It is not necessarily only husbands, wives or children who are bereaved, although one's immediate reaction is to think of these close relatives. So intense is the emotion of grief that it affects even those sometimes wrongly assumed to be untouched by loss: the very young and the very old, the mentally ill and the mentally disabled. 'The bereaved' are, by definition, those who suffer loss and grief in response to a death; those who were, in some important way, committed to the person who died.

Jacob (1993) maintains that, although grief is one of the most universal human responses encountered by nurses, it is a concept which is still poorly understood. From a review of the literature and a concept analysis, Jacob's paper provides insight into the complexity of grief and, interestingly, she draws attention to the fact that there may be positive outcomes of a grief experience (i.e. personal growth and new relationships) as well as negative ones (i.e. depression, morbidity and mortality).

Bereavement

To be bereaved means, literally, to be deprived. Although feelings of loss and grief are almost universal responses in bereavement, many other reactions can occur. Shock, disbelief, anger, denial, shame, guilt, resentment, anxiety, fear, depression and despair are among the emotional reactions which may be experienced by the bereaved to

a varying degree and at different times throughout the grieving process. However, sometimes a death brings relief to those left behind and this may be the case, for example, if the family has had to watch suffering in someone they love, and bear the burden of care during a prolonged terminal illness.

The classic research of Kubler-Ross in the 1960s provided an understanding of the stages of dying and this also served as a means of understanding the experience of bereavement as a *process.* Murray Parkes (1972) later outlined the stages of bereavement.

Initially there is usually a short period of intense grief when the bereaved person suffers profound despair and sorrow and openly mourns. Shock and total disbelief can be experienced at this time, especially in the case of sudden death, and the experience may seem unreal. Then there is a long period of sadness. Pining for the dead person is common, indeed normal, and often this takes the form of 'searching behaviour' involving attachment to places and objects associated with the dead person's life and their relationship.

While grieving, a sense of the persisting presence of the dead person appears to be a comforting phenomenon and illusions, hallucinations and dreams may occur. Such events seem to help to compensate for the reality of the loss, and the loneliness felt. Sometimes the bereaved person experiences intense anxieties for the future and feels totally incapable of taking decisions and coping with everyday demands.

Depression is not uncommon and, even long after the death, episodes of intense grief and despair may return. Restitution from bereavement involves adaptation to a new life as the death of a significant person inevitably alters the role and function of the bereaved; a widow is no longer a wife and a son may now be the head of the household. The old identity must be given up and a new one evolved. Usually, the new life is moulded gradually and some significant milestones include events such as returning to work, moving house and making new friends.

Bereavement can be a long, painful and lonely process. Although it is probably true that time heals, a person seldom remains unaffected by a bereavement even after a long time lapse. It is not that they forget the dead person, but perhaps time gives them practice in adapting to living in changed circumstances.

Lifespan: relationship to the AL of dying

The model (see Figure 15.3) includes the lifespan as one of its components; birth is the lifespan's starting point and death is its endpoint. However death can occur at any age

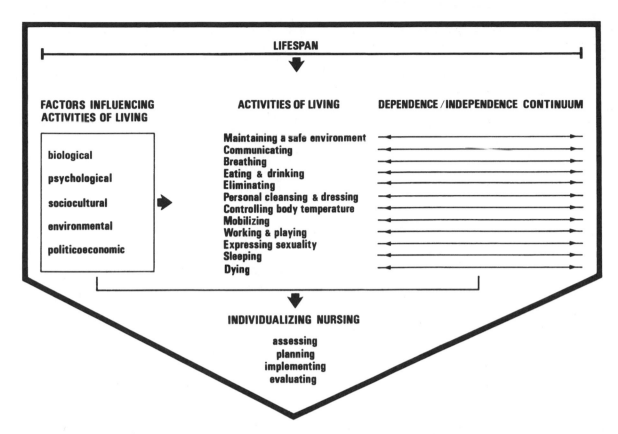

Fig. 15.3 The AL of dying within the model for nursing

and when it comes, it determines the length of an individual's lifespan. When the lifespan of groups of individuals is investigated, it is possible to detect trends in death rates within and between the groups and as most countries maintain population statistics, international comparisons can be made about average age of death and life expectancy.

A century ago in most industrialized countries the life expectancy was around 40 years, slightly higher for females; nowadays, it is nearer 80 years, women still living longer than men on average. The lengthening of life in the latter half of this century reflects:

- greater prosperity generally
- consequent improvements in diet
  and living conditions
- medical advances
- better health care.

There is, however, considerable variation across the world in average life expectancy (see Figure 15.4), and even between closely related countries (e.g. the four countries of the UK). The relatively low life expectancy in Scotland has been attributed, at least in part, to that country's relatively poor health status (HMSO, 1992). There are other European countries where health is poor and, in Hungary, for example, average age of death has actually been falling over the past decade.

Average age of death is important to understand when considering the relationship of the lifespan to the AL of dying. Most deaths, of course, occur in old age. In Figure 15.5 deaths by age distribution in England and Wales are shown (in the form of a histogram) and in Figure 15.6 the very similar distribution in Scotland is illustrated (this time in the form of a pie chart). The circumstances of death and dying will now be reviewed in relation to the different age groups.

Prenatal death

Death can occur even before birth. Death during early uterine existence may be associated with a spontaneous abortion, when the products of conception are expelled or may have to be removed. Or the fetus may die at a late stage in pregnancy and the mother knows that the period of labour will produce only a dead child. Or some babies may die during the process of birth. A 'still birth' is the legal term applied in the UK when death occurs after the 24th week of gestation.

It is not possible to know the 'reaction' of the child in these circumstances, but it is possible to observe the desolation experienced by parents who, of course, are the most directly affected. The sense of loss and despair, and even failure or guilt, is the very antithesis of all their

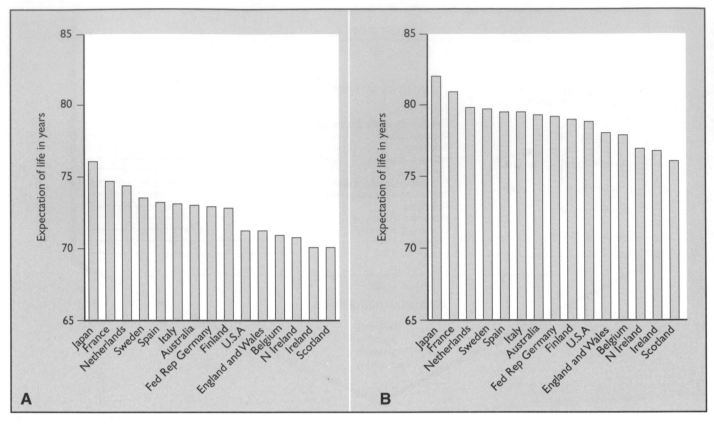

Fig. 15.4 Life expectancy at birth (A) Males (B) Females (Source: HMSO (1992))

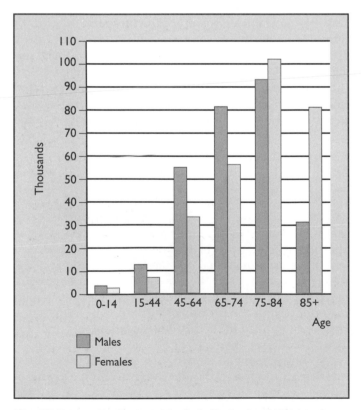

Fig. 15.5 Age distribution of deaths in England and Wales in the late 1980s (Source: OHE (1991) Fig. 3, p. 11)

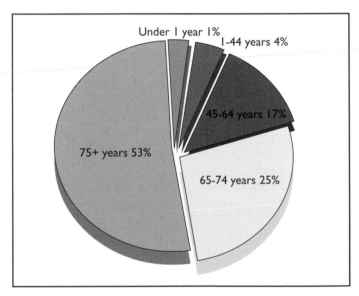

Fig. 15.6 Age distribution of deaths in Scotland in 1990 (Source: HMSO (1992) p. 28)

expectations, and alien to the usual atmosphere of a maternity ward if the mother is delivered in hospital; it is probably the hardest place in which to mourn a lost baby.

The importance of allowing the parents to see and even hold their stillborn baby became recognized in the 1980s (e.g. Mallinson, 1989), and in some hospitals a photograph is taken. Despite the obvious distress, this is thought to help with the grieving process. As Symes (1991) points out, perinatal death is also hard for health care staff and sometimes the parents' hurt and anger can be directed at doctors and nurses. She emphasizes, therefore, the importance of understanding and patience; and the particular need for staff to break the news of the baby's death in the kindest possible way, but without platitudes or inappropriate reassurances.

Infancy

Some babies die during the early weeks of life and so-called 'cot death' — the sudden infant death syndrome — has been the subject of intense media interest and extensive research in recent years. Explanation of cot death has been forwarded in various theories about, for example, overwhelming stress; functional or anatomical defects; maturation failure; and critical phases of development, but the reason for these distressing sudden deaths in apparently thriving babies was not often detectable (Barker, 1987; Milner, 1987). Then it was shown in a small study in Portsmouth that the incidence of cot deaths fell by 30% when health visitors had identified babies at risk on a 'birth score' (based on factors such as low birth weight, smoking during pregnancy, young or single motherhood, unemployment and multiple birth) and had made structured extra visits (Pope, 1988).

Subsequently, in the late 1980s, a review of published studies on SID (sudden infant death) identified that the prone sleeping position was linked with increased risk (Beal, 1988). In 1991, the UK's Health Department issued guidelines on how to reduce the risk of cot death, including the advice that babies should be put to sleep on their backs. Other advice recommended protection from cigarette smoke and from over-wrapping or overheating infants. In 1993, statistics were released which showed that cot deaths in the UK had been more than halved following the Government's campaign (from 912 deaths in 1991 to 456 in 1992). There is, of course, the need for the advice to be reiterated for new parents and Buckley (1993) describes the steps taken in her maternity unit to ensure that this happens: i.e. by operating a standard that 'all mothers will be aware of the measures to be taken to reduce the risk of cot death in the light of recent research'. A sound overview of the research into cot death is provided in the accompanying article by Mitchell (1993).

Sudden infant death syndrome has been one of the major causes of infant mortality in industrialized countries but, if infants survive the first year, they have a good life expectancy. There are, of course, parts of the developing world where infant mortality remains high.

Childhood

During the early decades of this century, childhood deaths were relatively common, often associated with infectious disease. Now in industrialized countries, deaths during childhood are rare, for example in the UK, they account for less than 1% of all deaths and the most common cause is accidents; theoretically accidents are preventable, a topic which is discussed in Chapter 4, Maintaining a Safe Environment.

Children do become aware of death and dying at quite an early age and it is interesting to note the findings of studies which have been conducted to ascertain what young children think about death. One of the earlier studies was carried out by Nagy in Hungary following the Second World War. A group of 378 children aged 3–10 years from different socioeconomic backgrounds and religions, and of varying intellectual ability were asked to express death-related thoughts verbally, in drawing and in writing. Nagy categorized the findings in three stages. In Stage I (3–5 years) there was no clear distinction between living and lifeless. The dead person was 'less alive' or asleep or had gone away and would return. In Stage II (5–6 years) death was personified as a death-man or skeleton who carried away living people and there was no return. In Stage III (9–10 years) death was inevitable and permanent; it was a termination of life.

In more recent studies mentioned by Boston & Trezise (1987) the distinctions made by under-5s and those in the age group 5–9 years seem to be similar. Even although children seem to enjoy the 'experience' of death through war games and fantasies, and inevitably nowadays see it depicted on television often associated with violence, the reality can be bewildering.

For a young child, the death of a parent is a devastating and tragic event. Couldrick (1993) explains the importance of preparing a child for the death of a parent who is terminally ill (see Box 15.2).

And if, for some reason, a sibling dies, it is equally important to talk with children about their feelings and reactions. They can be angry — or even feel guilty — with a brother or sister for dying and leaving them; Vas Dias (1987) mentions a 7-year-old after his brother's death, asking 'Mummy do you think Adam knew I loved him even if I didn't like him being ill?'

Preparing a child for his or her own death is probably the most difficult task of all. In the past it was common to try to conceal the fact, thinking this to be less distressing. Nowadays, it is generally agreed that children with a life-

Box 15.2 The death of a parent is a devastating and tragic event for a young child

Key points from:
Couldrick A 1993 'Do you mean that Mummy is going to die?': Caring for bereaved children. Professional Nurse 9(3): 186–189

1. Children need to be prepared for a terminally ill parent's death. It is important that they are told what is happening.
2. The child should be separated from the family for as little as possible. Their fantasies about what is happening may be much more terrifying than the reality.
3. Children who are included in the parent's care and are given information in a way that could be understood appear to value this experience.
4. After the death, the child's carer appears to feel more confident if they are supported by health professionals in handling uncertaintities (e.g. whether it is helpful for the child to see the body and/or attend the funeral) and understanding and responding to the child's expressed grief.

threatening illness tend to have insight into their predicament, even at an early age; and, therefore they need to be able to discuss their fears and feelings (Purssell, 1993).

Adolescence

Although the teenager understands intellectually about the finality of life, time is a sort of insulation between the adolescent and eventual death. So the dying adolescent who is just beginning to enjoy independence and self-confidence does not want to end what has just begun, and in the confusion and distress and often anger, may feel isolated from both parents and peers.

The death of an adolescent is devastating, especially to parents. In industrialized countries, parents do not expect to outlive their offspring and it is very difficult to comfort them after such a loss. Such premature death may be greatly resented. They have been cheated of time together which they had the right to expect; their adolescent child still had so much to give and so much to live for. Hopes and faith about life are dealt a severe blow which can have a lifelong effect on the family. However many bereaved parents consider that although the loss leaves a permanent scar, it is possible to grow because of the experience and help others in similar circumstances: and, as a result, they are often active members of self-support groups which exist for parents

who have lost an adolescent child, whether through illness or accident or suicide.

It is a sad indictment on modern, industrialized society that the suicide rate in this age group has been steadily increasing over the past 20 years in the USA and in almost all European countries. In their book *Suicide in Adolescence*, Dickstria & Hawton (1987) discuss the epidemiology of adolescent suicide and highlight some of the possible causes. They emphasize unemployment, above average intelligence, and loss of a parent through death or marital separation as important factors in the context of a society which lacks social cohesiveness, and which values material and technological possessions at the expense of the individual's emotional wellbeing.

Adulthood

During early adulthood, people are considered to be in the 'prime of life' and a consideration of personal death and dying is almost totally alien, at least in industrialized countries where long life is now a reasonable expectation. Sudden death, therefore, perhaps as a result of a road accident, comes as a shock to the family. There has been no time to contemplate the event and no opportunity to begin the process of grieving in anticipation of death. There has been no chance to say goodbye, and often there is an aura of unreality in the immediate post-death period. For the bereaved family there is an untimely change in status; perhaps a young family bereft of a parent, perhaps a sudden termination of a promising career. And, of course, nowadays there are added stresses when the death is the result of AIDS because the secrecy and social stigma which tends to be associated with this disease may complicate reactions to a death with revelations of undisclosed lifestyles, such as drug use or homosexuality (Miller et al, 1993).

In later adulthood, however, the physical and other changes associated with ageing probably serve to remind the individual of man's mortality; and an increasing incidence of disease in this age group, either personally or observed in friends and colleagues, make the possibility of death and the process of dying more of a reality. For a spouse or partner who is bereaved at this stage in life it can mean intense loneliness despite the support of family and friends; and for the young adults of the family, it may mean the loss of a supportive parent and perhaps taking on increasing responsibility for the remaining parent or younger siblings.

Old age

For the elderly there is the constant realization that they are approaching the end of the lifespan and they are made aware of this by an increasing number of deaths in their peer group. The majority of elderly people are healthy and retain their independence and may die suddenly or have a very short terminal illness. For some however, if they are ill and dependent, death may be welcomed as a release from pain and discomfort; for a few, the process of dying can be a long, courageously endured struggle to cherish their dignity and self-esteem despite a frail and failing body.

A long terminal illness of an elderly person may cause great difficulties for relations also. Although able to prepare themselves for the bereavement they have, in addition to their anxieties and fears, the burden of care at home, or hospital visiting, over a long period of time. For those who are bereaved by the death of an elderly person, it may mean the loss of a spouse with whom they have spent a lifetime, and for the younger generation it may mean the loss of a much-loved elderly parent or lifelong grandparent.

Perhaps because death in old age is viewed as 'natural', few studies of grieving have concentrated on the elderly age group. However, Garrett (1991) suggests that the grieving process may differ: extreme outbursts of overt grief are less common, but denial is often a prominent feature (the survivor speaking and behaving as if nothing has happened) and depression may be long lasting.

Indeed, the centrality of loss in the lives of elderly people and the frequency of depression may be reasons, coupled with social isolation and poverty, for the high suicide rate among the elderly. This fact has already been noted (see Figure 15.2, p. 397). Bowles (1993) summarizes the risk factors which have been identified from studies of suicide among older people (see Box 15.3) and she appeals for greater understanding of the hopelessness which affects many of the elderly in Western society which still perpetuates negative views of the expectations and status of old age.

Box 15.3 Suicide among older people

Risk factors:-

- Bereavement
- Care givers (especially those caring for a cognitively impaired dependent and those without psychological or financial support or opportunity of respite)
- Disabling conditions (e.g. CVA, Parkinson's disease, Huntingdon's disease and Alzheimer's)
- Severe medical illness
- Alcoholism
- Previous history of depression.

(Bowles, 1993)

Dependence/ independence in the AL of dying

Death is universal and inevitable, and apart perhaps from suicide, there is little personal independence about the time of death although there are some who maintain that individuals 'have turned their face to the wall' and willed themselves to die.

In the presence of general weakness and disease, the dying person is often aware that, with the passing of each day, there is some slight erosion of independence in the physical aspects of ALs. However at home and in hospital, as well as in a hospice, carers can encourage the person to continue exercising their independence for as long as possible and remain in control of pain relief (if pain is present), in control of quality of living, and in control of the immediate environment. Self-esteem can remain intact and even with increasing physical dependence, there can be independence of spirit. So while preserving the right to live independently to the optimum for the circumstances, the care providers have to help the dying person to balance the degree of personal dependence/ independence in the Activities of Living up until the time of death.

For the family of the dying person, there will probably be varying degrees of dependence on others during the terminal illness prior to death when family, friends, neighbours and colleagues often offer to assist with, for example, family transport and shopping as well as visiting the dying person. In the period of grieving, the presence and thoughtfulness of others can be comforting and supportive although the bereaved person knows that this is a transient phase until physical and emotional strength is renewed, and they return to their previous level of independent living.

Factors influencing the AL of dying

Apart from the differences associated with the various stages of the lifespan, as already discussed, a number of factors influence death and dying. The various factors are discussed under the headings biological, psychological, sociocultural, environmental and politicoeconomic factors, as in the model.

BIOLOGICAL

In old age, it is normal for all systems of the body to become less efficient and to undergo a gradual process of degeneration. The process of dying is not dissimilar except that the progressive decline is brought about by disease, and the nature of the particular pathology involved determines the course and speed of the irreversible degeneration of biological functioning. It is therefore difficult to diagnose the onset of 'dying' as a biological process.

Terminal illness

However, as already defined (p. 395), a terminal illness begins when medical treatment cannot halt the course of a disease, and can only alleviate the symptoms of the fatal illness. Recognition of the importance of treating the symptoms has led to the introduction of the term 'palliative care' in preference to the term 'terminal care'. Indeed, palliative medicine is now regarded as a medical specialty in its own right. Although palliative care was pioneered by the hospice movement (p. 409), and has tended to be associated with cancer, this approach is gradually being adopted throughout the health service and for terminally ill and chronically sick people with many different kinds of disease. In many instances a considerable length of time may elapse between the medical diagnosis of fatal illness and the onset of rapid physical decline in the very terminal stages of the illness which precede the event of death.

Dying, as a physical process, is a very complicated phenomenon and it is important to appreciate that it is seldom possible for doctors to diagnose the exact time of its onset or to give a precise prognosis of when death will occur.

Death

In contrast, it is usually possible to determine with accuracy the time at which death ultimately occurs. For most purposes it can be assumed that death has occurred when a person's pulse and respiration have ceased. But sometimes a much more elaborate diagnosis of death is required especially if there has been admission to hospital and sophisticated, artificial, 'life-support systems' are being used to maintain vital body functions. The concepts of 'clinical death' (death of the person), 'biological death' (death of the tissues) and 'brain death' (irreversible brain damage) reflect the different interpretations.

Although not spelled out in legal terms, there is medical agreement about the criteria indicating complete and irreversible brain death, requiring confirmation by at least two experienced doctors. The criteria include fixation of pupils, absence of corneal and of vestibulo-ocular reflexes; absence of response within the cranial nerve distribution to sensory stimuli; no response to bronchial stimulation when a catheter is passed into the trachea; no spontaneous breathing movement when the patient is disconnected from a mechanical ventilator (Allan, 1987; Simpson, 1987).

Agreed criteria for the definition of brain stem death are essential when removal of organs for transplant surgery is being considered, and they are strictly applied by a medical team quite separate from the transplant team. In the UK, a standard code of practice is observed and O'Brien (1990) demonstrated how the agreed criteria for diagnosing brain death could be set out clearly in a proforma for inclusion in the patient's notes.

Many patients who die in hospital are suitable candidates for organ donation and yet there is a critical shortage of donors. Shyr (1993) argues that this is partly due to the fact that the relatives are not routinely offered the chance of donating their loved one's organs even although it can often be a rewarding act at an otherwise sad time.

After death

After death, the body cools, the tissues and muscles lose their tone and rigor mortis (stiffening of the body) sets in after 2 or 3 hours.

Bereavement

There are also biophysical factors which are relevant in relation to bereavement. For those who are bereaved, there is usually extreme physical exhaustion. Unless the death is sudden and unexpected, there will probably have been a period of time prior to the death when it was necessary either to pay frequent visits to the hospital or to provide 24-hour care at home. Perhaps also there is a young family to be looked after, or full-time employment to be carried on during the terminal illness of the family member and immediately after, and inevitably there is accompanying stress and anxiety.

The bereaved seem to be more susceptible to physical illness. It has been recognized for some years that a bereaved spouse is admitted to hospital more frequently than married persons of the same age, and that elderly bereaved people are more likely to become physically ill than those in a younger age group. The elderly person is often in a poor physical state anyway, and the stress of the death of a spouse may exacerbate physical weakness.

Some writers do not hesitate to refer to the 'broken heart syndrome' and studies have shown that significantly more spouses die within a year of their wives' or husbands' death than others in the same age group over the same period. It is thought that the intensity of the trauma of grief has a direct effect on the body's physical function. The immune system is affected so the response to infection and neoplastic disorders is suppressed and as a consequence physical disease processes become evident; and this leads to further stress and a downward spiral in terms of health status.

PSYCHOLOGICAL

It is much less easy to describe psychological aspects of dying and bereavement because individuals do not respond in the same way and because any one person's reaction is influenced by personality, personal beliefs and total life experience. However, some of the generalities can be described.

Beliefs

Most people have some kind of personal belief about the meaning of death and often this is based on the philosophy of a particular religion. Most religions have some strong belief about the fate of man's spirit and soul after death. For example Christianity purports that there is life after death; Roman Catholics, Protestants and Jews believe that death marks the beginning of an afterlife with God, some being convinced that this existence is everlasting and will hold greater joy and peace than life on earth. Within such a philosophy then, the purpose of dying is to allow progression from life on earth to the afterlife.

Some religious and ideological groups believe that one can triumph over death by giving up life when and how one chooses, for example in highjacking episodes or war activities for ideological causes; meaning is given to death by the meaningfulness of the cause. Such people willingly sacrifice their lives for the 'idea', and may believe it stands them in good stead for the afterlife.

For those who do not hold such religious or ideological beliefs, dying may be seen to have no purpose other than to bring an inevitable end to living; a coming to terms with the finiteness of life. So, for some, death is a beginning; for some a transition; and for others, an end. And perhaps, albeit subconsciously, some of the grieving in bereavement is a form of grief for oneself; another's death is a reminder of one's own death, a reminder of the transience of life and the fact that the lifespan is not never ending.

Knowledge

Whether or not the person suspects or knows for certain that he is dying is an important factor. It is no virtue in itself that all people should be told they are dying, or discover the fact for themselves. However, the person's understanding of the prognosis will affect their attitude, mood and behaviour. Those with experience of caring for dying people tend to agree that they usually *are* aware, without needing to be told, of their fatal prognosis.

After all, the person is able to feel and see the symptoms and signs of the disease and to realize that there is decline rather than improvement; to consider the possibilities and probabilities of recovery; and most of all, to become aware of the altered way in which others begin to behave. Although at one time it tended to be thought kinder to patients to conceal information about a fatal illness, it is now generally acknowledged that patients should be told what they want to know. This change of view has resulted from research findings which have shown that the majority of dying patients *do* want to know the absolute truth about their prognosis (Dunlop & Hockley, 1990, p. 8).

Feelings

For some people, awareness of impending death may be accompanied by intense fear. Of course, the psychological changes which take place are not the same for any two individuals, but it appears that there are certain kinds of reactions which commonly occur in the dying person. As already mentioned, insight into people's feelings about dying was provided by the in-depth research interviews in North America with dying patients which Kubler-Ross (1969) conducted and analyzed.

She described that, on realizing what is happening, most people pass through a phase of *'denial and isolation'* in which they refuse to accept that they are dying. As denial lessens, the common reaction is one of *'anger'* and the person will ask 'Why me?' . . . 'What have I done to deserve this?' Sometimes attempts to cope with the situation then involve a stage of *'bargaining'*. The person tries to find ways of believing that a miracle recovery will happen or that they might be given more time and they make 'bargains' with the doctor or with God. When these fail and the imminent loss of life and loved ones becomes a reality, *'depression'* is experienced and this is an almost universal feature of the dying process. There is profound regret over missed opportunities and failures of the past and an overwhelming sadness engulfs the dying person.

With sensitive support the person can be helped through this experience by being reminded of the achievements of life, by being shown respect and love, and reassured that care will be provided right to the end and that what is important is to cope with each day at a time, to make the most of what is left, and to make any arrangements for the future which are important to set in place.

It should be realized, however, that these phases are not necessarily a linear progression; there is overlap and movement back and forth. Indeed, more contemporary writings tend to view grief (both in dying and bereavement) as a dynamic process rather than a progression through stages (Jacob, 1993). 'Stage theories' are criticized by Mak (1992) in a critique of writings on the psychological reactions of dying patients, and she points out that theories, such as Kubler-Ross's, have only limited empirical evidence to support them. Nevertheless it is useful to appreciate the various reactions so that the person can be helped to deal with these powerful emotions; and each individual has a unique way of dealing with them.

It does seem that dying need not be the terrible nightmare which many people fear so much. There can be serenity and composure in dying and many people die peacefully in their sleep with no apparent struggle or distress. In an article by Jones (1987a), for example, the story is told of a patient who was enabled to live out his last days at home, free of pain and spared the suffering of an isolated, agonizing demise and who maintained, 'I want my dying to be not all doom and gloom, but a celebration of my life'. In 1994 in the UK, widespread publicity was given to a much-loved TV star, Roy Castle, who had expressed just the same sentiment. Even in the final months of illness due to lung cancer (which, as a non-smoker, he maintained had been caused by years of showbiz work in smoky night clubs), he remained in the public eye, ceaselessly raising money for charities and, without doubt, displaying to the public that dying need not be a lonely and wholly depressing business. The possession of both a positive personality and a strong Christian faith enabled this sense of optimism to be maintained to the end and shared by his wife.

Loss

For those left behind, however, the loss of a loved one is almost always a psychologically traumatic event. Even before the death, the immediate family and friends of the dying person are often under great stress, concerned about the discomforts and pain of a loved one and also about the impending loss of someone who is significant to them.

When the death occurs, there is inevitably acute emotional upset reflecting the sense of desolation and loss. As memories flood back, those who are grieving may find it difficult to concentrate on other activities, often there is tearfulness, and there may be loss of appetite and loss of weight. These are expected symptoms of grief and are usually relatively transient; the person usually uses coping mechanisms to resume at least a semblance of normal Activities of Living. However there may be more prolonged psychological dysfunction related to grief.

Occasionally, the feelings of helplessness and hopelessness prove too much and the grief reaction is so intense and prolonged that the bereaved person suffers a mental breakdown which requires specialized medical treatment. This is more likely to happen to women than to men, to those of unstable personality, and to those bereaved by a sudden death, the death of a child or death as a result of suicide.

SOCIOCULTURAL

Social customs

Each society has its own way of treating death according to its culture. In societies where care of the dying is still very much a family responsibility, the social customs which surround death tend to be elaborate. The various rituals and the ceremonies performed are designed to encourage the bereaved to mourn openly and to seek the sympathy and support of members of their community.

Social customs throughout the world vary markedly. In the Middle East some funeral rituals involve prolonged and public exhibition of grief; and in some African societies mourners gather together to 'drown their sorrows' publicly in drinking ceremonies. Although the rituals differ, the common element is the emphasis on the importance and necessity of communal and overt mourning.

In Western societies elaborate ritual surrounding death is fast disappearing. In Victorian times, funerals were grand occasions and the whole community engaged in mourning. Death was an event to be shared. Families were large, but close-knit, units; mourners wore black and withdrew to the confines of their home, ceasing for a while to participate in any social activities and centering life around opportunities to share their sorrow and grief and show respect to the dead.

Modern society

Nowadays, with small nuclear families, often scattered over a wide geographical area, and with everyone 'in a hurry', sadness almost tends to be seen as getting in the way of our busy lives rather than being a necessary part of them. Moreover, death has become almost a taboo subject and people feel they must mourn discreetly and 'get over it' quickly. Norbert (1985) made the comment that 'dying has been removed so hygienically behind the scenes of social life … and expedited … with technical perfection from deathbed to grave!'

Cremation is now much more popular than burial; the cremation service is brief and there is not even a grave to remind the community of the death and allow the bereaved to maintain some kind of visible, physical contact with the memory of the dead person.

Burial practices

Of course although in Western culture the choice of cremation may seem to sever the final link, for other cultures it is the norm. The Navajo Indians for example, after elaborate mourning rituals, *must* burn the body in a special house or 'hogan'. Hindus and Sikhs must also be cremated, although they consider that children who are stillborn or under the age of 4 years should be buried — 'they cannot stand the heat of cremation and have no awareness of their past actions'. Muslims, on the other hand, must be buried, and although they have no special formalities for babies and small children it should be noted that 'for 40 days after the delivery, the mother is considered unclean and may not touch a dead body' (Black, 1987).

Religion

Many of the social customs surrounding death have their origin in religion and involve a ceremonial which ensures proper disposal of the dead body. For the Muslim there are strict religious practices. Every Muslim believes that the time of his death is predetermined and nobody can do anything to alter it. While dying, the family and friends recite parts of the Koran so that these are the last words heard. After death, perfumes are applied to the body, it is wrapped in a special cloth, then placed in a grave facing Mecca. In the Islamic view, a Muslim is not the owner of his own body; it is held in trust from God. Suicide is therefore forbidden; a post-mortem removal of organs for transplant is not allowed, and cremation is not permitted (Walker, 1982).

The practice of Orthodox Jews also requires that a dying person has a fellow Jew in attendance to read scriptures and recite prayers during his last hours. There is also a special way of laying out the corpse and similarly, mutilation of the body is forbidden. The ritual purification is a reflection of the belief that death is not the end, but the beginning of an afterlife with the Almighty. For the Hindu, too, death is not an end. Their faith is centred on the transmigration of souls with indefinite reincarnation, and the form of the new body depends on the type of life the person has led (Green, 1989); and the Dayak tribe of Borneo (Kastenbaum, 1981) believe the soul stays in heaven for a period of seven generations then is reborn on earth.

It is essential that health care professionals, especially in a multiracial society such as the UK, understand and respect the various cultural and religious beliefs associated with death and dying. House (1993) surveyed community nurses in an area of the South of England and, finding widespread concern about lack of knowledge, she produced a leaflet (included with the article) which explains clearly the main cultural and religious beliefs of members of the Hindu, Jewish and Muslim communities.

ENVIRONMENTAL

In urbanized, industrialized countries there has been a clear trend towards death in *institutions* rather than at home as once was the case. Figure 15.7 shows the increasing number of deaths in hospital and the decreasing

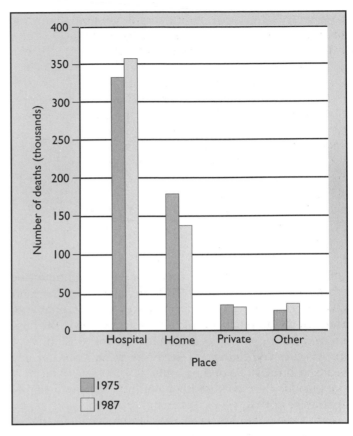

Fig. 15.7 Where people die: place of death in England and Wales in 1975 and 1987 (Source: OHE (1991) p. 6)

number of deaths at home between 1975 and 1987 in England and Wales. It has been suggested that, if this trend continues, the situation in the UK may approach that of Scandinavia where 90% of all deaths occur in hospitals (OHE, 1991 p. 7).

Home

It tends to be assumed that most people, given the choice, would prefer to die at home. However, there has been little research until relatively recently which has explored people's own preferences. Townsend et al (1990) interviewed patients (*n* = 84) who had cancer and were expected to die within a year, and they found that:-

- 58% wished to die at home
- 20% wished to receive terminal care in hospital
- 20% wished hospice care
- 2% had other preferences.

Later, the researchers established that:-

- 69% of the patients who died in hospital had stated a preference to die elsewhere
- 94% of patients who died at home had wished to do so.

Reviewing this and one or two other similar studies, Thorpe (1993) draws out the paradox:-

- most dying people would prefer to remain at home, but most of them die in institutions.

And he examines the question: 'Can more dying people remain at home?', identifying the necessary conditions for this to happen, as follows:-

- adequate nursing care
- provision of a night sitting service
- good symptom control
- confident and committed GPs
- access to specialist palliative care
- effective coordination of care
- financial support for carers.

It is important to recognize, however, that home care may not always be possible, however desirable. The carer may be elderly or frail; or, if young, may be unable to combine the care with employment and a career; the family may be unwilling to undertake the responsibility; or the procedures needed and/or the emotional burden may be beyond the skills of the family.

Hospital care, on the other hand, is seldom a highly desirable option.

Hospital

Apart from the unsuitable environment and pace of a general ward, almost all writers on the subject do not hesitate to point out that ours is a death-denying, death-defying culture and it is not surprising that health care staff who are educated with an explicit commitment to life, find it difficult to feel positive about the care of those who are dying. Many doctors still do feel powerless when cure is out of the question, and it is only relatively recently that explicit discussion of death and dying, and teaching about methods of palliative care, have been introduced to the nursing and medical curriculum.

The apparent failure of hospitals to meet the physical, emotional and social needs of dying patients was highlighted in a nursing research study conducted by Mills in Scotland in the early 1980s and, when published in 1994 (Mills et al, 1994), the findings were given widespread media publicity. There were practical reasons for delay in publishing, but the propriety of publicizing such old data relating to an issue of public concern, and when palliative care has been much developed in the interval, is perhaps questionable. Nevertheless, the findings of this research must serve to stimulate review of current practice in care of dying patients in the hospital sector of the health service.

The methods of this study are outlined in Box 15.4. Some of the findings are listed below:-

---

Box 15.4 Dying in hospital — a research study

Setting — Four teaching hospitals in the west of Scotland, 13 wards (6 surgical, 6 medical, 1 specialist unit).

Methods — Data collected mainly by observation (non-participant) — between 0730 and 1300 hours and 1700 and 2100 hours for 4 days or until the death of the patient being observed.

Interactions monitored between 23 dying patients and 190 nurses (48 qualified, 142 unqualified) — which nurses, care given and length of interactions were noted.

Ward rounds (91) were attended — content and length of consultations with a further 27 dying patients were noted.

Ward report sessions were attended and nursing reports and clinical records were read.

Patients — Of the 50 patients, 29 were women and 21 were men; their mean (average) age was 66 years (range 40–89). Fifteen had been admitted for terminal care, the other 35 had not been expected to die during hospitalization. The final period of hospital care lasted from 6 hours to 24 weeks.

Findings — see text (below)

(Mills, Davies & Macrae, 1994)

- Nursing care was provided predominantly by junior nursing staff
- Patients were usually alone (8 of the 23 were alone for at least 90% of the observation period and all but one were alone for at least three-quarters of the time. As death approached, their isolation increased
- The dying patients had many symptoms but nursing care was inadequate, e.g. the oral hygiene of 82% of patients was poor and thirst was not quenched for 56% of patients
- Although some consultants were caring, some concentrated on the patient's disease and made no reference in ward rounds to psychosocial needs.

Several 'case reports' are included in the published account of the study findings and one of these is reproduced in Box 15.5. In concluding, the authors state:

Box 15.5 Death in hospital — a case report (Mills et al, 1994)

A 56 year old man was admitted to die. He looked dishevelled, neglected and miserable. He was seen to smooth his hair with his hand and feel his rough skin. He received no attention to his oral hygiene, bathing or care of pressure areas during two days of observation. The nurses responsible for his care noted that the tasks had been done, though in fact he had received no attention.

' . . . dying patients are an integral part of the population of general hospitals. Their death should not be considered a failure; the only failure is if a person's death is not as comfortable as possible.'

That is perhaps the most important message of this research and it has to be borne in mind, as already discussed, that dying in *hospital* is not generally a person's preference.

Hospice

Because of the difficulties inherent in both home and institutional care for the dying, a new development emerged — the hospice movement. The idea itself is not really new. Boston & Trezise (1987) record that in the mid-19th century Mary Aikenhead founded in Dublin an order of nuns, one of whose duties was to care for the dying; and some decades later the order inaugurated a similar service in London.

The hospice movement as we know it today, however, was really started in the 1950s. There were two main originators. One was an organization, the Marie Curie Foundation, which raised funds to establish special residential homes for cancer sufferers. As well as providing skilled nursing it was intended to 'save much mental suffering, stress and strain for the relatives'. The other was an individual, Dr Cicely Saunders, who eventually opened St Christopher's in 1967, the first hospice 'planned on an academic model of care, research and teaching' and involving not only the patient but the family.

Hospices are designed as small, homely places to care for people during the final stages of terminal illness, and to provide expert palliative care. Patients are encouraged to maintain their normal lifestyle and enjoy living to the optimum level for them according to their abilities, with effective symptom control, and with maximum family cooperation, and support for family members as well as the patient.

The hospice movement in the UK continues to provide inpatient facilities but, increasingly, it has embraced the ideals of care in the community. Home care nurses and symptom control teams provide support for patients and their families who wish to manage the terminal illness at home, but with the expert help of hospice staff. And, more and more, the ethos and expertise of the hospice movement is spreading into hospitals. Dunlop and Hockley (1990) describe the 'hospital-hospice' interface in their book on 'Terminal Care Support Teams'.

POLITICOECONOMIC

In Western society, the commemoration of death is often an occasion when economic distinctions are emphasized. The type of funeral, the type of ceremony, whether or not there are commemorative plaques or headstones are activities which may reflect the economic status of the dead person's family.

Economic factors

The economic status of a country is reflected in the causes of death and the life expectancy of the population. The most important causes of death in industrialized countries, as already mentioned, are heart disease, cancer and stroke. There are links between these diseases and socioeconomic status, both between and within countries. In the UK, social class differences (i.e. the less good mortality rates in the lower social classes) were highlighted in a Report 'Inequalities in Health' (Black, 1980) and these persisted into the 1980s (Whitehead, 1987). In many developing countries, the picture reflects the lower economic status overall; infant mortality rates are high, preventable infectious diseases claim many lives, people still die from starvation and even those who manage to remain relatively healthy have a much shorter life expectancy than in the Western world.

The economic status of a country to some extent influences what can be done to prevent the circumstances which lead to avoidable early deaths, but the political decisions determine how much of the national budget can be relegated for health services.

Political factors

Political decisions also determine how much will be spent on costly hospital life-saving procedures which reach such a small percentage of the population, and how much will be used in the community rectifying the conditions which are the cause of so many deaths.

Political decisions also influence the provision made by the state for funeral costs and financial assistance to dependants in the form of death grants, widows' pensions, widowed mother's allowances, or their equivalents, and such financial support certainly helps the bereaved. The politicoeconomic status of a country is also reflected in the availability of schemes for private insurance cover against death, although in fact, government employers and large multinational companies may provide compensation to families following major disasters where the employee is killed or severely injured, irrespective of the employee's private insurance arrangements. Money and state support do not solve the problems of grief, but poverty can certainly make them worse.

Individualizing nursing for the AL of dying

Each individual has personal beliefs about life, and about death and dying. The experience of death is unique to each person, and drawing on the information given in relation to the components of the model already discussed, it is possible to identify not only the problems related to dying, but also the wishes of the individual and his/her family during this terminal Activity of Living. A résumé of the main points of the preceding discussion is contained in Box 15.6, this serving to draw attention to dimensions of individuality in the AL of dying.

Not all dying people require, or even wish, the help of a nurse, but for many people at the endpoint of the lifespan, some of their problems can at least be alleviated with skilled and sensitive nursing. Individualized nursing can only be carried out if the nurse knows about the patient's (and family's) problems, and about personal wishes (and those of the family) related to this last Activity of Living.

ASSESSING THE INDIVIDUAL IN THE AL

Knowledge about the patient's and family's problems and preferences is obtained through assessment, and understanding their *individual* circumstances and anxieties is of the utmost importance (see Box 15.6). This may take the form of a systematic nursing assessment on the patient's admission to hospital for terminal care. Alternatively, it may be a re-assessment of a patient whose condition in hospital has worsened and for whom terminal care must now be planned. Or, in other circumstances of a prolonged terminal illness at home, assessment and re-assessment at intervals may be undertaken by the community nurse (or hospice home care support nurse) as the patient's condition changes and new problems emerge.

Whatever the circumstances, assessing the individual and significant others is undertaken with the purpose of identifying individuality and problems relating to the AL of dying in order that individualized nursing can be planned. While observing and while conversing with the patient and the family, the nurse would be seeking answers to the following sorts of questions:

Box 15.6 Assessing the individual for the AL of dying

Lifespan: relationship to dying
- Age group of dying person and family/friends

Dependence/independence in dying
- Status in relation to all ALs
- Status during grieving and bereavement

Factors influencing dying
- Biological
  - terminal illness/cause of death
  - diagnosis of death
  - effects on other ALs
  - effect on physical and mental health of family/friends
- Psychological
  - beliefs about death and dying
  - knowledge and awareness of approaching death
  - whether or not significant others know of prognosis
  - fears, anxieties and feelings
  - effect of loss on family/friends
- Sociocultural
  - social customs surrounding death and dying
  - religious/cultural rituals
- Environmental
  - home/hospital/hospice
- Politicoeconomic
  - causes of death and life expectancy as indicators of socioeconomic status
  - state support for the dying and the bereaved

- what does the individual (and family) know about the prognosis?
- what are the individual's beliefs about dying and death?
- when is the individual likely to die?
- what factors will influence the way the individual is dying?
- what effect does the dying process have on the family and how does this affect the individual?
- what do the patient and family want the nurse to do when the death occurs?
- does the patient or family wish to consider organ donation?

- what effect will bereavement have on the family and/or significant others?
- what problems do the individual and family have at present or seem likely to develop?

IDENTIFYING ACTUAL AND POTENTIAL PROBLEMS

Information collected in the process of assessment and reassessment provides the basis for identification of the patient's and family's problems in relation to the AL of dying. The general principles which have been applied to all other ALs are relevant to this AL. Potential problems should be identified and prevented when possible; and actual problems should be solved or alleviated; or the patient should be helped to cope with them. When possible, the patient and family should be involved in the process of assessment and problem identification and should help to set realistic goals.

In many instances, review will have to be done daily because although, in the process of dying, there is often a gradual erosion of independence in all ALs, this may fluctuate from day to day, and the person who is dying should be helped to live to the optimum for that day. Cure is not the objective so palliative care is the appropriate approach; comfort and well-being are of paramount importance.

Of course, a multidisciplinary team may often be involved in assisting with the problems of a dying person and it is important that the individualized nursing plan is congruent with the team's mutually agreed objectives, so that the patient can be helped to be as comfortable as possible for as long as possible, and can die with dignity, and that the family members also receive appropriate and adequate support.

Against the background of the general discussion already provided in this chapter, 'problems' relating to the AL of dying are discussed under the following headings:

- physical problems associated with dying
- psychological problems associated with dying
- the family's problems.

This discussion by no means provides a comprehensive account of the nursing of dying patients. Rather, it aims to introduce student nurses to the range of issues and practices which are involved in individualizing nursing for the AL of dying.

PHYSICAL PROBLEMS ASSOCIATED WITH DYING

Physical discomforts can be so insistent. The psychological, sociocultural, environmental and economic factors influencing each AL must of course be considered by the nurse, but more time and effort can be given to those less

Table 15.1 Discomforts suffered by terminally ill patients (from Hockley et al 1988 British Medical Journal 296 (June 18): 1715–1717 reproduced by kind permission of the authors and editor of the British Medical Journal)

Symptoms	No. patients (n = 26)	Symptoms	No. patients (n = 26)
Anorexia	24	Pressure sores	16
Insomnia	23	Constipation	14
Immobility	23	Nausea	14
Malaise	23	Oedema	11
Sore mouth	21	Confusion	9
Cough	20	Incontinence	8
Dyspnoea	18	Vomiting	7
Pain	18	Malodorous wounds	2

tangible aspects of nursing if the individual can be helped to be physically comfortable in the process of dying. The person who is overwhelmed by distressing physical symptoms does not have the energy to engage in interpersonal relationships or benefit from the support they can offer. As a result, the quality of remaining life is often poor (Cartwright et al, 1973).

The range and frequency of physical problems suffered by dying patients have been identified in various surveys. Hockley et al included 26 terminally ill patients in their study and the range of discomforts reported by the patients to the researcher is given in Table 15.1. Almost all are physical discomforts.

Many patients had multiple symptoms. Reflecting on the apparent lack of effective symptom control, Dunlop and Hockley (1990) suggest that this may be the result of a variety of factors, including:-

- patients frequently accept symptoms as inevitable and do not complain
- professionals fail to recognize the symptoms, particularly the less obvious ones (e.g. nausea, pain and constipation)
- responses to symptoms are often inadequate (e.g. inattention to mouth care, infrequent/inadequate provision of medications such as analgesics and laxatives).

Thorough assessment is, therefore, crucial.

In order to identify whether or not a patient is experiencing any of these problems, or may be likely to, the nurse needs to carry out an assessment of all the ALs so that relevant nursing interventions can be planned. Some of the nursing interventions which can alleviate physical problems are mentioned below, and to reduce excessive repetition, cross references are given to more detailed, earlier discussions of these topics in relation to other ALs.

Pain

Pain (pp. 130–136) is probably what people fear most

about the process of dying, and although it is experienced at other times throughout life, it can be of particular distress to dying people. As long ago as 1972, Hinton reported that about one in eight people suffered pain during terminal illness; and these findings are corroborated in more recent studies such as Hockley et al (1988). Table 15.1 shows that 18 out of 26 patients reported pain.

For a long time it seemed to be assumed that the pain of dying could not be controlled and had to be endured. The work of Dr Cicely Saunders and others has radically altered medical thinking about this and it is now quite clear that with prudent use of analgesic drugs, control of terminal pain can and should be achieved.

The basic principle of pain management is that sufficiently potent analgesics are given *regularly* so that pain is not only relieved, but prevented and if pain does occur, then the dose should be increased or the drug changed.

The prescribing of drugs is of course a medical responsibility but it is one which relies on competent nursing assessment of pain (p. 132) and regular evaluation of the effectiveness of the pain control methods employed. Very often nurses do patients a disservice by being reluctant to give p.r.n. analgesics unless the patient's pain is obvious and debilitating, thinking that the drugs may not be effective if given too often or too early in the terminal phase. In fact, routine administration of analgesics can be effective for months in the majority of cases and in some instances are administered via infusion to provide a regulated and constant level in the blood. Preparing the patient and/or family to self-administer medications for pain relief, thus providing a much appreciated opportunity for the person to remain at home, and even at work during a protracted period of dying, was innovatory in the 1980s (Harris, 1988a) but since has become quite common.

New technology for pain control has been developing rapidly in recent years. Oncology services and pain clinics have demonstrated that expert management of pain in terminal illness can be achieved. Dunlop and Hockley (1990) classify the specialized techniques for pain control into two groups:-

● techniques which interrupt the pain pathway, either *peripherally* (with a 'nerve block' such as a neurolytic agent, phenol and alcohol being most frequently used) or *centrally* (e.g. by cordotomy).
● techniques which relieve pain by stimulation of the peripheral and central nerve systems (e.g. acupuncture, transcutaneous nerve stimulation and implanted stimulators).

In addition to pain caused by the terminal illness, the patient may suffer from other types of pain too. If confined to bed, pain may be experienced due to pressure or lack of movement. Joint pains and muscular tension can be alleviated with careful positioning, massage and the application of local heat.

Anorexia, nausea and vomiting

When someone has a lengthy, terminal illness, one of the most distressing aspects is watching them almost literally fade away and this is particularly common in people who have certain types of cancer. Along with obvious weight loss, there is muscle wasting, skin breakdown, impaired wound healing, decreased immunocompetence; and the general debility, weakness and malaise lead to a further lack of interest in food and a further decline in nutritional status (Holmes, 1988).

Some would say that in terminal illness nutritional support is not necessary; and clearly at some point in the process of dying, nutrition is not the paramount concern. But while the individual can enjoy meals — and food has a social function as well as the obviously physical one — everything should be done to provide small, easily digested meals which are appetizing; and this is achieved in some units, even in large, busy general hospitals.

Patients should be encouraged and helped if necessary, to clean their teeth or dentures, in the hope that it will be refreshing and encourage the inclination to eat. A coated tongue reduces any enjoyment of food flavour and a frank thrush infection may be painful, so mouth care every 2–4 hours may be required perhaps along with antifungal agents if thrush is present. Pineapple contains a proteolytic enzyme, ananase, which helps to clean the mouth and, if the patient enjoys the flavour, sucking a pineapple sweet, may be a welcome adjunct to organized mouth care. Iced tonic water to suck has a similar effect as do iced lemon and glycerine Q-tips which are commercially produced.

The presence of nausea and vomiting (p. 185) also serve to disincline interest in eating as well as being extremely unpleasant symptoms for a terminally ill person to cope with. Persistent nausea can be relieved by the use of antiemetic medications.

Difficulty in swallowing, and dehydration

Swallowing (p. 185) can be difficult if there is any obstruction in the upper alimentary tract such as a malignant growth, or pressure on the tract from growths or inflammation in neighbouring tissues. It may also occur when radiotherapy is administered to the upper trunk area, for example for lung cancer.

Dysphagia (p. 185) makes eating and drinking uncomfortable so a local anaesthetic in gel form given before food, or food given in semi-solid form may ease the patient's difficulty. Ice to suck, covered in gauze, sometimes helps to reduce the fear of choking, and can be soothing and refreshing, as well as helping to keep the buccal mucosa moist.

In addition in order to prevent dehydration, frequent small drinks of the patient's choice should be made available and help may be needed if the patient is weak or unable to sit up. Adequate hydration is by far the best way of preventing a 'dirty' mouth (p. 244). The nurse may find, however, that it is fear of urinary incontinence which causes the patient to reduce fluid intake. With dehydration, however, urine output is decreased and, indeed, dehydration may hasten death. Malone (1994) examines the ethical issues and legal considerations which surround decisions about rehydration therapy and its withdrawal for terminally ill patients.

Difficulty with eliminating

The dying person can be extremely distressed by urinary incontinence (p. 212), and it is necessary for the nurse to approach this problem with sympathy and tact. Despite its hazards, catheterization may be the best solution in these circumstances.

Faecal incontinence (p. 218) may be equally distressing, although constipation (p. 210) is more likely especially when opioid drugs are being used to provide analgesia. Irrespective of drugs, the lack of exercise, and reduced fluid and food intake also contribute to constipation and prophylactic treatment using laxatives may be necessary to prevent the potential problem of faecal impaction.

Pressure sores

General debility, reduced movement, reduced food intake and lack of vitamin C, and impaired sensation may cause pressure sores (pp. 245–251) to develop more readily in the dying person. Regular turning to relieve prolonged pressure on any one part may be carried out, but if this is too disturbing, bed appliances alone should be used.

Although prevention of pressure sores is important, it is more important to allow the dying person as much comfort and peace as possible in the absolutely final stages of life. Dying patients often seem to become very sensitive to pressure, such as from bedclothes, and great patience and skill may be needed to help the patient to be comfortable in bed during the last days or hours of life.

Difficulty in breathing, coughing

The patient and the family can be very distressed by dyspnoea (p. 155). Chemotherapy may be prescribed to reduce inflammation of the bronchial mucosa and relieve laboured breathing in a prolonged terminal illness but administration of oxygen is seldom helpful because use of the mask often merely increases the feeling of suffocation.

Ventilating the room, placing the bed near a window even if only for the psychological effect, and being with the patient may ease the sense of panic and fear. The very noisy breathing known as the 'death rattle' can be subdued by using drugs which dry up the excessive secretions in the respiratory tract.

Any dyspnoea will be exacerbated by a persistent cough (p. 150) which may be dry (for example caused by mechanical irritation of the respiratory tract or diaphragm) or moist (for example caused by infection, chronic obstructive airways disease, asthma or heart failure). Cough may be treated by providing a simple linctus or humidifying the air to provide peripheral suppression of the cause of the cough. When such measures are unsuccessful it may be possible to alleviate the cough by using medications which have either a peripheral or central suppression action.

Eye discomfort

In the final stages of terminal illness, the person may be fully alert, or may have long, drowsy periods or may be drifting in and out of consciousness. Whatever the circumstances, it is usually soothing to bathe the eyes to prevent encrustation and inflammation around the eyelids.

Unpleasant odour

Unless the nurses are meticulous in carrying out nursing activities related to such conditions as incontinence or discharging wounds, an unpleasant smell can result and it is distressing to all concerned. Hormones or other medications can be used to reduce the smell from a fungating lesion, such as may occur in advanced cancer of the breast. Good ventilation of the room and discreet use of deodorizers can be helpful and the patients will appreciate any attempt to minimize what for them and their family is a distressing problem.

Nursing activities

The kinds of nursing activities aimed to promote physical comfort for the dying are not substantially different from those applicable to problems already described in each of the AL chapters and cross-referenced above. However, greater skill and patience are often demanded of the nurse because 'minor' discomforts can assume major proportions as the patient's independence and strength diminish.

Dying patients can be encouraged to participate in their care when they feel able to do so, and nursing routines should be flexible enough to allow attention to be given at times when the patient can cope with the disturbance involved, and when pain control is at its optimum.

More and more nurses believe that complementary therapies, such as aromatherapy, can have great benefits for seriously ill or dying patients (Tattam 1992). There may be a place, therefore, for the more conventional nursing activities to be complemented by aromatherapy or massage. Although these therapies may be employed to relieve physical discomforts, they also often contribute to a sense of psychological well-being too.

As mentioned earlier, when physical discomforts receive adequate attention, more time and energy can be devoted to increasing the quality of life before death and, in this respect, attending to psychological problems is integral to the ideals of palliative care.

PSYCHOLOGICAL PROBLEMS ASSOCIATED WITH DYING

Although there are some almost universal features of the human response to impending death, and these have been outlined (p. 405), for purposes of individualizing nursing it is vital to understand that each dying patient and those close to him will react to the approaching death in a very individual way. The emotional reactions will vary as will the nature of the problems experienced. Likewise, cultural influences (including ethical, spiritual and religious) will vary. There will be differences too according to whether the dying person is cared for at home or in a hospital or hospice; and whether either or both parties are aware of the prognosis and the likely course of the terminal illness.

Fear and anxiety

There are so many things about which the dying person may feel apprehensive and afraid: for example, fear of death, fear of pain, fear of the process of dying, fear of loss of control and dignity, fear of being alone or of being rejected and fearful for those being left behind.

The knowledge that death will mean parting from family and friends obviously is a source of great sadness to the dying person and often there is considerable anxiety about their future and about how they will cope with their bereavement. The onset of depression, described earlier as a common feature of the dying process, is sometimes mistaken as a physical symptom, but probably is more often caused by the dying person's feelings of sadness, fear and regret.

The nurse may not be able to remove these fears and anxieties but, nevertheless, she may be able to provide comfort to a dying patient in simple ways, such as showing concern, listening to worries and providing company.

In gaining strength and courage to face death without fear many people find their religious beliefs an invaluable resource. Knowing this, the nurse who is involved in the care of a dying patient, whether at home or in hospital, can ensure that religious beliefs and practices are respected, and appropriate support is available. The

hospital chaplain (or the representative of any faith) who is a welcome visitor for the patient should be made to feel welcome in the ward by the nursing staff. With their religious knowledge and ability to give spiritual guidance, chaplains have a particular contribution to make to the care of the dying patient. Often they become the person in whom the patient confides innermost fears and anxieties; sometimes the chaplain helps the dying patient to understand the significance of death and to accept it with dignity and without fear.

Loneliness

According to many writers, such as Kastenbaum (1981) and Norbert (1985), one of the greatest concerns among people who are dying is that they will be left alone. People who die in hospital sometimes can experience an overwhelming sense of loneliness; although they are not 'alone', they are without close companionship.

The contact which the nurse has with the patient who is dying should be frequent and, if allowed, can become the basis of a trusting relationship which will help to reduce loneliness and isolation. There is probably no patient who is more in need of 'tender loving care' than the patient who is nearing death yet Norbert (1985) went so far as to say that while still alive, the dying are physically deserted. Indeed, the research reported by Mills et al (1994), and outlined earlier in this chapter, did show that dying patients in hospital *were* alone most of the time.

On the other hand, the patient may be surrounded by professionals and still *feel* alone, and deserted. This is understandable given that a patient dying in hospital is separated from family and the comfort and familiarity of home.

Separation from home

When dying people are nursed in their own home setting, at least they are surrounded by family, friends, neighbours and their personal possessions. The individual can retain at least some control over the immediate environment. When people are admitted to hospital or hospice to die, they are totally separated from familiar surroundings. There will come a moment when they realize that they will not again see their own home and their worldly possessions. This very final separation from family life and home environment must be coped with as well as the other fears and anxieties and physical discomforts of dying.

Most of the points about anxiety arising from a change of environment which were made when discussing other ALs are pertinent, and, indeed, are augmented when the person appreciates that death will take place within the restricted personal living space of the hospital. The patient who is dying may be particularly upset by hospital routines which are unfamiliar, especially those associated with washing and toileting when privacy may be threatened; eating and drinking likes and dislikes may not be given consideration; ward temperature and humidity may be uncomfortable; noise levels and the presence of other people will disturb periods of sleep; if bedfast, the capacity to mobilize will be out of personal control; there will be difficulty communicating with staff and other patients who are all strangers. All of these potential problems created by the change of environment may be exacerbated if the person comes from a different cultural group, especially if there are strict religious/cultural practices associated with dying and death, some of which may be difficult to continue in the hospital environment or simply not understood by the staff.

In Western culture, because hospitals are so geared to 'cure', it is not surprising that the experience of dying and death in a hospital environment can create such problems for the patient and family. Hospitals may be lonely places in which to die, yet paradoxically it is all too rare for relatives to be given the facilities to be alone with the dying person, free from interruptions.

It was the result of appreciating the shortcomings of hospitals in compensating for the dying person's separation from family and home, that the hospice movement placed such emphasis on providing calm, relaxed surroundings where care and concern for the wishes of the patient and family are paramount, and this permeates the environment.

Difficulty in facing the truth

The terminally ill person may not find it easy to seek a supportive relationship with nurses, and other care givers, and the nurse may not find it easy to offer involvement. Sometimes this is because nurses do not understand that reactions such as anger and depression are 'normal' in the process of dying. Often it is because they are afraid of being faced with the question 'Am I dying?'

In fact, this direct question is not often asked but, if it is, it means patients want to talk about their fears and uncertainties. Nevertheless, there are people who continue to use denial, and they should not be assaulted with truths they are unwilling, or not yet ready, to face. In many instances, however, dying patients *are* aware of their prognosis. Even though the patient has not been told explicitly there are many subtle ways in which the information may be transmitted by doctors and nurses. Sometimes both the patient and family choose not to admit openly that they know the prognosis; in other cases the knowledge is frankly shared. Whether or not dying patients should be told of their prognosis is a complex and delicate question.

There are good reasons on practical, psychological and spiritual grounds for adopting a policy in favour of telling the truth, and supporting the patient in the search for coping strategies. But equally, on occasions, there may be reasons for withholding this information: indeed, in some religions, it is anathema to tell patients they are dying. In practice, the decision should not be difficult if dying patients are given time and opportunity, with someone they can talk to and trust, to explore their fears and suspicions and to indicate what they want (and don't want) to know. What is important is for the nurse to be sensitive to the patient's own awareness of the situation and to know what has already been said by the doctor and relatives. Farrar (1992) maintains that nurses must be 'ready to detect cues that can lead to an open dialogue' (see Box 15.7).

The nurse will learn what she needs to know by listening carefully and observing astutely. Once she knows what the patient feels and understands about the situation, she can gain confidence to form a close relationship and show the patient that she is willing to listen. A dying person, feeling lonely and afraid, will gain comfort from companionship and closeness. Spending time with him, talking or sharing in his silence, can restore tranquillity to an existence which in so many ways is in turmoil. Showing sympathy and compassion are important aspects of nursing a dying patient and essential if the nurse is to help with the various psychological problems which may arise in the dying process.

However, before nursing staff can give support to patients and families, they must come to terms with their own attitudes about death and dying and most nursing programmes now provide opportunities for students to explore this important aspect of professional preparation and practice.

Box 15.7 Communicating with dying patients — 'How much do they want to know?'

- Many health care professionals either feel too inhibited to talk about death to a dying patient or believe it will undermine wellbeing
- In fact, most dying patients know they are dying and talking about it (*if the patient wants to*) is more likely to be helpful than harmful
- It is not a case of what to *tell* dying patients, but, rather, what they indicate (verbally or non-verbally) they want to know or discuss
- Take cues from the patient which allow open dialogue
- Talk at the patient's pace and in terms which *they* use (avoid referring directly to 'cancer' or 'dying' if the patient hasn't used these words).

(Based on Farrar, 1992)

THE FAMILY'S PROBLEMS

When discussing problems which relate to the AL of dying, it is essential to consider the *family's* problems as well as those of the patient. It is useful here to reiterate that the word 'family' has a wide interpretation and can include relatives, friends or partners, or indeed anyone else who is a 'significant other' in the dying person's life and terminal illness.

Fear and anxiety

Just as the dying person can be overwhelmed by fears and anxieties, so too can the family. They find it hard to watch if their loved one is suffering and find it difficult to understand the fluctuating moods, and sometimes unpredictable reactions. They may fear their own ability to cope with the event of death, to control their emotions and to face the future alone.

If the person is being looked after in hospital, the family may feel cut off and unable to find ways of expressing their love and concern; and in the publicity of an open ward they may find that maintaining their close relationship becomes difficult. In caring for a dying person at home the family faces other stresses arising from the total involvement of that situation. Their ability to cope emotionally may be eroded by the exhaustion of providing for all the needs of the dying person in the last stages of illness.

The positive value of establishing a supportive and humane relationship with the relatives of a dying patient was emphasized by one of the early writers on the subject, McNulty (1974):

'Nurses have a lot to answer for in their apparent insensitivity to the needs of relatives . . . I think that we are sometimes afraid to stop for fear we might not be able to answer the questions asked; afraid because we cannot give the so much wanted good news; afraid because we might have to say 'I don't know'. If only we could realize that just by stopping for a moment and sharing our presence, we may have to some degree lightened the family's burden.'

Being available is the essential point. Often, too, allowing close relatives to help in the patient's care, for example by helping the patient to wash or have a meal, may be greatly appreciated as this gives a purpose to visits, provides the opportunity for affection and concern to be expressed and may help to alleviate fears and anxieties.

Distress over protracted death

It is particularly distressing for a family when the patient is 'brain-dead' and no matter what they do and how often they visit, there is no obvious sign from the patient that there is any response. Although the development of

multisystem life support for critically ill patients has brought hope of recovery for many, inevitably it leads in some cases to a protracted death and, for the family, eventual disappointment follows initial hope.

It has been mentioned already (p. 404) that relatives of patients who are pronounced brain dead may gain some comfort from agreeing to organ donation. Shyr (1993) suggests that it first must be decided who is the best person to approach the relatives, and that this person must communicate understanding and concern, and not be afraid to show their own sadness as this may be a source of comfort to the relatives.

The final decision to withdraw life-supporting therapy, in which doctors must involve close relatives (Fulbrook, 1992), is obviously a distressing time for the family. The final hours are precious ones, often for the staff as well as for the family. Alderman (1993), writing about the death of Tony Bland (p. 397), describes the last few days of his life as follows:-

'. . . the nurses increased their input into his nursing care and he always had somebody with him. When his parents took a break, a nurse was constantly at his bedside — something they had expressed a desire to do.'

Tony's parents were at his bedside when he died. Some of the nurses, at his parents' request, joined the chaplain in prayer. The Blands also invited the staff to the funeral and many attended. 'His parents appreciated this support very much', Alderman was told.

Burdens of care-giving

Although having a dying relative in hospital is stressful and tiring for the family, providing care at home also makes great demands on relatives. It is generally agreed that home is the best place to die (and studies which support this claim were mentioned earlier in the Chapter, p. 407); but, at the same time, the likely strains on the family should not be underestimated. Care-giving throughout a terminal illness, especially for an elderly person, can be exhausting and emotionally draining. It is well recognized that carers must be provided with adequate support, both physical and emotional.

Community health services have greatly extended such support over recent years, and hospice support teams and specialist nurses (p. 409) are increasingly available to provide expert help for dying patients and their carers. Indeed, in a study conducted in three health districts in the south of England in the late eighties (Jones et al, 1993), it was found that the majority of carers had not had difficulty in getting help from health care professionals when it was urgently required. Overall, 150 of the 207 carers (who were interviewed 2–4 months after the death) considered that the support given had been 'excellent' and a further 45 rated it as 'good'.

However, although the patients' pain generally had been well controlled, 25% of the patients had not had relief of other symptoms. In addition, carers often needed domestic help earlier and, in general, they were considered to have required more advice than supplied about help available other than health services.

Berenthal (1994) rightly contends that statutory services and voluntary agencies should be working in partnership in caring for dying people. She considers that community nurses are ideally placed to assess needs; identify shortfalls and gaps in statutory service provision; and inform carers of the local voluntary services which can provide help to families who want to enable their loved one to die at home and who are willing to shoulder the burden of care which otherwise would fall to hospitals.

The shock of bad news

Being given bad news, especially if it is unexpected, is always upsetting and sometimes wholly shocking. The worst news we can ever be given is news of the death (or expected death) of a loved one. Without doubt, one of the most stressful of nursing duties is breaking the news of the actual event of death to a patient's next-of-kin and this is a task which must be done as sensitively and compassionately as possible (see Box 15.8).

The nurse can do little to ease the relative's distress; what is important is that she is prepared for the fact that reactions to news of a death cannot be predicted. The relative may appear totally inconsolable or almost unconcerned; sometimes anger is directed at the nurse or doctor. If the death is sudden (the family member recently saw them alive and well) the reaction might be one of disbelief. If the death is in strange surroundings such as overseas or on holiday — or in dramatic circumstances, such as following a fire, car or drowning accident — the family members (particularly if they are survivors of the accident) are shocked and numb, and often cannot even remember familiar phone numbers or addresses to seek help from relatives and friends.

Box 15.8 Breaking news of a death

'Unfortunately there is no easy way of giving the news of a death. It seems that a gentle, forthright announcement, followed by information about contributing causes, in a warm and sympathetic tone is most helpful. If this is done thoughtfully, showing concern, it does not appear to be cold and distant, and contributes to the event being accepted as reality.'

(Thayre & Hadfield-Law, 1993)

Breaking the news of sudden or accidental death is something which has to be done with particular frequency in any Accident and Emergency Department. In that nursing setting, there is the added disadvantage of having had no prior contact with the relatives, and the nurse's first communication may be to explain that death is imminent or, indeed, has already occurred. Ways in which bereaved relatives can be better supported in this situation are described by Burgess (1992) in her account of the benefits of a 'support nurse system' which was introduced, and later shown (by audit) to be providing appreciated support.

Demands in the immediate aftermath of death

In the first few hours and days after the death, the family members have to make many decisions and to deal with many practicalities. This, therefore, can be a demanding time — physically and emotionally exhausting, especially for the elderly and others who have been constant caregivers in the last weeks of the terminal illness.

Immediately after death, the family members must decide if they want to see the body. This can be important in confirming the reality and allowing the saying of a final farewell; and it is thought to help in the grieving process (Cathcart, 1988). The question of whether or not it is advisable for children to see the body of a parent who has died has already been raised (p. 402) as has the increasingly common practice of offering newly bereaved parents the opportunity to hold their stillborn baby (p. 401).

Beyond this, practical advice regarding what needs to be seen to after a death can be offered by the nurse (see Box 15.9).

Before relatives finally leave the hospital, if the death has occurred there, usually the nurse also returns the deceased person's effects to the next-of-kin. This should be done sympathetically, making sure that the person has some means of transport home.

The way in which nurses deal with the family at this final contact with the hospital is very important. Kindness and practical help will be remembered with gratitude whereas a casual or uncaring approach may well contribute to a lingering bad memory of the patient's time in hospital. The importance of providing practical comfort and support at the time of death is now recognized to be of such benefit that in some hospitals a specially designated liaison nurse is appointed to guide relatives through the immediate ordeal.

The problems of bereavement

Following the funeral, there are many problems which may face bereaved people as they attempt to accept and cope with the loss. There are emotional problems of grief,

---

Box 15.9 What to do after a death

Registering a death

- It is important that what is written on the death certificate is explained to the next-of-kin, and that he/she knows how to register the death.
- Deaths must be registered within 5 days at the offices of the Registrar of Births, Marriages and Deaths for the district where the death occurred or the body was found.
- The informant must take the notice given by the doctor and also, unless forwarded by the doctor, the medical certificate of cause of death.
- The Registrar will need to know the deceased person's full name, maiden name (if applicable), sex, date and place of birth, last employment and marital status. For this reason, the deceased's birth and marriage certificates are useful to have to hand.
- The Registrar issues a certificate of registration of death (free) and death certificate (charged) and these are needed later for various purposes (e.g. claiming benefits).

Arranging the funeral

- A Funeral Director will make all the arrangements although the decisions (e.g. cremation or burial) are made by the family.
- Costs are determined by the choice of coffin and headstone (if required), the venue and form of ceremony, the distances involved, notification procedures and any gathering after the funeral. Relatives should request an estimate of costs before agreeing arrangements.

(Farrell, 1990)

---

the difficulties of social adjustment and sometimes there are economic strains too, if the deceased person was the family breadwinner. In the immediate bereavement period there may be death grants and widow's pensions to claim; insurance policies to negotiate; the children's future to be reconsidered; mortgage payments to renegotiate; a rerouting of financial resources. Often quite crucial decisions have to be made at a time when those most affected by the death are least able to cope.

The early stage of acute grief can be particularly distressing and sometimes involves feelings of self-criticism and guilt, the person wondering if the death could have been prevented. Acute reactive depression and even suicidal thoughts may occur. Sometimes the problem is that the grief reaction may be delayed, particularly if

the bereaved had much to do with the practicalities of the funeral or if the death was very sudden or totally unexpected. Then they may wonder why they do not feel shocked and sad, only later having to cope with these intense feelings.

Some people find it distressing to mourn openly and find the funeral traumatic; others may be worried by the intensity of their emotions when alone and wonder if they might be on the verge of a complete mental breakdown. Most people appear to be surprised by just how long their feelings of loss and sadness last and begin to wonder if they will ever readjust and resume a normal life again. Bereavement is probably the most devastating experience which is faced in life and disrupts every Activity of Living. It is difficult for the person concerned to accept that it is a recognized process and a normal reaction to the loss of someone precious to them. However, although there are some 'standard' patterns of bereavement, as previously outlined (p. 398), the process of grieving is a very individual one and this must be recognized by nurses (and others) who play a supportive role at this time.

Perhaps the most helpful contribution the nurse can make is to help the bereaved person to face up to and work through the emotional difficulties. This means that they must be given time: time to grieve, time to talk, to reminisce, to express openly their fears and worries and to begin to plan a new future. The community nurse is in an ideal position to assess the needs and problems of a bereaved person. An elderly man now on his own could be encouraged to cope positively with the domestic tasks previously done by his wife. A bereaved parent left to bring up young children might be given help to consider how to support them in their grief, this most difficult of situations (both for the parent and the children) already have been highlighted (p. 402).

For people bereaved after a death from AIDS, Miller et al (1993) consider that nurses have a special role to play in bereavement counselling. Some of the main tasks for nurses include, they suggest:-

- to accompany relatives to view the body if requested or required
- to answer questions/give information about AIDS as a cause of death, remembering that the survivors may have fears for others or themselves
- to be available and provide an atmosphere for feelings to be openly expressed
- to assist in 'working through' loss
- to help identify who can be turned to for support
- to offer follow-up contact or referral to other counsellors.

And, as they note, nurses who work in the field of HIV/AIDS care may lose many patients of about their own age. They, too, need support and understanding.

In fact helping bereaved people is a communal responsibility; a basic human concern which can be shared by both professionals and the public. Bereavement is not an illness but a life event with which most people need the help of others. Giving help to the bereaved needs to begin before the death if this is possible, so that grief can be anticipated and preparations made for readjustment.

Grief cannot be cured, but it can be shared. Showing compassion to bereaved people will be a reminder that, despite their loss and feelings of intense loneliness, they are not entirely alone and that there is some reason to renew their sources of faith and hope, and have the courage to begin again; that there is the possibility of being and feeling happy again without being disrespectful to the person who has died.

Some bereaved people find it helpful to attend organized groups which have been created to provide an opportunity to share and talk through feelings of grief and thereby derive consolation, and in some instances, practical help from, for example, The Bereaved Parents Helpline; The Compassionate Friends; Cruse; The National Organization for the Widowed and Their Children; Age Concern; The Gay Bereavement Project. After national disasters, a multiprofessional counselling team is sometimes involved to assist bereaved families both in the immediate aftermath and with follow-up services over a period of time.

PLANNING AND IMPLEMENTING NURSING ACTIVITIES AND EVALUATING OUTCOMES

It is clear, then, that caring for the dying and bereaved is an important aspect of nursing. The emphasis of all nursing is on helping people to cope with the Activities of Living; dealing with death is no different. Caring for the dying is concerned with life before death and helping the bereaved is about life after death.

In the course of describing the problems which dying patients and their families commonly experience, many different kinds of nursing activities have been mentioned. Some are aimed at preventing problems (e.g. unpleasant physical symptoms of terminal illness, such as constipation); others are implemented to alleviate or solve actual problems (e.g. pain control); and many (including giving time and companionship) are concerned with helping patients and their families to cope with the demands and stresses of dying and grieving.

Many of the nursing activities which are relevant to this AL are carried out in much the same way whether care is being provided at home or in a hospital or hospice. The nurse's role varies, however, depending on whether the death is sudden or preceded by terminal illness, and depending on the age groups of the dying person and significant others. Planning and implementing individualized nursing care, therefore, must take account of the individual circumstances and all of the different factors (as previously discussed) which may influence the AL of dying.

Individualizing nursing is thought of in the context of this model in terms of the four phases of the process of nursing — assessing, planning, implementing and evaluating (Fig. 3.9). These phases can be worked through rapidly in an emergency or quickly-changing situation (e.g. a sudden, life-threatening condition) whereas, with more time, assessing and planning can be carried out comprehensively and with full negotiation with patients and relatives (e.g. when requirements are being worked out for what is likely to be a lengthy period of terminal care). In the process of planning nursing, all of the Activities of Living must be considered collectively (i.e. because of their interrelationships) although there may be some nursing goals which are specific to the AL of dying.

Some kind of statement of goals is needed if the outcomes of nursing are to be evaluated. In general terms, the goals of nursing in relation to the AL of dying are closely aligned with the overall goals of palliative care (see Box 15.10). Palliative care has been a fast-growing area, and it is a distinctly multidisciplinary area of health care. There is, however, nothing novel about *nursing's* involvement in palliative and terminal care.

The role of the nurse in caring for the dying was mentioned in Virginia Henderson's famous definition of the function of nursing (Henderson, 1960). She wrote:

Box 15.10 Palliative care — Definition

Palliative care is the active total care of patients whose disease is not responsive to curative treatment. Control of pain, of other symptoms, and of psychological, social and spiritual problems is paramount. The goal of palliative care is achievement of the best possible quality of life for patients and their families.

Palliative care:

- affirms life and regards dying as a normal process;
- neither hastens nor postpones death;
- provides relief from pain and other distressing symptoms;
- integrates the psychological and spiritual aspects of patient care;
- offers a support system to help patients live as actively as possible until death; and
- offers a support system to help the family cope during the patient's illness and in their own bereavement.

(WHO, 1990)

'Nursing is primarily assisting the individual (sick or well) in the performance of those activities contributing to health, or its recovery (*or to a peaceful death*) that he would perform unaided if he had the necessary strength, will or knowledge . . .'

Nursing is concerned with helping people, both in living and in dying.

REFERENCES

Alderman C 1993 A family loss. Nursing Standard 7(27): 18–19

Allan D 1987 Criteria for brain stem death. The Professional Nurse 2(11) August: 357–359

Barker W 1987 Close encounters of a preventive kind. Senior Nurse 7(1) July: 13–15

Black D 1980 Working group on inequalities in health. HMSO, London

Black J 1987 Broaden your mind about death and bereavement in certain ethnic groups in Britain. British Medical Journal 295 August 29: 536–539

Beal S 1988 Prone or supine for preterm babies? Lancet (2): 512

Berenthal J A 1994 A welcome break for carers? The role of voluntary services in caring for dying people. Professional Nurse 9(4): 267–270

Boston S, Trezise R 1987 Merely mortal: coping with dying, death and bereavement. Methuen, London

Bowles L 1993 Logical conclusion? (suicide among older people). Nursing Times 89(31): 32–34

British Medical Association 1988 The Euthanasia Report. BMA, London

Buckley R 1993 Reducing the risk (cot death). Nursing Times 89(43): 28–30

Burgess K 1992 Supporting bereaved relatives in A&E. Nursing Standard 6(19): 36–39

Bypass R 1988 Soothing body and soul. Nursing Times 84(24) June 15: 39–41

Cartwright A, Hockey L, Anderson J 1973 Life before death. Routledge and Kegan Paul, London

Cathcart F 1988 Seeing the body after death. British Medical Journal 297(6655) October 22: 997–998

Conboy-Hill S 1987 Dying people — how do nurses feel and what training do they want? Paper presented to British Psychology Society (London) Conference

Couldrick A 1993 'Do you mean that Mummy is going to die?' caring for bereaved children. Professional Nurse 9(3): 186–189

Dickstria R, Hawton K (ed) 1987 Suicide in adolescence. Dordrecht, Nijhoff. Distributed by MTP Press

Dunlop R J, Hockley J M 1990 Terminal care support teams: the hospital/hospice interface, Oxford University Press, Oxford

Ellis P 1991 Euthanasia: the way to a peaceful end? Professional Nurse 7(3): 157–160

Farrar A 1992 How much do they want to know? — Communicating with dying patients. Professional Nurse 7(9): 606–609

Farrell M 1990 What to do after a bereavement. Professional Nurse 5(10): 539–542

Fulbrook P 1992 Assessing quality of life: the basis for withdrawal of life-supporting treatment? Journal of Advanced Nursing 17: 1440–1446

Garrett G 1991 A natural way to go? Death and bereavement in old age. Professional Nurse 6(12): 744–749

Green J 1989 Death with dignity: Hinduism. Nursing Times 85(6) February 8: 50–51

Harris L 1988 Something to live for. Nursing Times 84(32) August 10: 25–28

Henderson V 1960 Basic principles of nursing care. International Council of Nurses, Geneva

Hinton J 1972 Dying. Penguin, Harmondsworth

HMSO 1992 Scotland's Health: A Challenge To Us All. The Scottish Office, Edinburgh

Hockley J, Dunlop R, Davies R 1988 Survey of distressing symptoms in dying patients and their families in hospital and the response to a symptom control team. British Medical Journal 296(6638) June 18: 1715–1717

Holmes S 1988 Nourishing with care. Community Outlook in Nursing Times 84(30 July 27: 24–28

Hope T 1992 Advance directives about medical treatment. British Medical Journal 304: 398

House N 1993 Palliative care for people from ethnic minority groups. Professional Nurse (Feb): 329–333

Jacob S R 1993 An analysis of the concept of grief. Journal of Advanced Nursing 18: 1787–1794

Johnson K 1993 A moral dilemma: killing and letting die. British Journal of Nursing 2(12): 635–640

Jones I 1987a A dignified death. Nursing Times 83(20) May 20: 50–52

Jones I 1987b Living after loss. Nursing Times 83(33) August 19: 45–46

Jones R V H, Hansford J, Fiske J 1993 Death from cancer at home: the carers' perspective. British Medical Journal 306: 249–251

Kastenbaum R 1981 Death, society and human experience. Mosby, St Louis

Kubler Ross E 1969 On death and dying. Macmillan, New York

Mak M H J 1992 Psychological responses to death and dying. Senior Nurse 12(3): 48–51

Mallinson G 1989 When a baby dies. Nursing Times 85(9) March 1: 31–34

Malone N 1994 Hydration in the terminally ill patient. Nursing Standard 8(43): 29–32

McNulty B 1974 The nurse's contribution in terminal care. Nursing Mirror 139(15) October 10: 59–61

Miller R, Goldman E, Bor R, Scher I 1992 Counselling in terminal care. Nursing Standard 6(26): 52–55

Miller R, Bor R, Goldman E et al 1993 Bereavement counselling in HIV disease. Nursing Standard 7(39): 48–51

Mills M, Davies H T O, Macrae W A 1994 Care of dying patients in hospital. British Medical Journal 309: 583–586

Milner A 1987 Recent theories on the cause of cot death. British Medical Journal 295(6610) November 28: 1366–1368

Mitchell A 1993 Tragic statictics (cot death). Nursing Times 89(43): 30–32

Murray Parkes C 1972 Bereavement: studies of grief in adult life. Penguin, Harmondsworth

Newsweek 1988 Correspondence on 'A right to die!' Newsweek CX1 (15) April 11: 5

Norbert E 1985 The loneliness of dying. Blackwell, Oxford, p 23, 85

O'Brien M D 1990 Criteria for diagnosing brain stem death. British Medical Journal 301: 108–109

OHE 1991 Dying with Dignity. Office of Health Economics, London

Pope N 1988 New hope on cot deaths? Nursing Times N 84(33) August 17: 21

Purssell E 1994 Telling children about impending death. British Journal of Nursing 3(3): 119–120

Robertson G S 1995 making an advance directive. British Medical Journal, 6974, 310, 236–238

Shyr S 1993 Nurse's role in encouraging organ donation. British Journal of Nursing 2(4): 236

Simpson A 1987 Brain stem death. Nursing Times 83(8) February 25: 41–42

Symes J 1991 What comfort this grief? Coping with perinatal bereavement. Professional Nurse (May): 437–441

Tattam A 1992 The gentle touch. Nursing Times 88(32): 16–17

Thayre K, Hadfield-Law L 1993 Never going to be easy; Giving bad news. RCN Nursing Update. Nursing Standard 8(12): 3–8

Thorpe G 1993 Enabling more dying people to stay at home. British Medical Journal 307: 915–918

Townsend J, Frank A O, Fermont D et al 1990 Terminal cancer care and patients' preference for place of death: a prospective study. British Medical Journal 301: 415–417

Vas Dias S 1987 Psychotherapy in special care baby units. Nursing Times 83(23) June 10: 50–52

Walker C 1982 Attitudes to death and bereavement among cultural minority groups. Nursing Times 78(50) December 15: 2106–2109

Ward B J, Tate P A 1994 Attitudes among NHS doctors to requests for euthanasia. British Medical Journal 308: 1332–1334

Whitehead M 1987 The health divide: inequalities in health in the 1980s. Health Education Council, London

WHO 1990 Cancer pain relief and palliative care. Report of a WHO Expert Committee (Technical Report Series No 804). World Health Organization, Geneva

WHO 1991 WHO annual statistics. World Health Organization, Geneva

Appendix 1

Example of a patient/client assessment form and nursing plan

The type of information appropriate for patient assessment and for devising a nursing plan has already been discussed, generally, in the chapter about the Model for Nursing; and in more detail, in each AL chapter.

It cannot be emphasized too strongly that this proforma is only a guideline. Many agencies have already devised a proforma which suits their particular circumstances and this example merely provides a guideline which could be helpful to some units which use our model.

It is worth making a few points about this particular document:

- Page one of the document includes biographical and health data elicited at the first assessment and does not usually change over a particular episode when nursing is required.
- Page two includes information about the person's ALs (insofar as they reflect the person's stage on the lifespan; their dependence/independence status; and are influenced by biological, psychological, sociocultural, environmental and politicoeconomic factors). There is a reminder list of the 12 ALs but it may not be relevant to collect information about all of them; the choice is a matter for the nurse's professional judgement as discussed in Chapter 3.

  The phrase 'usual routines' reflects our model's concept of individuality. The phrases 'what can/cannot be done independently' and 'previous coping mechanisms' particularly reflect the dependence/independence concept. The person's actual problems are recorded on the R. hand side of Page two with potential problems designated as (p).

- Page three is for the Nursing Plan and forms the R. side of a double fold so that problems identified at the initial assessment do not need to be recorded a second time. Goals are stated in outcome terms and a date for evaluation of the selected nursing interventions can be entered.

  Once recorded, the Nursing Plan only needs additional information when:

  * a goal has been achieved
  * a nursing intervention has to be changed to achieve the already set goal
  * the goal has to be modified
  * the date of evaluation has to be changed
  * the person develops further problems.

- Page four makes provision for interventions which may be medically prescribed or initiated by another member of the health team. Such information would not necessarily be documented in AL format.

The 'other notes' section could be used for recording e.g. clinic appointments or loans of equipment, emphasizing the fact that early planning is needed for the person's discharge from hospital.

However, if a lengthy rehabilitation period in the community setting were planned, a more detailed section might be required as e.g. on Page five and Page six.

Patient Assessment Form: Biographical and health data

Date of admission   Date of assessment   Nurse's signature

_____   _____   _____

                                 Surname   Forenames

Male ☐   Age [   ]   _____   Prefers to be addressed as

Female ☐   _____   _____

              Date of birth
              Single/Married/Widowed/Other

Address of usual residence   _____

Type of accommodation   _____
(incl. mode of entry if relevant)

Family/Others at this residence _____

Next of kin   Name   Address

                                 Relationship   Tel. no.
                                 _____

Significant others
(incl. relatives/dependants
visitors/helpers/neighbours)

Support services   _____

Occupation
                                 _____

Religious beliefs and relevant practices

Recent significant life events/crises

_____

Patient's perception of current health status

                                 _____

Family's perception of patient's health status

                                 _____

Reason for admission/referral

                                 _____

Medical information (e.g. diagnosis, past history, allergies)

_____

GP Address Tel. no. | Consultant Address Tel. no.

_____

Plans for discharge

Patient Assessment Form: Assessment of ALs

Date

Usual routines:
what can/cannot be done independently

**Activity of living
AL**

previous coping mechanisms

Patients problems:
actual/potential (p)

Reminder of
the 12 ALs

Maintaining a
    safe environment
Communicating
Breathing
Eating and drinking
Eliminating
Personal cleansing and
    dressing
Controlling body
    temperature
Mobilizing
Working and playing
Expressing sexuality
Sleeping
Dying

Nursing Plan: Related to ALs

Goals	Nurse-initiated nursing interventions related to ALs	Evaluation

Nursing Plan: Derived from medical/other prescription

Nursing interventions derived from medical/other prescription	Goals	Evaluation

Other Notes

Medications Prescribed

Date	Prescription	Dose	Route	Frequency	Discontinued

Treatment Prescribed

Date	Prescription	Frequency	Response	Discontinued

Equipment on Loan

Date	Article	Source	Returned

Appointments

Date	Place	Reason	Conveyance	Arranged

Supportive Services

Service	Date	Remarks	Discontinued
Social worker			
Meals on wheels			
Home help			
Marie Curie Foundation			
Twilight/night nursing			
Physiotherapy			
Occupational therapy			
Speech therapy			
Chiropody			
Day hospital			
Voluntary services			
Other			

Index